Atlas of Bladder Disease

Atlas of
Bladder Disease

Editor

David R. Staskin, MD

Associate Professor of Urology
Tufts University School of Medicine
Caritas-St. Elizabeth's Medical Center
Boston, Massachusetts

With 46 contributors
Current Medicine Group LLC, part of
Springer Science+Business Media LLC

Springer

CURRENT MEDICINE GROUP LLC, PART OF
SPRINGER SCIENCE+BUSINESS MEDIA LLC
400 MARKET STREET, SUITE 700•PHILADELPHIA, PA 19106

Developmental Editor..Stephanie Brown
Senior Developmental Editor ....Elizabeth Orthmann
Editorial Assistant...Juleen Deaner
Design and Layout ....Dan Britt
Illustrators ....Marie Dean, Heather Hoch, Sara Krause, Wieslawa Langenfeld, Jacqueline Leonard, Maureen Looney, and Giovanna Santoni
Managing Editor ....Megan Charlton
Production Coordinator......................................Carolyn Naylor
Indexer ....Holly Lukens

Library of Congress Cataloging-in-Publication Data

Atlas of bladder disease / editor, David R. Staskin.
p. ; cm.
Includes bibliographical references.
ISBN 978-1-57340-307-8 (alk. paper)
1. Bladder--Diseases--Atlases. I. Staskin, David.
[DNLM: 1. Urinary Bladder Diseases--Atlases. 2. Urinary Bladder--pathology--Atlases. WJ 17 A8615 2009]
RC919.A85 2009
616.6'200222--dc22

2009029143

ISBN 978-1-4939-3945-9

www.springer.com

For more information, please call 1 (800) 777-4643
or email us at orders-ny@springer.com

www.currentmedicinegroup.com

10 9 8 7 6 5 4 3 2 1

Preface

The study of the bladder is inseparable from its structural relationships to other pelvic organs and function in the lower urinary tract. The choice of topics and the content of the chapters in this edition of the *Atlas of Bladder Disease* justly reflect these associations. The atlas includes information about specific disease states and disorders, evaluation and classification, and conservative and operative therapy. A spotlight on recent advances in pharmacology, tissue engineering, and robotic surgical techniques highlights the expanding science and technology available to researchers, clinicians, and surgeons.

The *Atlas of Bladder Disease* reflects the high quality of the internationally-based group of authors from diverse specialties, who have accepted the invitation to contribute and furnish these chapters, and the publisher, who has assisted in fashioning these presentations into a high-quality textbook. The purpose of this endeavor was to create a highly illustrated volume of tables, diagrams, and photographs that would graphically span a selected portion of both the academic and the practical, the established and the "cutting edge," and the art and the science of the bladder, in a format that is eye-catching, well organized, and highly informative. Authors were asked to "organize and write the chapter as if it was a lecture and you were narrating your slides."

So much of what we academically produce and consume, and rightfully so, is the product of "work" and "dedication," and that is obvious in the final product. However, on occasion we are able to not only enjoy the completion of the task, but can also enjoy reading and absorbing the material in a clear, concise, and well-illustrated format. The contributors to this volume have exceeded our expectations. Thank you—job well done.

David R. Staskin, MD
Editor, and for the Authors
Boston, MA

Contributors

E. Jason Abel, MD
Fellow
Department of Urologic Oncology
University of Texas MD Anderson Cancer Center
Houston, Texas

Anthony Atala, MD
W. Boyce Professor and Chair
Department of Urology
Director
Wake Forest Institute for Regenerative Medicine
Wake Forest University School of Medicine
Winston-Salem, North Carolina

Bary Berghmans, PhD, MSc, PT
Pelvic Care Center
University Hospital Maastricht
Maastricht, The Netherlands

Nol Bernards, MD
Department of Research and Development
Dutch Institute for Allied Health Care
Amersfoort, The Netherlands

Jerry G. Blaivas, MD
Clinical Professor of Urology
Weill Medical College of Cornell University
New York, New York
Adjunct Professor of Urology
SUNY Downstate Medical School
Brooklyn, New York

Travis L. Bullock, MD
Center for Continence Care and Pelvic Medicine
Urology Consultants, Ltd
Saint Louis, Missouri

Linda Cardozo, MD, FRCOG
Professor
Department of Urogynecology
King's College Hospital
London, United Kingdom

George K. Chow, MD
Department of Urology
Mayo Medical School
Mayo Clinic
Rochester, Minnesota

Doreen E. Chung, MD, FRCSC
Brady Urologic Health Center
Weill Cornell Medical College
New York, New York

Craig V. Comiter, MD
Associate Professor
Department of Urology
Stanford Medical School
Stanford, California

Anurag K. Das, MD, FACS
Assistant Professor
Department of Surgery
Harvard Medical School
Director
Center for Neuro-urology and Continence
Division of Surgery/Urology
Beth Israel Deaconess Medical Center
Boston, Massachusetts

Prokar Dasgupta, MD, FRCS Urol
Consultant Urologist and Reader in Urology
Guy's and St. Thomas' NHS Foundation Trust
School of Medicine
Kings College London
London, United Kingdom

Juan J. de Benito, MD
Department of Urology
William Beaumont Hospital
Royal Oak, Michigan

Mario De Gennaro, MD, FEAPU
Head
Paediatric Neurourology and Urodynamics
"Bambino Gesu" Children's Hospital, Research Institute
Rome, Italy

Roger R. Dmochowski, MD
Department of Urology
Vanderbilt Medical Center
Vanderbilt University
Nashville, Tennessee

Daniel S. Elliott, MD
Department of Urology
Mayo Medical School
Mayo Clinic
Rochester, Minnesota

Benjamin J. Girdler, MD
Chief Urology Resident
Department of Urology
William Beaumont Hospital
Royal Oak, Michigan

Erik Hendriks, PhD, MSc, PT
Department of Epidemiology
Maastricht University
Maastricht, The Netherlands

Sender Herschorn, MD
Division Chair and Professor
University Division of Urology
Director of Continuing Professional Development for the University
Department of Surgery
Sunnybrook Health Sciences Centre
Toronto, Ontario, Canada

Jay K. Jhaveri, MD
Research Associate
Robotic Prostatectomy and Urologic Oncology Outcomes Program
James Buchanan Brady Foundation
Department of Urology
Weill Cornell Medical College
New York Presbyterian Hospital
New York, New York

Ashish M. Kamat, MD
Director
Urologic Oncology Fellowship Program
Assistant Professor and Attending Surgeon
Departments of Urology and Cancer Biology
The University of Texas MD Anderson Cancer Center
Houston, Texas

Simon Y. Kimm, MD
Resident Physician
Department of Urology
Stanford Medical School
Stanford, California

L. Spencer Krane, MD
Department of Urology
Wake Forest University
Winston Salem, North Carolina

Brett D. Lebed, MD
Fellow/Clinical Instructor
Department of Urology
Medical University of South Carolina
Charleston, South Carolina

Courtney L. Lee, MD
Urology Resident
Department of Urology
SUNY Downstate Medical Center
Brooklyn, New York

Scott A. MacDiarmid
Alliance Urology Specialists
Greensboro, North Carolina

Shawn M. McGee, MD
Department of Urology
Mayo Medical School
Mayo Clinic
Rochester, Minnesota

Declan G. Murphy, MB, FRCS Urol
Consultant Urologist
Guy's and St. Thomas' NHS Foundation Trust
School of Medicine
Kings College London
London, United Kingdom

Jørgen Nordling, Dr Med Sci, MD
Professor of Urology
University of Copenhagen
Copenhagen, Denmark
Consultant Urologist
Department of Urology
Herlev Hospital
Herlev, Denmark

Kenneth M. Peters, MD
Department of Urology
William Beaumont Hospital
Royal Oak, Michigan

Dudley Robinson, MD
Kings College of London
University of London
London, United Kingdom

Eric S. Rovner, MD
Professor
Department of Urology
Medical University of South Carolina
Charleston, South Carolina

Maura Seleme, PhD, MSc, PT
Associação Brasileira de Ajuda e Formação sobre Incontinência Urinária (ABAFI)
Curitiba, Brazil

Steven W. Siegel, MD
Metropolitan Urologic Specialist
Center for Continence Care and Female Urology
Adjunct Associate Professor
Department of Urology
University of Minnesota
Saint Paul, Minnesota

Christopher P. Smith, MD, MBA
Associate Professor
Scott Department of Urology
Baylor College of Medicine
Houston, Texas

David R. Staskin, MD
Director
Center for Pelvic Health
Division of Urology
St. Elizabeth's Medical Center
Associate Professor of Urology
Tufts University School of Medicine
Boston, Massachusetts

Gerald Y. Tan, MB, ChB (Ed),
Associate Consultant
Department of Urology
Tan Tock Seng Hospital
Singapore

Alexis E. Te, MD
Brady Urologic Health Center
Weill Cornell Medical College
New York, New York

Ashutosh K. Tewari, MD, MCh
Ronald P. Lynch Professor of Urologic Oncology
Director, Lefrak Institute of Robotic Surgery
Director, Prostate Cancer Institute
Department of Urology
James Buchanan Brady Foundation
Weill Cornell Medical College
New York Presbyterian Hospital
New York, New York

Andrea Tubaro, MD, FEBU
Associate Professor of Urology
Second School of Surgery
Sant'Andrea Hospital
La Sapienza University
Rome, Italy

Marijke Van Kampen, PhD, MSc, PT
Faculty of Kinesiology and Rehabilitation Science
Katholieke Universiteit Leuven
Leuven, Belgium

Arndt van Ophoven, MD, PhD
Professor of Neuro-Urology
Department of Urology
University of Bochum
Bochum, Germany
Director
Division of Neuro-Urology
University Hospital Marienhospital Herne
Herne, Germany

Jack R. Walter, MD
Urology Service
Brooke Army Medical Center
Fort Sam Houston, Texas

George D. Webster, MBFRCS
Professor of Urology
Department of Surgery
Division of Urology
Duke University Medical Center
Durham, North Carolina

Alan J. Wein, MD, PhD (Hon)
Professor
Surgery/Urology Department
University of Pennsylvania School of Medicine
Chair
Division of Urology
Penn Medicine, Hospital of the University of Pennsylvania Health System
Philadelphia, Pennsylvania

Jeffrey P. Weiss, MD
Professor of Urology
Associate Program Director
Department of Urology
SUNY Downstate Medical School
Brooklyn, New York

Contents

Chapter 1
Classification of Lower Urinary Tract Dysfunction in the Female Patient 1
David R. Staskin and Alan J. Wein

Chapter 2
Neurogenic Bladder 11
Anurag K. Das

Chapter 3
Nocturia: Diagnosis and Management 23
Courtney L. Lee, Jeffrey P. Weiss, and Jerry G. Blaivas

Chapter 4
Bladder Pain Syndrome 35
Jørgen Nordling and Arndt van Ophoven

Chapter 5
Urodynamics 51
Sender Herschorn

Chapter 6
Bladder Ultrasound in Voiding Dysfunction 81
Andrea Tubaro and Mario De Gennaro

Chapter 7
Pelvic Floor Rehabilitation 97
Bary Berghmans, Maura Seleme, Erik Hendriks, Nol Bernards, and Marijke Van Kampen

Chapter 8
Pharmacology and Pharmacologic Treatment of the Male Bladder Outlet 127
Doreen E. Chung and Alexis E. Te

Chapter 9
Uropharmacology: Botulinum Neurotoxin 147
David R. Staskin and Christopher P. Smith

Chapter 10
Urinary Stress Incontinence 159
Dudley Robinson and Linda Cardozo

Chapter 11
Simple and Complex Urethral Diverticula 179
Eric S. Rovner and Brett D. Lebed

Chapter 12
The Male Sling and Artificial Urinary Sphincter I 189
Simon Y. Kimm and Craig V. Comiter

Chapter 13
Artificial Urinary Sphincter II . . . 201
George D. Webster and Jack R. Walter

Chapter 14
Bladder Tissue Engineering . . . 209
L. Spencer Krane and Anthony Atala

Chapter 15
Bladder Cancer . . . 221
E. Jason Abel and Ashish M. Kamat

Chapter 16
Robotic-Assisted Laparoscopic Radical Cystectomy . . . 239
Declan G. Murphy and Prokar Dasgupta

Chapter 17
Robotic Sacrocolpopexy: Suspension of the Bladder and Vagina . . . 251
Shawn M. McGee, George K. Chow, and Daniel S. Elliott

Chapter 18
Bladder Neck Reconstruction Following Minimally Invasive Radical Prostatectomy . . . 259
Jay K. Jhaveri, Gerald Y. Tan, and Ashutosh K. Tewari

Chapter 19
Sacral Neuromodulation for Voiding Dysfunction . . . 267
Travis L. Bullock and Steven W. Siegel

Chapter 20
Percutaneous Tibial Nerve Stimulation and Overactive Bladder . . . 279
Scott A. MacDiarmid and David R. Staskin

Chapter 21
Lumbar to Sacral Ventral Nerve Rerouting . . . 289
Benjamin J. Girdler, Juan J. de Benito, and Kenneth M. Peters

Chapter 22
Overactive Bladder: Physiology of Normal and Abnormal Urinary Storage and Basis for Pharmacological Therapy . . . 305
Roger R. Dmochowski and David R. Staskin

Index . . . 313

1

Classification of Lower Urinary Tract Dysfunction in the Female Patient

David R. Staskin and Alan J. Wein

The classification of lower urinary tract (LUT) dysfunction has been presented in various forms based on different criteria—for example, those that are primarily neurologic [1–3]—and in expanded form based on function by the authors [4–6]. For the purpose of this chapter, LUT function is divided into two functions, storage and emptying, and two functional areas, bladder and bladder outlet. During the storage phase, the bladder (detrusor) accommodates urine at low intravesical pressure and a competent outlet (sphincter) prevents urinary leakage. During the emptying phase, the bladder contracts and is preceded by a coordinated and sustained relaxation of the bladder outlet to allow unobstructed and complete bladder emptying. The LUT is under neurologic control, a complex interaction of afferent (sensory input) and efferent (motor output) interactivity that is functionally divided into three zones (intracranial, spinal, and peripheral). The LUT in the female patient is a complex interaction of anatomy, physiology, and function. Anatomic support of the bladder and bladder outlet and interaction with the pelvic floor structures is critical to normal voiding function. Classification of LUT dysfunction in the female patient can be categorized by applying these factors to logically group findings for the purpose of communicating pathophysiology, diagnosis, and treatment.

Following is the classification of LUT dysfunction: filling and emptying phases (*see* Fig. 1); afferent and efferent control (*see* Fig. 2); mixed conditions of bladder and outlet dysfunction (*see* Fig. 3); bladder/outlet and storage/emptying (including bladder activity and outlet activity [*see* Fig. 4], symptomatic descriptions [*see* Figs. 5 and 6], and common conditions [*see* Figs. 5 and 6]); neurologic activity (*see* Fig. 7); urodynamic studies (*see* Fig. 8); treatment (*see* Fig. 9); and complex descriptive classification (*see* Fig. 11). In classifying LUT dysfunction, the presumption is that incontinence or any "wetness" experienced by the patient is urine and that the source of egress is the urethra; rule out wetness secondary to perspiration, inflammation, or discharge, or from vaginal and/or rectal sources. For example, specific to the differential diagnosis of "wetness" is the importance of ruling out vesico-vaginal or uretero-vaginal fistula (*see* Fig. 10).

The overactive bladder. The symptoms of overactive bladder syndrome (OAB) are currently defined as urgency, with or without urge incontinence, usually with frequency and nocturia [7–9]. The etiology of OAB is considered "idiopathic" and a neurologic (clinically apparent) etiology is classified independently. An understanding of urgency incontinence and OAB symptoms requires an appreciation of the complex relationships between afferent and efferent neurologic pathways from the bladder mucosa and musculature, the bladder neck and sphincter, and the pelvic floor, in addition to central and peripheral pathways, although definitive reflex arcs in the human may not have been identified [10].

The underactive bladder. Emptying failure secondary to bladder dysfunction may be a result of either detrusor smooth muscle pathology or insufficient neural stimulation. Insufficient neural stimulation may occur at the neuromuscular level (molecular pharmacology), with nerve impairment (neuropathy), or with alterations in central control of micturition. For this reason, an underactive bladder secondary to an overactive sphincter and/or pelvic floor should be considered, since the initiation of voiding requires both pelvic floor and urethral sphincter relaxation in the absence of anatomic obstruction. During the initial phase of bladder emptying, the detrusor contraction is preceded by pelvic floor and sphincteric relaxation, which continues until voiding is completed. A lack of pelvic floor relaxation may be implicated in many voiding disorders [10–13].

The underactive outlet. Stress urinary incontinence (SUI) is the involuntary loss of urine per urethra, which occurs when intravesical pressure overcomes the urethral resistance owing to an increase in intra-abdominal pressure or the loss of urethral resistance in the absence of a true bladder contraction. Urethral closure pressure is maintained by preserving or augmenting anatomic support and by maintaining and increasing the intrinsic activity of the external sphincter complex. It is reasonable to assume that the complex etiology of SUI is a mixture of anatomic support abnormalities and intrinsic sphincter abnormalities. Therapy may be directed toward correcting the defect or toward compensating for the deficiency by increasing the function of another component that contributes to urethral resistance. In fact, the most common operation for SUI is a midurethral sling. The mechanism of action has been described as a "kinking" or "backboard" effect that in fact does not correct the common finding of bladder neck hypermobility but does increase urethral resistance to leakage and compensate for defects in anatomic support and intrinsic urethral deficiency [14–16].

The overactive outlet. Failure to empty the bladder may be due to elevated outlet resistance or to impaired contractility of the bladder. The most commonly observed clinical etiology of elevated outlet resistance is iatrogenic obstruction following incontinence surgery [17]. Other forms of anatomic urethral obstruction are less common. Neurogenic outlet obstruction, commonly seen following injury to the suprasacral spinal cord, is due to a loss of coordination between the bladder and sphincter (detrusor sphincter dyssynergia). The paradoxical failure of the outlet to relax during voiding may result in anatomic obstruction to flow or to inhibition of the initiation or completion of the detrusor contraction. Contraction of the pelvic floor or sphincter is a normal response for bladder inhibition, but when pathologic may be classified as pseudodyssynergia (voluntary or behavioral) or true dyssynergia (neurogenic) [10–13].

Mixed-combined disorders. Disorders of the bladder and outlet during storage and emptying may occur alone and in combination. The most common mixed storage disorder in the female patient is underactive outlet (SUI) and OAB [18,19].

Sensory disorders. Many sensory disorders may be a result of "amplified sensation" with hypersensitivity of normal pathways and activation of normally dormant pathways. Afferent neurons from the bladder and urethra are of major importance during both the storage and emptying phases, both initiating the voiding reflex and sustaining the voiding drive during bladder emptying. Somatic activity may inhibit the emptying reflex by voluntary contraction of the external sphincter or pelvic floor; although not established in humans, it may provide inhibitory activity during bladder filling. The pudendal nerve is responsible for the innervation of pelvic floor structures, as well as the genital skin, urethral mucosa, and anal canal. Proprioceptive information of the periurethral musculature and sensory innervation of the levator ani muscles are also mediated by the pudendal branches. Increased sensation or pain attributed to the bladder is a major clinical challenge [20–22].

Pathophysiology, symptoms, and conditions. A direct correlation between the underlying pathophysiology, the presenting symptoms, and the actual condition is difficult due to complex etiologies and overlapping presentations [23–25]. However, the ability to correlate LUT symptoms (see Fig. 6) or neurologic lesions (see Figs. 3 and 4) with the appropriate working diagnosis for evaluation and therapy is possible. An expanded classification (see Fig. 7C) is more comprehensive but not without clinical exceptions, alternative constructs, and the need for further research and iterations.

The classification of voiding dysfunction has been presented with the major focus incorporating the division of the LUT into the bladder and the bladder outlet, and the "activity" during storage/filling and emptying/voiding. These systems can be clearly illustrated with the functional areas of the bladder and outlet on the vertical axis and the functions of filling/storage and voiding/emptying on the horizontal axis. These graphic representations can be used to correlate functional anatomy, LUT function, urodynamic testing, etiology, and therapy.

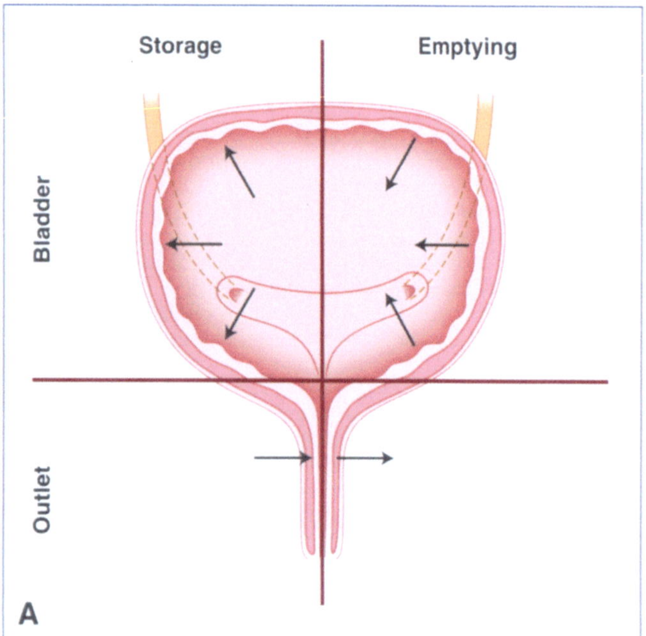

Figure 1-1. A, Function and activity classification divides the lower urinary tract into its two anatomic areas: the bladder (detrusor) and bladder outlet (sphincter) during the physiologic functions of storage (filling) and emptying (voiding). The bladder or outlet activity is described as "overactive" or "underactive."

Continued on the next page

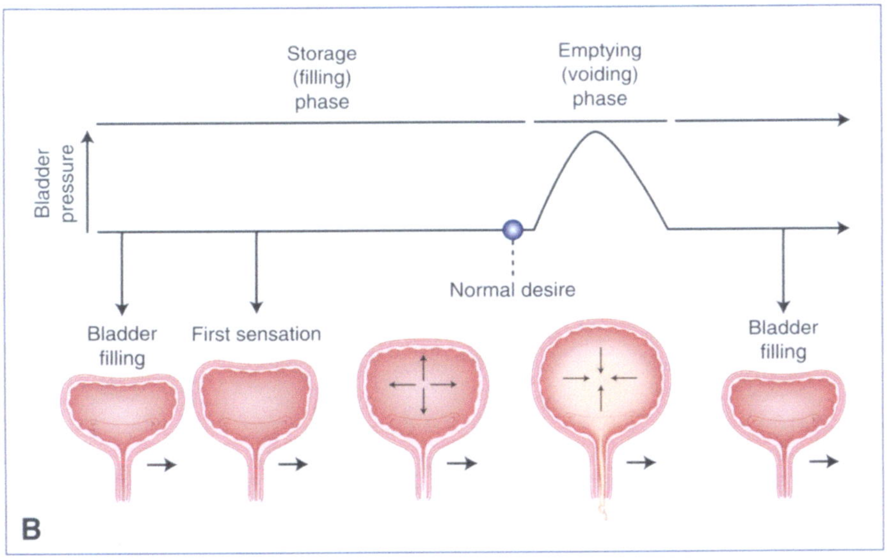

FIGURE 1-1. *(Continued)* **B,** In storage the bladder accommodates urine low pressure with competent outlet. In emptying the bladder contracts to completion with unobstructed outlet.

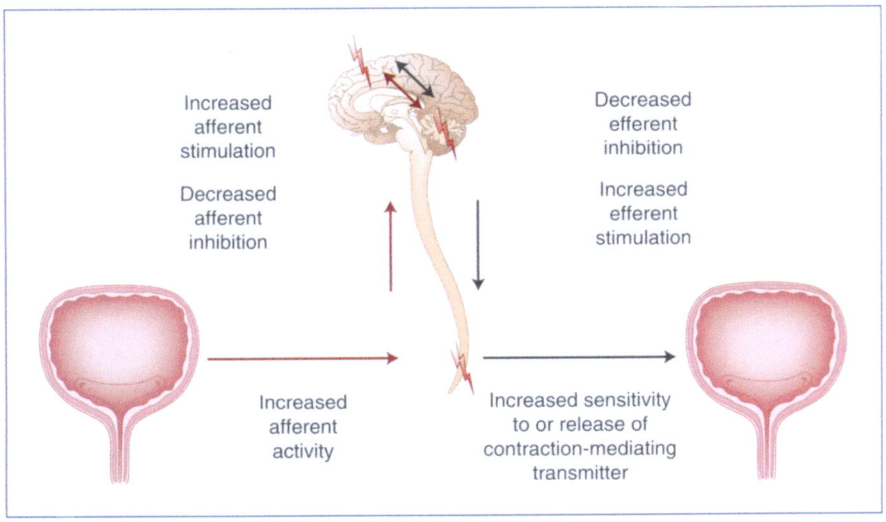

FIGURE 1-2. Neuro-urologic control: efferent and afferent balance from central nervous system to lower urinary tract (LUT). Abnormalities at any of multiple interactive levels may result in LUT symptoms.

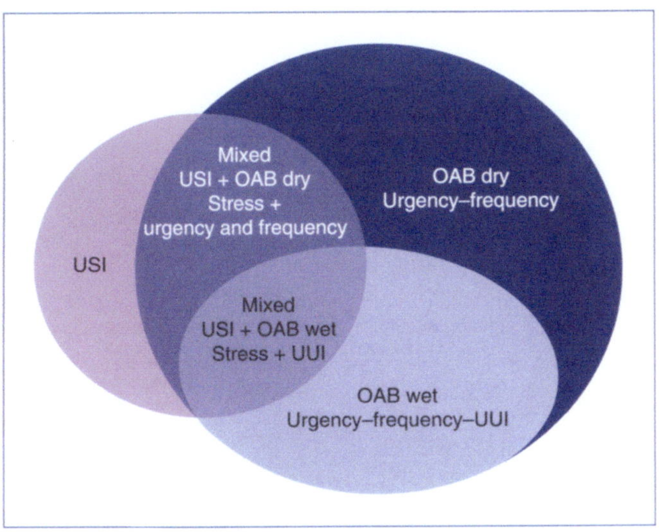

FIGURE 1-3. Mixed symptoms: overactive bladder (OAB) equals urgency with or without incontinence, frequency, and nocturia. Underactive outlet symptoms (stress or stress urinary incontinence) equal loss with effort and may occur alone or in combination. USI—urodynamic stress incontinence; UUI—urgency urinary incontinence. (*Adapted from* Wein and Rackley [26].)

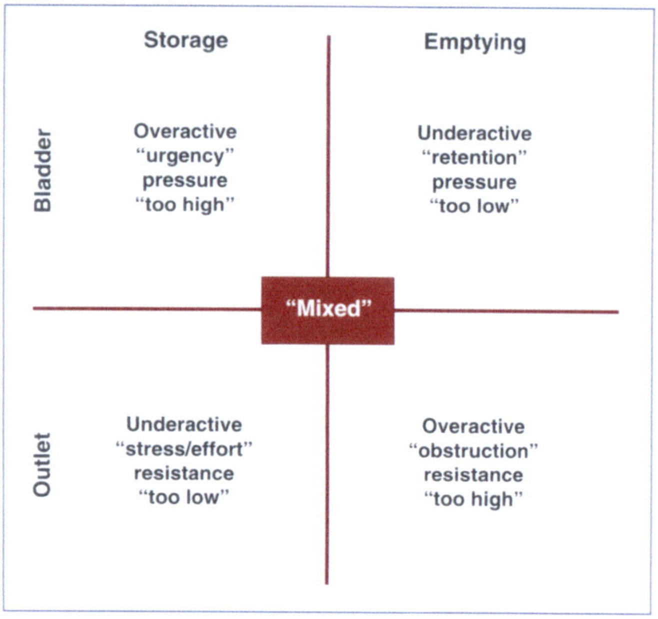

FIGURE 1-4. The four squares depict bladder, outlet, storage, and emptying, as well as the function, primary symptom, and urodynamic finding.

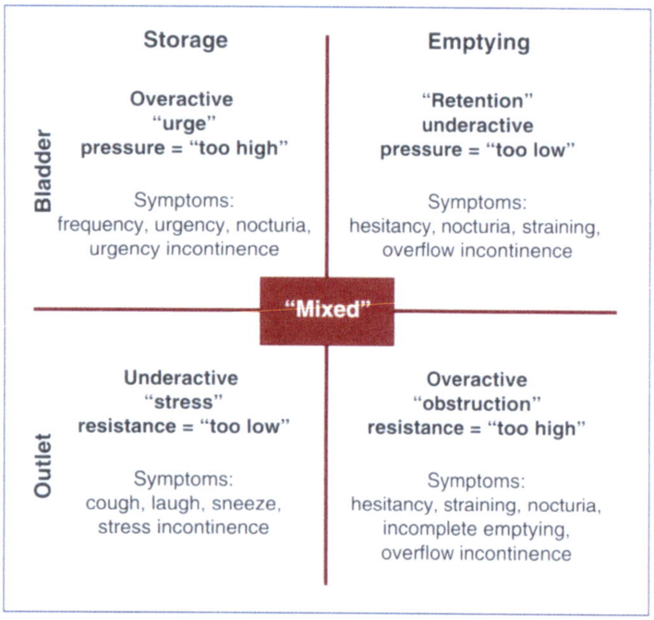

FIGURE 1-5. The four squares depict bladder, outlet, storage, and emptying, including expanded description of symptoms.

Classification by Symptoms

Stress urinary incontinence (SUI)	
Symptom:	the involuntary loss of urine on effort or exertion (lift, strain, cough, sneeze)
Activity:	underactive outlet
Condition:	urodynamic stress incontinence—the involuntary loss of urine resulting from an increase in intra-abdominal pressure that overcomes the resistance of the bladder outlet in the absence of a true bladder contraction. The decrease in bladder outlet or urethral resistance may result from poor anatomic support of the bladder neck (urethral hypermobility/SUI-A) or a loss of urethral function (intrinsic sphincter deficiency [ISD] [SUI-ISD]) or, most commonly a mixture.
Clinical confusion:	the patient describes the symptom of urinary loss with "activity" but the etiology of involuntary leakage is actualy an uninhibited bladder contraction. SUI should have urinary loss synchronous with "effort"; similarly, many patients will describe SUI as a sensation, which is confused with "urgency"; finally, stress and urgency incontinence may coexist.
Urgency urinary incontinence (UUI)	
Symptom:	the loss of urine with the sensation of urgency, voiding before the ability to toilet
Activity:	overactive bladder (OAB wet)—detrusor overactivity
Condition:	UUI (urodynamic)—the involuntary loss of urine resulting from an increase in bladder pressure secondary to detrusor overactivity (an uninhibited bladder contraction or unstable bladder). Detrusor overactivity may be the result of a suprasacral spinal or intracranial neurologic lesion that results in uncontrolled reflex contractions (detrusor hyperreflexia) or may be idiopathic. Patients may demonstrate other symptoms associated with "urgency" (frequency, urgency, nocturia) without urinary loss (OAB dry).
Clinical confusion:	the patient has decreased sensation and loses urine from motor activity of the detrusor without the feeling of "urgency." OAB is a syndrome consisting of the symptoms "urgency, with or without urgency incontinence, usually with frequency and nocturia," suggestive of urodynamic bladder overactivity but inclusive of "urgency and frequency without incontinence" OAB dry (vida infra) or the sensation of urgency (desire to void in the absence of a detectable rise in detrusor pressure–sensory urgency).
Mixed urinary incontinence (MUI)	
Symptom:	mixed symptoms of UUI and SUI, urinary loss with effort and with urgency
Activity:	OAB wet detrusor overactivity and underactive sphincter
Condition:	a mixture of the conditions described above as SUI and UUI
Clinical confusion:	urinary loss may be from SUI or UUI but the predominance and bother resulting from one condition or the other may not be discernable from the history and physical examination alone, thus creating difficulty in choosing treatment for the "primary" symptom.
Urgency and frequency without incontinence	
Symptom:	urgency and frequency without urinary loss
Activity:	detrusor overactivity with compensatory sphincter activity or no detrusor activity or abnormal afferent activity or processing (sensory)
Condition:	Urgency is the complaint of a sudden compelling desire to pass urine that is difficult to defer and frequency is the complaint by the patient who considers that she voids too often by day or at night (going to bed and arising), whereas nocturia is waking at night one or more times to void preceded by and followed by sleep. "Sensory urgency" is a term that has been removed from the International Continence Society (ICS) lexicon and was used to describe the sensation of urinary urgency without a detectable rise in detrusor pressure.
Clinical confusion:	the classification of a moderate or strong "desire to void" without true "urgency" is unresolved. "Sensory urgency–desire to void" is not in the current ICS lexicon.
Overflow incontinence	
Symptom:	the involuntary loss of urine resulting from urinary retention with bladder overdistention. The retention (failure to empty) may result from inadequate bladder contractility or outlet obstruction (or both).
Activity:	underactive bladder (retention)/overactive outlet (obstruction)
Condition:	Urinary loss occurs when the intravesical pressure overcomes the urethral resistance as a result of bladder contractility and increases in intra-abdominal pressure or urethral relaxation.
Clinical confusion:	the symptoms that are described may be a mixture of stress (SUI) and urgency (OAB) complaints.
Altered bladder sensation and pain	
Symptom:	frequent voiding with or without pain; conversely, a loss of sensation
Activity:	no detrusor contraction/alteration in afferent input or processing
Condition:	Bladder pain, discomfort, and pressure can be characterized by type, frequency, duration, location, and precipitating and relieving factors. Bladder sensation can be described as increased, normal, reduced, absent, or nonspecific (neurologic). Increased or decreased voiding may be correlated with the sensation.
Clinical confusion:	Urinary urgency and frequency without incontinence may be a product of abnormal sensation or bladder contractile activity. The source of pelvic pain may not be the lower urinary tract. Interstitial cystitis or chronic urethritis remain diagnoses of exclusion.
Functional incontinence	
Symptom:	the involuntary loss of urine resulting from a deficit in the ability to perform toileting functions secondary to physical or mental limitations
Activity:	abnormal lower urinary tract function usually coexists with functional issues.
Clinical confusion:	the underlying pathophysiology of stress, urge, or overflow incontinence may coexist, as well as difficulty in eliciting an accurate history. The patient's primary "functional" issue may be dementia, delirium, or other forms of altered cognition; physical disability may prevent easy and rapid toilet access. These conditions often exist alone or in combination with lower urinary tract dysfunction.

Figure 1-6. Symptomatic classification is based on the concept that symptoms may suggest inclusively the underlying abnormal activity, pathophysiology, and condition. Since the patient's symptoms may be extremely useful or misleading due to overlapping findings in lower urinary tract conditions [8–10], an illustrative differential diagnosis of common conditions is also presented.

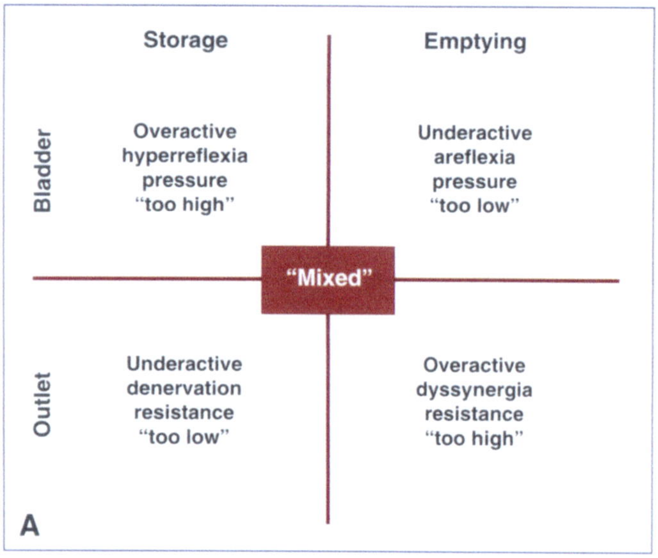

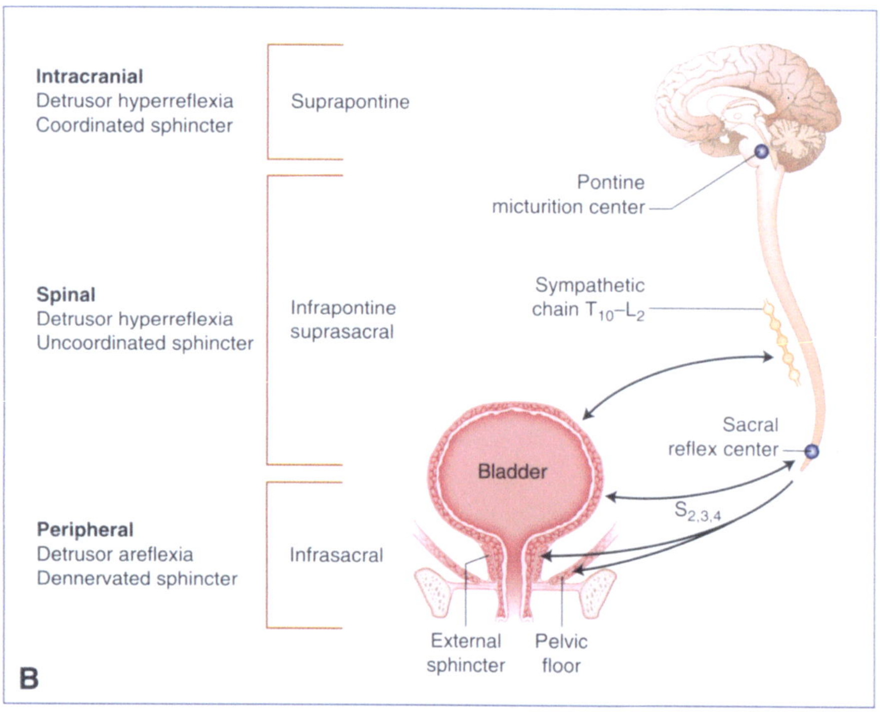

Classification by Neurologic Activity*

Lesion location	Bladder	Internal (smooth muscle) sphincter	External (skeletal) sphincter
Peripheral	Hypo-areflexic, underactive	Denervated (+/–)	Denervated (+/–)
Infrasacral	Areflexic, underactive	Innervated	Denervated, underactive
Spinal	Hyperreflexic, overactive	Uncoordinated if T6 or above	Dyssynergic, overactive
Suprapontine	Hyperreflexic	Coordinated	Coordinated

*Expected behavior of the bladder, internal sphincter, and external sphincter based on location of the lesion.

C

Figure 1-7. **A**, The four squares depict bladder, outlet, storage, and emptying: neurourologic terminology.

B, Neurourologic control: intracranial, spinal, and peripheral zones are illustrated. Hyperreflexia is seen with lesions above the sacral reflex center. Sphincter coordination is lost with spinal lesions (pontine coordination) and is preserved with intracranial lesions. Denervation is expected with infrasacral lesions.

C, Neurogenic voiding dysfunction classification. The nature of the lesion and the expected behavior of the detrusor and sphincter can be correlated with symptoms. The neurologic terms of *detrusor hyperreflexia* and *areflexic* and the outlet descriptors of *dyssynergic* or *denervated* are used and correlate with the type of function/activity.

	Storage	Emptying
Bladder	**Overactive "urge" pressure = "too high"** Specific urodynamic studies Cystometrogram (filling) Detrusor leak point pressure (fluoroscopy)	**"Retention" underactive pressure = "too low"** Specific urodynamic studies Residual urine Cystometrogram (voiding) Pressure flow (Pdet flow; fluoroscopy)
Outlet	**Underactive "stress" resistance = "too low"** Specific urodynamic studies Urethral pressure profile Valsalva leak point pressure (fluoroscopy)	**Overactive "obstruction" resistance = "too high"** Specific urodynamic studies Residual urine Pressure flow (Pdet flow) EMG MUPP (fluoroscopy)

FIGURE 1-8. The four squares depict bladder and outlet and storage and emptying: urodynamic tests that are used to objectify storage capacity and emptying ability, and bladder pressure and outlet resistance. EMG—electromyelogram; MUPP—maximal urethral pressure profile.

	Storage	Emptying
Bladder	**Overactive "urge" pressure = "too high"** Surgical treatment, neuromodulation, augmentation, botulinum toxin (unapproved)	**"Retention" underactive pressure = "too low"** Surgical treatment, CIC/urethral/suprapubic catheter, neuromodulation, neural transposition
Outlet	**Underactive "stress" resistance = "too low"** Surgical treatment, periurethral injection, suspension sling, artificial sphincter	**Overactive "obstruction" resistance = "too high"** Surgical treatment, incision or resection of obstructing sling, urethroplasty urethrolysis, neuromodulation, botulinum toxin (unapproved)

FIGURE 1-9. The four squares depict bladder, outlet, storage, and emptying: common surgical procedures used to correct, compensate, or circumvent pathology. CIC—clear intermittent catheterization. Unapproved—not approved by the US Food and Drug Administration.

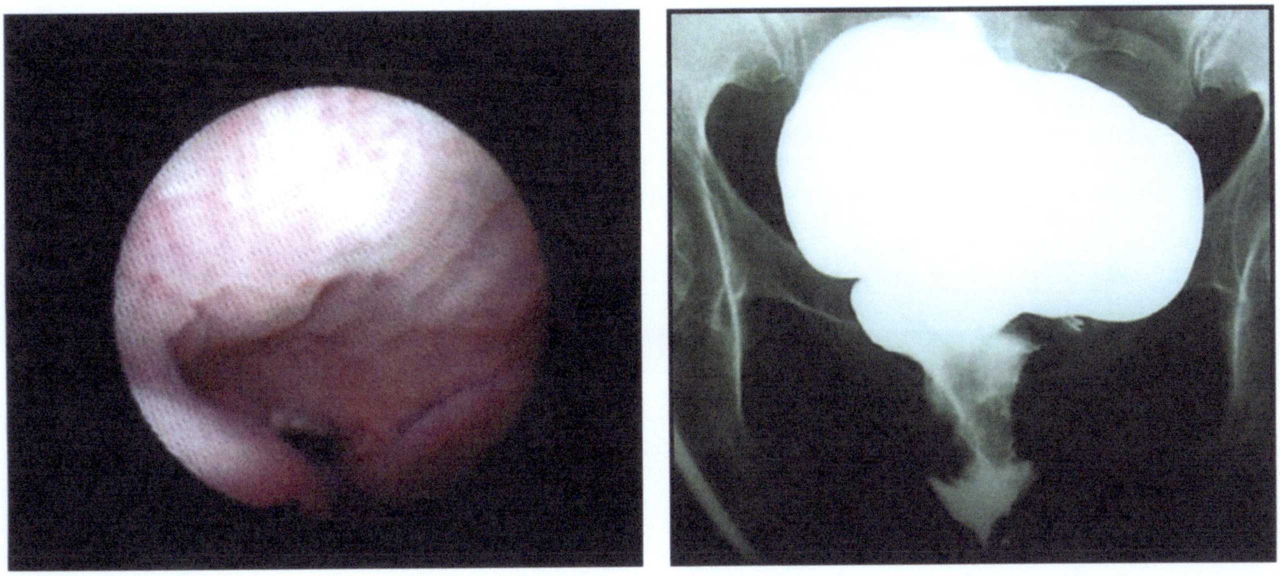

FIGURE 1-10. Vesicovaginal fistula: cystoscopic view of fistula left of midline on posterior wall *(left)* and cystogram with contrast filling the vagina *(right)*. In the United States, fistulas are associated with hysterectomy in 50% of cases.

Outlet Dysfunction: Bladder Outlet and Pelvic Floor

A. Underactive outlet (decreased urethral resistance)

Symptomatic: stress urinary incontinence (SUI)

1. Anatomic support defects (SUI-A) (types I and II SUI):

   Pathophysiology: anatomic motion creates inequities in transmission pressures to bladder and outlet, overcoming urethral resistance, and conformational changes caused by vaginal wall motion disrupt outlet integrity

   a) anatomic defects of fascia, muscles, ligaments, and bony pelvis

   b) functioning support: muscular contraction—denervation or loss of identification, strength, or coordination of levator musculature

   c) degree of intrinsic sphincter deficiency (ISD) (see 2) that, in combination with SUI-A I or II, contributes to critical decreases in resistance during an effort to permit urinary leakage

2. ISD (SUI-ISD) (type III) (low urethra)

   Pathophysiology: deficiency of the urethral closure mechanism secondary to decreased innervation, vascularization, or trauma to mucosa, submucosa, or smooth nonstriated skeletal or skeletal musculature of urethra—intrinsic deficiency of the closure mechanism

   a) proximal urethral sphincter: bladder neck (smooth muscle) and proximal urethra (SUI-ISD-p)

   b) external sphincter: denervation or loss of resting tone, voluntary or reflex contraction (SUI-ISD-d)

   c) combined or total proximal and external sphincter deficiency (SUI-ISD-t)

3. Combined SUI (SUI-A-ISD)

   Pathophysiology: a degree of both anatomic motion and sphincter dysfunction

   a) leakage from ISD may exist without hypermobility

   b) hypermobility alone without a degree of ISD is not sufficient to result in urinary loss

4. *Failure to inhibit the detrusor: decreased pelvic floor inhibitory activity of bladder (etiology for OAB; see C)*

   Pathophysiology: failure to contract the pelvic floor releases detrusor reflex and decreases ability to inhibit active contraction

   a) neurologic: (infrasacral) denervation (areflexia of the pelvic floor)

   b) behavioral: failure to contract the pelvic floor (lack of identification/strength/coordination)

   c) mechanical: damage to pelvic floor structures with intact innervation

B. Overactive outlet (increased urethral resistance)

Symptomatic: overflow incontinence/retention; frequency–urgency

1. Anatomic obstruction (physical blockage)

   Pathophysiology: increased outlet resistance secondary to compression or narrowing

   a) iatrogenic: surgical (eg, for urinary incontinence)

   b) other: congenital, inflammatory, neoplastic, traumatic

2. Functional obstruction (failure of relaxation)

   Pathophysiology: increased outlet resistance, inappropriate contraction or failure of normal relaxation

   a) neurogenic: detrusor sphincter dyssynergia (skeletal musculature)

   b) behavioral: failure to relax pelvic floor musculature or the external sphincter

3. Combined anatomic and functional obstruction

4. *Inhibition of detrusor activity: increased pelvic floor activity*

   Pathophysiology: failure to relax the pelvic floor inhibits the initiation of detrusor activity and inhibits the ability to develop or continue a sustained detrusor contraction

   a) neurologic: (suprasacral) overactivity/hyperreflexia (dyssynergic pelvic floor activity)

   b) behavioral: failure to relax the pelvic floor (learned, acquired, maladaptive, psychogenic)

   c) situational: "voluntary" inhibition secondary to environment or pain

Italics indicate pelvic floor activity.

A

FIGURE 1-11. Descriptive classification. An expanded functional classification of voiding dysfunction including bladder afferents and the pelvic floor activity is given. Function, anatomy, and disease are combined to explain the observed behavior and to understand pathophysiology. In addition to the effects of bladder and outlet on storage and emptying, the interaction of structure and function is considered. **A** lists outlet dysfunction, **B** lists bladder dysfunction, and **C** lists disorders of sensation. A combination of **A** and **B** is also possible.

Continued on the next page

Bladder Dysfunction

A. Detrusor overactivity (increased intravesical pressure)

Symptomatic: urgency incontinence (with or without sensation), overactive bladder (OAB) wet

1. Involuntary detrusor contractions: detrusor overacitivty (motor urgency)

   Pathophysiology: increased detrusor (intravesical) pressure overcomes urethral resistance or causes the sensation of urinary urgency

   a) detrusor overactivity: primary = idiopathic, subclinical neurologic, or symptomatic phasic detrusor activity; secondary = obstruction, reflex urethral relaxation, increased detrusor/mucosal afferent activity; OAB urgency, with (OAB wet) or without (OAB dry) incontinence, usually with frequency and nocturia (absence of other pathology)

   b) detrusor overacitvity (hyperreflexia): supraponitne (intracranial) neurologic lesion (with or without sphincter control); spinal (suprascral) neurologic lesion (with or without sphincteric dyssynergia)

2. Decreased compliance

   Pathophysiology: increased intravesical pressure secondary to decreased accommodation of the detrusor

   a) fibrosis: radiation, inflammation, immune response

   b) neurologic: loss/reversal of accommodation reflex—conus medullaris or peripheral

3. Combined detrusor contractions and decreased compliance

4. Pelvic floor underactivity *(see I.A.4)—decreased pelvic floor inhibition*

B. Underactive bladder (decreased intravesical pressure)

Symptomatic: overflow incontinence/retention

1. Peripheral denervation or neuropathy

   Pathophysiology: decreased contractility—neural efferent or myogenic/decreased afferent stimulation

   a) congenital, inflammatory, neoplastic, or trauma lesion to peripheral nerves

   b) diabetes or other metabolic cause

2. Detrusor myopathy

   Pathophysiology: decreased contractility secondary to smooth muscle damage

   a) fibrosis/collagen deposition

   b) inflammation/obstruction/overdistension

3. Pharmacologic inhibition

   Pathophysiology: decreased contractility secondary to receptor blockade of neural efferents or afferents

   a) antimuscarinics

   b) smooth muscle relaxants/spasmolytics /membrane stabilizers

4. Pelvic floor overactivity *(see I.B.4)*

Italics indicate pelvic floor activity.

B

Disorders of Sensation

A. Decreased sensation

1. Decreased bladder sensation

   Pathophysiology: denervation, myopathy, behavioral, pharmacologic

   a) decreased sense of fullness and normal urge response

   b) loss of sense of fullness/urge warning only with active contraction

   c) loss of sense of fullness/urge incontinence without an appreciation of "desire to void"

   d) urinary retention without an appreciation of distension

2. Decreased bladder outlet and pelvic floor sensation

   Pathophysiology: denervation, myopathy, behavioral, pharmacologic causing decreased ability to identify/contract/coordinate

   a) bladder overactivity (see I.A.4): failure to inhibit?

   b) bladder underactivity (myogenic or mucosal) (see II.B.4): failure to initiate?

   c) contributory to decreased bladder sensation? (see III.A.1.a d)

   d) sexual dysfunction—anorgasmia

B. Increased sensation

1. Increased sensation of the bladder/bladder outlet

   Pathophysiology: neuropathic, inflammatory, mucosal permeability defect, psychogenic, afferent amplification

   a) frequency–urgency symptoms

   b) suprapubic and pelvic pain syndromes

2. *Increased sensation of the pelvic floor/bladder outlet*

   Pathophysiology: neuromuscular myalgia, neuropathic, inflammatory, psychogenic

   a) levator myalgia

   b) frequency–urgency and pelvic pain syndromes

3. *Combined deficit*

Italics indicate pelvic floor activity.

C

Figure 1-11. *(Continued)*

References

1. Lapides J: Neuromuscular, vesical and ureteral dysfunction. In *Urology*. Edited by Campbell MF and Harrison JGH. Philadelphia: WB Saunders; 1970:1343–1279.
2. Hald T, Bradley WE: *The Urinary Bladder: Neurology and Dynamics*. Baltimore: Williams and Wilkins; 1982.
3. Krane RJ, Siroky MB: Classification of voiding dysfunction: value of classification systems. In *Controversies in Neuro-Urology*. Edited by Barrett and Wein AJ. Churchill Livingston; 1984: 223–238.
4. Staskin DR, Zimmern PE, Hadley HR, Raz S: The pathophysiology of stress incontinence. *Urol Clin North Am* 1985, 12:271–280.
5. Staskin DR, Wein AJ: Classification of voiding dysfunction in the female patient. In *Textbook of Female Urology and Urogynecology*, edn 2. Edited by Cardozo L and Staskin DR. Oxon, UK: Informa Healthcare; 2006:173–184.
6. Wein AJ: Pathophysiology and classification of voiding dysfunction. In *Campbell-Walsh Urology*, edn 9. Edited by Wein AJ, Kavoussi LR, Novick AC, *et al*. Philadelphia: Elsevier Science (Saunders); 2007:1973–1985.
7. Abrams P, Cardozo L, Fall M, *et al*.: The standardisation of terminology of lower urinary tract function: report from the Standardisation Sub-committee of the International Continence Society. *Neurourol Urodyn* 2002, 21:167–178,
8. Sand P, Dmochowski R: Analysis of the standardisation of terminology of lower urinary tract dysfunction: report from the Standardisation Sub-committee of the International Continence Society. *Neurourol Urodyn* 2002, 21:167–178.
9. Homma Y: Lower urinary tract symptomatology: its definition and confusion. *Int J Urol* 2008, 15:35–43.
10. Birder L, Drake M, De Groat, *et al*.: Neural control. In *Incontinence: 4th International Consultation on Incontinence*, edn 4.Edited by Abrams P, Cardozo L, Khoury S, Wein AJ. Paris: Health Publications Editions 21, Committee 3; 2009:167–254.
11. Gunnarsson M, Mattiasson A: Female stress, urge, and mixed urinary incontinence are associated with a chronic and progressive pelvic floor/vaginal neuromuscular disorder: an investigation of 317 healthy and incontinent women using vaginal surface electromyography. *Neurourol Urodyn* 1999, 18:613–621.
12. Bø K.: Pelvic floor muscle training is effective in treatment of female stress urinary incontinence, but how does it work? *Int Urogynecol J Pelvic Floor Dysfunct* 2004, 15:76–84.
13. Messelink B, Benson T, Berghmans B, *et al*.: Standardization of terminology of pelvic floor muscle function and dysfunction: report from the pelvic floor clinical assessment group of the International Continence Society. *Neurourol Urodyn* 2005, 24:374–380.
14. Petros PE, Ulmsten UI: An integral theory and its method for the diagnosis and management of female urinary incontinence. *Scand J Urol Nephrol Suppl* 1993, 153:1–93.
15. Plzak L 3rd, Staskin D: Genuine stress incontinence theories of etiology and surgical correction. *Urol Clin North Am* 2002, 29:527–535.
16. DeLancey JO, Trowbridge ER, Miller JM, *et al*.: Stress urinary incontinence: relative importance of urethral support and urethral closure pressure. *J Urol* 2008, 179:2286–2289.
17. Leng WW, Chancellor MB: Recognition and treatment of bladder outlet obstruction after sling surgery. *Rev Urol* 2004, 6:29–33.
18. Tyagi R, Staskin DR: Mixed incontinence: the misclassification of patients and limitations of clinical trials. *Curr Urol Rep* 2005, 6:424–428.
19. Brubaker L, Stoddard A, Richter H, *et al*.: Mixed incontinence: comparing definitions in women having stress incontinence surgery. *Neurourol Urodyn* 2009, 28:268–273.
20. Birder LA: More than just a barrier: urothelium as a drug target for urinary bladder pain. *Am J Physiol Renal Physiol* 2005, 289:F489–F495.
21. Yoshimura N: Lower urinary tract symptoms (LUTS) and bladder afferent activity. *Neurourol Urodyn* 2007, 26(6 Suppl):908–913.
22. Wyndaele JJ, De Wachter S: The sensory bladder (1): an update on the different sensations described in the lower urinary tract and the physiological mechanisms behind them. *Neurourol Urodyn* 2008, 27:274–278.
23. Bergman A, Bader K: Reliability of the patient's history in the diagnosis of urinary incontinence. *Int J Gyneaecol Obstet* 1990, 32:255.
24. Versi E, Cardozo L, Anand D, Cooper D: Symptoms analysis for the diagnosis of genuine stress incontinence. *Br J Obstet Gynaecol* 1991, 98:815.
25. Holroyd-Leduc J, Tannenbaum C, Thorpe H, *et al*.: What type of urinary incontinence does this woman have? *JAMA* 2008, 299:1446–1456.
26. Wein AJ, Rackley RR: Overactive bladder: a better understanding of pathophysiology, diagnosis and management. *J Urol* 2006, 175:S5–S10.

2 Neurogenic Bladder

Anurag K. Das

Neurogenic bladder is a term used to describe voiding dysfunction due to neurologic disease. Common neurologic diseases that cause bladder dysfunction include multiple sclerosis, Parkinson's disease and other movement disorders, and traumatic spinal cord injuries. Although there are multiple classification systems for neurogenic voiding dysfunction, the most clinically useful classifications are functional and divide the problems into disorders of storage and of emptying. These can then be further subdivided into storage disorders due either to the bladder or outlet, or emptying failure due either to the bladder or outlet. Of course, the entire bladder and outlet constitutes a unit, the vesico-urethral unit, and in many cases disorders include a combination of the bladder and the outlet, making it difficult to determine a precise cause and effect relationship.

Treatment of neurogenic bladder can be directed toward preserving the upper tract renal function and social continence. This may be accomplished initially with anticholinergic medications, clean intermittent catheterization, or other simple measures. Some patients may require more aggressive measures such as augmentation enterocystoplasty and many women who are in wheelchairs and have limited mobility may require a continent catheterizable stoma.

In this chapter, we will explore cystometrogram tracings, voiding cystourethrogram images, and operative pictures of common findings and procedures related to neurogenic bladder.

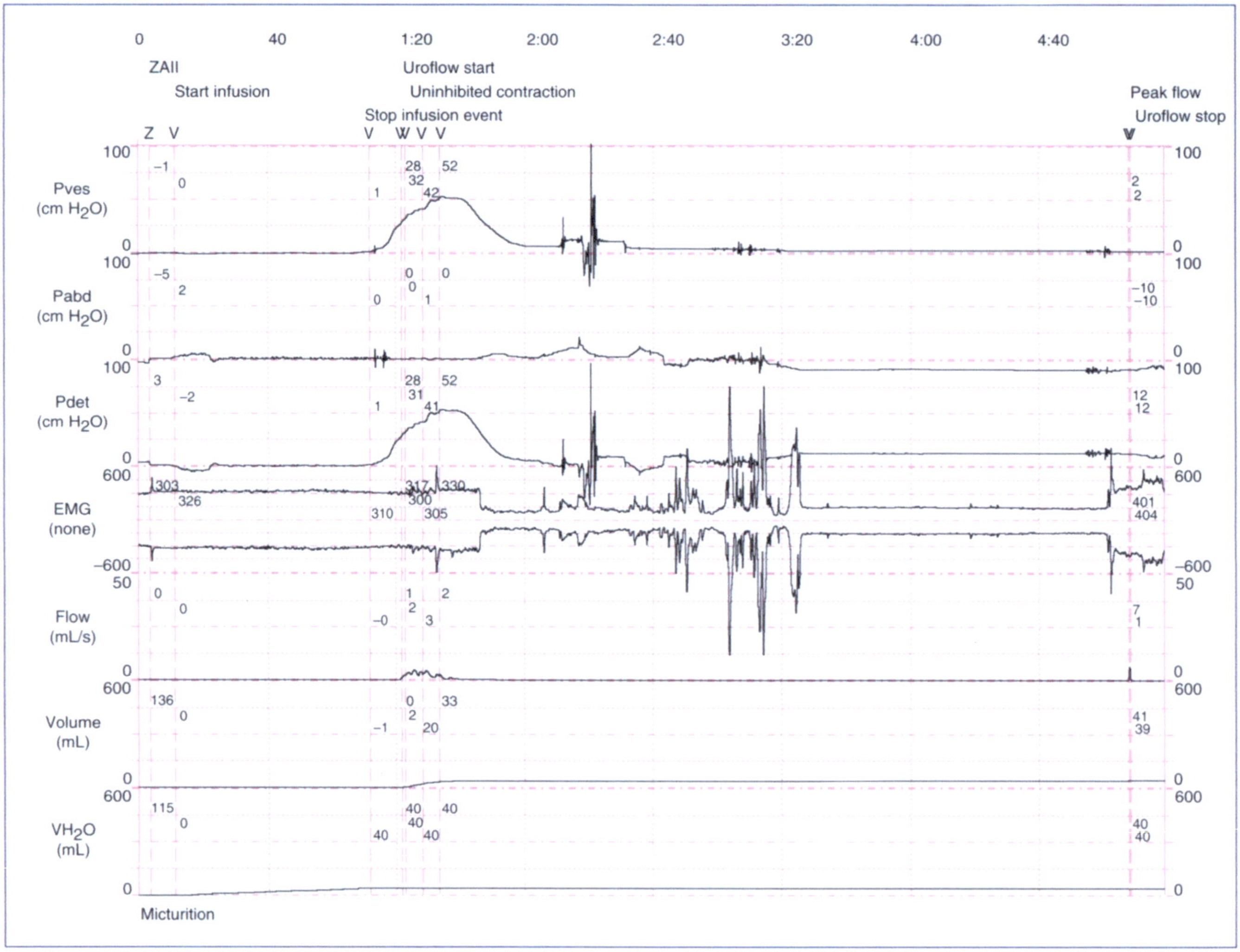

FIGURE 2-1. A 75-year-old man with multiple systems atrophy (Shy-Drager syndrome) presents with significant frequency, urge incontinence, and incontinence without awareness. Cystometrography reveals detrusor overactivity (neurogenic) at low volumes with incomplete emptying.

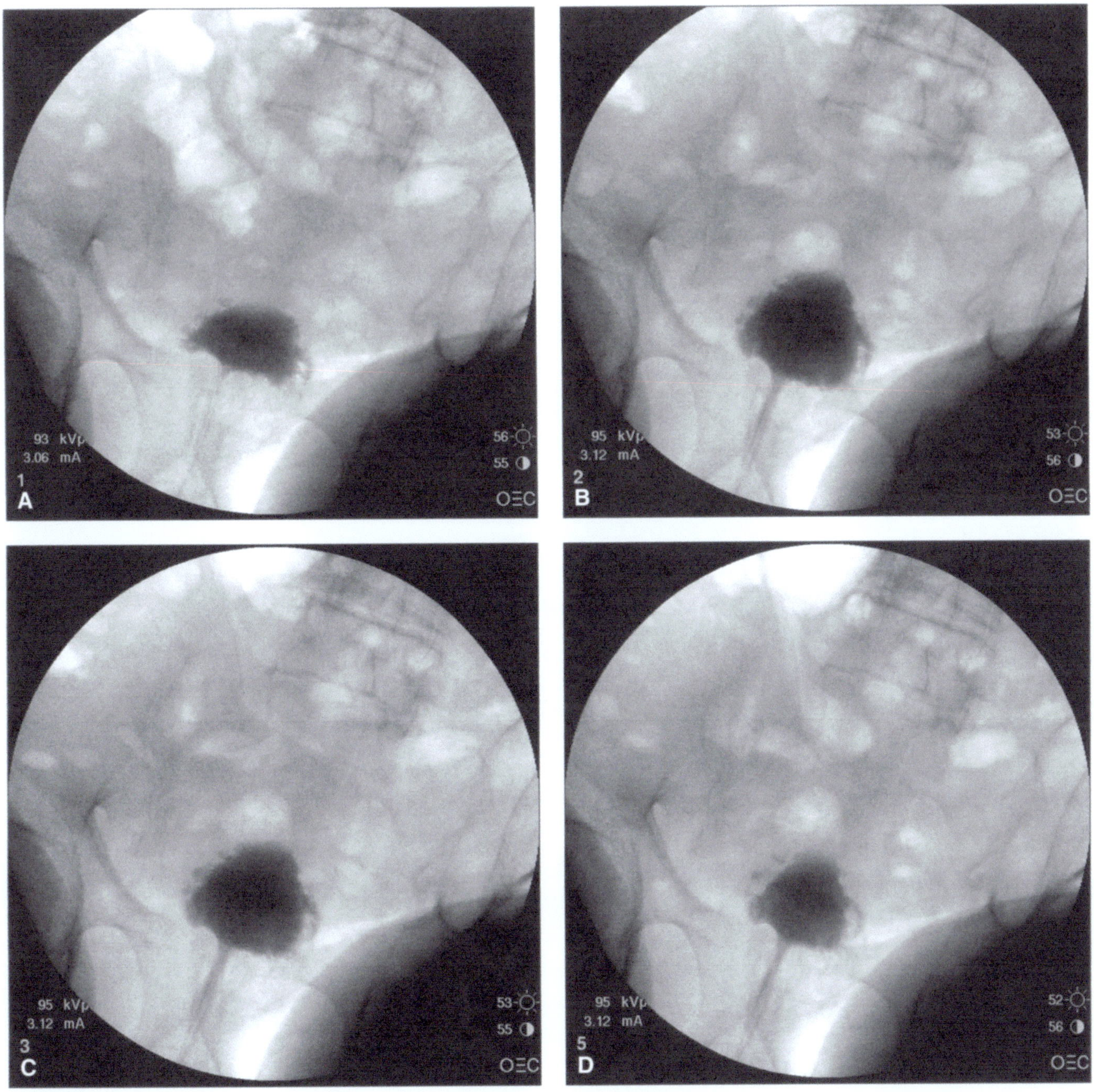

FIGURE 2-2. A–D, Voiding cystourethrography reveals a small-capacity, thick-walled bladder with multiple diverticula, an open bladder neck, and prostatic urethra.

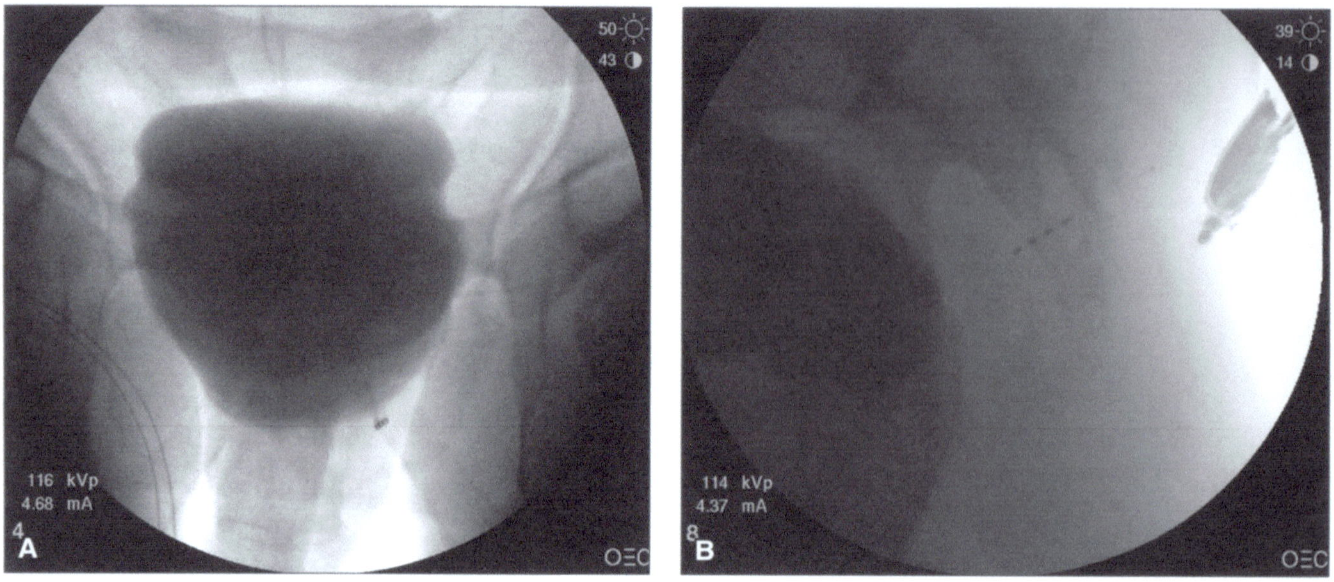

FIGURE 2-3. A 45-year-old man with nonobstructive retention of unclear etiology is treated with sacral neuromodulation. **A**, Voiding cystourethrography showing a smooth, larger capacity bladder and **B**, the lateral view showing quadripolar tined lead at the S3 location, attached to an implantable pulse generator.

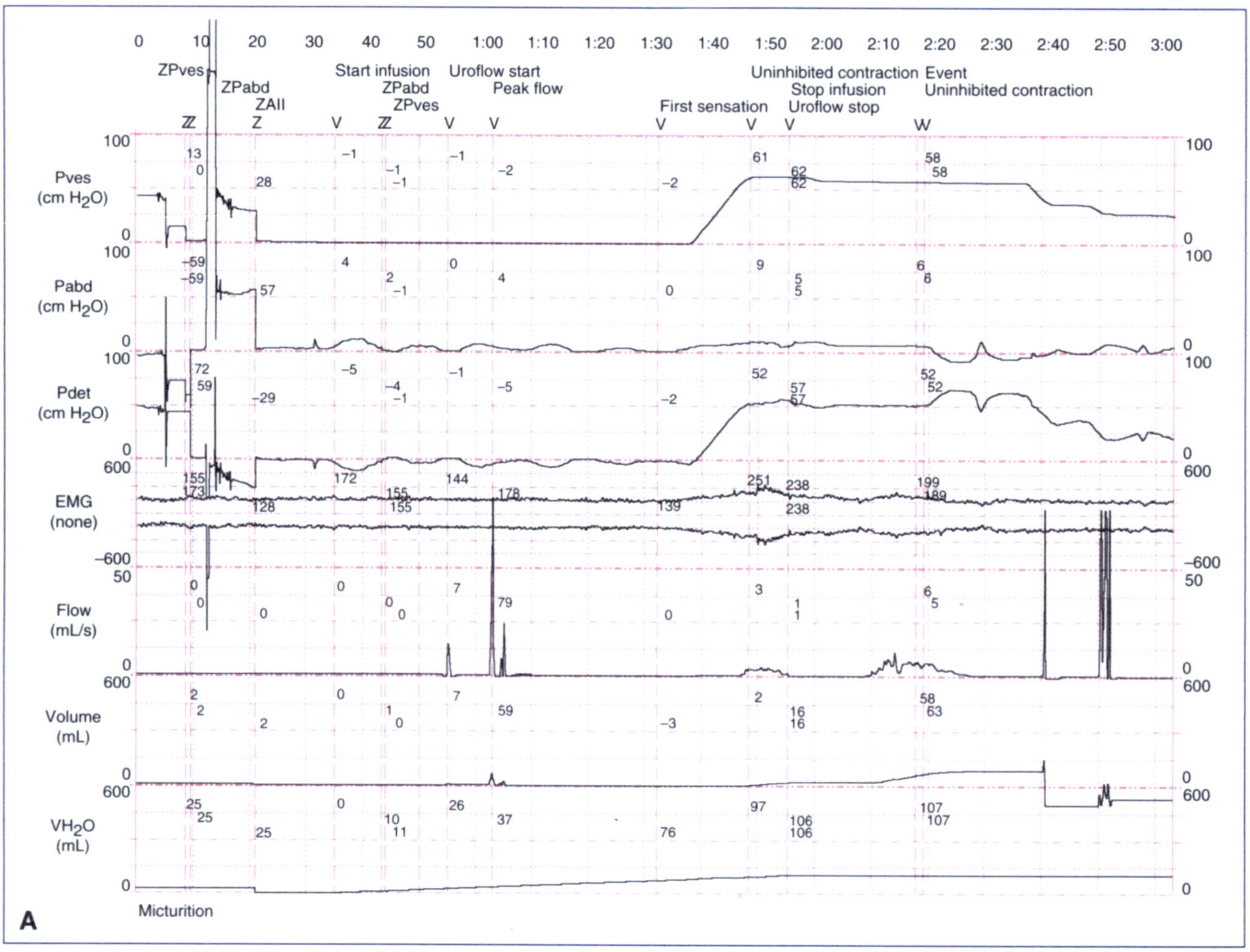

FIGURE 2-4. A 79-year-old woman with Parkinson's disease presents with significant frequency, urge incontinence, and incomplete bladder emptying (**A**). A cystometrogram and pressure–flow studies reveal detrusor overactivity with incomplete emptying and likely detrusor–sphincter dyssynergia or poor sphincteric relaxation.

Continued on the next page

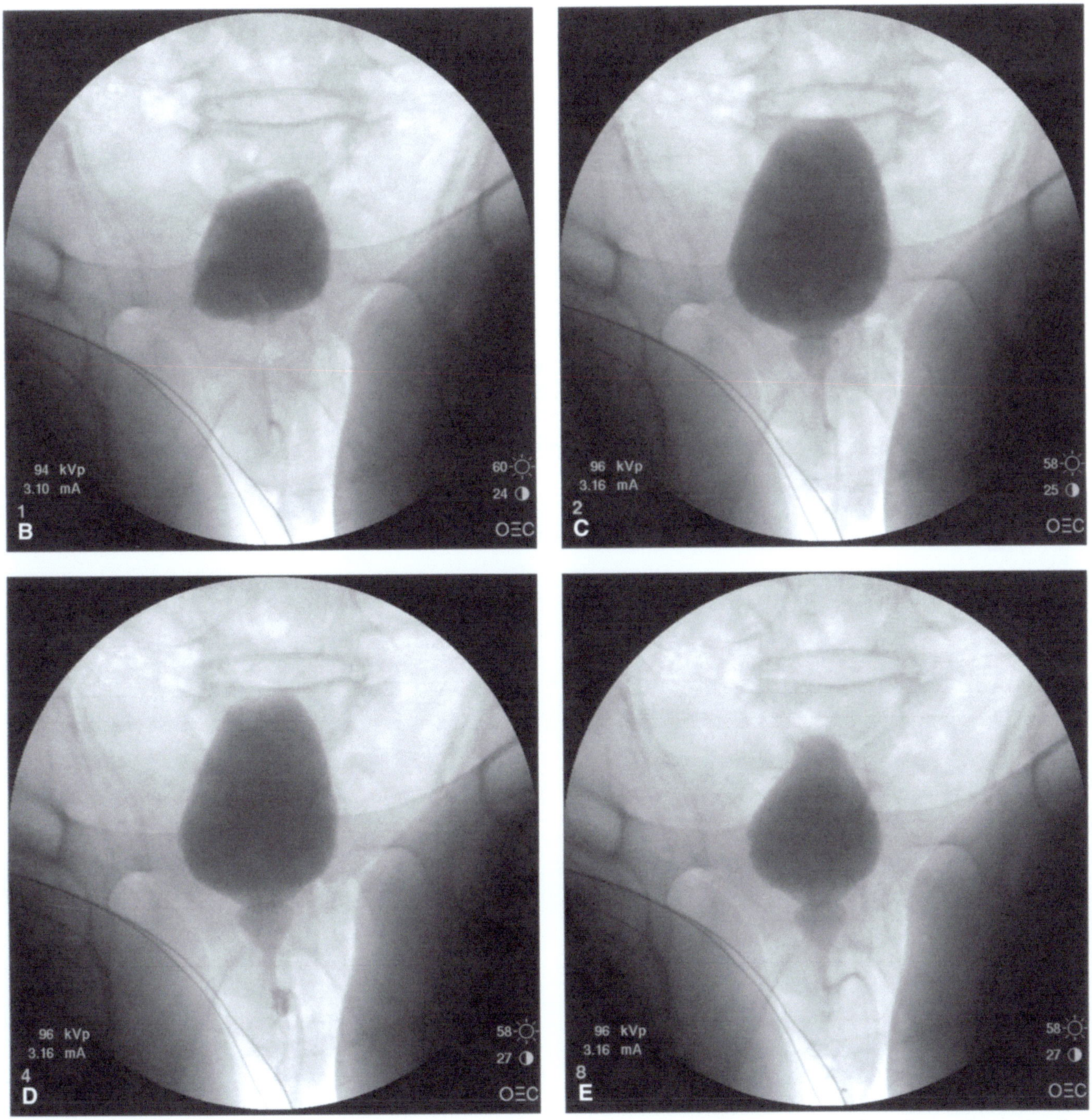

FIGURE 2-4. *(Continued)* Voiding cystourethrography (**B–E**) reveals a somewhat vertically oriented bladder and a "spinning top urethra" with open bladder neck, dilation of the posterior urethra, and poor relaxation of the external sphincter. Cystoscopy did not reveal any strictures.

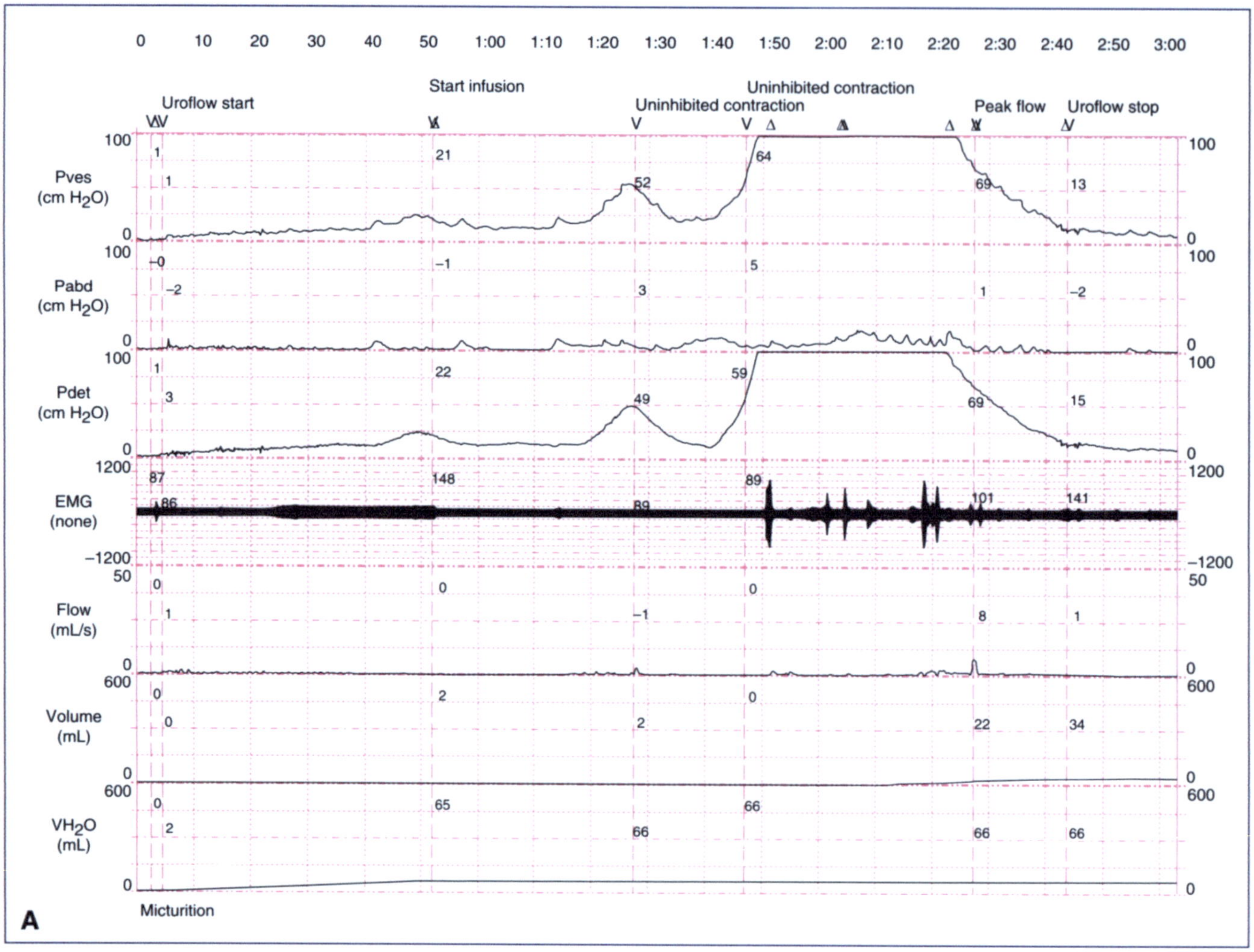

FIGURE 2-5. A 59-year-old man with gait disorder and a history of previous stroke presents with slow stream, a feeling of incomplete emptying, and urge incontinence. A cystometrogram reveals detrusor overactivity starting at low volumes. A voiding pressure–flow study reveals high-grade obstruction with low flow and high detrusor pressures (**A**).

Continued on the next page

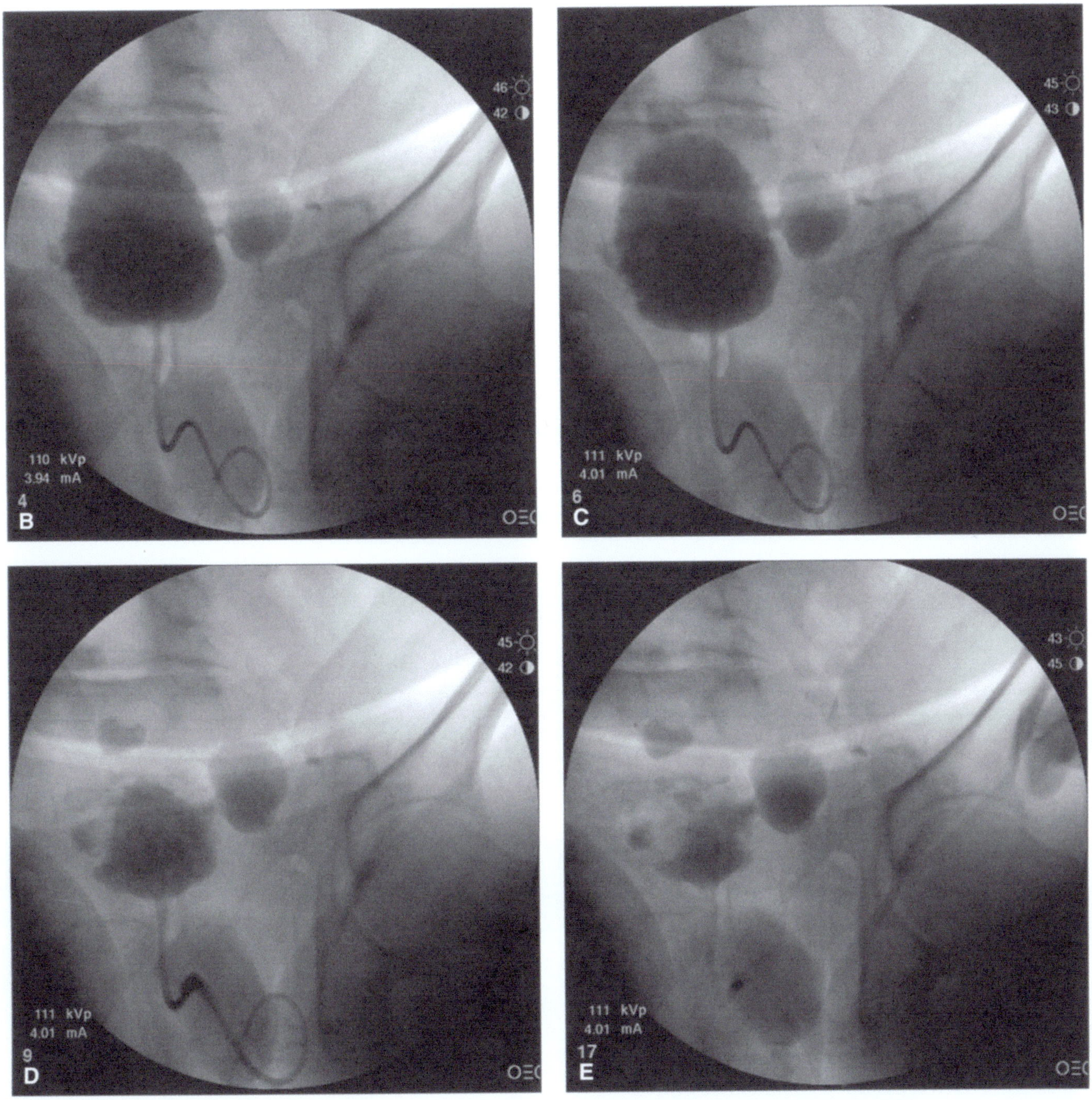

Figure 2-5. *(Continued)* Voiding cystourethrography (**B–E**) reveals a small-capacity, vertically oriented, thick-walled bladder with multiple diverticula. The bladder neck reveals poor funneling and the prostatic urethra is narrow. Such cases present a perplexing clinical scenario, as it is very difficult to determine whether the detrusor overactivity is secondary to chronic high-grade obstruction or is of neurogenic etiology. If the patient can sense the overactive contraction, the etiology is less likely to be neurogenic.

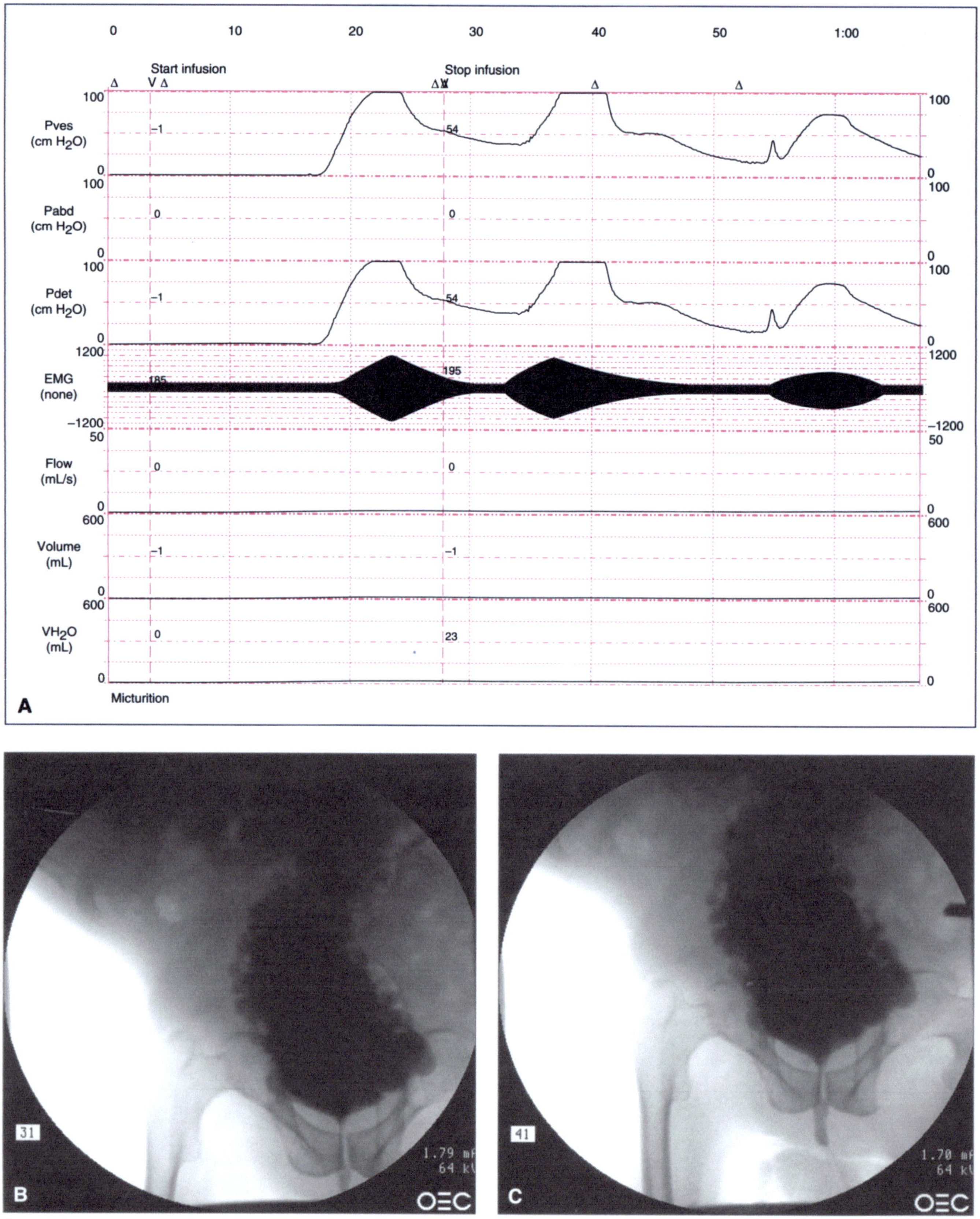

FIGURE 2-6. A 32-year-old man with a spinal cord injury and paraplegia managed with anticholinergics and clean intermittent catheterization every 4 hours undergoes a routine urodynamic study. A cystometrogram reveals very limited capacity with detrusor overactivity and detrusor–sphincter dyssynergia (**A**). Voiding cystourethrography reveals a vertically oriented bladder with multiple diverticulae and a closed bladder neck (**B** and **C**). Maximally tolerated antimuscarinics fail to improve compliance significantly with detrusor pressures over 40 cm of water at a volume of 140 mL.

Continued on the next page

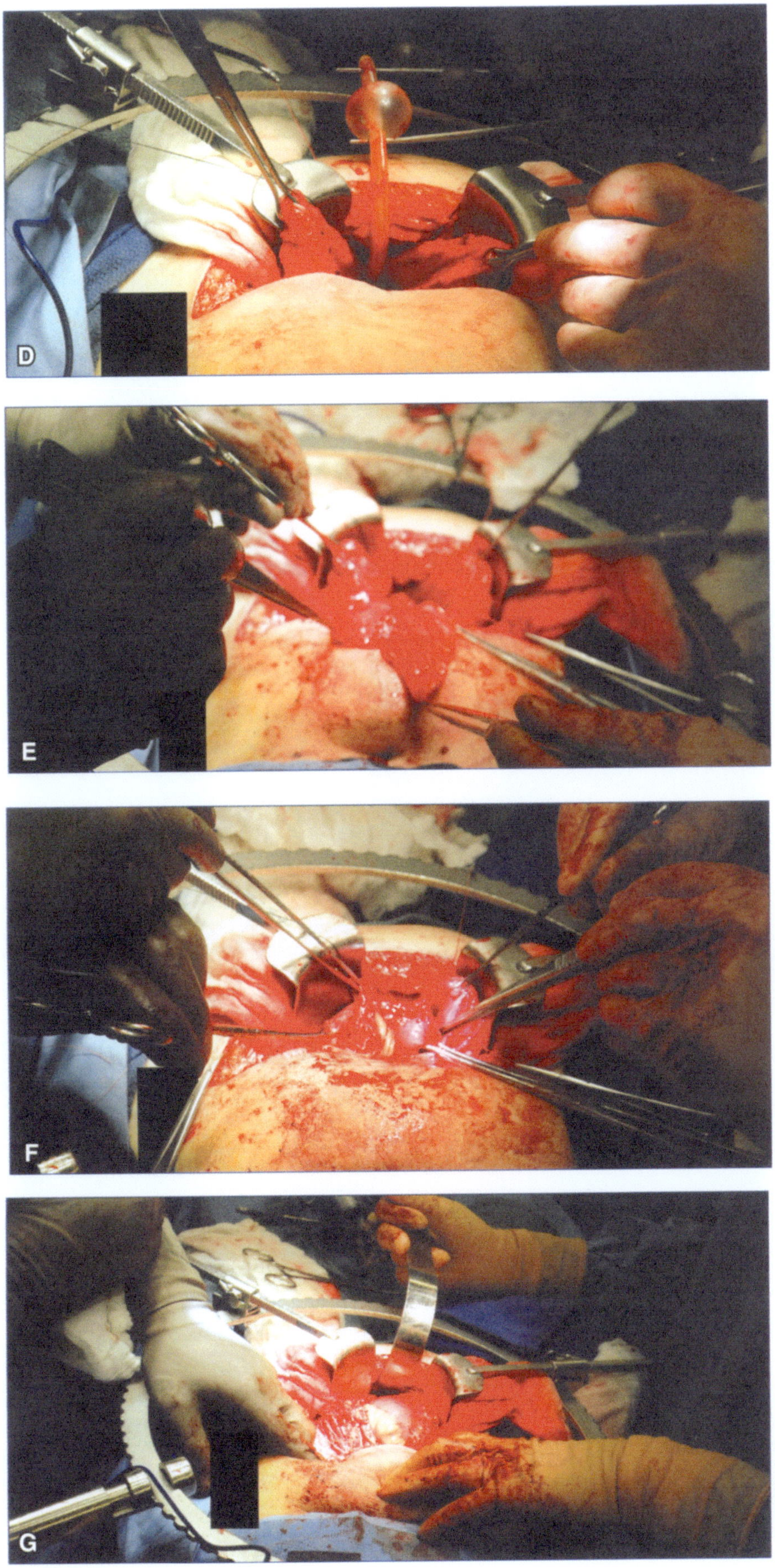

FIGURE 2-6. *(Continued)* The patient undergoes augmentation ileocystoplasty. The bladder is bivalved (**D**); a 12-cm piece of ileum is isolated on its mesentery and the bowel is closed with a side-to-side stapled anastomosis. The isolated patch of ileum is opened and patched onto the bladder (**E–G**).

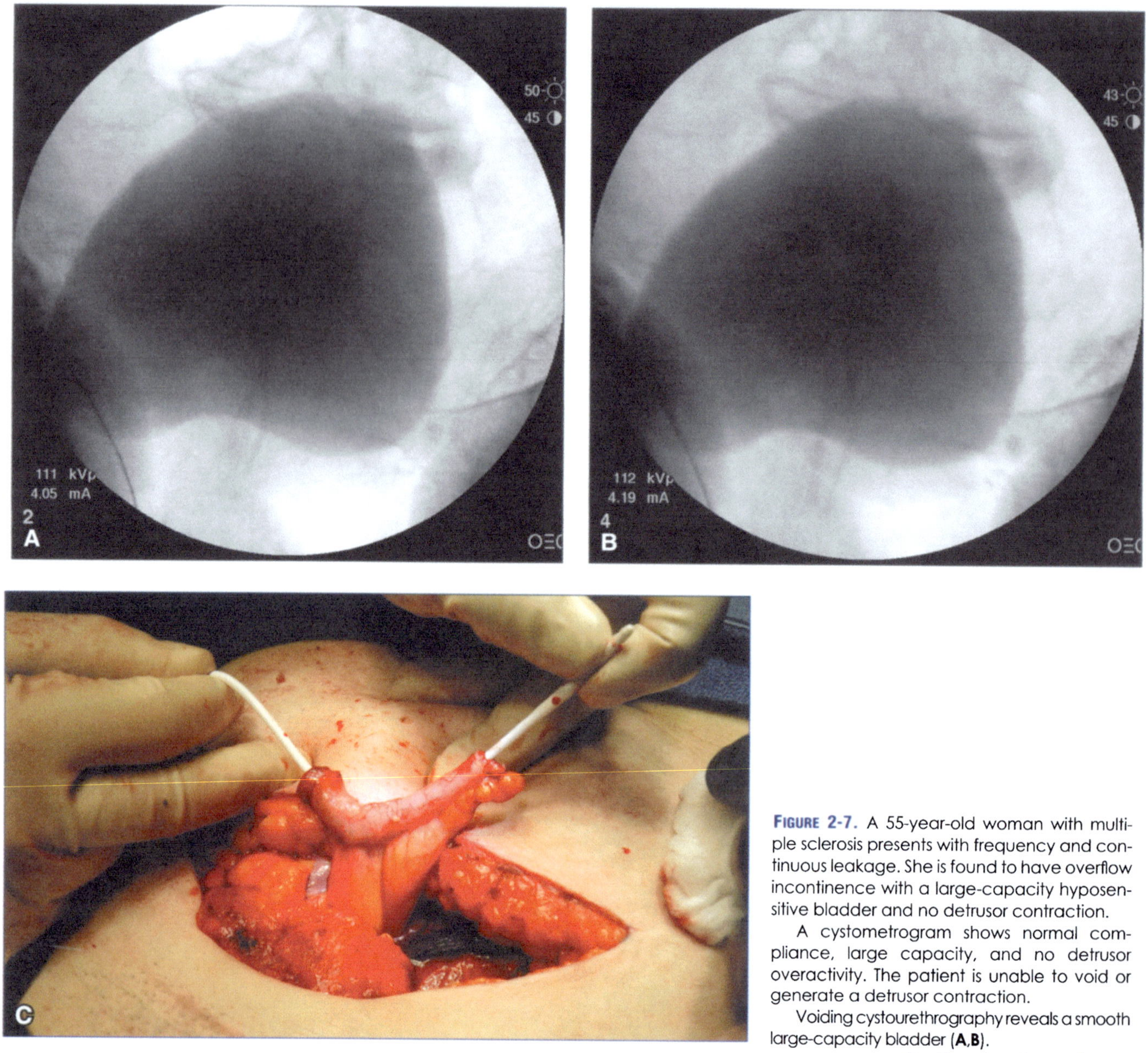

FIGURE 2-7. A 55-year-old woman with multiple sclerosis presents with frequency and continuous leakage. She is found to have overflow incontinence with a large-capacity hyposensitive bladder and no detrusor contraction.

A cystometrogram shows normal compliance, large capacity, and no detrusor overactivity. The patient is unable to void or generate a detrusor contraction.

Voiding cystourethrography reveals a smooth large-capacity bladder (**A**,**B**).

Continued on the next page

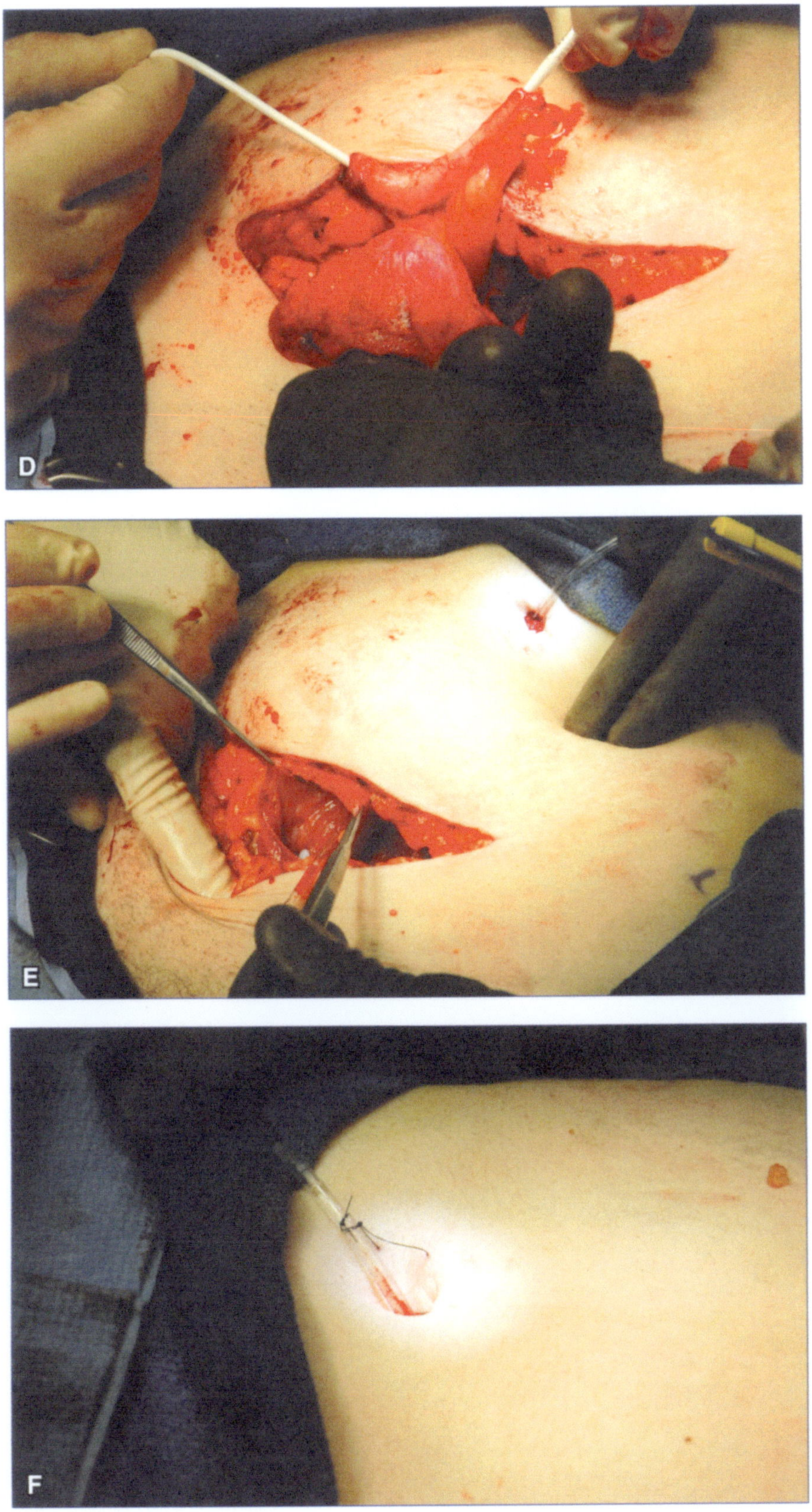

FIGURE 2-7. *(Continued)* The patient is initially taught self-intermittent catheterization. However, due to anatomy and the inability to adduct hips, she is unable to do so.

An appendicovesicostomy is created as a continent catheterizable stoma (**C**–**F**).

Initially, the appendix is isolated from its blood supply and detached from the colon. The closed (noncolonic) end is opened and the bladder is mobilized and opened. The noncolonic end is implanted at the most cephalad portion of the bladder, utilizing a nonrefluxing anastamosis. The colonic end is attached to the umbilicus.

3

Nocturia: Diagnosis and Management

Courtney L. Lee, Jeffrey P. Weiss, and Jerry G. Blaivas

One of the most common reasons for interrupted sleep in the general adult population is nocturia, waking (at least once) during the night to urinate [1]. Sleep is important for both physical and mental well being. It is generally thought that adults need around 7 to 8 hours of sleep per night and that adequate sleep has a restorative effect. Insufficient or disrupted sleep has commonly been linked with excessive daytime sleepiness, leading to both poor motivation and job performance and physical and mental disorders, particularly depression and altered mood [2–5].

Various studies have shown that patients who have nocturia are more likely to have depression and anxiety, and to miss more days from work due to sickness [6]. They also have a lower overall satisfaction with daily life, a worse general state of health, and an increase in mortality compared with those having fewer episodes of nocturia [6–8].

The prevalence of two or more nocturnal voids ranges from 11% to 28% in various population studies, including adults of all ages [9–12]; 38% to 60% of men and 36% to 55% of women are estimated to void at least once per night [10–12].

The International Continence Society (ICS) defines nocturia as waking during the night at least once to urinate, irrespective of bother [1]. Additionally, the ICS suggests that a nocturic void is preceded and followed by sleep [1].

There are numerous conditions that are associated with nocturia. The etiology of nocturia falls into five broad categories: 1) nocturnal polyuria (NP); 2) low nocturnal bladder capacity (NBC) despite normal global bladder capacity; 3) diminished global bladder capacity; 4) mixed (a combination of NP and low bladder capacity); and 5) global polyuria. These categories are derived from the 24-hour voiding diary wherein each voided volume and its corresponding time is entered (see Figure 3-1). An algorithm for evaluation analysis of nocturia is presented in Figure 3-2 and categories and causes related to nocturia are listed in Figure 3-3.

On the basis of the voiding diary, the patient is categorized as having NP, low nocturnal or global bladder capacity, a mixed disorder, or polyuria by using a few simple equations (see Figure 3-4).

Nocturia is evaluated in multiple questionnaires that evaluate lower urinary tract symptoms (see Figure 3-5) [13]. Question 7 of the International Prostate Symptom Score is used in numerous studies of nocturia to quantify the amount of nocturia. However, this correlates poorly with the objective measurement of nocturnal voids per night on frequency/volume charts [14].

An example of bladder diary analysis for a patient with nocturnal polyuria is seen in Figure 3-6 and causes and treatments of nocturnal polyuria are listed in Figure 3-7. An example of diary analysis for a patient with decreased NBC is seen in Figure 3-8. Causes and treatments of decreased NBC are listed in Figure 3-9. An example of a bladder diary analysis for a patient with mixed nocturia is seen in Figure 3-10 and an example of a bladder diary analysis for a patient with global polyuria is seen in Figure 3-11. Causes and treatments of global polyuria are listed in Figure 3-12. An illustration of the workup of global polyuria can be seen in Case Study 1, Figures 3-13 to 3-17. Other investigational treatments for nocturia are listed in Figure 3-18. More research will be needed to assess their true role in the treatment of nocturia.

VOIDING DIARY

PATIENT NAME ______________________ LAST 4 ________

DATE __________________ TIME DIARY STARTED ________

BEDTIME ______ TIME YOU GOT UP FOR THE DAY ________

Time of urination	Amount (mL or ounces)
1	
2	
3	
4	
5	
6	
7	
8	
9	
10	
11	
12	
13	
14	
15	
16	
17	
18	
19	

Figure 3-1. Twenty-four-hour voiding diary. The evaluation of nocturia begins with a focused history and physical examination considering aspects such as sleep, urinary complaints, fluid intake, cardiac problems, medication, prior lower urologic tract surgery, and other comorbidities that may account for excessive nocturnal urine output, detrusor overactivity, or sensory urgency. Of paramount importance is a frequency/volume chart, also known as a voiding diary. The voiding diary includes the volume and time of each urine void, the time of retiring for sleep, and the time of rising during a 24- to 72-hour period. The patient is instructed to record the diary on a typical day and inform the doctor whether the night measured was representative of a normal sleep cycle.

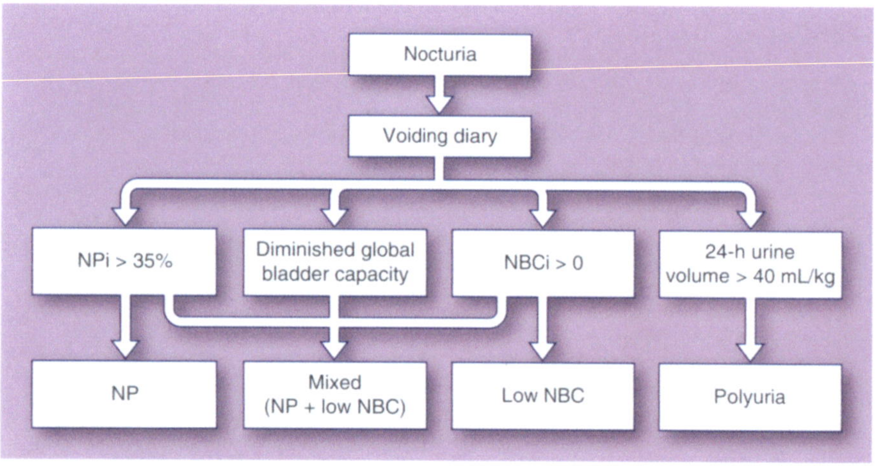

Figure 3-2. Evaluation of nocturia. The etiology of nocturia falls into five broad categories: 1) nocturnal polyuria (NP); 2) low nocturnal bladder capacity (NBC) despite normal global bladder capacity; 3) diminished global bladder capacity; 4) mixed (a combination of NP and low bladder capacity at day or night); and 5) global polyuria. These categories are derived from the 24-hour voiding diary wherein each voided volume and its corresponding time is entered. Formulas for diary-derived nocturia parameters are explained in Figure 3-4. NBCi—nocturnal bladder capacity index; NPi—nocturnal polyuria index.

Causes of Nocturia

Nocturia category	Causes
Nocturnal polyuria	Congestive heart failure
	Diabetes mellitus
	Obstructive sleep apnea
	Peripheral edema
	Venous stasis
	Nephrotic syndrome
	Hepatic failure
	Hypoalbuminemia
	Excessive nighttime fluid intake
Diminished NBC or global bladder capacity	Prostatic obstruction
	Nocturnal detrusor overactivity
	Neurogenic bladder
	Cancer of the bladder, prostate, or urethra
	Learned voiding dysfunction
	Anxiety disorders
	Pharmacologic agents
	Bladder calculi
	Ureteral calculi
Global polyuria	Diabetes mellitus
	Diabetes insipidus
	Primary polydipsia

FIGURE 3-3. Causes of nocturia. Pathologic conditions that cause nocturia include cardiovascular disease, diabetes mellitus and insipidus, lower urinary tract obstruction, and awaking to void for other reasons such as anxiety or primary sleep disorders [2,9,15]. Behavioral and environmental factors that contribute to nocturia include the consumption of a diuretic medication, caffeine, alcohol, or excessive fluid shortly before retiring for the night [16]. Commonly prescribed medications such as beta blockers and selective serotonin reuptake inhibitors are associated with an increase in nocturia [17,18]. Prostate disease and neurogenic and overactive bladders have reportedly led to frequent nocturnal rising [9,16,19]. Nocturia may additionally result from stroke, congestive heart failure, peripheral edema (eg, owing to venous insufficiency or nephrotic syndrome), and myeloneuropathy secondary to vertebral disc disease or spondylosis [20].

Formulas for the Evaluation of Nocturia

Formula	
Ni	Ni > 1: nocturia is due to NUV exceeding MVV
Ni = NUV ÷ MVV	
NPi	NPi > 0.35: Dx is nocturnal polyuria
NPi = NUV ÷ 24 hV	
NBCi	NBCi > 0: nocturia occurring at volumes < MVV
Ni − 1 = PNV (round up to the next highest integer if it is a mixed number)	
NBCi = ANV − PNV	

FIGURE 3-4. Formulas for the evaluation of nocturia. Nocturnal urine volume (NUV) is the volume of urine voided throughout the night and includes the volume of the first morning void. The maximum voided volume (MVV) is defined as the largest volume of urine voided throughout the 24-hour period. The nocturia index (Ni) is calculated by dividing NUV by MVV [21]. When the Ni is greater than 1, the NUV exceeds the bladder maximal storage capacity and nocturia occurs (enuresis will occur instead of nocturia if the patient does not awaken). The nocturnal polyuria index (NPi) is defined as NUV divided by the 24-hour urine volume. When NPi is greater than 0.35, a patient has nocturnal polyuria [1]. The Ni minus 1 equals the predicted number of nightly voids (PNV). If the PNV is not an integer, it must be rounded up to the next highest integer. The nocturnal bladder capacity index (NBCi) is the difference between the PNV and the actual nightly voids (ANVs). The greater the NBCi, the more nocturia may be attributed to diminished nocturnal bladder capacity owing to urologic as opposed to medical disorders.

Instruments to Evaluate Nocturia

Type of Instrument	Questionnaire
Condition-specific questionnaires evaluating LUTS	Bristol Female LUTS Questionnaire [25]
	Incontinence Impact Questionnaire [26]
	Incontinence Quality of Life Questionnaire [27,28]
	ICSmale Questionnaire [29,30]
	International Prostate Symptom Score [31]
	Kings Health Questionnaire [32]
	Urogenital Distress Inventory [26]
General quality-of-life instruments	EuroQOL Index [33]
	Medical Outcomes Study 36-Item Short Form Health Survey (SF-36) [34]
	Nottingham Health Profile [35]
	Short Form (SF-12) [36]
	Sickness Impact Profile [37]
Sleep-related quality-of-life instruments	Basic Nordic Sleep Questionnaire [38]
	Epworth Sleepiness Scale [39,40]
	Medical Outcomes Study Sleep Scale [41]
	Pittsburgh Sleep Quality Index [42]
	NNES-Q [22]
	N-QOL [23,24]

Figure 3-5. Instruments to evaluate the severity and impact of nocturia. Until recently, instruments that evaluated lower urinary tract symptoms (LUTS), general health, or sleep were used to evaluate the impact of nocturia on quality of life. Two nocturia-specific instruments have recently been developed. The Nocturia, Nocturnal Enuresis, and Sleep-Interruptions Questionnaire (NNES-Q) was validated to evaluate the severity and impact of nocturia and nocturnal enuresis. In addition to 10 questions assessing the occurrence and impact of nocturia and nocturnal enuresis, the 12-question questionnaire has two questions that look at the occurrence of sleep disturbance secondary to factors other than nocturia and the bother associated with sleep interruptions in general [22]. The 13-item Nocturia Quality-of-Life (N-QOL) questionnaire evaluates the impact of nocturia. Twelve of the questions are directly related to nocturia and are divided into sleep/energy and bother/concern domains. The final question assesses global quality of life. This questionnaire does not quantify nocturia; it only evaluates the quality of life associated with nocturia [23]. The N-QOL questionnaire is validated in both male and female patients who have nocturia [23,24].

Nocturnal Polyuria

Example of Diary Analysis for NP

NUV = 750 mL
24-h volume = 1500 mL
NPi = NUV/24 h = 0.5 (NPi > 0.35; therefore, nocturia is related to nocturnal polyuria.)

Figure 3-6. Example of diary analysis for nocturnal polyuria (NP). NP is the increased production of urine at night, which is offset by lowered daytime urine production, resulting in a normal 24-hour urine volume [43]. The NP index (NPi) is defined as the nocturnal urine volume (NUV) divided by the 24-hour urine volume. Normally, urine is produced in a circadian pattern that is age dependent. In young people (< 25 y), mean NPi is .14 as compared with older people (> 65 y) whose mean NPi is .34 [44]. Therefore, NP exists when the 24-hour urine production is within normal limits and NPi is greater than 0.35.

Causes of and Treatments for NP

Causes	Treatment
Congestive heart disease	Diuretics
Peripheral edema	Compressive stockings
	Leg elevation
OSA	CPAP
Other	Desmopressin (nocturnal antidiuretic therapy)
	NSAIDs

Figure 3-7. Treatment of nocturnal polyuria (NP). In patients who have congestive heart disease or peripheral edema, compressive stockings may prevent fluid accumulation and help to diminish nocturnal urinary output. Late afternoon naps with elevation of the legs simulate sleep during the day and may diminish the burden of nocturnal fluid excretion. If edema is present either in the legs or presacral area, diuretics administered in the mid to late afternoon may help diminish this third spacing.

Continuous positive airway pressure (CPAP) has been shown to decrease nighttime voids in patients with obstructive sleep apnea (OSA) [45–47]. Desmopressin is one of the best-studied single pharmacologic treatments for nocturia. This ADH analogue has been proven to be an effective and well-tolerated treatment throughout several randomized tablet studies. Nocturnal urine volume and actual nocturic voids decrease in adults whose nocturia is treated with desmopressin; this reduction is more marked in patients with greater degrees of pretreatment nocturnal diuresis [48–50]. Desmopressin is approved to treat nocturia in many nations worldwide.

Since nonsteroidal anti-inflammatory drugs (NSAIDs) have been shown to reduce renal plasma flow, glomerular filtration rate, and urine output, they have also been evaluated to treat NP [51]. Several studies have found statistically significant decreases in nocturia with NSAID treatment [45–46,52–55].

Diminished Nocturnal Bladder Capacity

Example of Diary Analysis for Diminished NBC

NUV = 750 mL

MVV = 250 mL

Ni = NUV/MVV = 3

PNV = Ni − 1 = 3 − 1 = 2

ANV = 7

NBCi = ANV − PNV = 7 − 2 = 5 (NBCi > 2; therefore, nocturnia is strongly related to low NBC.)

Figure 3-8. Example of diary analysis for diminished nocturnal bladder capacity (NBC). There are two types of nocturia due to diminished bladder capacity: a global decrease in bladder capacity as expressed by low maximum voided volume (MVV) and decreased NBC. In both conditions, nocturnal urinary volume (NUV) exceeds bladder capacity and the patient is awakened by the need to void because the bladder does not hold enough. Urologic causes of both low nocturnal and global bladder capacity include infravesical obstruction, idiopathic nocturnal detrusor overactivity, neurogenic bladder, cystitis, bladder calculi, ureteral calculi, and neoplasms of the bladder, prostate, or urethra. A urologic workup for etiology of diminished NBC includes cystoscopic and urodynamic techniques for diagnosing these disorders. ANV—actual nightly void; NBCi—nocturnal bladder capacity index; Ni—nocturia index; PNV—predicted number of nightly voids.

Causes of and Treatments for NBC

Causes	Treatments
BPH	Alpha-blockers [56,58]
	5-alpha reductase inhibitors [58]
	Transurethral or open prostatectomy [57]
OAB	Anticholinergics [59–63]
	Botulism-A [67]
	Sacral neuromodulation [66]

Figure 3-9. Treatment of diminished nocturnal bladder capacity (low NBC). Although some studies show a statistically significant improvement in nocturia after medical and surgical treatment for benign prostatic hyperplasia (BPH), the clinical significance is unclear [56–58]. In one evaluation of men with BPH who had nocturia refractory to medical treatment, all patients had nocturnal polyuria [52]. Therefore, it is important to consider all etiologies of nocturia when treating men who have nocturia, even when there is an accompanying diagnosis of BPH.

Several studies have evaluated the efficacy of antimuscarinics in the treatment of nocturia associated with overactive bladder (OAB) as a secondary endpoint in OAB trials, demonstrating modest improvement in nocturia [59–63]. Although some of the studies reached statistical significance, the clinical significance of the results are uncertain. Antimuscarinics should be reserved as a treatment of nocturia in patients with concomitant OAB. Two studies found tolterodine extended release produced a statistically significant reduction in the median percent change of OAB-related nocturic episodes, but had no effect on normal non-OAB nocturic voids [64,65].

Studies of cystoscopic detrusor injections of botulinum A and sacral neuromodulation for OAB refractory to medical therapy have shown a decrease in nocturic events after treatment [66,67].

Mixed Nocturia

Example of Diary Analysis for Mixed Nocturia

24-h volume = 2500 mL (no polyuria)

NUV = 1500 mL

MVV = 500 mL (normal global bladder capacity)

Ni = NUV/MVV = 3

PNV = Ni − 1 = 3 − 1 = 2

ANV = 6

NBCi = ANV − PNV = 6 − 2 = 4 (NBCi > 2, indicating low NBC)

NPi = 1500/2500 = 60% (NPi > 0.35, indicating nocturnal polyuria)

Figure 3-10. Example of diary analysis for mixed nocturia. An example of nocturia times six in a patient with normal bladder capacity (NBC), nocturnal polyuria, and diminished NBC is provided. ANV—actual nightly void; MVV—maximum voided volume; NBCi—nocturnal bladder capacity index; Ni—nocturia index; NPi—nocturnal polyuria index; NUV—nocturnal urine volume; PNV—predicted number of nightly voids.

Global Polyuria

Example of Diary Analysis for Global Polyuria
24-h volume = 5000 mL
NUV = 1500 mL
MVV = 500 mL
Ni = NUV/MVV = 3
PNV = Ni − 1 = 3 − 1 = 2
ANV = 2
NBCi = ANV − PNV = 2 − 2 = 0 (nocturic voids at capacity)
NPi = 1500/5000 = 30% (normal)

FIGURE 3-11. Example of diary analysis for global polyuria. Polyuria is defined as a 24-hour urine output greater than 40 mL/kg that causes both daytime urinary frequency and nocturia owing to a general increase in urine output, outstripping even normal bladder capacity. This contrasts with nocturnal polyuria, in which 24-hour urine volume remains normal but there is increased production of urine throughout the night. The inappropriate excretion of water in polyurics leads to polydipsia to prevent circulatory collapse. ANV—actual nightly void; MVV—maximum voided volume; NBCi—normal bladder capacity index; Ni—nocturia index; NPi—nocturnal polyuria index; NUV—nocturnal urine volume; PNV—predicted number of nightly voids.

Causes of and Treatments for Global Polyuria

Causes	Treatment
DM	Decrease serum glucose
DI	
Primary polydipsia	
Dipsogenic polydipsia	No known treatment
Psychogenic polydipsia	Behavioral modification to reduce fluid intake
Central diabetes insipidus	Desmopressin replacement therapy
Nephrogenic diabetes insipidus	Withdraw external causes of ADH insensitivity such as tetracyclines, litium, and electrolyte disorders where applicable

FIGURE 3-12. Treatment of global polyuria. Uncontrolled diabetes mellitus (DM) leads to hyperglycemia and an osmotic diuresis that predisposes patients to nocturia. Treatment decreases the serum levels of glucose with diet, oral hypoglycemics, and insulin when indicated. Primary polydipsia is either dipsogenic or psychogenic.

Dipsogenic polydipsia is associated with a history of a central neurologic abnormality such as prior brain trauma, radiation, or surgery. Psychogenic polydipsia is a long-term behavioral or psychiatric disorder treated with behavioral modification to reduce fluid intake, although unfortunately many patients are resistant to such changes. There is no specific treatment available for dipsogenic polydipsia.

Diabetes insipidus (DI) is a disorder of water balance: central DI is caused by deficient synthesis of an antidiuretic hormone secondary to the loss of neurosecretory neurons in the hypothalamus or posterior hypophysis and nephrogenic DI is due to an inability of the kidneys to respond to ADH.

Case Study

7/22/07, 11:35 AM

CC: "I am waking up to pee all the time."

HPI: This is a 62-year-old female with no significant medical comorbidities complaining of nocturia × 3 and suprapubic cramping. Upon further questioning, she admits to daytime frequency, but denies urgency, incontinence, dysuria, hematuria, and any obstructive voiding symptoms.

PMH: Denies HTN, DM, CAD, and COPD
PSH: Tubal ligation at the age of 30 y
GYN: G_1P_1 NSVD
Meds: Denies
All: PCN
SH: Denies tobacco and alcohol consumption

PE: No CVAT
Abdomen soft, nontender, nondistended
GYN: Mild cystocele, no rectocele, no evidence of urethral masses
Extremities: no peripheral edema
Neurological evaluation: WNL

PVR: 0

Figure 3-13. Physician records from an initial visit for a 62-year-old woman who has polyuria. CAD—coronary artery disease; CC—chief complaint; COPD—chronic obstructive pulmonary disease; CVAT—costovertebral angle tenderness; DM—diabetes mellitus; G_1P_1—gravida 1, para 1; GYN—gynecologic history; HPI—history of the present illness; HTN—hypertension; NSVD—normal spontaneous vaginal delivery; PCN—penicillin; PE—physical examination; PMH—past medical history; PSH—past surgical history; PVR—postvoid residual urine volume; SH—social history; WNL—within normal limits.

7/29/07, 12:15 PM

Urine Analysis: No blood
Urine culture: negative

Cystoscopy: Unremarkable

Voiding frequency chart:

24-h voided volume:	*5190 mL*
Usual voided volume:	*300 mL*
Functional bladder capacity (MVV):	*1200 mL*
Awake hours—number of voids:	*14*
Sleep hours—number of voids:	*3*
NUV:	*1530 mL*
Nocturia index (NUV/MVV):	*1.2*
Nocturia polyuria index (NUN/total):	*29%*
NBC index:	*2*

Figure 3-14. Physician records from a followup visit for a 62-year-old woman who has polyuria. MVV—maximum voided volume; NBC—nocturnal bladder capacity; NUV—nocturnal urine volume.

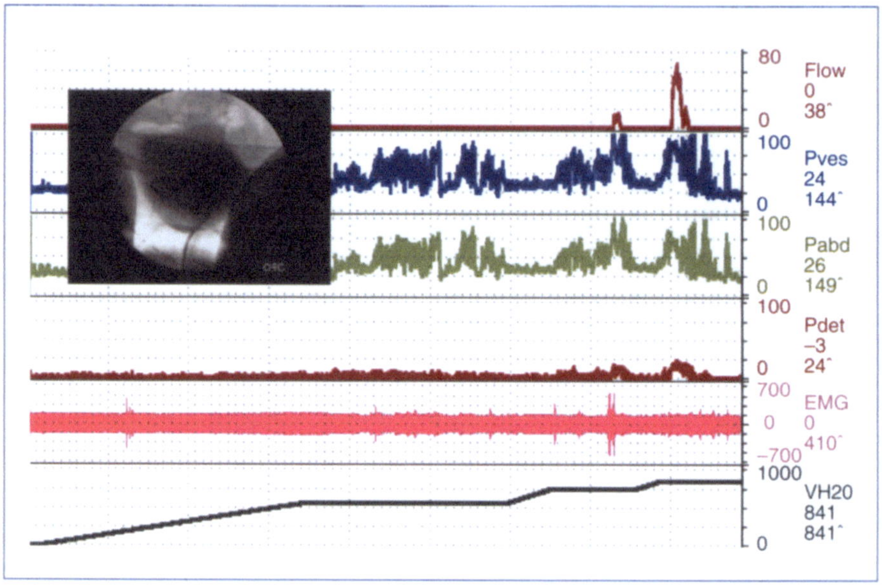

FIGURE 3-15. Videourodynamic study (cystometric capacity = 800 mL; Qmax = 38 mL/s; no involuntary bladder contractions; cystocele). This case evaluates a patient who complains of nocturia and suprapubic cramping associated with polyuria. She has no relevant endoscopic or urodynamic abnormalities. Her lower urinary tract symptoms are secondary to global polyuria. EMG—electromyograph; Pabd—abdominal pressure; Pdet—detrussor pressure; Pves—vesical pressure; VH_2O—volume of infused water.

FIGURE 3-16. Overnight water deprivation test (WDT). When polyuria is demonstrated using the voiding diary, a WDT must be employed to distinguish between diabetes insipidus (DI) and polydipsia [68]. When performing this test, the patient refrains from drinking throughout the night. The first morning void is checked for osmolality. If the first morning void urine osmolality is greater than 800 mOsm/kg H_2O, there is normal ADH secretion and normal renal response to ADH; polyuria is due to primary polydipsia.

If the WDT is abnormal, a renal concentrating capacity test (RCCT) distinguishes between central and nephrogenic DI. Either 40 μg intranasal or 0.4 mg oral desmopressin is administered and water intake is restricted for the first 12 hours after drug administration. The bladder is emptied and a urine sample for osmolality is obtained 3 to 5 hours

Overnight WDT

	Baseline	After overnight fast
Serum osmolality (mOsm/kg)	286	288
Urine osmolality (mOsm/kg)	203	697

9/15/07, 10:25 AM

Voiding Frequency Chart	
24-h voided volume:	*2490 mL*
Usual voided volume:	*350 mL*
Functional bladder capacity (MVV):	*950 mL*
Awake hours—number of voids:	*8*
Sleep hours—number of voids:	*0*
NUV:	*730 mL*
Nocturia index (NUV/MVV):	*0.77*
Nocturia polyuria index (NUV/total):	*29%*
NBC index:	*0*

FIGURE 3-17. Diary following behavior modification. After an overnight fast, the patient's urine osmolality was close to normal (> 800 mOsm/kg in an ideal case), excluding diabetes insipidus as a cause for polyuria. Therefore, the water deprivation test shows primary polydipsia. The differential diagnosis includes psychogenic versus dipsogenic polydipsia. Since the patient had no history of head trauma or radiation therapy, the diagnosis is psychogenic polydipsia and he or she is treated with behavior modification. Symptoms of both nocturia and suprapubic cramping were resolved with near-resolution of the polyuria and blood pressure and serum sodium levels remained normal. MVV—maximum voided volume; NBC—nocturnal bladder capacity; NUV—nocturnal urine volume.

Novel Treatments for Nocturia

Novel Treatments for Nocturia

Treatment	Author	Parameter evaluated	Pretreatment	Posttreatment	P values	Time of treatment	Outcomes instrument
Estrogen therapy [58]	Long *et al.* [69]	Incidence of nocturia	Estrogen tablets: 59%	Estrogen tablets: 37%	Estrogen tablets: $P < 0.05$	3 mo	Bristol Female LUTS Questionnaire
			Estrogen cream: 43%	Estrogen cream: 10%	Estrogen cream: $P < 0.01$		
Pelvic floor exercises	Johnson *et al.* [70]	Mean number of episodes of nocturia per night	1.9 ± 0.8	1.4 ± 0.6	$P < 0.001$ (compared to the placebo)	8 wk	Bladder diary
Physical exercise	Sugaya *et al.* [71]	Mean number of episodes of nocturia per night	3.3 ± 0.7	1.9 ± 0.8	$P < 0.001$	8 wk	Not reported
Peripheral afferent nerve stimulation	Congregado *et al.* [72]	Mean number of episodes of nocturia per night	2.9 ± 2.2	1.4 ± 1.1	$P < 0.001$	10 wk	Bladder diary
Melatonin	Drake *et al.* [73]	Mean number of episodes of nocturia per night	3.1 ± 0.8	2.8 ± 0.7	$P = 0.07$ (compared to the placebo)	4 wk	Bladder diary
	Sugaya *et al.* [74]	Mean number of episodes of nocturia per night	3.4 ± 0.8	2.6 ± 0.9	$P < 0.001$	4 wk	IPSS
Sedatives	Song *et al.* [75]	Median number of episodes of nocturic events per night	3	2	$P = 0.001$	8 wk	IPSS
	Sugaya *et al.* [74]	Number of episodes of nocturia per night	3.5 ± 0.9	2.5 ± 1.1	$P < 0.001$	4 wk	IPSS

FIGURE 3-18. Other treatments for nocturia. Numerous investigators have evaluated several ways to treat nocturia including behavioral therapy, exercise, acupuncture, and sedatives. These treatments need to be studied further in order to elucidate their role in treating nocturia. IPSS—International Prostate Symptom Score; LUTS—lower urinary tract symptom.

Case Study 2

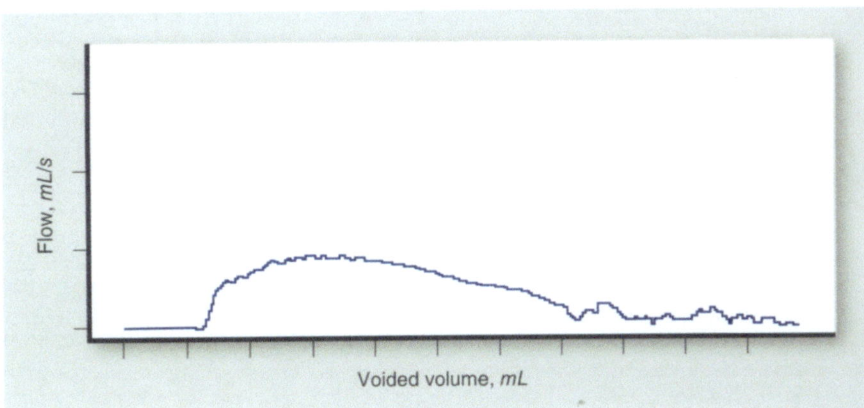

FIGURE 3-19. Uroflow. This is a case of an 80-year-old retired man who presents with frequency, urgency, and nocturia × 8. He also complains of occasional hesitancy, weak stream, and intermittency. He denies straining, incontinence, the sensation of incomplete emptying, hematuria, and dysuria. His examination is only significant for a smooth 30-gram prostate with no nodules. His American Urological Association symptom score is 22 and his prostate-specific antigen is 4.2. Uroflow revealed that Qmax is 9 mL/s, the voided volume is 150 mL, and the pattern plateau is PVR = 0.

Voiding Frequency Chart

24-h voided volume: *	*1300 mL*
MVV:	*200 mL*
Awake hours—number of voids:	*6*
Sleep hours—number of voids:	*8*
NUV:	*600 mL*
Nocturia index (NUV/MVV):	*3*
Nocturia polyuria index (NUV/total):	*46%*
NBC index:	*6*

FIGURE 3-20. Voiding diary. This patient has an elevated nocturnal bladder capacity (NBC) index and nocturnal polyuria index. Therefore, he has mixed nocturia secondary to both decreased NBC and nocturnal polyuria. MVV—maximum voided volume; NUV—nocturnal urine volume.

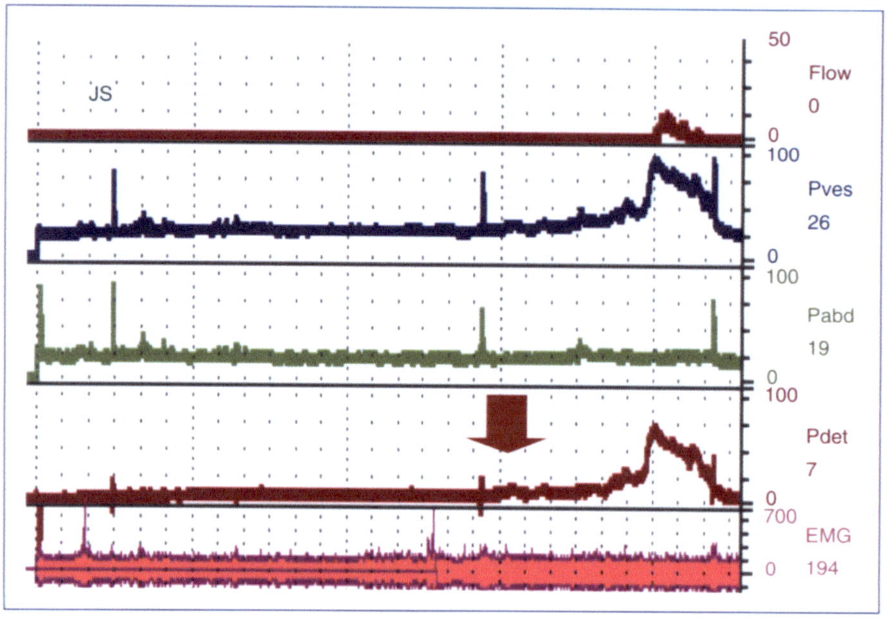

FIGURE 3-21. Urodynamic study. Cystoscopy revealed a trabeculated bladder with tri-lobar "obstructing" prostatic enlargement. A urodynamic study demonstrated a small bladder capacity with detrusor overactivity (*arrow*). The Qmax was 10 mL/s and pdet Qmax was 58 cm H_2O. EMG—electromyograph; Pabd—abdominal pressure; Pdet—detrusor pressure; Pves—vesical pressure.

Voiding Frequency Chart	
24-h voided volume:	*1276 mL*
MVV:	*300 mL*
Awake hours—number of voids:	*5*
Sleep hours—number of voids:	*3*
NUV:	*450 mL*
Nocturia index (NUV/MVV):	*1.5*
Nocturia polyuria index (NUV/total):	*35%*
NBC index:	*2*

FIGURE 3-22. Posttransurethral resection of the prostate (TURP) voiding diary. The patient underwent TURP to relieve prostatic obstruction. At his 6-month followup visit, the American Urological Association symptom score decreased from 22 to 7 and his nocturia deceased from eight to three voids per night. His voiding diary at this time showed resolution of the decreased nocturnal bladder capacity (NBC), but persistence of (mild) nocturnal polyuria. Nocturnal polyuria might be addressed for further improvement of his nocturia. MVV—maximum voided volume; NUV—nocturnal urine volume.

References

1. Van Kerrebroeck P, Abrams P, Chaikin D, *et al.*: The standardisation of terminology in nocturia: report from the Standardisation Sub-committee of the International Continence Society. *Neurourol Urodyn* 2002, 21:179–183.
2. Naitoh P, Kelly TL, Englund C: Health effects of sleep deprivation. *Occup Med* 1990, 5:209–237.
3. Hetta J, Rimon R, Almqvist M: Mood alterations and sleep. *Ann Clin Res* 1985, 17:252–256.
4. Lindberg E, Janson C, Gislason T, *et al.*: Sleep disturbances in a young adult population: can gender differences be explained by differences in psychological status? *Sleep* 1997, 20:381–387.
5. Broman JE, Lundh LG, Hetta J: Insufficient sleep in the general population. *Neurophysiol Clin* 1996, 26:30–39.
6. Asplund R, Aberg H: Nocturnal micturition, sleep and well-being in women of ages 40–64 years. *Maturitas* 1996, 24:73–81.
7. Van Kerrebroeck P: Nocturia and tamsulosin OCAS. *Eur Urol Suppl* 2007, 6:723–727.
8. Kujubu DA, Aboseif SR: Evaluation of nocturia in the elderly. *Permanente J* 2007, 11:38–40.
9. Yoshimura K, Terada N, Matsui Y, *et al.*: Prevalence of and risk factors for nocturia: analysis of a health screening program. *Int J Urol* 2004, 11:282–287.
10. Coyne KS, Zhou Z, Bhattacharyya SK, *et al.*: The prevalence of nocturia and its effect on health-related quality of life and sleep in a community sample in the USA. *BJU Int* 2003, 92:948–954.
11. van Dijk L, Kooij DG, Schellevis FG: Nocturia in the Dutch adult population. *BJU Int* 2002, 90:644–648.
12. Schatzl G, Temml C, Schmidbauer J, *et al.*: Cross-sectional study of nocturia in both sexes: analysis of a voluntary health screening project. *Urology* 2000, 56:71–75.
13. Donovan JL: Measuring the impact of nocturia on quality of life. *BJU Int* 1999, 84(Suppl 1):21–25.
14. Ku JH, Hong SK, Kim HH, *et al.*: Is questionnaire enough to assess number of nocturic episodes? Prospective comparative study between data from questionnaire and frequency-volume charts. *Urology* 2004, 64:966–969.
15. Gourova LW, van de Beek C, Spigt MG, *et al.*: Predictive factors for nocturia in elderly men: a cross-sectional study in 21 general practices. *BJU Int* 2006, 97:528–532.
16. Barker JC, Mitteness LS: Nocturia in the elderly. *Gerontologist* 1988, 28:99–104.
17. Asplund R, Johansson S, Henriksson S, *et al.*: Nocturia, depression and antidepressant medication. *BJU Int* 2005, 95:820–823.
18. Kaplan SA, Walmsley K, Te AE: Tolterodine extended release attenuates lower urinary tract symptoms in men with benign prostatic hyperplasia. *J Urol* 2005, 174:2273–2276.

19. Saito M, Kondo A, Kato T, *et al.*: Frequency-volume charts: comparison of frequency between elderly and adult patients. *Br J Urol* 1993, 72:38–41.

20. Van Cauter E, Plat L, Leproult R, Copinschi G: Alteration of circadian rhythm and sleep in aging: endocrine consequences. *Hormone Res* 1998, 49:147–152.

21. Weiss JP, Blaivas JG, Stember DS, *et al.*: Evaluation of the etiology of nocturia in men: the nocturia and nocturnal bladder capacity indices. *Neurourol Urodyn* 1999, 18:559–565.

22. Bing MH, Moller LA, Jennum P, *et al.*: Validity and reliability of a questionnaire for evaluating nocturia, nocturnal enuresis and sleep-interruptions in an elderly population. *Eur Urol* 2006, 49:710–719.

23. Abraham L, Hareendran A, Mills IW, *et al.*: Development and validation of a quality-of-life measure for men with nocturia. *Urology* 2004, 63:481–486.

24. Mock LL, Parmelee PA, Kutner N, *et al.*: Content validation of symptom-specific nocturia quality-of-life instrument developed in men: issues expressed by women, as well as men. *Urology* 2008, 72:736–742.

25. Jackson S, Donovan J, Brookes S, *et al.*: The Bristol Female Lower Urinary Tract Symptoms Questionnaire: development and psychometric testing. *Br J Urol* 1996, 77:805–812.

26. Shumaker SA, Wyman JF, Uebersax JS, *et al.*: Health-related quality of life measures for women with urinary incontinence: the Incontinence Impact Questionnaire and the Urogenital Distress Inventory. Continence Program in Women (CPW) Research Group. *Qual Life Res* 1994, 3:291–306.

27. Patrick DL, Martin ML, Bushnell DM, *et al.*: Quality of life of women with urinary incontinence: further development of the incontinence quality of life instrument (I-QOL). *Urology* 1999, 53:71–76.

28. Wagner TH, Patrick DL, Bavendam TG, *et al.*: Quality of life of persons with urinary incontinence: development of a new measure. *Urology* 1996, 47:67–72.

29. Donovan JL, Abrams P, Peters TJ, *et al.*: The ICS-'BPH' Study: the psychometric validity and reliability of the ICSmale questionnaire. *Br J Urol* 1996, 77:554–562.

30. Donovan JL, Brookes ST, de la Rosette JJ, *et al.*: The responsiveness of the ICSmale questionnaire to outcome: evidence from the ICS-'BPH' study. *BJU Int* 1999, 83:243–248.

31. Barry MJ, Fowler FJ Jr, O'Leary MP, *et al.*: The American Urological Association symptom index for benign prostatic hyperplasia. The Measurement Committee of the American Urological Association. *J Urol* 1992, 148:1549–1564.

32. Kelleher CJ, Cardozo LD, Khullar V, *et al.*: A new questionnaire to assess the quality of life of urinary incontinent women. *Br J Obstet Gynaecol* 1997, 104:1374–1379.

33. The EuroQol Group: EuroQol—a new facility for the measurement of health-related quality of life. *Health Policy* 1990, 16:199–208.

34. Ware JE Jr, Gandek B: Overview of the SF-36 Health Survey and the International Quality of Life Assessment (IQOLA) Project. *J Clin Epidemiol* 1998, 51:903–912.

35. Hunt SM, McEwen J, McKenna SP: Measuring health status: a new tool for clinicians and epidemiologists. *J R Coll Gen Pract* 1985, 35:185–188.

36. Gandek B, Ware JE, Aaronson NK, *et al.*: Cross-validation of item selection and scoring for the SF-12 Health Survey in nine countries: results from the IQOLA Project—international quality of life assessment. *J Clin Epidemiol* 1998, 51:1171–1178.

37. Bergner M, Bobbitt RA, Carter WB, *et al.*: The sickness impact profile: development and final revision of a health status measure. *Med Care* 1981, 19:787–805.

38. Partinen M, Gislason T: Basic Nordic Sleep Questionnaire (BNSQ): a quantitated measure of subjective sleep complaints. *J Sleep Res* 1995, 4:150–155.

39. Johns MW: A new method for measuring daytime sleepiness: the Epworth Sleepiness Scale. *Sleep* 1991, 14:540–545.

40. Johns MW: Reliability and factor analysis of the Epworth Sleepiness Scale. *Sleep* 1992, 15:376–381.

41. Lau DT, Morlock RJ, Hill CD: Psychometric evaluation of the medical outcomes study-sleep scale in persons with overactive bladder. *Clin Ther* 2006, 28:2119–2132.

42. Buysse DJ, Reynolds CF III, Monk TH, *et al.*: The Pittsburgh Sleep Quality Index: a new instrument for psychiatric practice and research. *Psychiatry Res* 1989, 28:193–213.

43. Asplund R: The nocturnal polyuria syndrome (NPS). *Gen Pharmacol* 1995, 26:1203–1209.

44. Kirkland JL, Lye M, Levy DW, *et al.*: Patterns of urine flow and electrolyte excretion in healthy elderly people. *Br Med J* 1983, 287:1665–1667.

45. Guilleminault C, Lin CM, Goncalves MA, *et al.*: A prospective study of nocturia and the quality of life of elderly patients with obstructive sleep apnea or sleep onset insomnia. *J Psychosom Res* 2004, 56:511–515.

46. Fitzgerald MP, Mulligan M, Parthasarathy S: Nocturic frequency is related to severity of obstructive sleep apnea, improves with continuous positive airways treatment. *Am J Obstet Gynecol* 2006, 194:1399–1403.

47. Margel D, Shochat T, Getzler O, *et al.*: Continuous positive airway pressure reduces nocturia in patients with obstructive sleep apnea. *Urology* 2006, 67:974–977.

48. Lose G, Lalos O, Freeman RM, *et al.*: Efficacy of desmopressin (Minirin) in the treatment of nocturia: a double-blind placebo-controlled study in women. *Am J Obstet Gynecol* 2003, 189:1106–1113.

49. Mattiasson A, Abrams P, Van Kerrebroeck P, *et al.*: Efficacy of desmopressin in the treatment of nocturia: a double-blind placebo-controlled study in men. *BJU Int* 2002, 89:855–862.

50. van Kerrebroeck P, Rezapour M, Cortesse A, *et al.*: Desmopressin in the treatment of nocturia: a double-blind, placebo-controlled study. *Eur Urol* 2007, 52:221–229.

51. Kinn AC, Elbarouni J, Seideman P, *et al.*: The effect of diclofenac sodium on renal function. *Scand J Urol Nephrol* 1989, 23:153–157.

52. Okada S, Watanabe H, Kojima Y, *et al.*: Loxoprofen sodium treatment for elderly men with refractory nocturia: effect on night-time urine production. *Int J Urol* 2008, 15:462–464.

53. Addla SK, Adeyoju AB, Neilson D, *et al.*: Diclofenac for treatment of nocturia caused by nocturnal polyuria: a prospective, randomised, double-blind, placebo-controlled crossover study. *Eur Urol* 2006, 49:720–725.

54. Araki T, Yokoyama T, Kumon H: Effectiveness of a nonsteroidal anti-inflammatory drug for nocturia on patients with benign prostatic hyperplasia: a prospective non-randomized study of loxoprofen sodium 60 mg once daily before sleeping. *Acta Medica Okayama* 2004, 58:45–49.

55. Falahatkar S, Mokhtari G, Pourreza F, *et al.*: Celecoxib for treatment of nocturia caused by benign prostatic hyperplasia: a prospective, randomized, double-blind, placebo-controlled study. *Urology* 2008, 72:813–816.

56. Vallancien G, Emberton M, Alcaraz A, *et al.*: Alfuzosin 10 mg once daily for treating benign prostatic hyperplasia: a 3-year experience in real-life practice. *BJU Int* 2008, 101:847–852.

57. Margel D, Lifshitz D, Brown N, *et al.*: Predictors of nocturia quality of life before and shortly after prostatectomy. *Urology* 2007, 70:493–497.

58. Johnson TM II, Jones K, Williford WO, *et al.*: Changes in nocturia from medical treatment of benign prostatic hyperplasia: secondary analysis of the Department of Veterans Affairs Cooperative Study Trial. *J Urol* 2003, 170:145–148.

59. Cardozo L, Lisec M, Millard R, *et al.*: Randomized, double-blind placebo controlled trial of the once daily antimuscarinic agent solifenacin succinate in patients with overactive bladder. *J Urol* 2004, 172:1919–1924.

60. Abrams P, Swift S: Solifenacin is effective for the treatment of OAB dry patients: a pooled analysis. *Eur Urol* 2005, 48:483–487.

61. Chapple CR, Cardozo L, Steers WD, *et al.*: Solifenacin significantly improves all symptoms of overactive bladder syndrome. *Int J Clin Pract* 2006, 60:959–966.

62. Rudy D, Cline K, Harris R, *et al.*: Multicenter phase III trial studying trospium chloride in patients with overactive bladder. *Urology* 2006, 67:275–280.

63. Zinner N, Gittelman M, Harris R, *et al.*: Trospium chloride improves overactive bladder symptoms: a multicenter phase III trial. *J Urol* 2004, 171:2311–2315.

64. Nitti VW, Dmochowski R, Appell RA, *et al.*: Efficacy and tolerability of tolterodine extended-release in continent patients with overactive bladder and nocturia. *BJU Int* 2006, 97:1262–1266.

65. Rackley R, Weiss JP, Rovner ES, *et al.*: Nighttime dosing with tolterodine reduces overactive bladder-related nocturnal micturitions in patients with overactive bladder and nocturia. *Urology* 2006, 67:731–736.

66. Wallace PA, Lane FL, Noblett KL: Sacral nerve neuromodulation in patients with underlying neurologic disease. *Am J Obstet Gyn* 2007, 197:96.e1–5.

67. Schmid DM, Sauermann P, Werner M, *et al.*: Experience with 100 cases treated with botulinum-A toxin injections in the detrusor muscle for idiopathic overactive bladder syndrome refractory to anticholinergics. *J Urol* 2006, 176:177–185.

68. Adam P: Evaluation and management of diabetes insipidus. *Am Fam Physician* 1997, 55:2146–2153.

69. Long CY, Liu CM, Hsu SC, *et al.*: A randomized comparative study of the effects of oral and topical estrogen therapy on the lower urinary tract of hysterectomized postmenopausal women. *Fertil Steril* 2006, 85:155–160.

70. Johnson TM II, Burgio KL, Redden DT, *et al.*: Effects of behavioral and drug therapy on nocturia in older incontinent women. *J Am Geriatr Soc* 2005, 53:846–850.

71. Sugaya K, Nishijima S, Owan T, *et al.*: Effects of walking exercise on nocturia in the elderly. *Biomed Res* 2007, 28:101–105.

72. Congregado Ruiz B, Pena Outeirino XM, Campoy Martinez P, *et al.*: Peripheral afferent nerve stimulation for treatment of lower urinary tract irritative symptoms. *Eur Urol* 2004, 45:65–69.

73. Drake MJ, Mills IW, Noble JG: Melatonin pharmacotherapy for nocturia in men with benign prostatic enlargement. *J Urol* 2004, 171:1199–1202.

74. Sugaya K, Nishijima S, Miyazato M, *et al.*: Effects of melatonin and rilmazafone on nocturia in the elderly. *J Int Med Res* 2007, 35:685–691.

75. Song YS, Ku JH: Zolpidem pharmacotherapy combined with alpha-blocker therapy for nocturia unresponsive to alpha-blocker monotherapy in men with lower urinary tract symptoms: a preliminary study. *Int Urol Nephrol* 2007, 39:1147–1152.

4 Bladder Pain Syndrome

Jørgen Nordling and Arndt van Ophoven

Pelvic pain syndromes are often related to the organ from which the pain is perceived to originate; *ie*, testicular pain syndrome, vulvar pain syndrome. Pain perceived by the patient to originate from the bladder may be caused by numerous disorders, such as simple bacterial cystitis, bladder stones, and cancer. After excluding well-known causes of bladder pain, a group of patients remain for which it has not been possible to diagnose such a cause. These patients have often been labelled as having interstitial cystitis (IC). However, as this disease or condition has no definition and varying diagnostic criteria, this chapter will discuss bladder pain syndrome (BPS).

The prevalence of BPS is reported to range from very rare to rather common, depending on variations in definition and study designs. The prevalence is likely between 0.2% and 2%, with a male-to-female ratio of 1:5 to 10.

The diagnosis is mostly a diagnosis of exclusion; therefore, patient evaluation focuses on diagnosis of exclusion with special emphasis on pelvic examination and the bladder. Basic evaluation should include the patient's history, as well as a focused physical examination including vaginal examination in women and digital rectal examination in men. Urine examination is mandatory to exclude infection. The attitude toward cystoscopy, especially in general anesthesia including hydrodistension and in some patients bladder biopsy, differs considerably around the world.

In Asia, the findings of glomerulations or Hunner's lesion is mandatory to have a diagnosis of IC. In Europe, cystoscopy with hydrodistension and in many institutions also bladder biopsy is performed to look for positive signs of bladder involvement and to classify the patients according to the European Society for the Study of BPS/IC classification system. Treatment is directed against local treatment with bladder irrigation and pain treatment, with visceral pain killers such as amitriptyline, gabapentin, and pregabalin.

BPS: Confusable Disease

Confusable disease	Excluded or diagnosed by*
Carcinoma and carcinoma in situ	Cystoscopy and biopsy
Infection with	
Common intestinal bacteria	Routine bacterial culture
Chlamydia trachomatis, Ureaplasma urealyticum	Special cultures
Mycoplasma hominis, Mycoplasma genitalium	
Corynebacterium urealyticum, Candida species	
Mycobacterium tuberculosis	Dipstick; if "sterile," pyuria culture for *M. tuberculosis*
Herpes simplex and human papilloma virus	Physical examination
Radiation	Medical history
Chemotherapy, including immunotherapy with cyclophosphamide	Medical history
Anti-inflammatory therapy with tiaprofenic acid	Medical history
Bladder-neck obstruction and neurogenic outlet obstruction	Uroflowmetry and ultrasound
Bladder stone	Imaging or cystoscopy
Lower ureteric stone	Medical history or hematuria: upper urinary imaging such as CT or IVP
Urethral diverticulum	Medical history and physical examination
Urogenital prolapse	Medical history and physical examination
Endometriosis	Medical history and physical examination
Vaginal candidiasis	Medical history and physical examination
Cervical, uterine, and ovarian cancer	Physical examination
Incomplete bladder emptying (retention)	Postvoid residual urine volume measured by ultrasound scanning
Overactive bladder	Medical history and urodynamics
Prostate cancer	Physical examination and PSA
Benign prostatic obstruction	Uroflowmetry and pressure-flow studies
Chronic bacterial prostatitis	Medical history, physical examination, culture
Chronic nonbacterial prostatitis	Medical history, physical examination, culture
Pudendal nerve entrapment	Medical history, physical examination, nerve block may prove diagnosis
Pelvic floor muscle–related pain	Medical history, physical examination

**The diagnosis of a confusable disease does not necessarily exclude a diagnosis of BPS.*

Figure 4-1. Bladder pain syndrome (BPS): definition. BPS is defined as chronic (lasting greater than 6 months) pelvic pain, pressure, or discomfort perceived to be related to the urinary bladder accompanied by at least one other urinary symptom, such as a persistent urge to void or frequency. Confusable diseases that may be the cause of the symptoms must be excluded. Further documentation and classification of BPS may be performed according to findings at cystoscopy with hydrodistension and morphological findings in bladder biopsies. The presence of other organ symptoms, as well as cognitive, behavioral, emotional, and sexual symptoms, should be addressed [1]. CT—computed tomography; IVP—intravenous pyelogram; PSA—prostate-specific antigen.

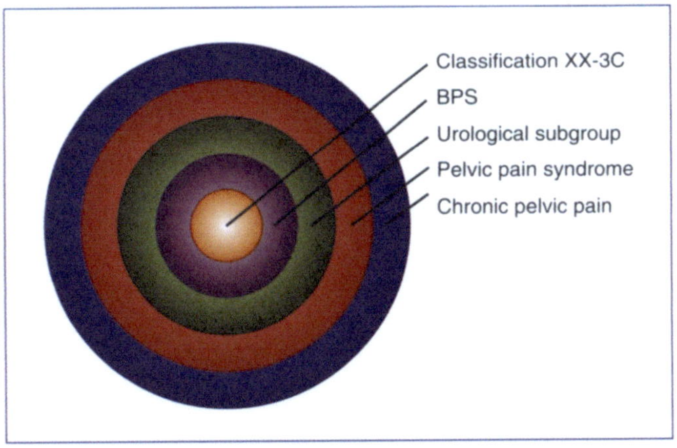

Figure 4-2. Bladder pain syndrome (BPS) classification. BPS is defined as pain with a collection of symptoms, the most important of which is pain perceived to be in the bladder. Interstitial cystitis (IC) is distinguished as an end-organ, visceral–neural pain syndrome, whereas BPS can be considered to be a pain syndrome that involves the end-organ (bladder) and neural–visceral (myopathic) mechanisms. In IC, end-organ primary pathology is expected; this is not necessarily the case in broader BPS.

Patient Evaluation: History

Special emphaisis should be given to

- Previous pelvic operations
- Previous UTI
- Bladder history/urological diseases
- Location of pelvic pain (referred pain) and relation to bladder filling/emptying
  - Characteristics of pain
    - Onset
    - Correlation with other events
    - Description
- Previous pelvic radation treatment
- Autoimmune diseases
- Presence of other pain syndromes

Figure 4-3. Patient evaluation: history. A general but thorough medical history should be taken. UTI—urinary tract infection.

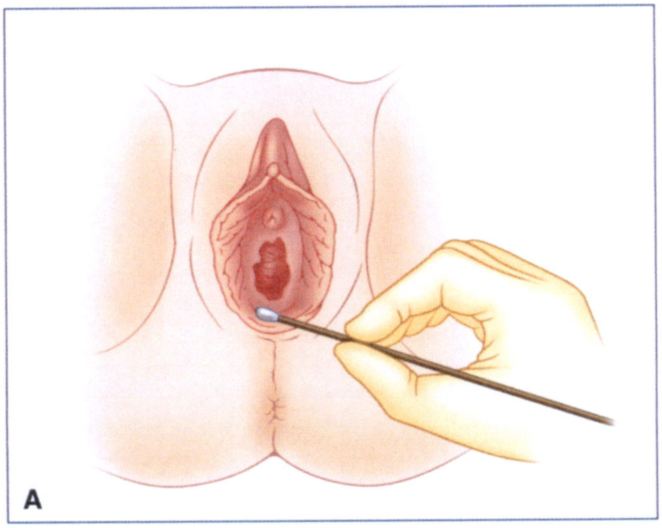

Physical Examination

A common physical examination should be performed, including

- Palpation of the lower abdomen for bladder fulness and tenderness
  - Standing: kyphosis, scars, hernia
  - Supine: abduction/adduction of the hips, hyperaesthetic areas

In females, a physical examination should include vaginal examination with pain mapping of the vulvar region and vaginal palpation for tenderness of the bladder, urethra, levator and adductor muscles of the pelvic floor. Tenderness might be graded as mild, moderate, or severe.

In males, DRE should be performed with pain mapping of the scrotal–anal region and palpation of tenderness of the bladder, prostate, levator and adductor muscles of the pelvic floor, and the scrotal content.

B

Figure 4-4. Patient evaluation and physical examination. A general physical examination should be performed (**A**), including the items outlined in **B**. DRE—digital rectal examination.

Laboratory Tests for Bladder Pain Syndrome

Urine dipstick (ABS, pH, leucocytes, nitrate), urine culture in all; if sterile, pyuria culture for TB

Urine cytology in risk groups

Investigations for vaginal ureaplasma and chlamydia in women and prostatitis in men are optional

Figure 4-5. Laboratory tests. Few laboratory tests provide information of value in patients with bladder pain syndrome; some are shown here. ABS—albumin, blood, sugar; TB—tuberculosis.

Voiding chart

Name: **Date:**

☐ Mo ☐ Tues ☐ Wed
☐ Thu ☐ Fri ☐ Sat
☐ Sun

Time getting up:
Time going to bed:

1	2	3	4	5	6	7	8	9
Time	Drink	Volume drank, *mL*	Void	Volume voided, *mL*	Bladder sensation, 0–5	Urine loss	Degree urine loss, 1–3	Woken up
	☐		☐			☐		☐
	☐		☐			☐		☐
	☐		☐			☐		☐
	☐		☐			☐		☐
	☐		☐			☐		☐
	☐		☐			☐		☐
	☐		☐			☐		☐
	☐		☐			☐		☐
	☐		☐			☐		☐
	☐		☐			☐		☐
	☐		☐			☐		☐
	☐		☐			☐		☐
	☐		☐			☐		☐
	☐		☐			☐		☐
	☐		☐			☐		☐
	☐		☐			☐		☐
	☐		☐			☐		☐
	☐		☐			☐		☐
	☐		☐			☐		☐
	☐		☐			☐		☐
	☐		☐			☐		☐
	☐		☐			☐		☐
	☐		☐			☐		☐
	☐		☐			☐		☐
	☐		☐			☐		☐
	☐		☐			☐		☐

A

Figure 4-6. Voiding diary. A voiding diary that records volume intake and output for 3 consecutive days is recommended at the initial evaluation (**A**). The voiding diary also records patient sensations at voiding [2].

Continued on the next page

Comments on the Voiding Charts

1. Before filling in the voiding charts, please postpone voiding for as long as possible (until a very urgent desire to void) on two separate occasions. Measure the volumes voided after refraining from voiding with a measuring cup in milliliters. During postponing, pay attention to the different sensations that may arise from the bladder. Write this information down on a separate sheet.

2. After measuring the postponed voiding, please fill out the voiding charts for three consecutive days (24 h/d), during which normal daily activities are continued. Please fill out your drinking and voiding habits as accurately as possible.

- Please note on each chart the date and the times of waking up and going to sleep.

- **Please note the time (hours and minutes) at each event (drinking, voiding, involuntary loss of urine–column 1) and mark the corresponding event column.** Mark column 2 for drinking, column 4 for voiding, column 7 for loss of urine, and column 8 if you wake up at night to void.

- Please **measure** the **volumes** you drank (at every event–column 3) and the volumes you voided (at every event–column 5). The volumes drunk can be estimated (*eg*, a large glass contains approximately 200 mL). However, the volumes voided have to be measured accurately by means of a measuring cup in milliliters.

- Continue to register events during the night. Start a new chart page when getting up and register the first void after getting up there.

- Register every time you go to the toilet to void (mark column 4, estimate the degree of bladder sensation in column 6, and measure the voided volumes with the measuring cup (column 5).

  Degrees of Desire to Void

  0. No bladder sensation at all.
  1. Some sensation of bladder filling, without a clear desire to void. Voiding can easily be delayed for more than 60 minutes.
  2. First desire to void. Voiding can be delayed for at least 30 minutes.
  3. Strong desire to void. Voiding cannot be delayed for more than 15 minutes.
  4. Urgent desire to void. Voiding cannot be delayed for more than 5 minutes.
  5. Pain in the lower abdomen.

- Please register every episode of urine loss in column 7 and estimate the amount of urine lost in column 8 according to the following definitions:

  1. Just a few drops or some spots in pad
  2. Underclothes are wet or protective pads are wet
  3. Both under- and outerclothes are wet

B

FIGURE 4-6. *(Continued)* Discriminating between overactive bladder syndrome and bladder pain syndrome depends on the quality of the sensation's desire to void. Therefore, recording sensations is desirable at each voiding (**B**).

Control Visit BPS Patient

Name: Date:

Number of voidings during 24 hours. Make a mark for each voiding (example: ~~IIII~~ ~~IIII~~ II for 12 voidings):

Daytime: Nighttime:

Please mark your degree of bladder/pelvic pain **during the last 24 hours** on the scale below.

Average pain during the last 24 hours:
No pain________________________________Intolerable pain

Worst pain during the last 24 hours:
No pain________________________________Intolerable pain

Least pain during the last 24 hours:
No pain________________________________Intolerable pain

A

	Delighted	Pleased	Mostly satisfied	Mixed—about equally satisfied and dissatisfied	Mostly dissatisfied	Unhappy	Terrible
If you were to spend the rest of your life with your urinary condition just the way it is now, how would you feel about that?	0	1	2	3	4	5	6

B

Figure 4-7. Overactive bladder syndrome vs bladder pain syndrome (BPS). During followup, a simpler voiding diary that includes a recording of bladder pain could be used (**A**). Recording the quality of life is important in patients with BPS, but a recommended quality of life questionnaire is not currently available.

Continued on the next page

Interstitial cystitis symptom index

1. During the past month, how often have you felt the strong need to urinate with little or no warning?
   0. ___Not at all
   1. ___Les than 1 time in 5
   2. ___Less than half the time
   3. ___About half the time
   4. ___More than half the time
   5. ___Almost always

2. During the past month, have you had to urinate less than 2 hours after you finished urinating?
   0. ___Not at all
   1. ___Less than 1 time in 5
   2. ___Less than half the time
   3. ___About half the time
   4. ___More than half the time
   5. ___Almost always

3. During the past month, how often did you most typically get up at night to urinate?
   0. ___Never
   1. ___Once
   2. ___2 times
   3. ___3 times
   4. ___4 times
   5. ___5 or more times

4. During the past month, have you experienced pain or buzzing in your bladder?
   1. ___Not at all
   2. ___Once
   3. ___A few times
   4. ___Fairly often
   5. ___Almost always
   6. ___Usually

Add the numerical values of the checked entries
Total score____

Interstitial cystitis problem index

During the past month, how much has each of the following been a problem for you?

1. Frequent urination during the day?
   0. ___No problem
   1. ___Very small problem
   2. ___Small problem
   3. ___Medium problem
   4. ___Big problem

2. Getting up at night to urinate?
   1. ___No problem
   2. ___Very small problem
   3. ___Small problem
   4. ___Medium problem
   5. ___Big problem

3. Need to urinate with little warning?
   1. ___No problem
   2. ___Very small problem
   3. ___Small problem
   4. ___Medium problem
   5. ___Big problem

4. Burning, pain, discomfort, or pressure in your bladder?
   1. ___No problem
   2. ___Very small problem
   3. ___Small problem
   4. ___Medium problem
   5. ___Big problem

Add the numerical values of the checked entries
Total score____

C

Figure 4-7. *(Continued)* Shown is the IPSS (**B**) and the O'Leary-Sant questionnaires (**C**) [8].

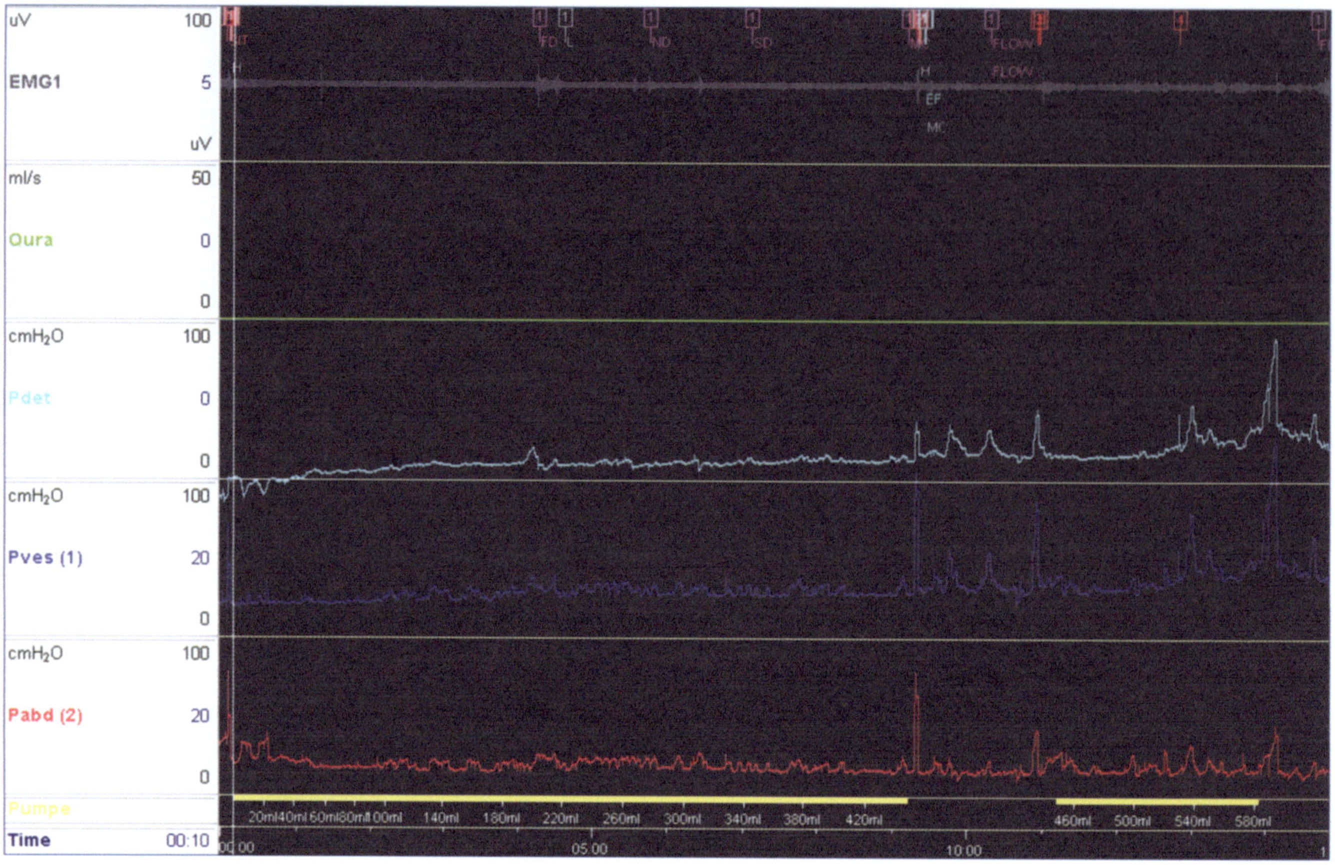

FIGURE 4-8. Detrusor overactivity may coexist with bladder pain syndrome, which could have implications for treatment. Therefore, it is recommended to perform filling cystometry to look for detrusor overactivity, volume at first desire to void, and cystometric bladder capacity. In women, flowmetry, postvoid residual urine volume, and pressure flow studies are optional [3]. EMG—electromyogram.

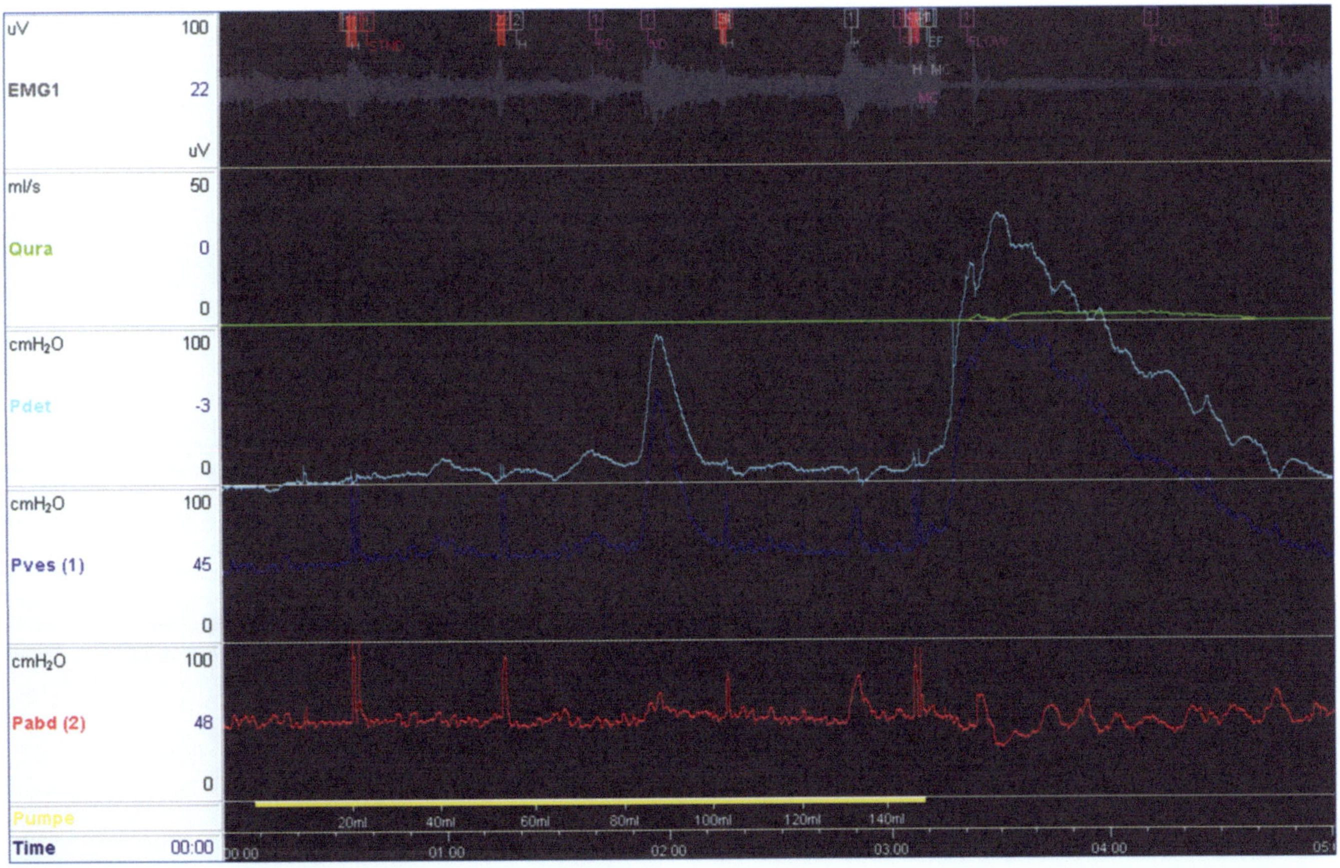

FIGURE 4-9. In men, bladder outlet obstruction may be a differential diagnosis and flowmetry should be performed in male patients. If the maximum flow rate is below 20 mL/s, a pressure flow study and measure of residual urine volume should be performed [3]. EMG—electromyogram.

Sensation results

Sensation	Bladder filling	Vesical pressure	Detrusor pressure
First sensation	104 mL	11 cmH_2O	5 cmH_2O
First desire	106 mL	11 cmH_2O	5 cmH_2O
Normal desire	115 mL	10 cmH_2O	3 cmH_2O
Strong desire	119 mL	10 cmH_2O	4 cmH_2O
Maximum cyst capacity	155 mL	11 cmH_2O	5 cmH_2O

Transducer information

P1 Pves (1) p1

P2 Pabd (2) p2

Detrusor-volume plot

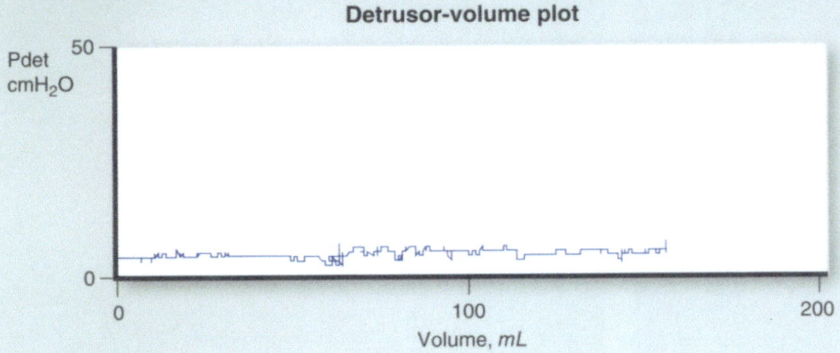

FIGURE 4-10. Potassium-sensitivity testing. Potassium-sensitivity testing is optional, but has shown prognostic value in bladder irrigation studies [4]. The modified potassium test described by Daha *et al.* does not produce the same degree of bladder pain as the original test [5]. Test results for a 34-year-old woman with Hunner's lesion at cystoscopy are shown. Filling cystometry with saline demonstrates a cystometric bladder capacity of 155 cc.

Sensation results

Sensation	Bladder filling	Vesical pressure	Detrusor pressure
First sensation	47 mL	8 cmH_2O	4 cmH_2O
First desire	48 mL	8 cmH_2O	4 cmH_2O
Normal desire	56 mL	8 cmH_2O	3 cmH_2O
Strong desire	64 mL	9 cmH_2O	2 cmH_2O
Maximum cyst capacity	68 mL	9 cmH_2O	2 cmH_2O

Transducer information

P1 Pves (1) p1

P2 Pabd (2) p2

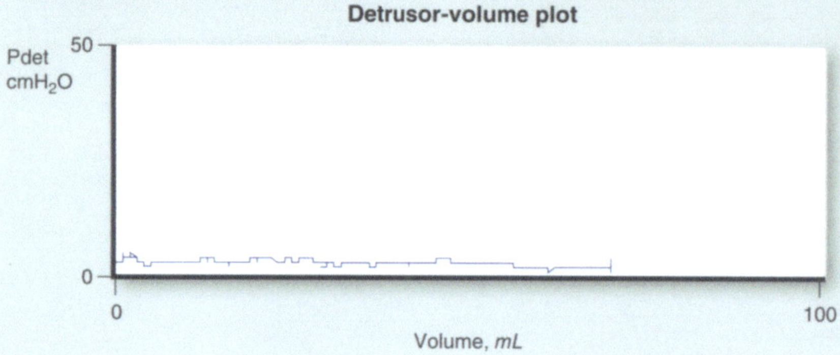

FIGURE 4-11. Potassium chloride (KCL)–sensitivity testing. Test results for the same patient as in Figure 10-10 are shown, using 0.2 M KCL as the filling medium. The cystometric bladder capacity is now 68 cc, or 44% of the capacity using saline as the filling medium. The modified potassium-sensitivity test is positive if the cystometric bladder capacity during infusion with 0.2 M KCL is 70% or less of the cystometric bladder capacity using saline as the filling medium, according to Daha *et al.* [5].

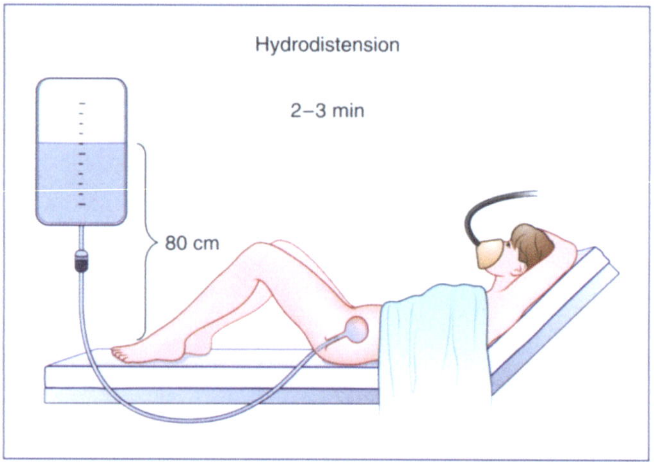

FIGURE 4-12. Cytoscopy. Bladder distension under general anesthesia has been a controversial issue. During this procedure, the bladder is distended for 3 minutes at a pressure of 80 cmH_2O. The bladder is emptied and the capacity is measured, providing important information about bladder fibrosis and possible contracted bladder. The bladder is refilled to about 30% to 50% of capacity and inspected for glomerulations, mucosal rupture, and Hunner's lesions. Biopsies may be obtained for excluding carcinoma in situ and looking for inflammatory infiltrates including mast cells in the submucosal and detrusor muscles.

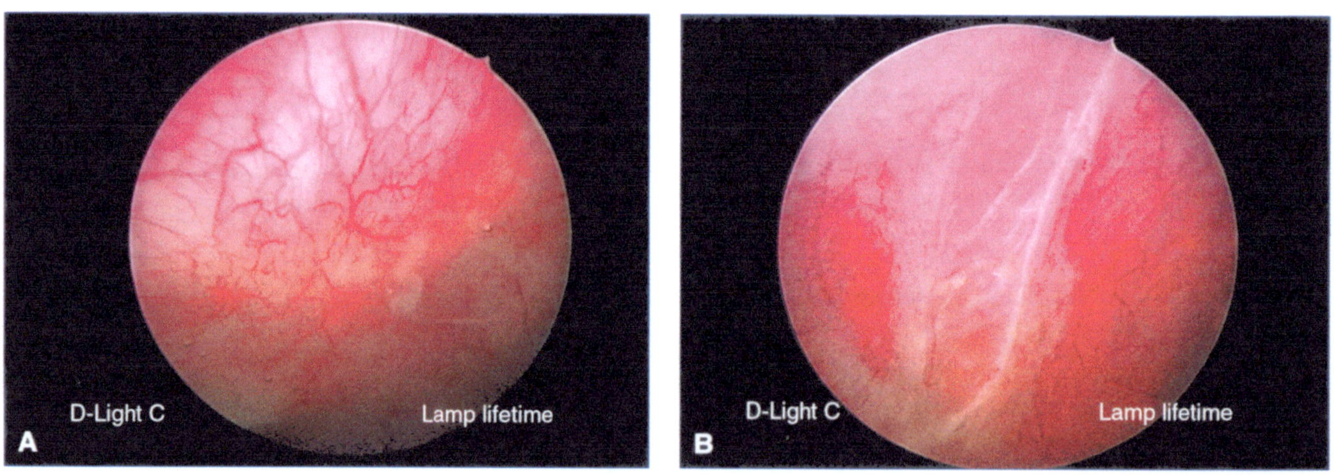

FIGURE 4-13. Hunner's lesion. A 64-year-old woman with bladder pain syndrome was studied for 20 years. **A** shows the cystoscopic finding of a Hunner's lesion at the start of cystoscopy under general anesthesia. **B** shows the patient after hydrodistension, with mucosal and submucosal rupture into the muscular layer, with blood oozing from the borders of the rupture. The patient became pain free after the resection and coagulation of this lesion and a large lesion in the top of the bladder.

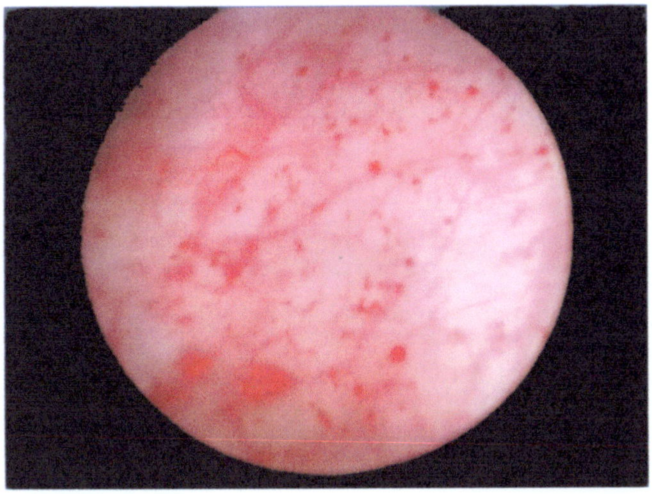

FIGURE 4-14. Glomerulations. Bladder glomerulations grade I after hydrodistension in a 41-year-old woman with bladder pain syndrome are shown. Glomerulations after hydrodistension of the bladder probably are largely unspecific [6,7]. The following is the grading system that is used: grade 0: normal mucosa; grade I: petechia in at least two quadrants; grade II: large submucosal bleeding (ecchymosis); grade III: diffuse global mucosal bleeding; grade IV: mucosal disruption, with or without bleeding/edema [3].

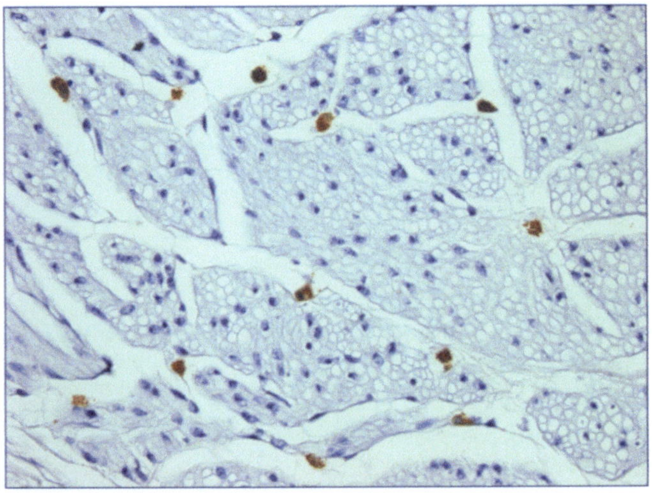

FIGURE 4-15. Morphology: mast cells. Mast cells in the detrusor muscle of the bladder in a patient with bladder pain syndrome are shown (tryptase staining). (*Courtesy of* T. Horn, Department of Pathology, Herlev Hospital, University of Copenhagen, Copenhagen, Denmark.)

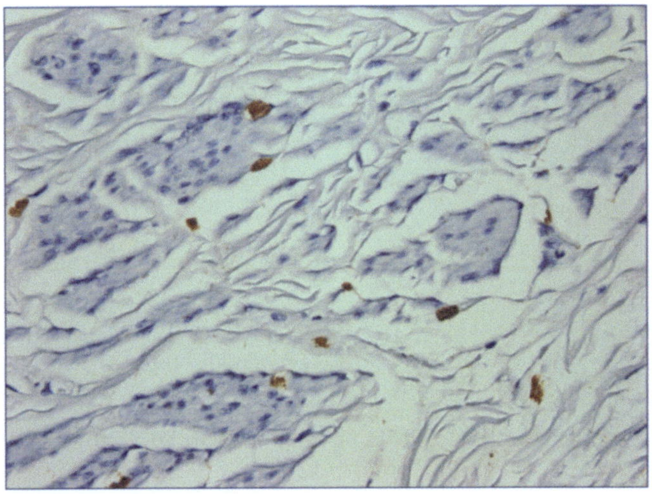

FIGURE 4-16. Fibrosis. Mast cells in a patient with bladder pain syndrome are shown (tryptase staining). It can be seen how the muscle bundles are split by large areas of fibrous tissue. (*Courtesy of* T. Horn, Department of Pathology, Herlev Hospital, University of Copenhagen, Copenhagen, Denmark.)

Cystoscopy with Hydrodistension

Biopsy	Not done		Glomerulations*	Hunner's lesion†
Not done	XX	1X	2X	3X
	XA	1A	2A	3A
Inconclusive	XX	1X	2X	3X
Positive‡	XC			

**Cystoscopy: glomerulations grades 2–3; †with or without glomerulations; ‡histology showing inflammatory infilatrates, detrusor mastocytosis, granulation tissue, or intrafascicular fibrosis*

FIGURE 4-17. Cystoscopic and morphologic changes. Cystoscopic and morphologic changes may be important for treatment or prognosis. The European Society for the Study of Bladder pain Syndrome/Interstitial Cystitis has, therefore, recommended this classification based on findings during cystoscopy with hydrodistension and morphological findings in bladder biopsies.

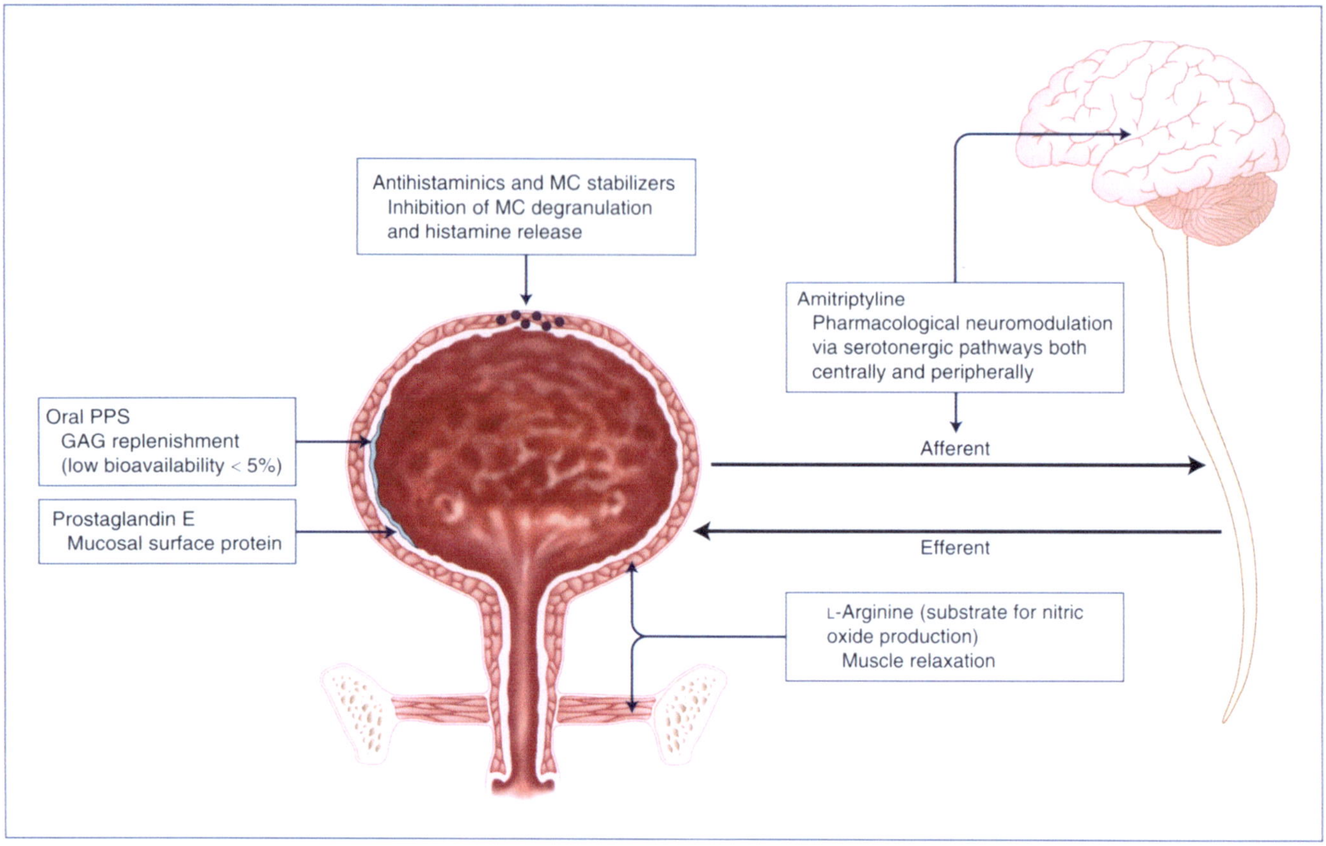

FIGURE 4-18. Treatment: basic therapeutic concept of oral treatment strategies. Basic therapeutic concepts of oral treatment strategies are shown. Only pentosanpolysulfate (PPS) is approved by the US Food and Drug Administration for the treatment of bladder pain syndrome/interstitial cystitis. However, amitriptyline was approved for chronic pain syndromes in European countries and has a well-established usefulness as a co-analgesic in pain therapy. Antihistaminics and mast cell (MC) stabilizers appear to be most useful in patients reporting symptom flares during allergy season. L-Arginine should not be recommended in high doses following acute myocardial infarction, because safety concerns arose from cardiovascular trials. GAG—glycosaminoglycan.

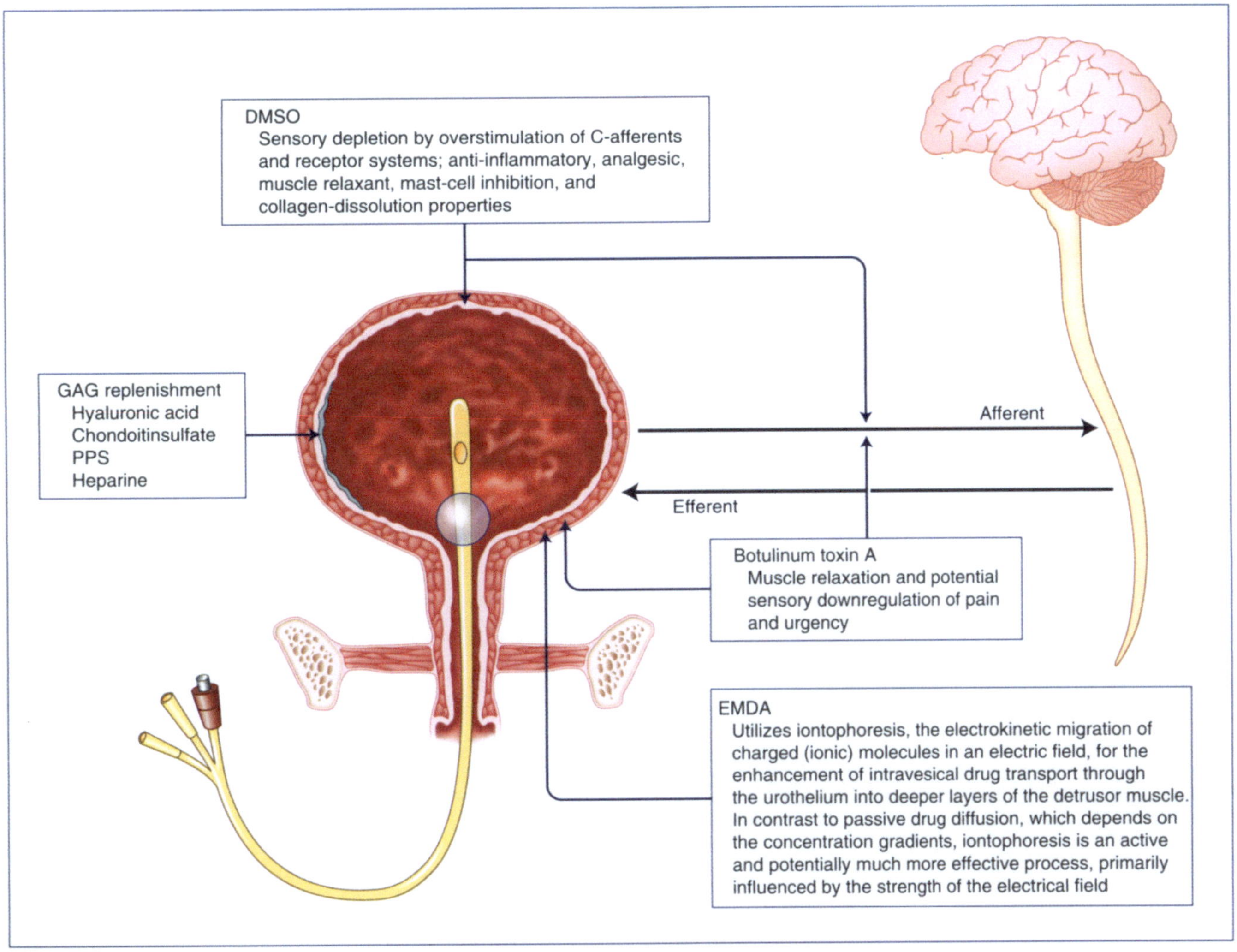

Figure 4-19. Basic therapeutic concept of intravesical treatment strategies. Dimethylsulfoxide (DMSO) 50% is approved by the US Food and Drug Administration for the treatment of bladder pain syndrome/interstitial cystitis. However, clinical data suggest that a 25% solution results in equal symptom reduction and comes with fewer side effects (eg, short-term postinterventional symptom increase). The mode of action regarding the sensory impact of botulinum toxin on chronic pelvic pain conditions is currently not fully understood. All available glycosaminoglycan (GAG) replenishment compounds are generally well tolerated by patients. The classic electromotive drug administration (EMDA) cocktail includes 100 mL lidocaine 2%, 2 mL epinephrine 1:1000, 20 mg scopolamine, and 40 mg dexamethasone. PPS—pentosanpolysulfate.

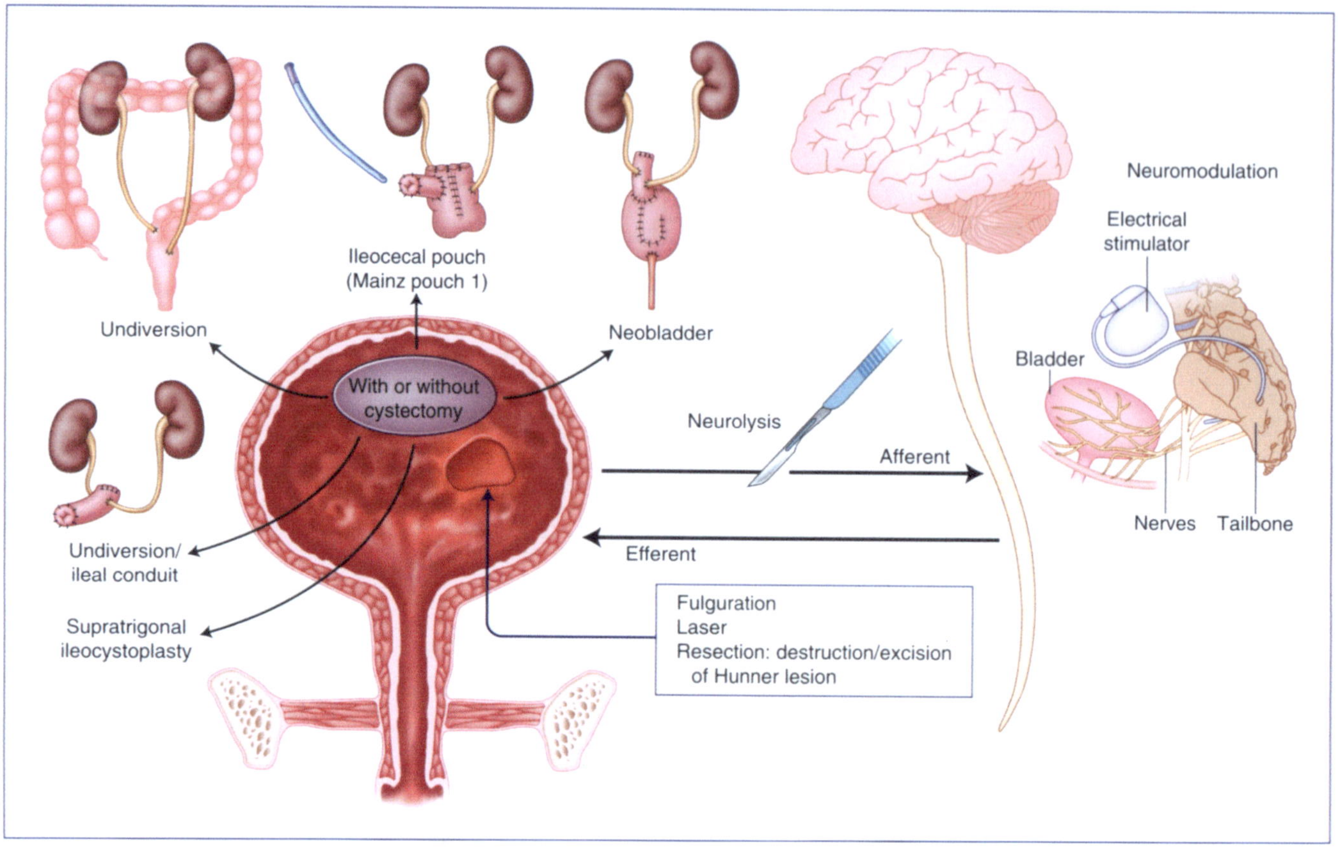

FIGURE 4-20. Basic therapeutic concepts of surgical treatment strategies. While neurolysis and neuromodulation focus on the interaction with efferent and afferent neuronal structures, open surgical interventions aim at the maximum removal of the affected vesical and urethral urothelium. Various surgical techniques for bladder substitution are available at the surgeon's preference. Undiversion techniques do not necessarily require bladder removal, because the drained bladder typically evokes only minor sensory input.

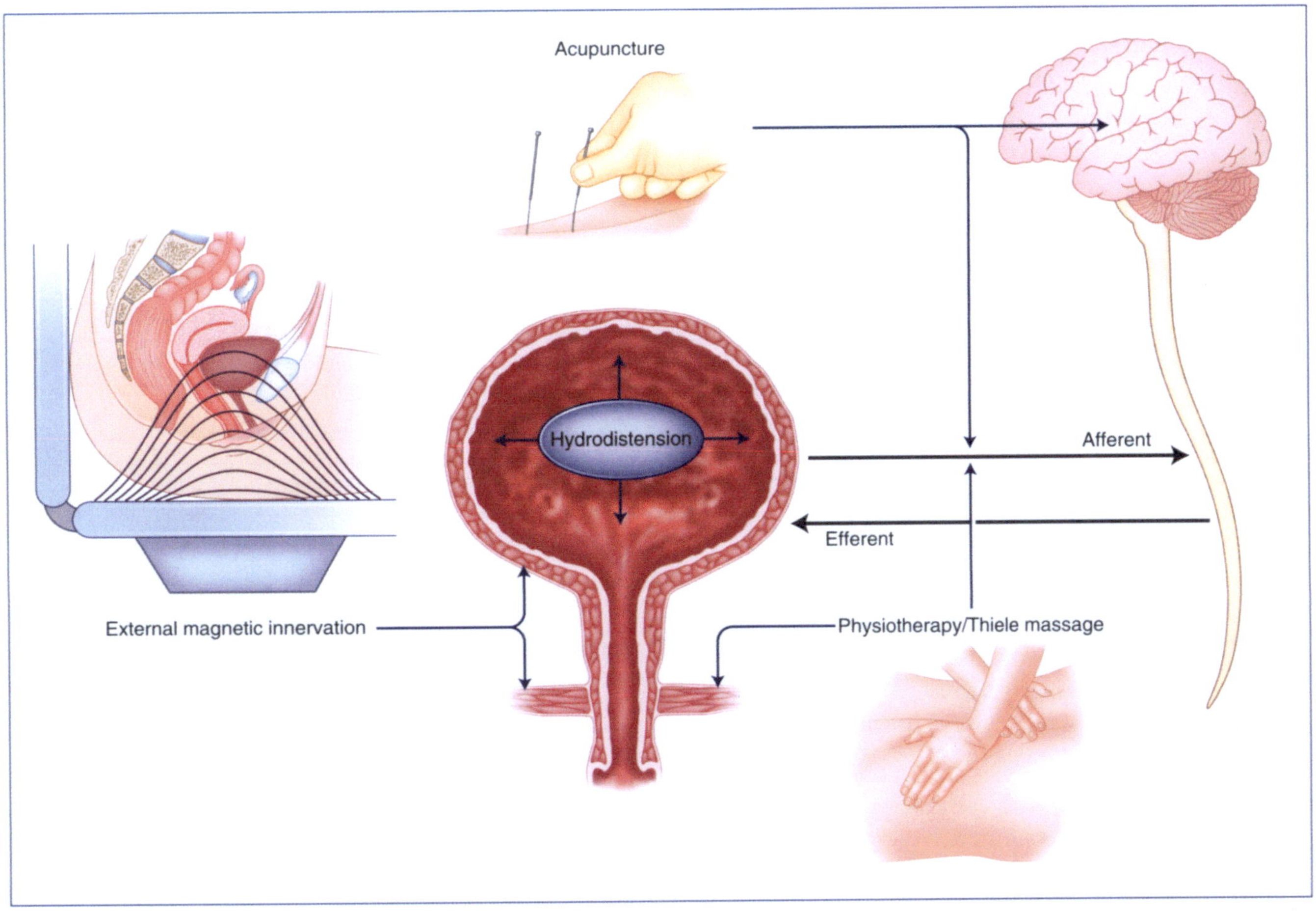

FIGURE 4-21. Basic therapeutic concepts of physical treatment strategies have gained increased attention by both patients and physicians over the past years. These interventions add valuable to classic, *eg*, oral, therapeutic approaches without interfering with them. Additionally, they typically show no side effects. Hydrodistension, however, is performed under anesthesia and might induce postinterventional gross hematuria due to the induction of urothelial cracking, *ie*, Hunner's lesions.

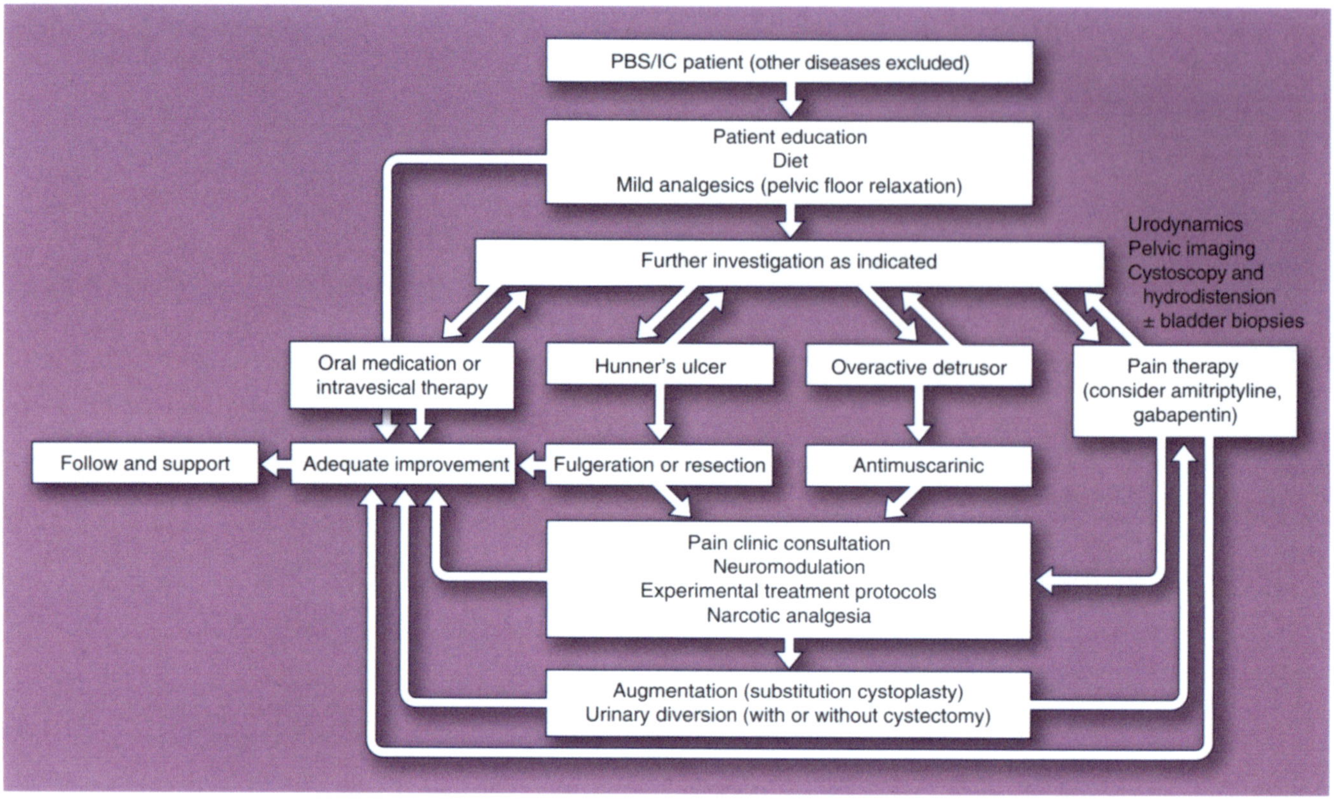

Figure 4-22. Bladder pain syndrome/interstitial cystitis (BPS/IC) treatment algorithm. The European Society for the Study of BPS/IC proposed the treatment algorithm for BPS shown here.

References

1. van de Merwe JP, Nordling J, Bouchelouche P, *et al.*: Diagnostic criteria, classification, and nomenclature for painful bladder syndrome/interstitial cystitis: an ESSIC proposal. *Eur Urol* 2008, 53:60–67.
2. Wyndaele JJ, De Wachter S: The basics behind bladder pain: a review of data on lower urinary tract sensations. *Int J Urol* 2003, 10(Suppl):S49–S55.
3. Nordling J, Anjum FH, Bade JJ, *et al.*: Primary evaluation of patients suspected of having interstitial cystitis (IC). *Eur Urol* 2004, 45:662–669.
4. Riedl CR, Daha KL, Pfluger H, Hohlbrugger G: Intravesical hyaluronic acid for the treatment of interstitial cystitis. *J Urol* 2003,169(Suppl).
5. Daha LK, Riedl CR, Hohlbrugger G, *et al.*: Comparative assessment of maximal bladder capacity, 0.9% NaCl versus 0.2 M KCL, for the diagnosis of interstitial cystitis: a prospective controlled study. *J Urol* 2003, 170:807–809.
6. Waxman JA, Sulak PJ, Kuehl TJ: Cystoscopic findings consistent with interstitial cystitis in normal women undergoing tubal ligation. *J Urol* 1998, 160:1663–1667.
7. Furuya R, Masumori N, Furuya S, *et al.*: Glomerulation observed during transurethral resection of the prostate for patients with lower urinary tract symptoms suggestive of benign prostatic hyperplasia is a common finding but no predictor of clinical outcome. *Urology* 2007, 70:922–926.
8. O'Leary MP, Sant G: The interstitial cystitis symptom and problem indices: rationale, development, and application. In: *Interstitial Cystitis*. Edited by Sant GR. Philadelphia: Lippencott-Raven; 1997:271–276.

5 Urodynamics

Sender Herschorn

In the initial assessment of patients with lower urinary tract (LUT) dysfunction, it is recommended that clinicians do a complete history and general assessment including a review of systems, past medical history, social history, and other treatment-planning issues such as a patient's goals, support, and cognitive function. A physical examination should include abdominal, pelvic, and rectal assessments, as well as neurologic testing if it is indicated. Urinalysis should be done. An estimation of postvoid residual should be done in individuals with suspected voiding dysfunction. Other tests such as imaging and endoscopy are not routinely recommended and depend on the clinical circumstances [1].

Urodynamic testing is not routinely recommended except when the results may change management techniques, such as prior to invasive treatment; after treatment failure, if more information is required to plan further therapy; as part of the initial and long-term monitoring of neurogenic bladder dysfunction; in complicated incontinence and complicated voiding dysfunctions; in young men with LUT symptoms (LUTS); and in children with daytime urgency and urgency incontinence, persistent diurnal enuresis, and spinal dysraphism [1,2].

The term "urodynamics studies" (UDS) was defined by the International Continence Society (ICS) in 1988 and involves an assessment of the function and dysfunction of the LUT by any appropriate method [3]. A more recent terminology report included the term "urodynamic observations," which are observations noted during UDS. An example is an involuntary bladder contraction that may have a number of possible causes but does not represent a definitive diagnosis of a disease or condition [4].

The current view is that UDS are a series of tests such as flow studies, filling cystometry, pressure-flow studies, or urethral function measurements. These can be combined with simultaneous electromyography (EMG) tracing, radiographic imaging, or ultrasound. The aim is to gain an understanding of the LUT behavior by using the observations recorded during the test [5].

If accurate, UDS will help the clinician to: identify or rule out factors contributing to the LUT dysfunction and assess their relative importance; obtain information about other aspects of LUT dysfunction; predict the consequence of LUT dysfunction for the upper urinary tract; predict the outcome of a contemplated treatment; confirm the effects of an intervention or understand the mode of action of a particular treatment, especially a new one; and understand the reason(s) for the failure of a previous treatment.

LUT symptoms can be grouped according to when they are thought to occur during LUT function (see Fig. 5-1). The three broad phases of LUT function are storage, voiding, and post-voiding or postmicturition phases. The actual tests can be selected on the basis of what will most likely explain or reproduce the patient's symptoms. The clinician must be aware of the limitations of testing due to mechanical and machine-related problems as well as patient factors such as cooperation and movement artifacts. Failure to demonstrate an abnormality does not necessarily exclude it and not all recorded abnormalities are clinically important. The performance and interpretation of the test should also be consistent with current standards [6].

This chapter will illustrate with examples how patients with LUT dysfunction can be evaluated with urodynamics and how the results can be used to recommend treatment.

Lower Urinary Tract Symptoms

Storage	Voiding	Postvoiding
Frequency	Slow stream	Feeling of incomplete emptying
Nocturia	Splitting or spraying	Postvoid dribble
Urgency	Intermittent stream	
Urinary incontinence	Hesitancy	
Stress	Straining	
Urgency	Terminal dribble	
Mixed		
Enuresis (nocturnal)		
Continuous		
Other types		

FIGURE 5-1. Symptoms associated with lower urinary tract (LUT). This table shows the symptoms associated with the phase of LUT function. The listed complaints are further defined [4].

Storage symptoms include the following: urinary frequency, voiding too often during the day; nocturia, waking up at night one or more times to void; urgency, a sudden compelling desire to void that is difficult to defer; stress urinary incontinence, involuntary leakage upon effort or exertion, or on sneezing or coughing; urge(ncy) urinary incontinence, involuntary leakage accompanied or immediately preceded by urgency; and mixed urinary incontinence, involuntary leakage associated with urgency and also with stress incontinence. Enuresis also means any involuntary leakage (nocturnal enuresis occurs during sleep). Continuous urinary incontinence is continuous leakage.

Voiding symptoms include the following: slow stream, the perception of reduced urine flow; splitting or spraying intermittent stream, describes urine flow during voiding; hesitancy, difficulty in initiating voiding resulting in a delay in starting; straining, muscular effort needed to initiate, maintain, or improve the urinary stream; and terminal dribble, the prolonged final part of voiding when the flow has slowed substantially.

Postvoiding symptoms include a feeling of incomplete emptying and postvoid dribble, which is a loss of finishing voiding.

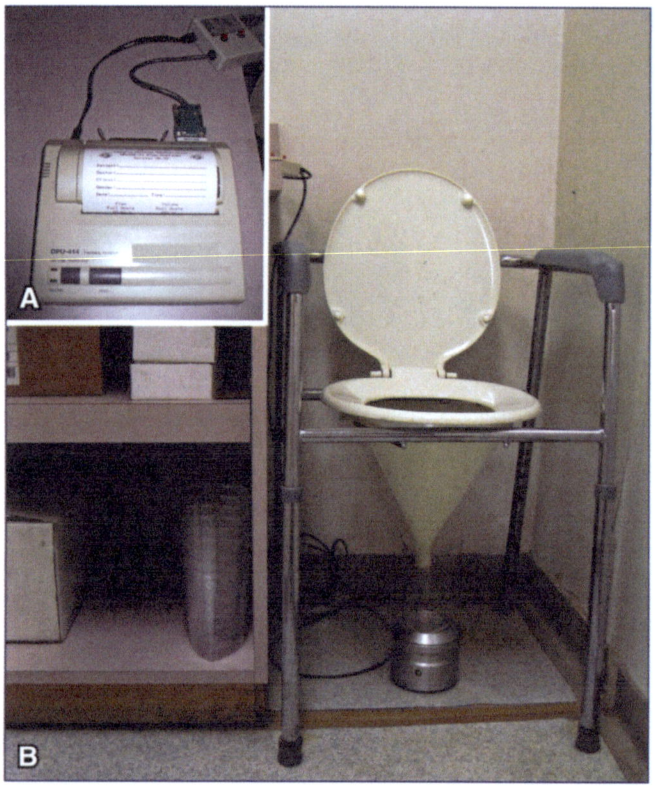

FIGURE 5-2. Flow meter. The apparatus for measuring free flow rate is shown. The recorder that measures the flow rate and computes the various parameters of the flow is shown in **A**. The patient sits or stands to void into the machine (**B**). The urine goes through the funnel into the collection beaker. The change in weight in the load cell is measured and converted to urine flow rate, volume, and other parameters, which are printed out automatically.

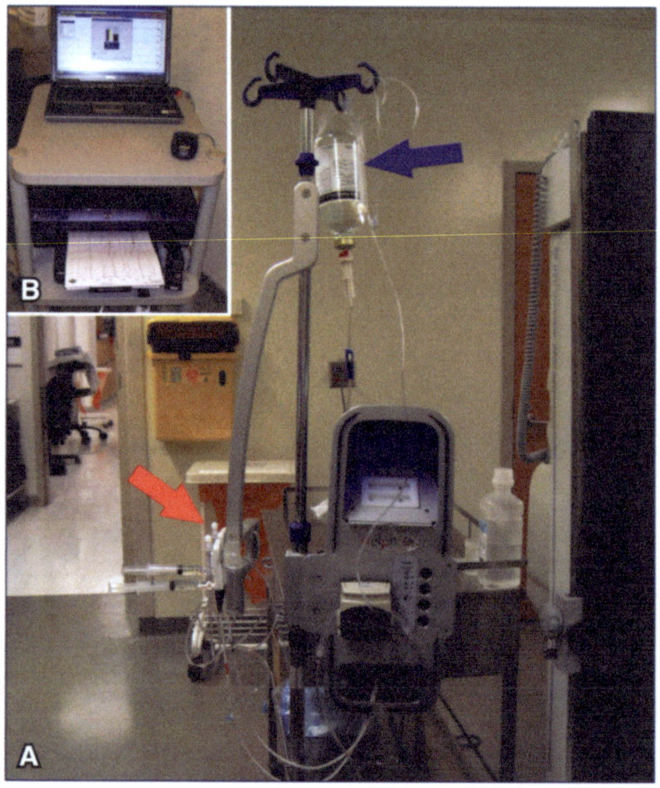

FIGURE 5-3. Multichannel urodynamic recorder. **A**, The pressures can be measured with external pressure transducers (*red arrow*) monitoring rectal (abdominal) pressure (Pabd) and total abdominal or intravesical pressure (Pves). The abdominal pressure is subtracted from the intravesical pressure to yield the subtracted detrusor pressure (Pdet). Filling of the bladder is accomplished through a separate catheter from the IV bag (*blue arrow*). Simultaneous flow rates can be measured with a similar load cell arrangement as in Figure 5-2. The results are transmitted to a computer and printed (**B**).

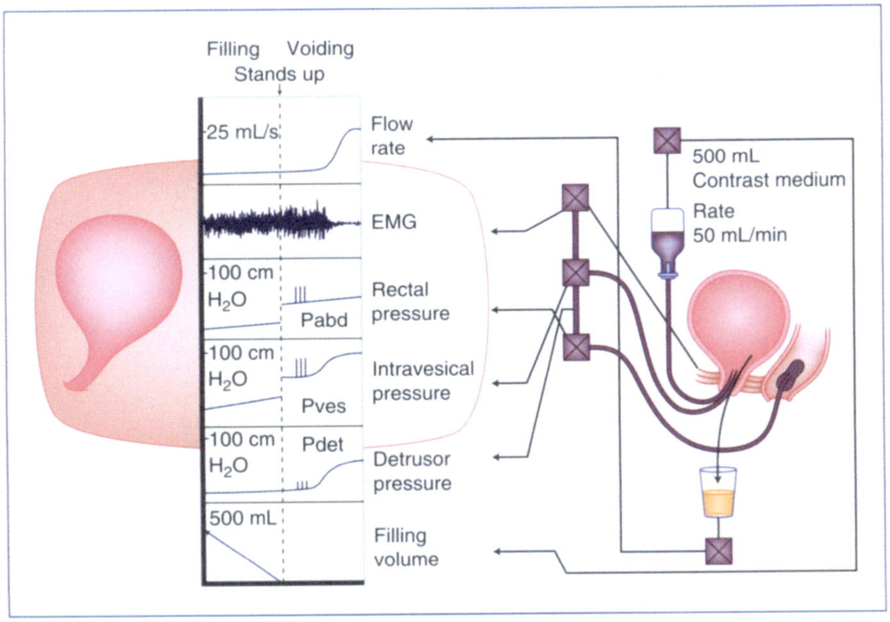

FIGURE 5-4. Videourodynamic setup. The catheters are inserted as follows: 8F polyethylene tube into the bladder for fluid infusion; another 8F tube for pressure measurement (Pves); and 10–12F plastic tube with covering of end holes for rectal pressure (Pabd) measurement. The bladder is filled and then the filling catheter is removed. Cough and Valsalva leak pressure measurements are taken, then the patient is asked to void. The pressure measurements and the flow rate are done during the voiding phase.

A videourodynamic study is indicated when a diagnosis cannot be made with certainty without simultaneous evaluation of the structure and function of the lower urinary tract [7]. Areas in which this study may be useful include complicated incontinence problems in men and women, voiding dysfunction to localize the site of obstruction, neurogenic bladder dysfunction, and in identifying other pathologic problems that may be associated. . EMG—electromyogram.

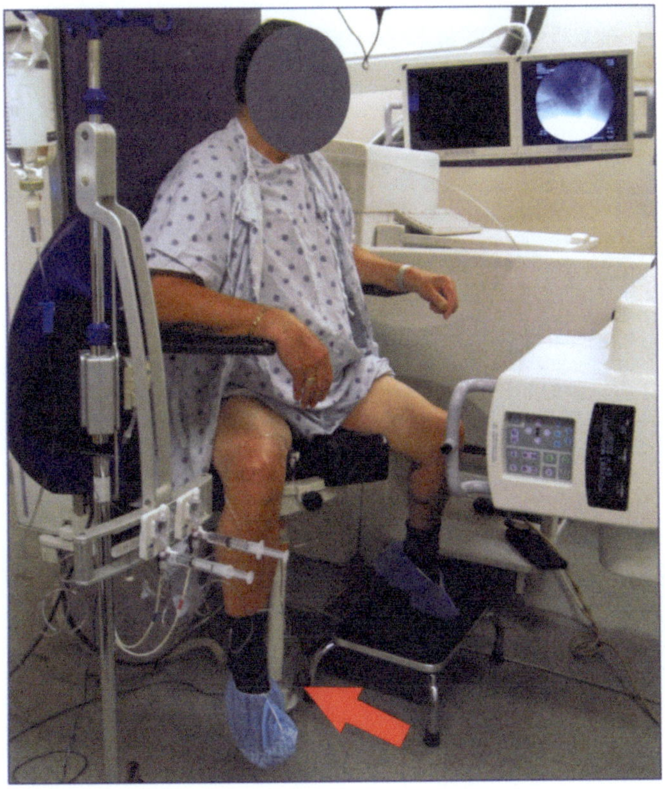

FIGURE 5-5. Videourodynamic study. The patient shown is undergoing a videourodynamic study. The fluoroscopic unit monitors the filling and voiding study. The patient is seated on the commode chair and will be able to do stress maneuvers to test for stress incontinence. The patient will also be asked to void in front of the camera to assess the posterior urethra. The flow meter (*red arrow*) is connected to the system and the flow tracing is integrated into the study.

Bladder Parameters Measured During Filling Cystometry	
Bladder sensation during filling cystometry	
Normal	Defined by three points: first sensation, first desire to void, strong desire to void
Increased	Early first sensation or other points
Reduced	Diminished throughout bladder filling
Absent	No sensation
Nonspecific	Abdominal fullness
Bladder pain	
Urgency	Sudden compelling desire to void
Detrusor function during filling cystometry	
Normal	Little or no change in pressure
DO	Involuntary contraction during filling (spontaneous or provoked)
Neurogenic DO	Neurological condition associated
Idiopathic DO	No defined cause
Phasic detrusor overactivity	Wave form +/– urinary incontinence
Terminal detrusor overactivity	Single involuntary contraction at capacity, resulting in bladder emptying
Detrusor overactivity incontinence	Incontinence due to a contraction
Provocative maneuvers	Techniques used to provoke DO
Bladder compliance	Calculated by dividing the volume change (ΔV) by the change in detrusor pressure (ΔPdet) during that change in bladder volume
Bladder capacity	
Cystometric capacity	Volume at end of filling
Maximal cystometric capacity	Volume at which the patient can no longer delay voiding

Figure 5-6. This table indicates the items to be measured during filling cystometry. The test measures the patient's bladder response to volume infusion. The International Continence Society (ICS) has defined the parameters that are to be measured and they consist of two parts: the patient's sensation of bladder filling and the urodynamic studies (UDS) observations and measurements during the test. Detrusor overactivity, uninhibited bladder contractions, used to be called *instability* or *hyperreflexia*, if they were associated with neurologic disease. Now, the terms used are simply *idiopathic* or *neurogenic detrusor overactivity* [4].

Compliance arises from the muscular, collagenous, and elastic components of the bladder wall. Smooth muscle has the ability to relax after stretching [8] and therefore complies with filling. Decreased compliance is thought to be due to bladder wall damage and an increase in connective tissue relative to smooth muscle [9]. The formula for computing compliance is in this table. The ICS recommends two standard points for compliance calculations: the detrusor pressure at the start of filling and the detrusor pressure at cystometric capacity or immediately before the start of any detrusor contraction. Both points are measured excluding any detrusor contraction [4].

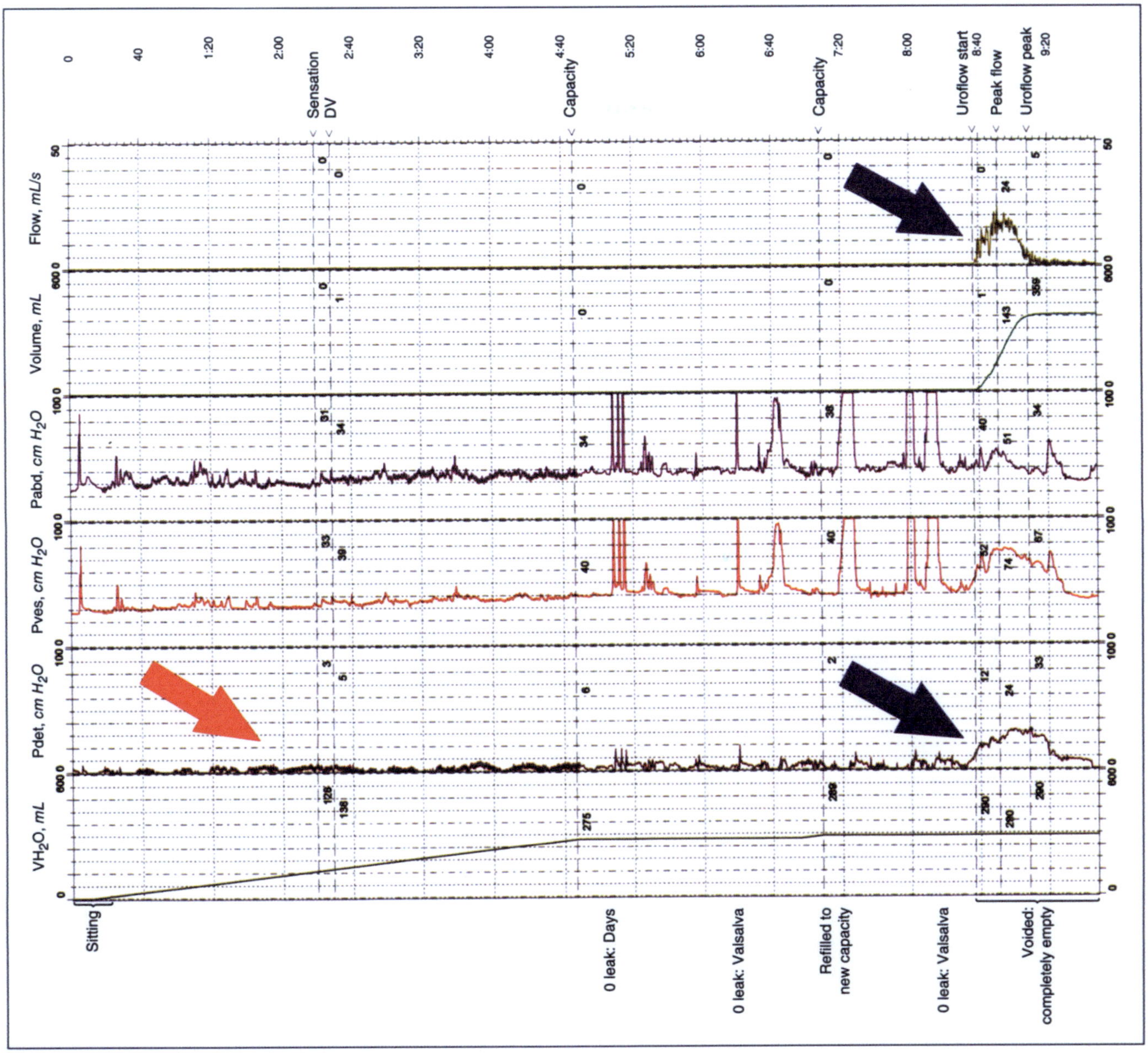

FIGURE 5-7. Multichannel urodynamics tracing. This 54-year-old gravida 2, para 2 woman is being evaluated for stress urinary incontinence (SUI). She voids every 2 hours during the day and does not have nocturia. She has a normal urinary flow and feels that she empties completely. She has occasional urgency and urgency incontinence. Past history includes a hysterectomy for menorrhagia and she takes a diuretic for hypertension.

This multichannel tracing shows that sitting fill cystometry is normal. Her first sensation is at 130 cc, first desire is at 150 cc, and her strong desire to void is at 275 cc. During the filling phase she has no detrusor contractions measured on subtracted detrusor (Pdet) monitoring (*red arrow*). Bladder compliance is normal. Provocative maneuvers to test for SUI were negative, as indicated by the handwriting on the tracing. She then voided with a voluntarily initiated detrusor contraction up to 20 cm H_2O (*lower blue arrow*) and a maximum flow of 20 cc/s (*upper blue arrow*), and emptied her bladder completely.

This study did not demonstrate her complaints. Since the testing circumstances can be uncomfortable for the patient, with an observer present and catheters in the urethra and rectum, the reported symptoms may not always be reproduced on the urodynamic studies.

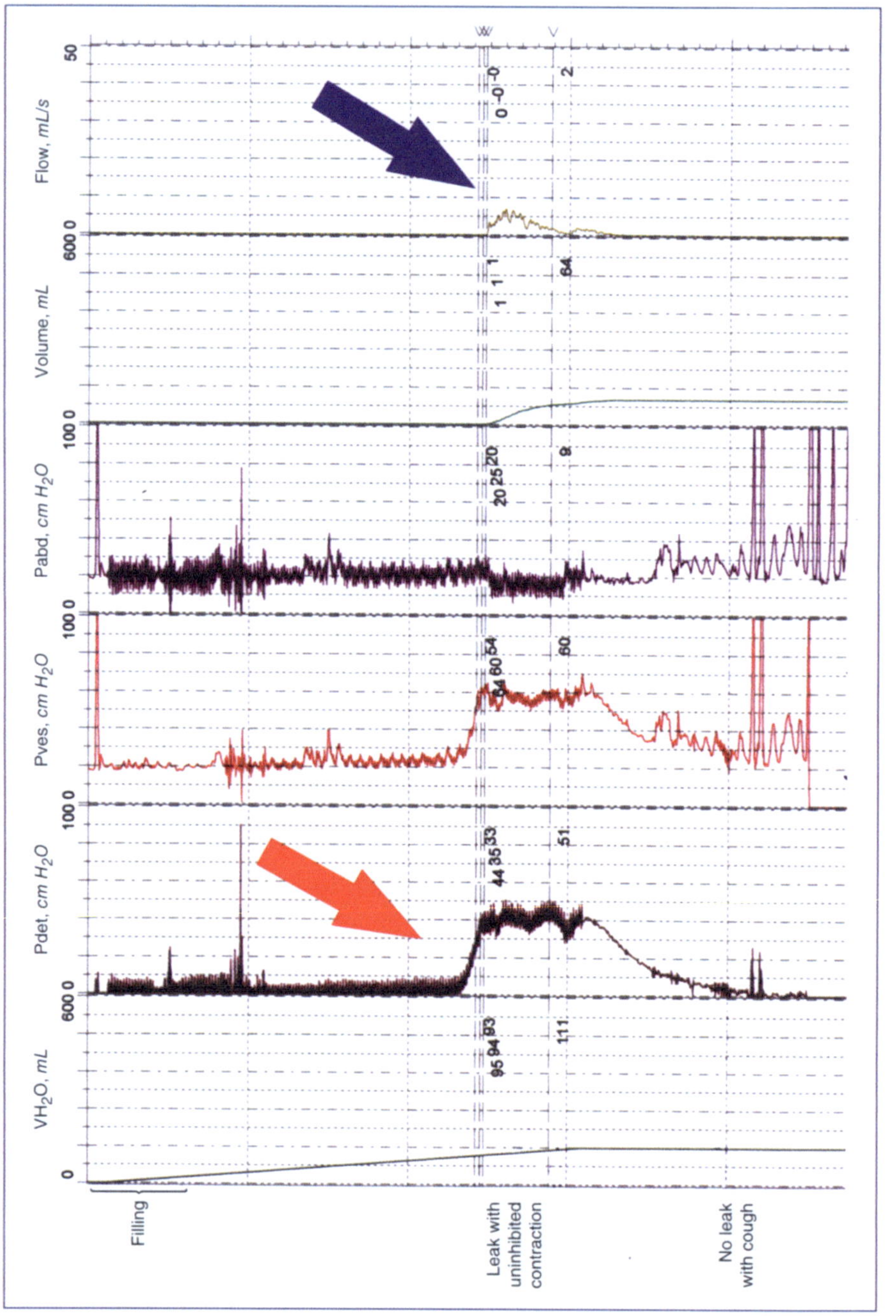

FIGURE 5-8. Idiopathic detrusor overactivity. This 56-year-old gravida 4, para 4 woman reports primarily of occasional stress incontinence and wears pads when she goes out of the house. She also has occasional urgency and urgency incontinence. She voids every 2 hours during the day and awakes to void twice at night. Her urinary flow is normal and she empties her bladder completely. Her past history includes a retropubic urethropexy and hysterectomy.

The filling phase of the multichannel urodynamics studies is shown here. The bladder is filled with the patient in the sitting position. After 95 cc, there is an uninhibited contraction up to 40 cm H_2O (*red arrow*) on Pdet with associated urinary incontinence (*blue arrow*). She actually voided a small amount into the flowmeter at the time (*blue arrow*). This is idiopathic detrusor overactivity.

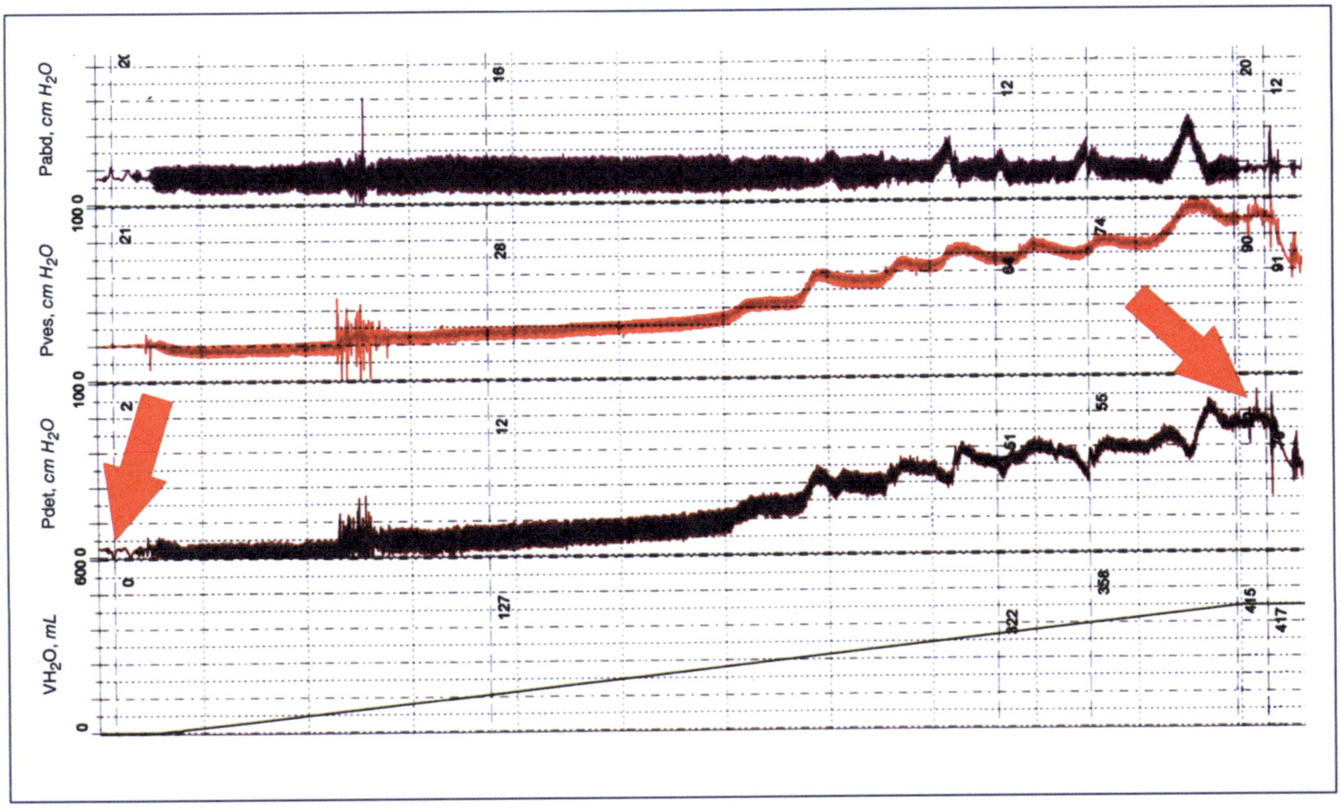

Figure 5-9. Low bladder compliance. This figure shows a filling cystometrogram on a 58-year-old man who had a spinal cord injury at T10–11 40 years ago. He manages his bladder with self-intermittent catheterization four times daily and wears a condom catheter for leakage in between. He also takes tolterodine extended release daily.

The maximal cystometric capacity is 415 cc and the subtracted detrusor pressure rise (Pdet) at that volume is 70 cm H_2O. The calculated compliance ($\Delta V/\Delta Pdet$) between the two *red arrows* is 5.9 cc/cm H_2O. This is low compliance [10]. His detrusor leak pressure was 70 cm H_2O, which means that the bladder storage pressure has the potential for reaching high levels if not treated. Since the patient catheterizes at lower volumes, he can keep his storage pressure low. Additionally, the poor compliance demonstrated on this examination may have been worsened by the rapid fill rate [2]. With poor compliance and high storage pressures, he is at risk of developing upper tract deterioration [11].

Assessment of Urethral Function During Filling Cystometry

Urethral pressure measurements	
Urethral pressure	Fluid pressure needed to open a closed urethra
Urethral pressure profile	Graph indicating the intraluminal pressure along the length of the urethra
Urethral closure pressure profile	Subtraction of intravesical pressure from urethral pressure
Maximum urethral pressure	Maximum pressure of the measured profile
MUCP	Maximum difference between the urethral pressure and the intravesical pressure
Functional profile length	Length of urethra along which the urethral pressure exceeds the intravesical pressure
Pressure "transmission" ratio	Increment in urethral pressure on stress as a percentage of the simultaneously recorded intravesical pressure
Abdominal/detrusor pressure measurements	
ALPP	Intravesical pressure at which urine leakage occurs due to increased abdominal pressure in the absence of a detrusor contraction
DLPP	Lowest detrusor pressure at which urine leakage occurs in the absence of either a detrusor contraction or increased abdominal pressure

Figure 5-10. Urethral function during filling. This table shows the different measures of urethral function during filling. Intraluminal urethral profilometry, characterized by maximal urethral closure pressure (MUCP), has been reported to have considerable overlap in normal (54–25 cm H_2O) and stress-incontinent (39–24 cm H_2O) women in multiple publications [5]. Furthermore, the value of MUCP is dependent on the type of catheter used, its orientation within the urethra, the degree of bladder fullness, and the position of the patient [12].

Abdominal leak point pressure (ALPP) is produced by coughing or Valsalva leak point pressure. However, the procedure is not consistently defined or standardized. Various studies have demonstrated a weak association between ALPP and the severity of incontinence. ALPP is also not helpful in predicting the outcome of sling procedures in women [5].

Both methods are not recommended as single tests, but to be interpreted within the context of filling cystometry and physical examination [5]. On the other hand, detrusor leak point pressure (DLPP) in neurologic disease is important to ascertain whether high pressures may cause renal damage [13]. Examples of abdominal/detrusor measurements to assess urethral function during filling will be given.

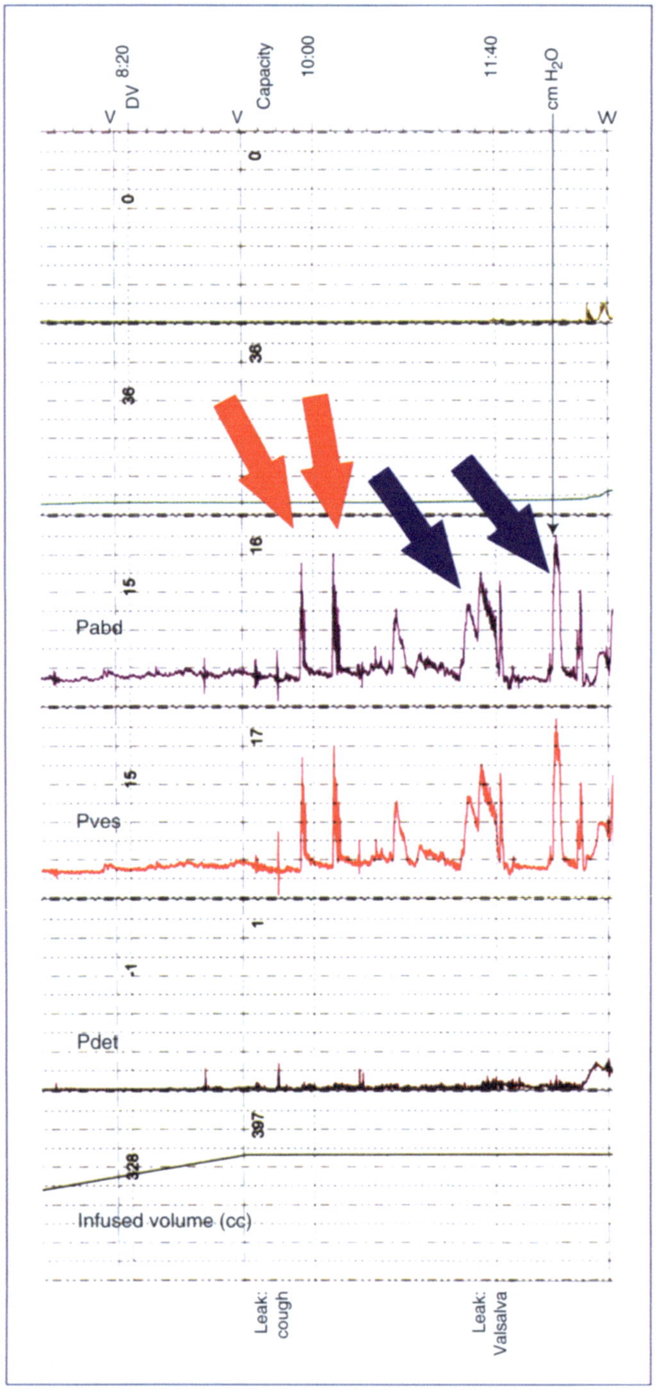

FIGURE 5-11. Urodynamic studies (UDS) of stress urinary incontinence (SUI). This UDS tracing is from the filling cystometry of a 73-year-old gravida 0, para 0 woman who reports SUI. She has no frequency, nocturia, urgency, or urgency incontinence. She voids normally. During cystometry, 400 cc of saline was infused into her bladder. She has normal sensation and no uninhibited detrusor contractions on Pdet (detrusor obstruction). Her SUI is tested with coughing (*red arrows*) and Valsalva (*blue arrows*). Her Valsalva leak point pressure is 83 cm H_2O and her coughing leak point pressure is at about the same level.

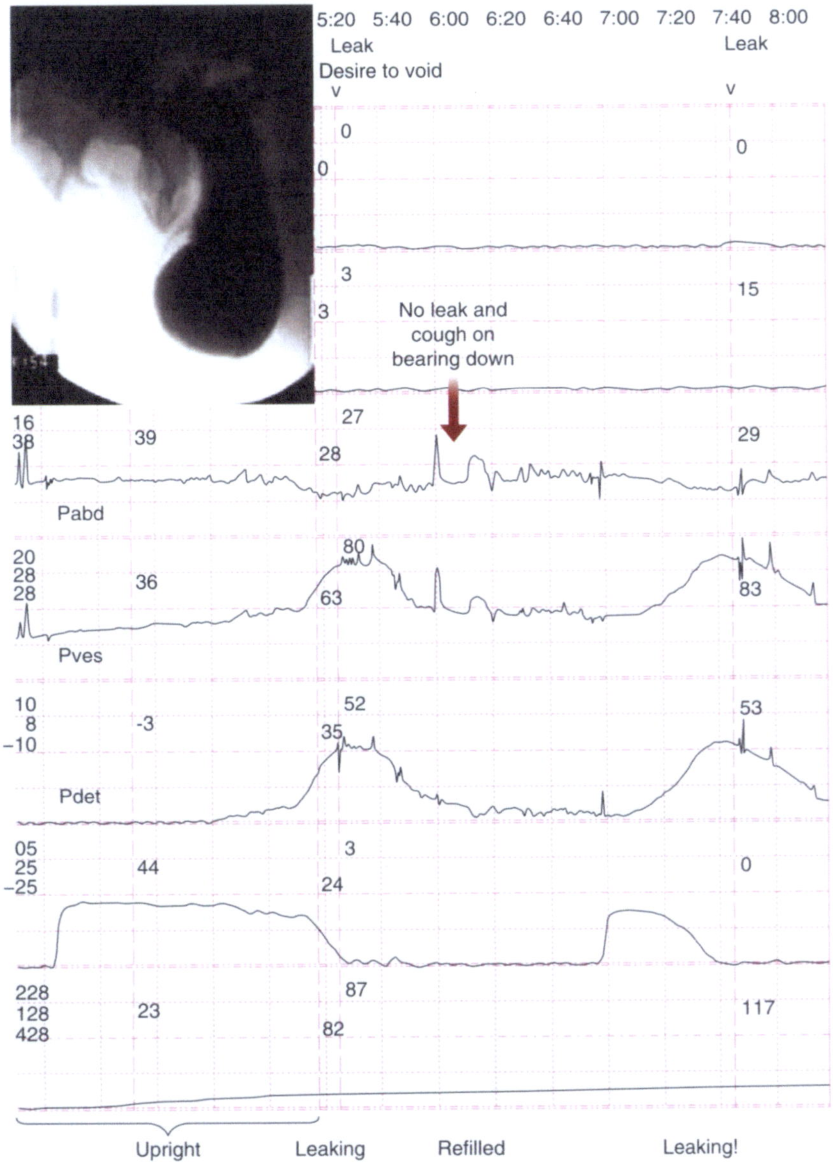

FIGURE 5-12. Occult stress incontinence. This urodynamics studies tracing from an 81-year-old gravida 4, para 4 woman who reports mixed urinary incontinence. Her filling cystometry shows marked detrusor overactivity incontinence (Pdet up to 50 cm H_2O). When the contraction settles, she is asked to strain (*red arrow*) but does not leak. A simultaneously cystogram demonstrates marked bladder prolapse, which is most likely preventing the leak with straining. This is an example of prolapse masking the leak. The test could be repeated with a tampon in the vagina.

On physical examination, reducing the prolapse resulted in marked stress urinary incontinence with coughing and straining. This is an example of one of the caveats of abdominal leak point pressure testing.

Measurements of the Voiding Phase	
Uroflowmetry	
Urine flow	Continuous, intermittent, smooth, fluctuating
Flow rate	Volume expelled per time unit (cc/s)
Voided volume	Total volume expelled (cc)
Maximum flow rate	Maximum measured value (after correction for artifacts) (Qmax)
	Normal for males is 15–20 cc/s; abnormal is < 5 cc/s. There is a decline with age [14]. Normal for women can be > 30 cc/s. There may be no decline with age [15].
Voiding time	Total duration of voiding including interruptions
Flow time	Time over which measurable flow occurs
Average flow time	Voided volume divided by flow time
Time to maximum flow	Elapsed time from onset to maximum flow
Pressure measurements during flow studies	
Premicturition pressure	Immediately before the initial isovolumetric contraction
Opening pressure	Recorded at the onset of urine flow
Opening time	Time from the initial rise in detrusor pressure to the onset of flow
Maximum pressure	Maximum value measured
Pressure at maximum flow (Pdet Qmax)	Lowest pressure recorded at the maximum measured flow rate
Closing pressure	Measured at the end of flow
Minimum voiding pressure	Minimum measured during flow
Flow delay	Delay between change in bladder pressure and change in the measured flow rate

FIGURE 5-13. This table shows the parameters that can be measured during the voiding phase: uroflowmetry and pressure flow studies [4]. The specific parameters measured are in the *left column* with the explanation in the *right column.*

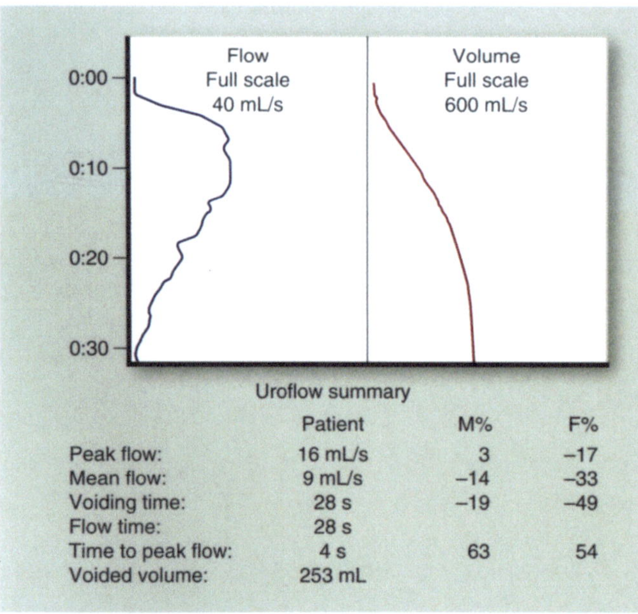

FIGURE 5-14. Normal male uroflow. This 50-year-old man complains of daytime urinary frequency and nocturia. He has no voiding symptoms and the voided volume is 253 cc. The shape of the curve is normal and the Qmax is 16 cc/s. The flow is continuous and the flow and voiding times are equal. His postvoid bladder scan is zero.

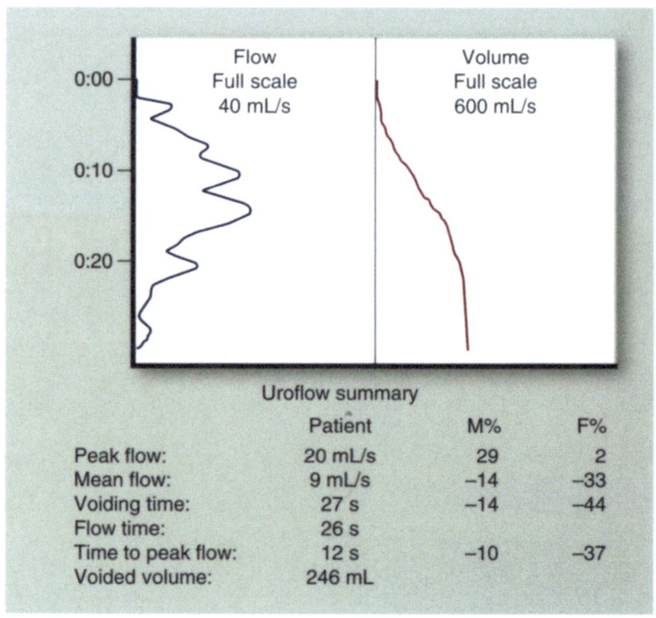

FIGURE 5-15. Straining uroflow in men. This 70-year-old man complains of having to strain to void. He has no daytime frequency, urgency, or nocturia and has to use manual compression to empty his bladder. His voided volume is 246 cc. Although the Qmax is normal, the curve is notched; this indicates that he is straining to void. His postvoid residual on bladder scan is zero.

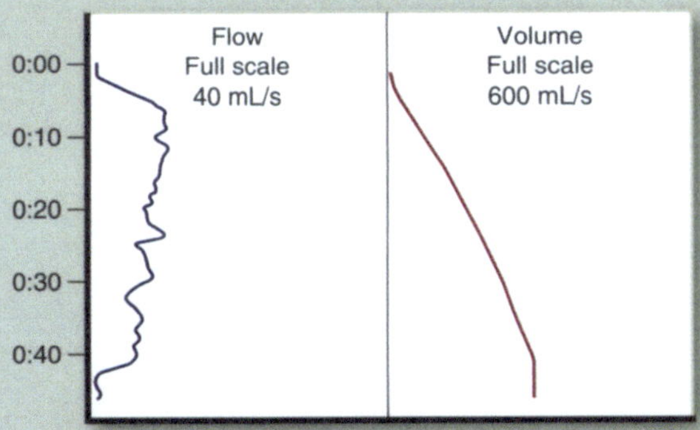

Uroflow summary

	Patient	M%	F%
Peak flow:	10 mL/s	–40	–52
Mean flow:	7 mL/s	–41	–53
Voiding time:	40 s	–59	–97
Flow time:	40 s		
Time to peak flow:	5 s	55	46
Voided volume:	304 mL		

FIGURE 5-16. Uroflow with urethral stricture. This 43-year-old man complains of urinary frequency, nocturia, slow stream, and hesitancy, which are storage and voiding symptoms. Eight years ago, he was involved in a motor vehicle accident that resulted in lumbosacral fracture. He had no neurological injury. The uroflow shows a voided volume of 304 cc, his Qmax is 10 cc/s, and there is a continuous curve. The curve is relatively flat throughout most of the voiding time, consistent with a urethral stricture, which was demonstrated on cystoscopy. His postvoid residual on bladder scan was 45 cc.

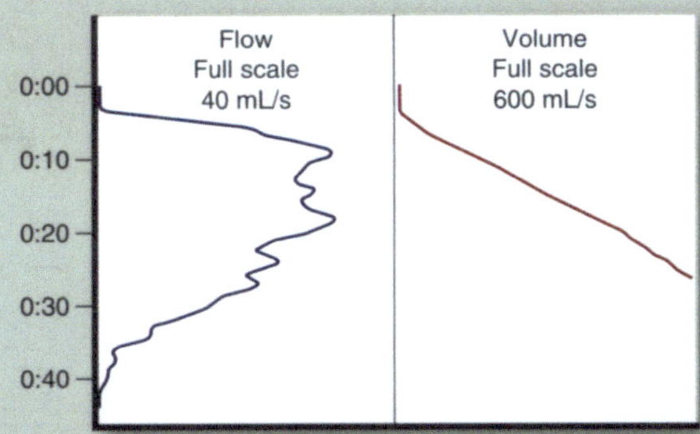

Uroflow summary

	Patient
Peak flow:	33 mL/s
Mean flow:	19 mL/s
Voiding time:	37 s
Flow time:	37 s
Time to peak flow:	15 s
Voided volume:	718 mL

FIGURE 5-17. Normal uroflow in a woman. This 62-year-old woman reports stress urinary incontinence and has no other storage or voiding symptoms. She has a large bladder capacity and voided 718 cc; her Qmax is 33 cc/s, a smooth, bell-shaped curve with normal parameters. Her postvoid residual on bladder scan is zero.

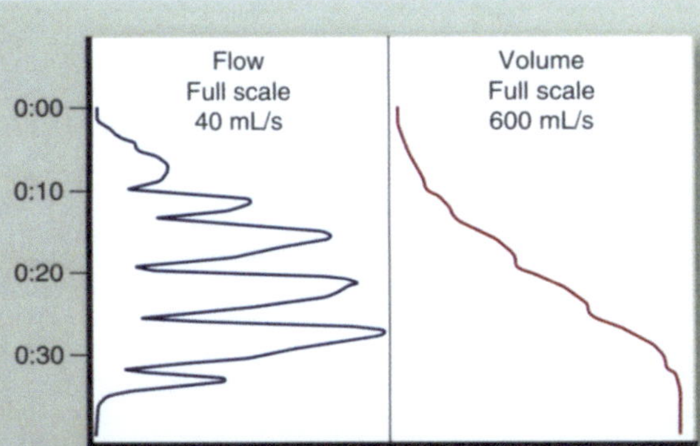

Uroflow summary

	Patient
Peak flow:	40 mL/s
Mean flow:	17 mL/s
Voiding time:	34 s
Flow time:	34 s
Time to peak flow:	25 s
Voided volume:	588 mL

FIGURE 5-18. Straining uroflow in a woman. This 67-year-old woman reports stress urinary incontinence. She has nocturia, no other storage symptoms, and has no voiding symptoms. Prior to the uroflow, she was asked to void normally without straining. She voided 588 cc with a Qmax of 40 cc/s and deep notches, which are consistent with straining. The flow time was less than 40 cc and she was not aware of having strained.

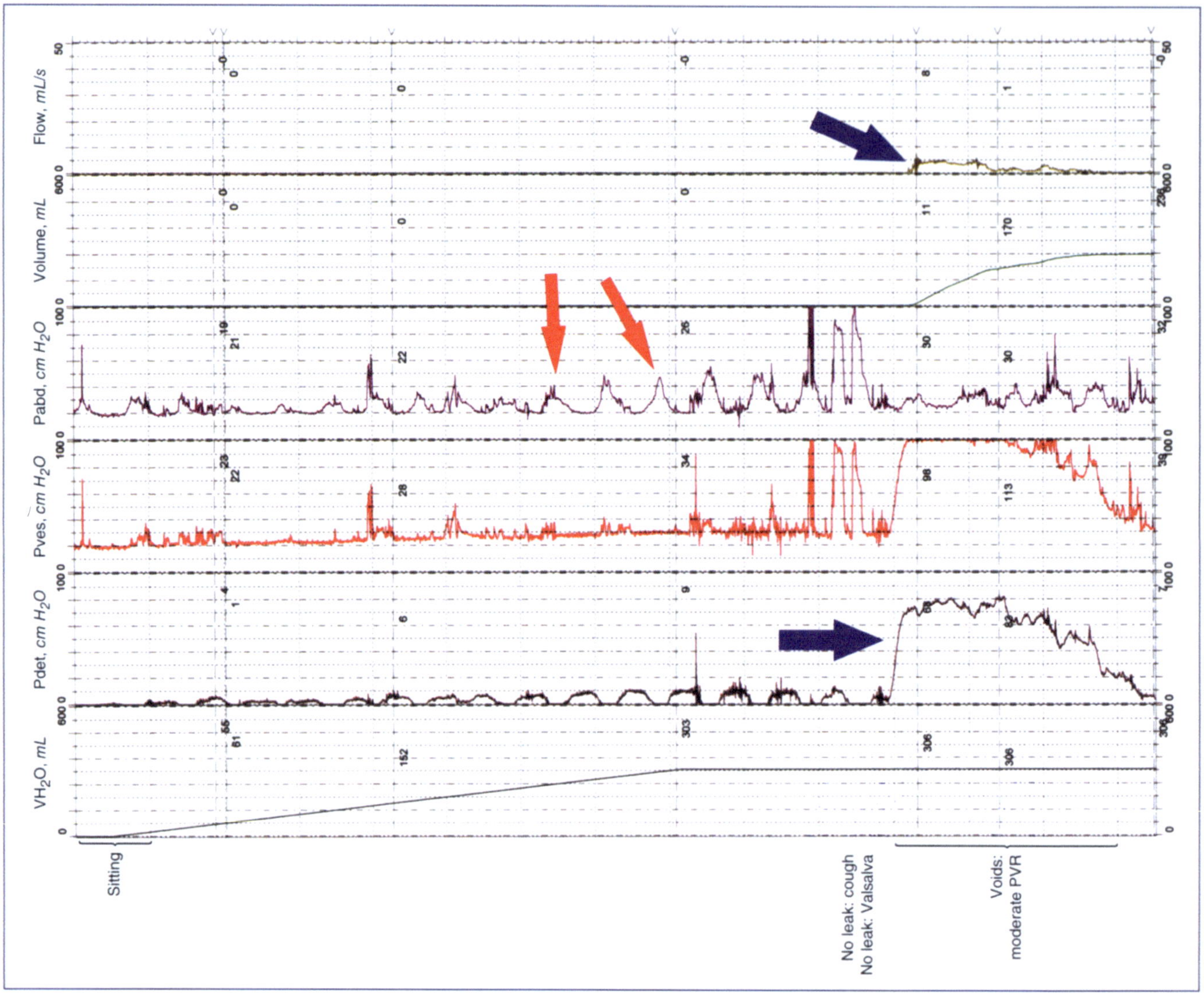

Figure 5-19. Pressure flow study on a man with lower urinary tract symptoms. This 62-year-old man reports urinary frequency of every 1.5 hours and nocturia two or three times nightly. He also has a slow urinary stream accompanied by hesitancy, and a history of one episode of retention. Despite therapy with alfuzosin and finasteride, his symptoms are quite troublesome.

His postvoid residual urine at the start of the test was 60 cc. His bladder was infused with saline at a moderate rate. His first sensation was at 55 cc, strong sensation at 155 cc, and his capacity was 303 cc. There were no uninhibited contractions (detrusor overactivity) on filling. Rectal contractions or peristaltic waves are noted in Pabd (*red arrows*) and are reflected as pressure drops on Pdet. His bladder filling is normal. He was asked to void and voluntarily initiated a detrusor contraction up to 68 cm H_2O (*lower blue arrow*) when flow began (*upper blue arrow*). His Qmax was 8 cc/s. The detrusor pressure was sustained and he voided 253 cc. The high pressure and low flow are consistent with outlet obstruction [16], most likely from his enlarged prostate.

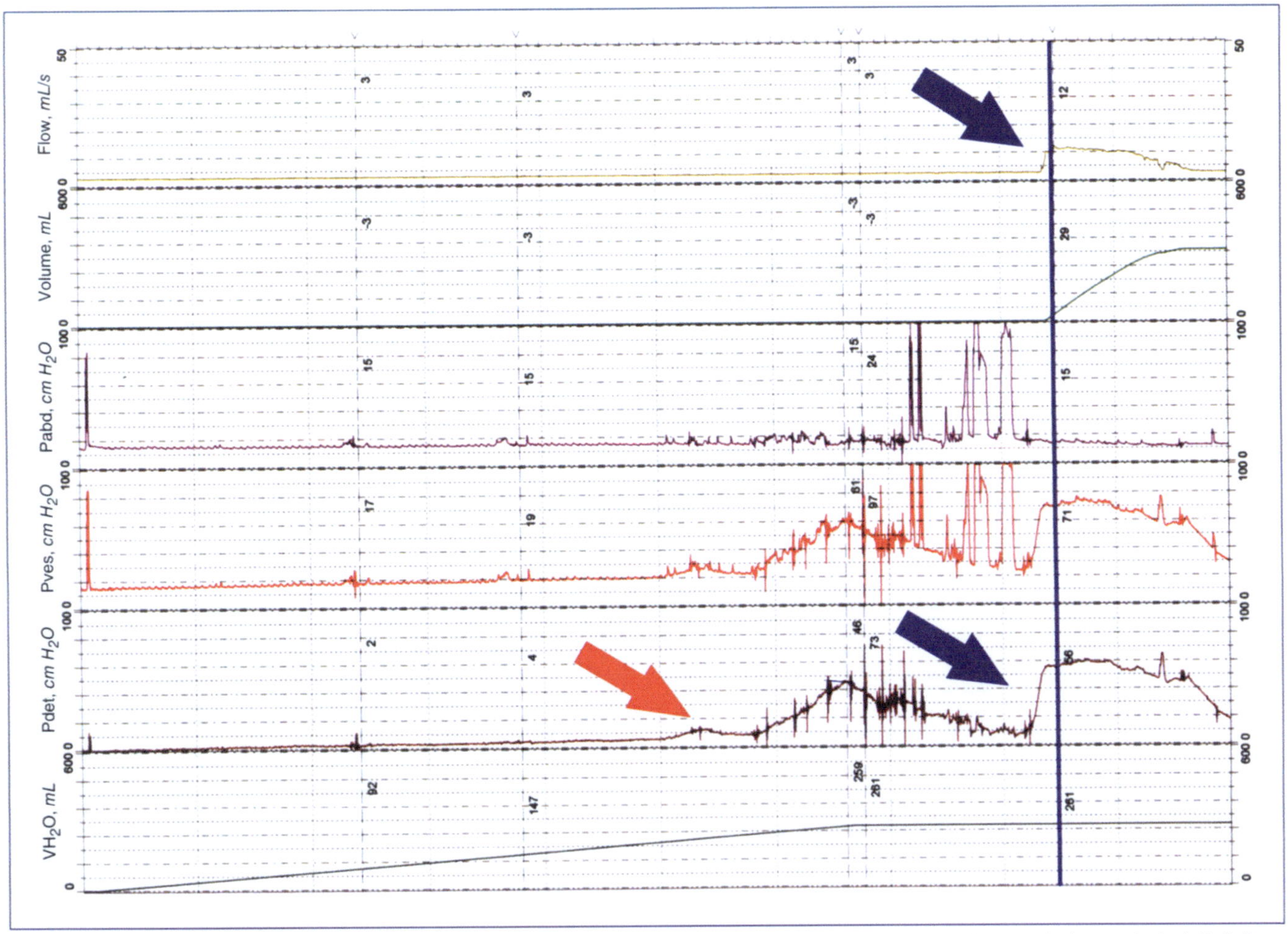

FIGURE 5-20. Pressure-flow study in a man with lower urinary tract symptoms. This 74-year-old man reports urinary frequency every 2 hours and daily urgency and urgency incontinence. He wakes up twice at night to void and has a weak urinary stream with hesitancy. According to the International Prostate Symptom Score that he completed, the storage symptoms are the most frequent. He is being treated with tamsulosin.

His filling phase shows marked detrusor overactivity (DO) with Pdet up to 48 cm H_2O (*red arrow*). No detrusor overactivity incontinence is noted. He is asked to cough and strain as noted by the pressure rises on the Pves and Pabd tracings, but no leakage is demonstrated. He is then asked to void, which voluntarily initiates a detrusor contraction (*lower blue arrow*). Flow is also initiated (*upper blue arrow*). His Pdet is 56 cm H_2O and Qmax is 12 cc/s. His detrusor contraction is sustained and he is able to empty his bladder completely. His results are consistent with bladder outlet obstruction with DO. Since he has troublesome and persistent storage symptoms despite an alpha blocker, he is a candidate for the addition of an antimuscarinic. The risk of urinary retention with this combination is low [17]. PVR—postvoid residual.

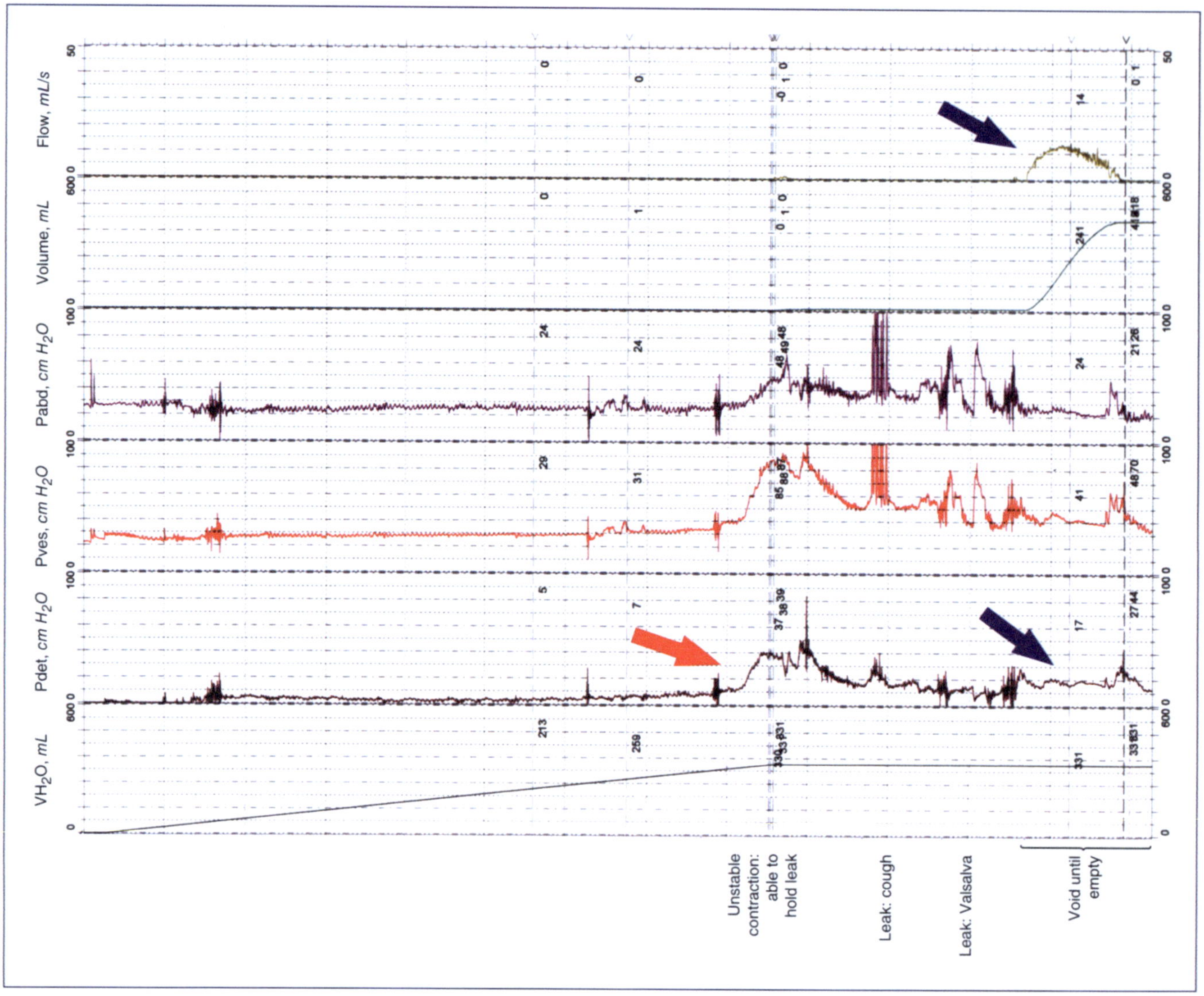

Figure 5-21. Pressure/flow study in a man with storage (overactive bladder [OAB]) symptoms. This 70-year-old man reports daytime frequency every 1 to 2 hours and nocturia ×1. He has urgency, daily urgency incontinence, a fair stream, and no other voiding symptoms. He has been treated with tamsulosin, finasteride, and solifenacin, but still has troublesome OAB symptoms.

His residual urine after voiding before the urodynamic studies was 25 cc. During the filling study, his first bladder sensation was at 213 cc. He had a first desire to void at 260 cc and after 300 cc he had a detrusor contraction up to 37 cm H_2O (*red arrow*) associated with some incontinence. He was able to suppress the contraction by contracting his pelvic floor muscles. He voided with a Pdet of 20 cm H_2O and a Qmax of 14 cc/s (*blue arrows*) and emptied his bladder completely. Since he is not obstructed, the major finding is the detrusor overactivity incontinence.

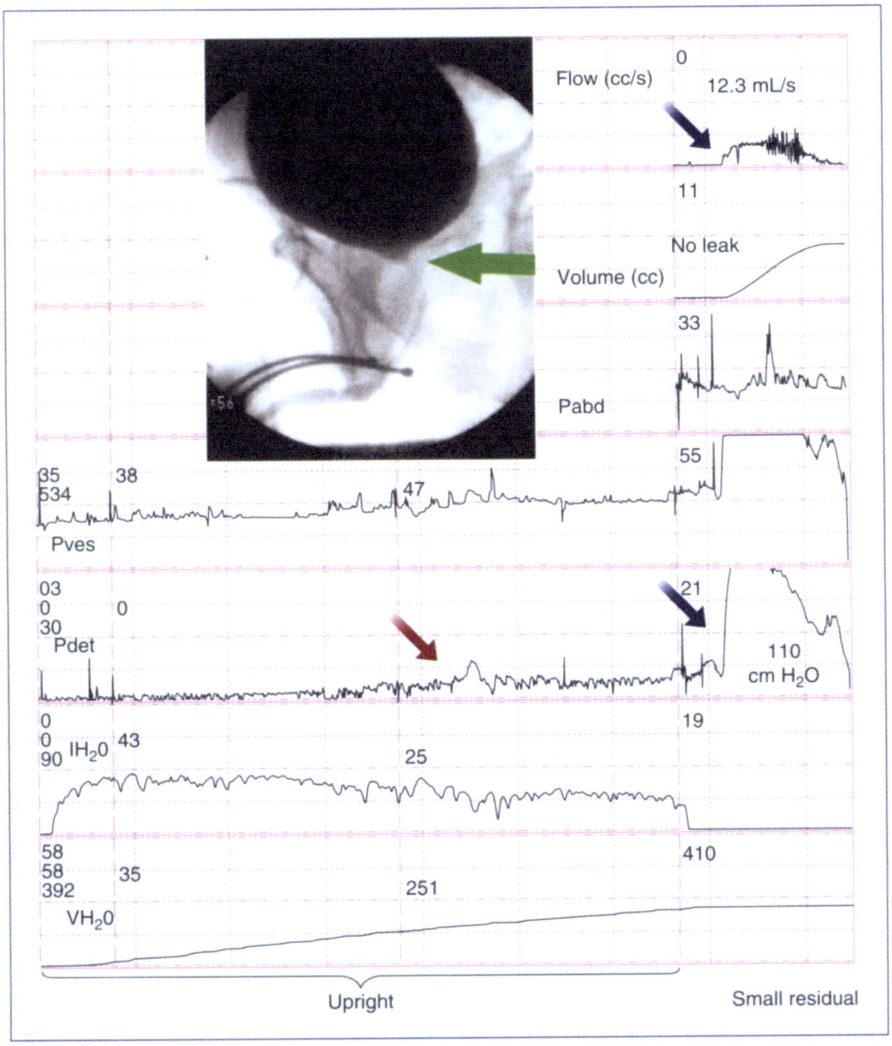

FIGURE 5-22. Videourodynamics for lower urinary tract symptoms in a man. This 67-year-old man complains of urinary frequency, nocturia, urgency, and slow stream. Bladder filling shows detrusor overactivity with a Pdet of 28 cm H_2O (*red arrow*) and a capacity of 410 cc. He voided with a Pdet of 110 cm H_2O (*lower blue arrow*) and had Qmax of 12 cc/s (*upper blue arrow*). This demonstrated outlet obstruction. Simultaneous fluoroscopic imaging during voiding demonstrated prostatic obstruction (*green arrow*). He also has a semirigid penile implant visible. He was treated with tamsulosin and finasteride, but after 6 years his symptoms worsened and he underwent a successful transurethral resection of the prostate.

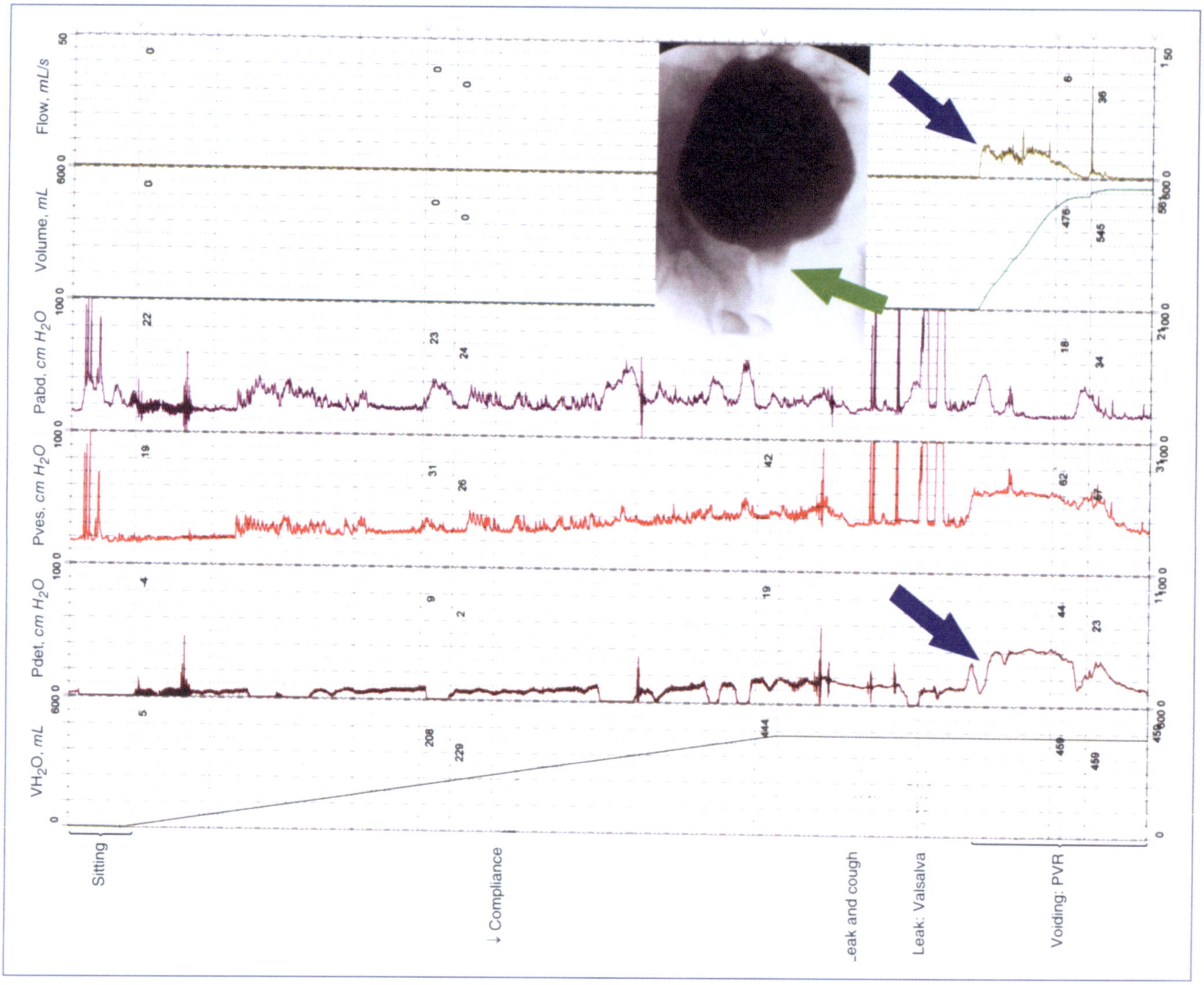

FIGURE 5-23. Videourodynamics in a man with recurrent lower urinary tract symptoms after transurethral resection of the prostate. The same man as discussed in Figure 5-21 is now 79 years old and reports frequency, nocturia, urgency, and occasional urgency incontinence. On bladder filling, first sensation was at 208 cc, first desire to void at 229 cc, and strong desire to void at 444 cc. There was a mild decrease in compliance. He voided with a Pdet of 44 cm H_2O (*lower blue arrow*) and Qmax of 12 cc/s (*upper blue arrow*) and emptied his bladder completely. On fluoroscopy during voiding, his bladder neck and prostate are wide open (*green arrow*). He has overactive bladder symptoms and no detrusor obstruction or obstruction. Since he also developed myasthenia gravis, he is not a candidate for anticholinergics.

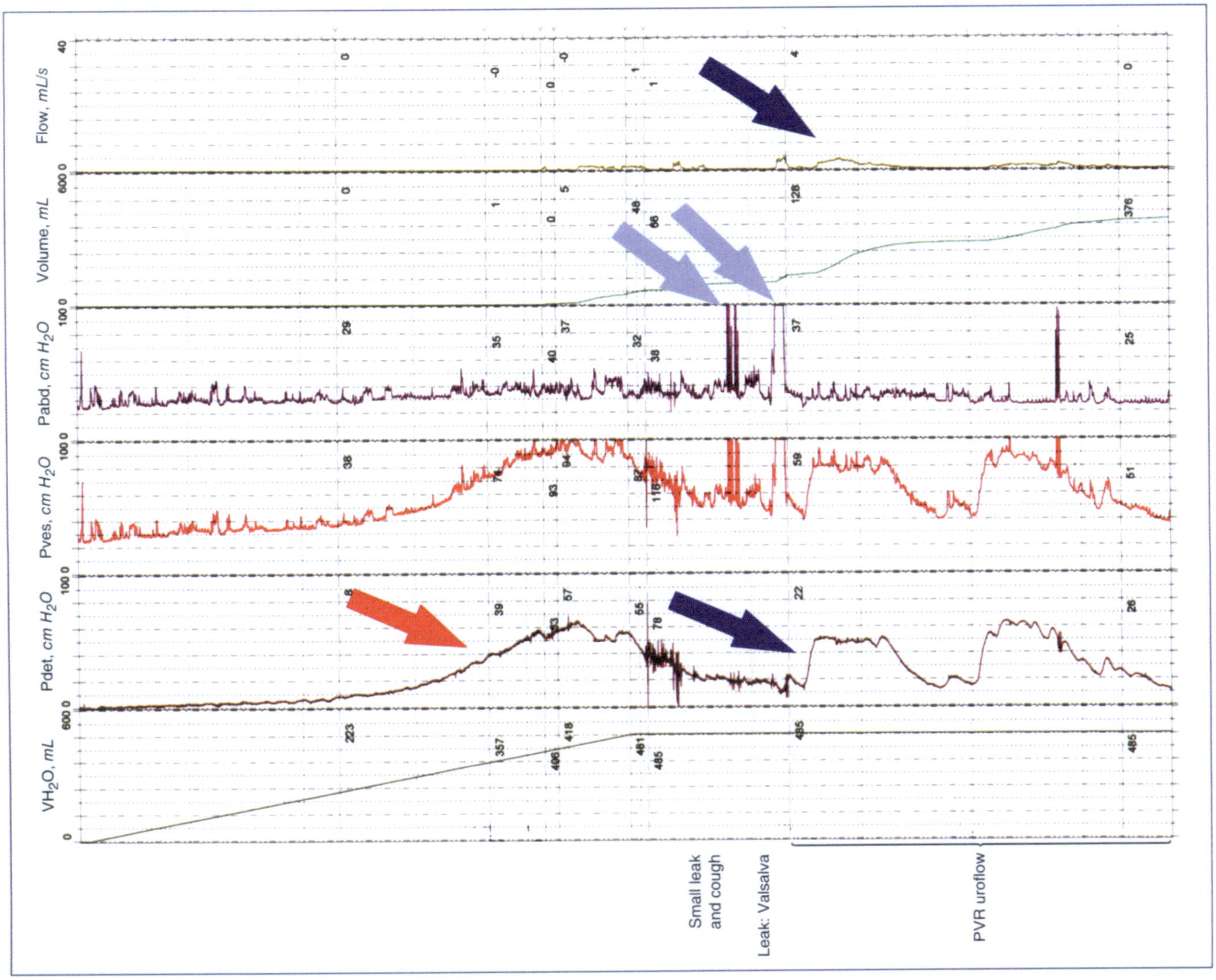

FIGURE 5-24. Multichannel study of a man with post-high–intensity focused ultrasound (HIFU) incontinence and stricture. This 70-year-old man reports stress incontinence. He voids every 2 hours and has nocturia ×1. He underwent HIFU for localized prostate cancer and has an undetectable prostate-specific antigen. He had a direct vision internal urethrotomy for a resultant stricture in the distal prostatic fossa and needs to use two to three incontinence pads daily.

On bladder filling his first sensation is at 223 cc and first desire to void at 357 cc. There was detrusor obstruction (DO) with a pressure rise up to 63 cm H_2O and urinary leakage (*red arrow*). His capacity was 485 cc. The pressure subsided to 20 cm H_2O and he leaked with coughing and straining (*light blue arrows*). His abdominal leak point pressure was 100 cm H_2O. He voided 376 cc with Pdet up to 50 to 60 cm H_2O (*lower dark blue arrow*) and a low flow rate (*upper dark blue arrow*). After the tubes were removed, he emptied into the flowmeter with a Qmax of 12 cc/s and a voiding time of 24 s.

Although he does not have urgency, urgency incontinence, or slow stream, the study showed DO and outflow obstruction. The findings may be explained by the stricture being occluded with the urodynamic study catheter.

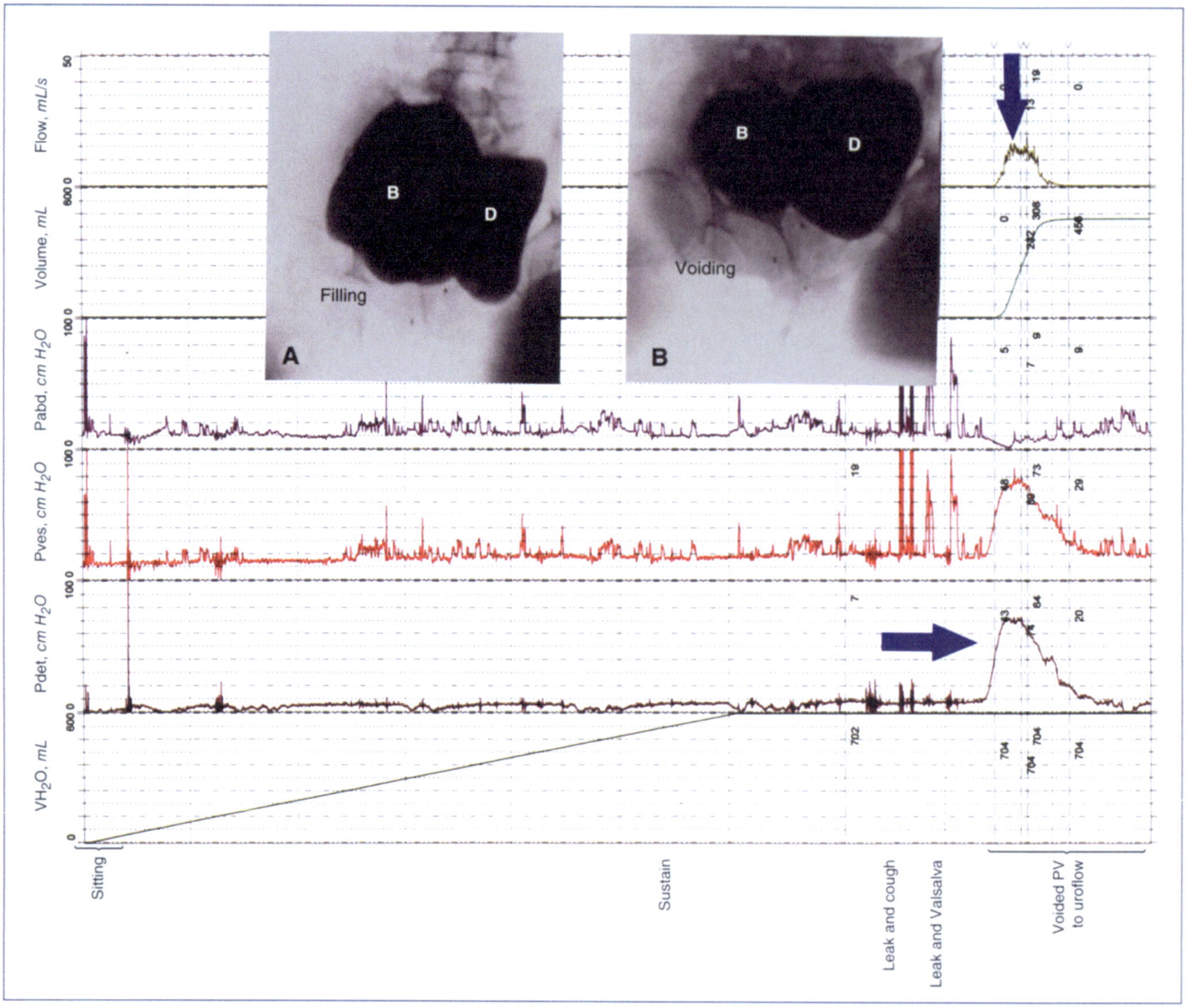

FIGURE 5-25. Videourodynamics of a man with a bladder diverticulum. This 71-year-old man has recurrent nonfebrile urinary tract infections. He has daytime frequency every 2 hours and nocturia three to four times each night. He has hesitancy, slow stream, and strains to void. He self-catheterizes twice daily. His postvoid residual prior to the study was 400 cc. On bladder filling, he has decreased sensation. He felt a desire to void at 700 cc and no detrusor obstruction was elicited. The filling fluoroscopy image (**A**) shows the bladder (*B*) and the diverticulum (*D*).

The patient was able to void voluntarily with a Pdet of 73 cm H_2O and Qmax of 13 cc/s. His voiding parameters are in the equivocal/obstructed zones. The voiding study image (**B**) shows that the bladder (*B*) is emptying into the diverticulum (*D*).

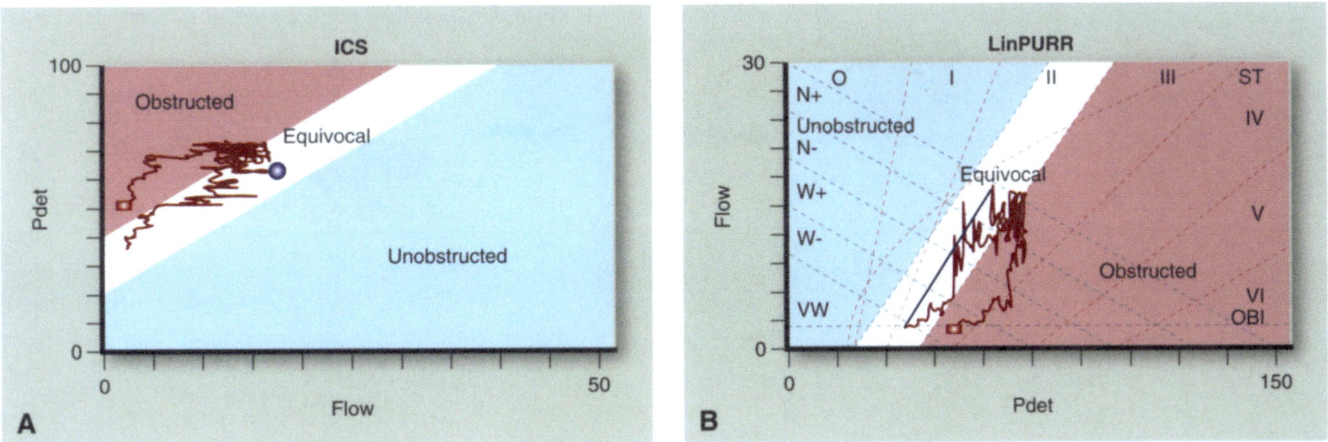

FIGURE 5-26. Pressure/flow nomograms. Pressure/flow nomograms have been designed to analyze results more completely when there is a question of whether or not the tracing indicates an obstruction. The pressure flow plot from Figure 5-24 is depicted on the following nomograms.

A, In the International Continence Society nomogram, the equivocal zone (*yellow band*) is between 20 and 40 cm H_2O for increasing flow rates [18]. Pressure is plotted against flow. The PdetQmax is indicated by the *blue dot*. The Bladder Outlet Obstruction Index (BOOI) can be calculated by the formula BOOI = PdetQmax − 2(Qmax). In this patient, it is 73 − (2 × 13) = 47, which is considered to be obstructed (unobstructed is less than 20).

B, The LinPURR (linearized passive urethral resistance ratio) or Schafer nomogram allows grading of the degree of obstruction from 0 (no obstruction) to 6 (severe obstruction) [19]. The linPURR line (*blue line*) of this patient links the relative lowest detrusor pressure at which flow starts or stops to the PdetQmax point. In this patient, it travels through band II, corresponding to slight obstruction.

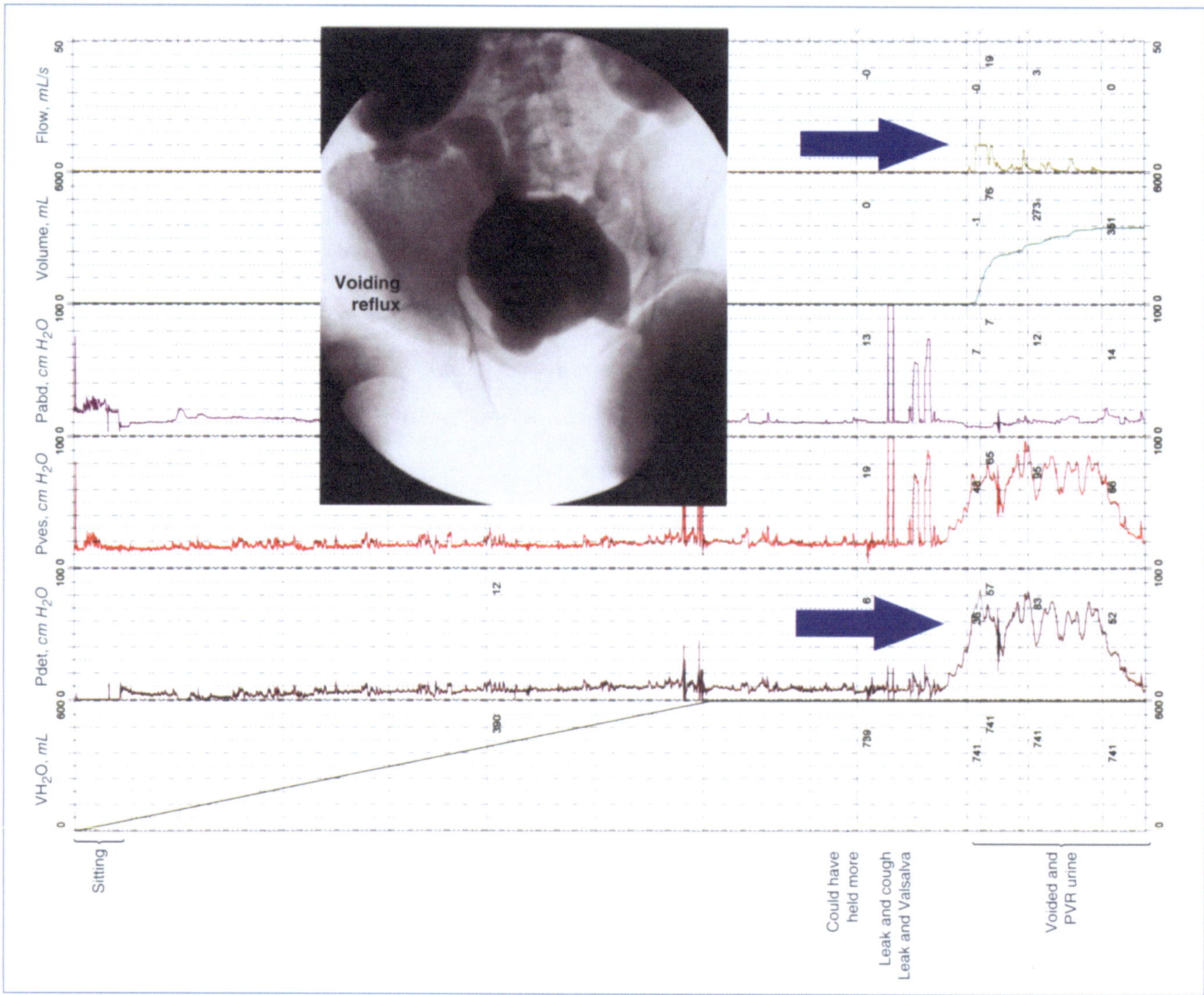

FIGURE 5-27. Videourodynamics in a man with outlet obstruction and reflux. This 36-year-old man has renal failure and bilateral hydronephrosis. He has no storage complaints, but voids with a slow stream and his postvoid residual is 400 cc.

During the bladder-filling phase, his first sensation was at 400 cc and he had a strong desire to void at 740 cc. There is no detrusor obstruction or poor compliance demonstrated. During the voiding phase, PdetQmax is 82 cm H_2O and Qmax is 12 cc/s (*blue arrows*). On the fluoroscopic image during voiding (*inset*), he has grade 4 to 5 bilateral vesicoureteral reflux. His bladder neck also appears not to open. He has bladder outlet obstruction and high voiding pressure that most likely led to his renal failure. The bilateral reflux has also most likely lowered the voiding pressure.

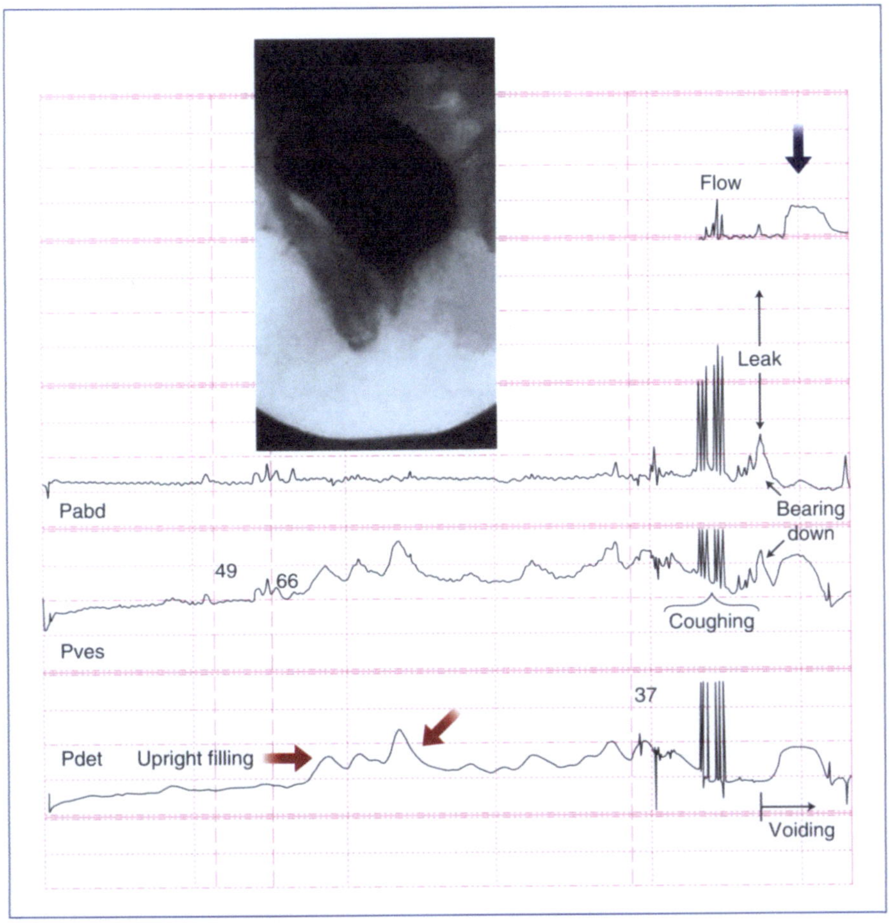

FIGURE 5-28. Videourodynamics in a man with postprostatectomy incontinence. This 67-year-old man had a radical prostatectomy and postoperative radiation therapy for prostate cancer. He reports storage symptoms including frequency, nocturia, urgency, urgency incontinence, and stress incontinence. He has no voiding difficulty and uses five large incontinence pads daily.

The bladder-filling study shows a decrease in compliance and multiple uninhibited contractions during the filling as well (*red arrows*). His first sensation was at 140 cc, desire to void at 175 cc, and a strong desire to void at 230 cc. He leaked with coughing and straining on a stress testing with a Valsalva leak point pressure of 75 cm H_2O (fluoroscopic image, (*inset*). He voided with a PdetQmax of 43 cm H_2O and Qmax of 12 cc/s (*blue arrow*).

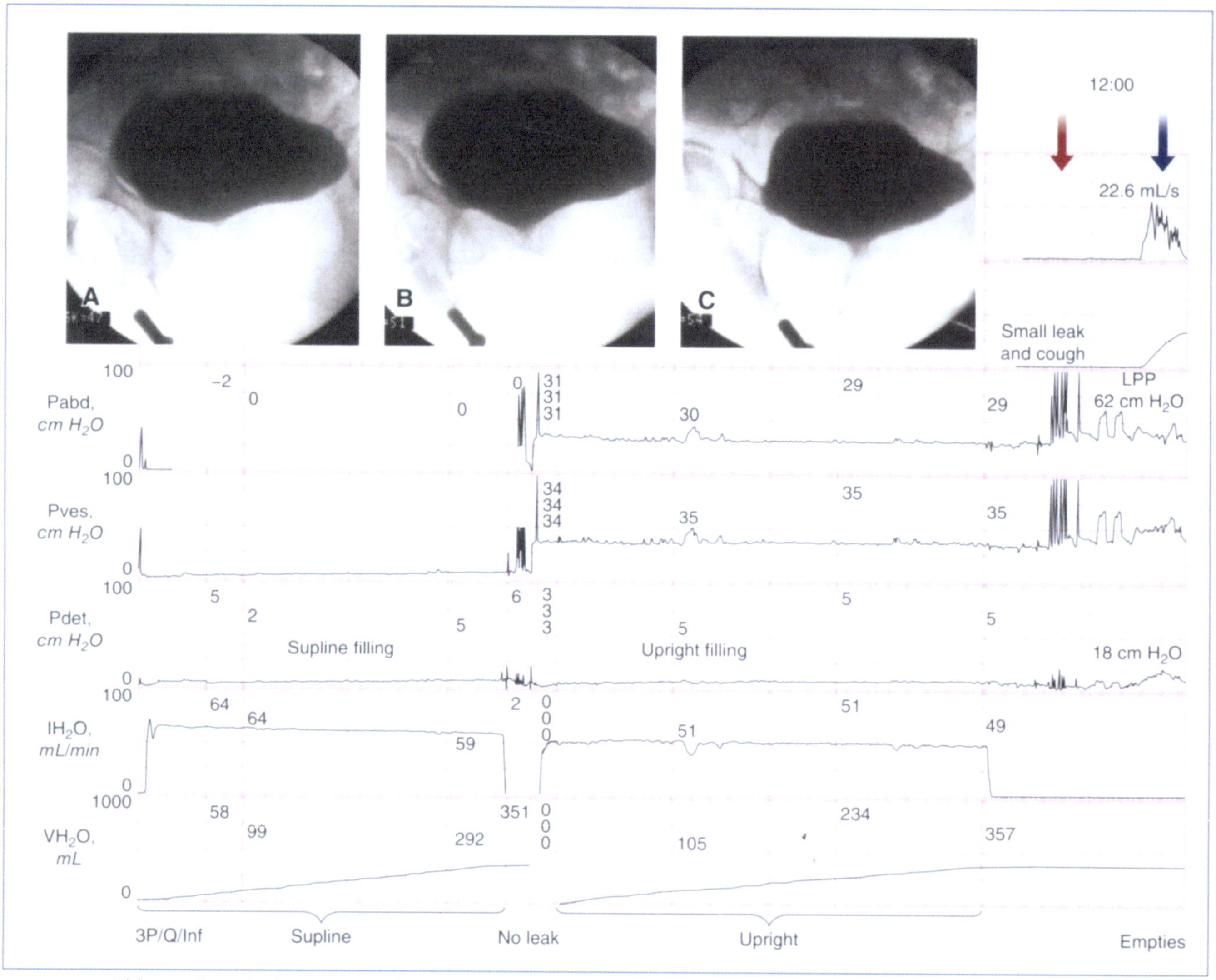

FIGURE 5-29. Videourodynamics in a woman with stress incontinence. This 64-year-old gravida 4, para 4 woman with the chief complaint of stress incontinence. She has no frequency or nocturia, but has occasional urgency and urgency incontinence. She has no voiding symptoms but wears one to two pads per day.

On upright filling, her first sensation is at 105 cc, first desire to void at 234 cc, and a strong desire to void at 357 cc. She has no detrusor obstruction and the compliance is normal. On upright fluoroscopy after filling at rest, her bladder neck is slightly open (**A**). With coughing, there is a small amount of descent or mild hypermobility (**B**; *red arrow*) and her Valsalva leak point pressure is 62 cm H_2O. She has no apparent cystocele (**B**) and her voiding phase is normal with a voiding pressure (Pdet) of 18 cm H_2O and Qmax of 23 cc/s (**C**; *blue arrow*).

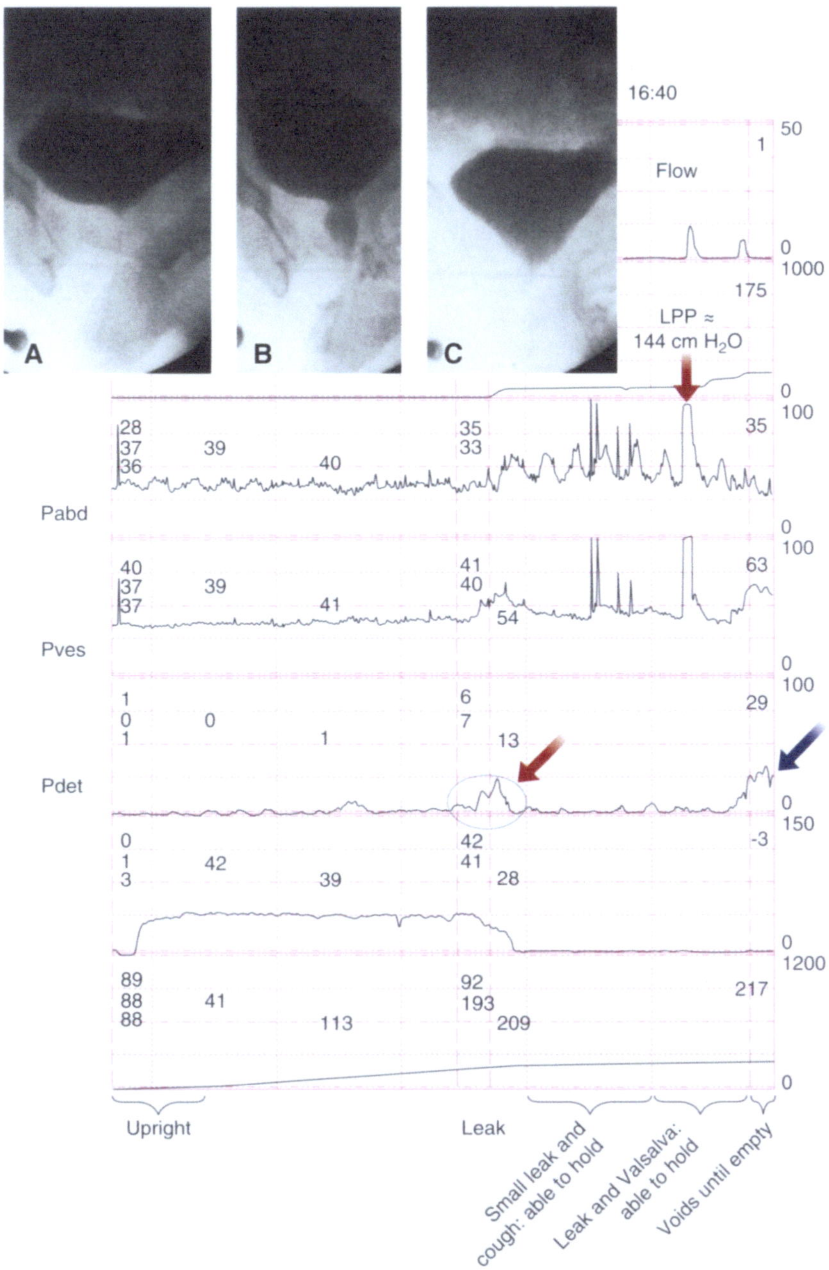

FIGURE 5-30. Videourodynamics in a woman with mixed incontinence. This 52-year-old gravida 2, para 2 woman reports both stress and urgency incontinence. She has daytime frequency and nocturia, as well as one to two daily episodes urgency incontinence. Her most bothersome symptom is the urgency incontinence.

Her postvoid residual at the start of the test was 10 cc. On upright filling, the bladder neck is slightly open at rest (**A**). The first sensation of filling is at 41 cc, first desire to void at 113 cc, and a strong desire to void at 209 cc when she has an uninhibited contraction (*lower red arrow*) that results in incontinence (**B**). With straining, she leaks with a high Valsalva leak point pressure of more than 140 cm H_2O (*upper red arrow*) (**C**). The hypermobility and descent of the bladder are also seen. She voluntarily initiated a detrusor to contraction to void (*blue arrow*) but is unable to empty during the test.

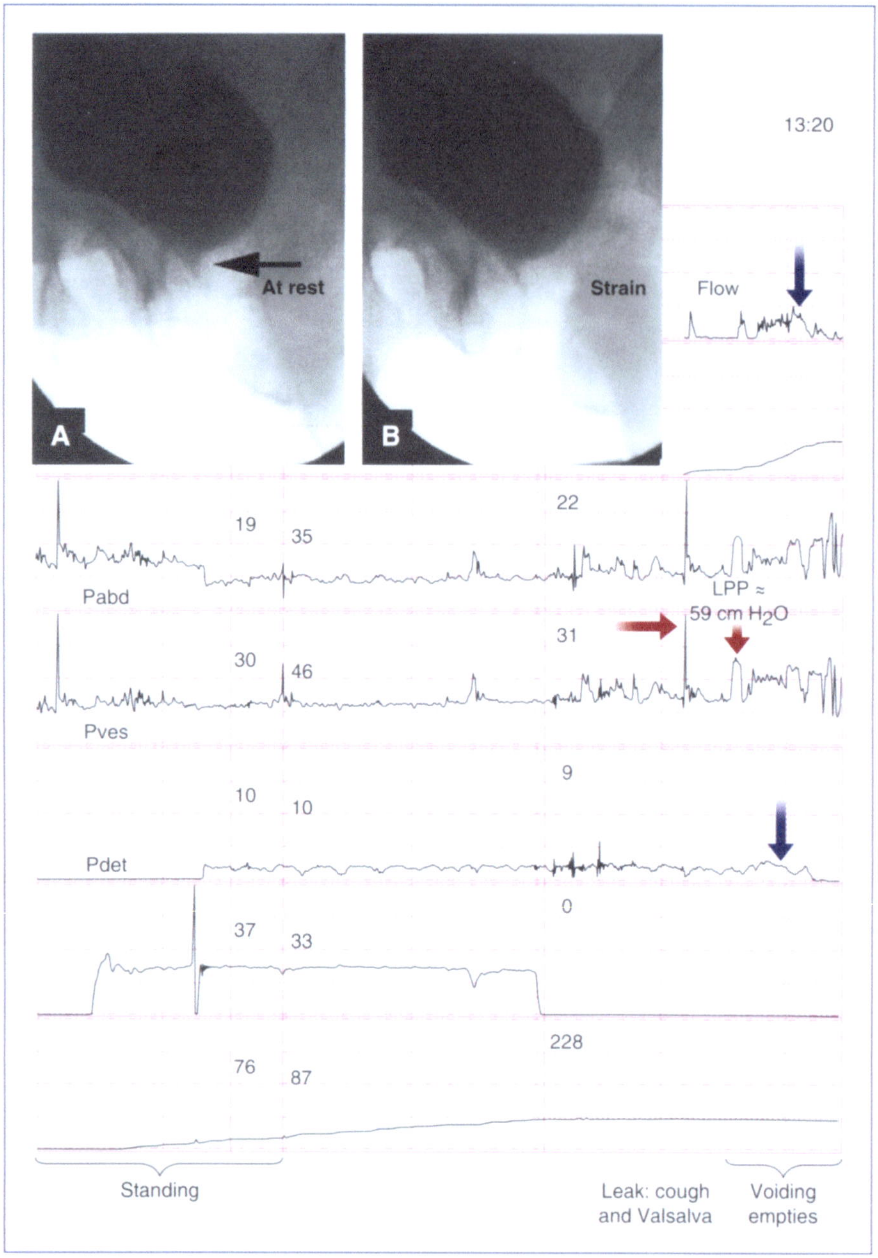

FIGURE 5-31. Videourodynamics in a woman with stress incontinence and previous surgery. This 69-year-old gravida 3, para 3 woman complains of recurrent stress incontinence after two previous stress-incontinence repairs. She has daytime frequency and nocturia ×1. She leaks with most types of exertion and wears four thick pads per day. She has no voiding difficulties.

Prior to the test, her postvoid residual urine was 10 cc. On upright bladder filling, her first sensation is at 76 cc, first desire at 87 cc, and strong desire to void at 228 cc. Her bladder neck is open at rest (**A**). With coughing and straining, she leaks (*red arrows*). On straining (**B**), there is almost no urethral movement and her Valsalva leak point pressure is 59 cm H_2O. She voids with a low Pdet of 12 cm H_2O and Qmax of 13 cc/s (*blue arrows*) and empties completely. The study demonstrates that her stress incontinence is not associated with hypermobility.

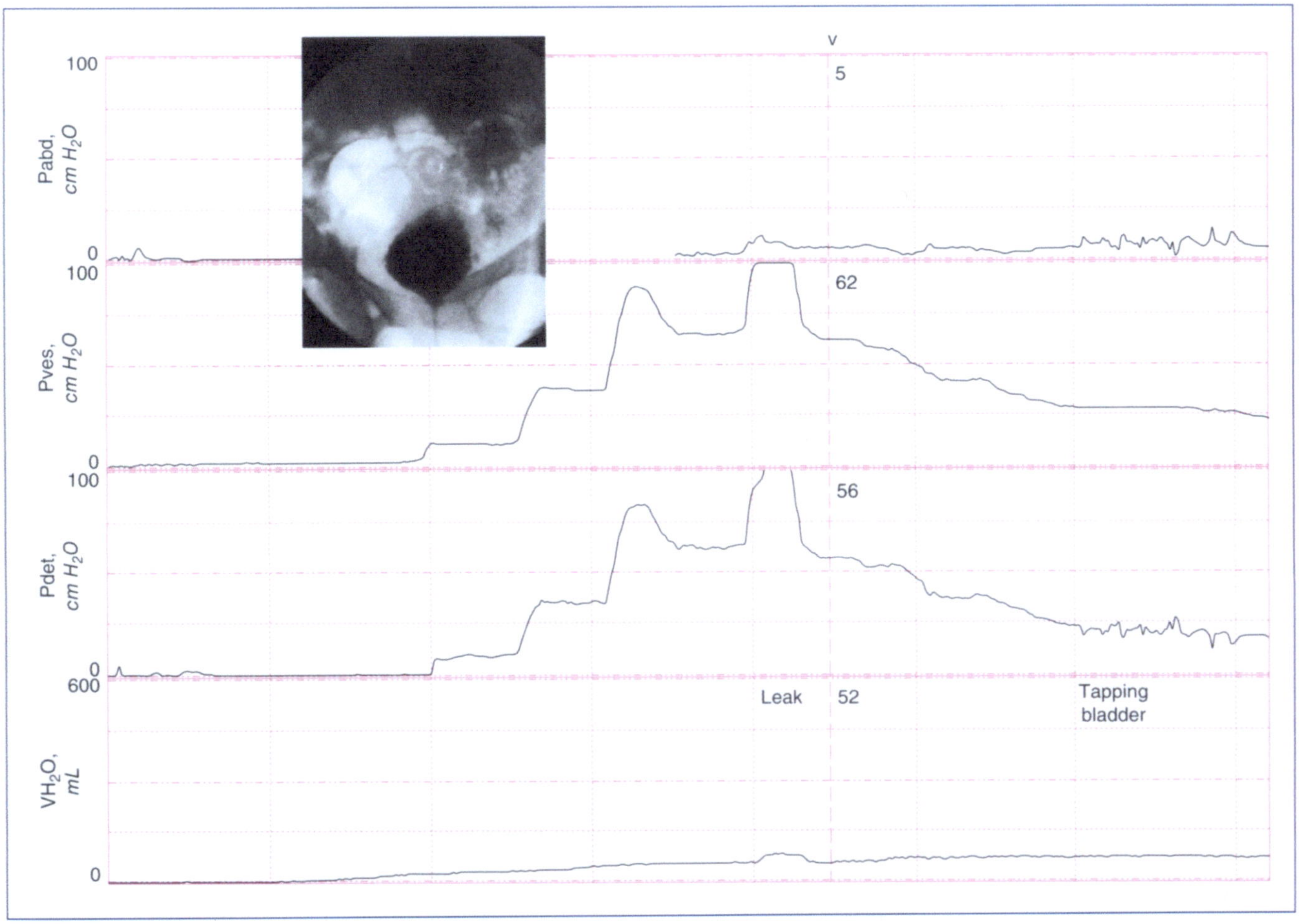

FIGURE 5-32. Videourodynamics in a woman after spinal cord injury. This 25-year-old woman has a C7–8 lesion 16 months after spinal cord injury following a motor vehicle accident. She needed an indwelling catheter for repeated attacks of autonomic dysreflexia and her upper tracts showed marked bilateral hydronephrosis on ultrasound.

She was given nifedipine just prior to the urodynamic studies. On bladder filling, there are contractions of greater than 75 to 100 cm H_2O after only 50 cc were instilled. The bladder capacity is 75 cc. On the fluoroscopic image (*inset*), her bladder is heavily trabeculated. The proximal urethra opens and the distal sphincter remain tight, consistent with detrusor sphincter dyssynergia.

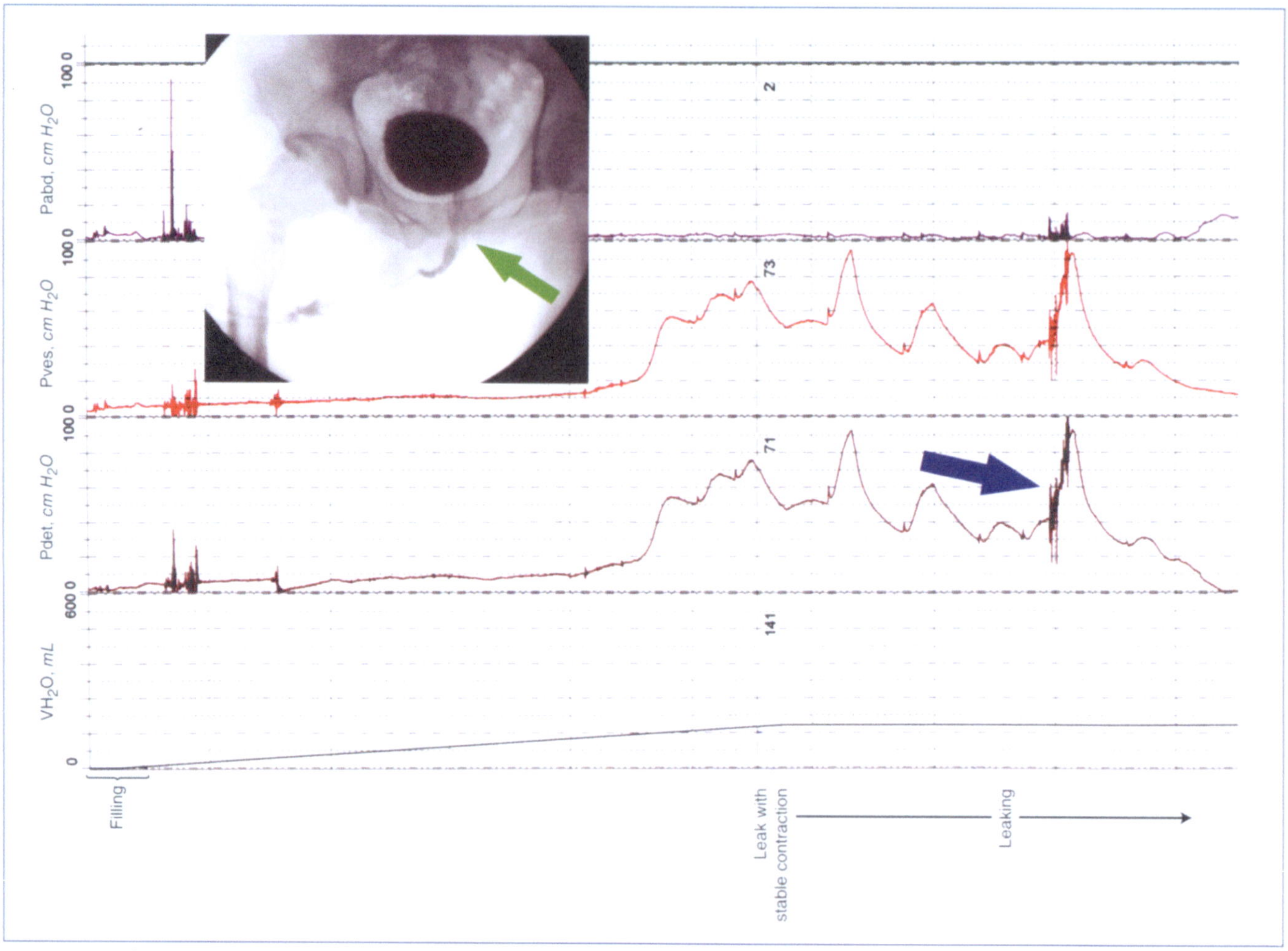

FIGURE 5-33. Videourodynamics in a man after spinal cord injury. This 29-year-old man had a T8–9 complete injury after a motor vehicle accident. He is 23 months after injury and manages his bladder with clean intermittent catheterization every 4 hours and condom catheter drainage in between catheterizations. He has occasional nonfebrile urinary tract infections and his renal ultrasound is normal.

On bladder filling, the compliance is normal. An uninhibited contraction is stimulated after 125 cc and the capacity is 140 cc. The contraction pressure is up to 71 cm H_2O. The fluoroscopic image during a contraction (*inset*) shows mild and intermittent external sphincter tightening, detrusor sphincter dyssynergia (DSD; *green arrow*). The patient's lower abdomen was tapped to stimulate voiding (*blue arrow*) and a contraction up to 90 cm H_2O was generated. This study shows that the patient has neurogenic detrusor overactivity with intermittent DSD.

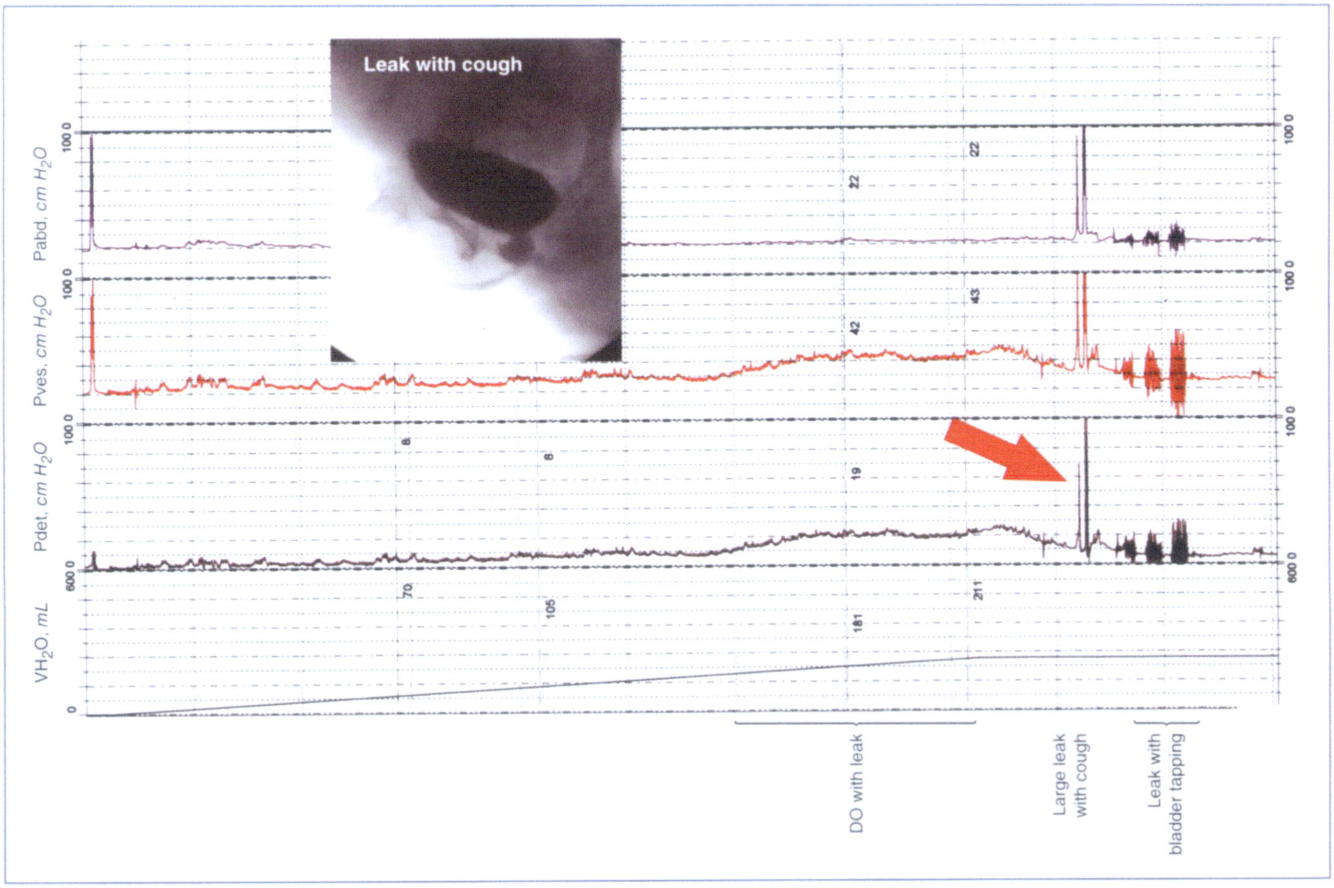

FIGURE 5-34. Videourodynamics in a man with spina bifida. This 43-year-old man was born with lumbosacral spina bifida and myelomeningocele. He manages his bladder with condom drainage for incontinence and strains to void. He has frequent, recurrent nonfebrile urinary tract infections. His renal function and upper tract appearance on ultrasound are normal.

On bladder filling, he has a first sensation after 80 cc and a desire to void at 105 cc. There is a decreased compliance curve with the pressure rising to 23 cm H_2O after 211 cc were instilled. His bladder neck is wide open at rest and he leaks with coughing and straining (*red arrow; inset*). The pressure falls as soon as he leaks and he is able to empty his bladder with abdominal straining.

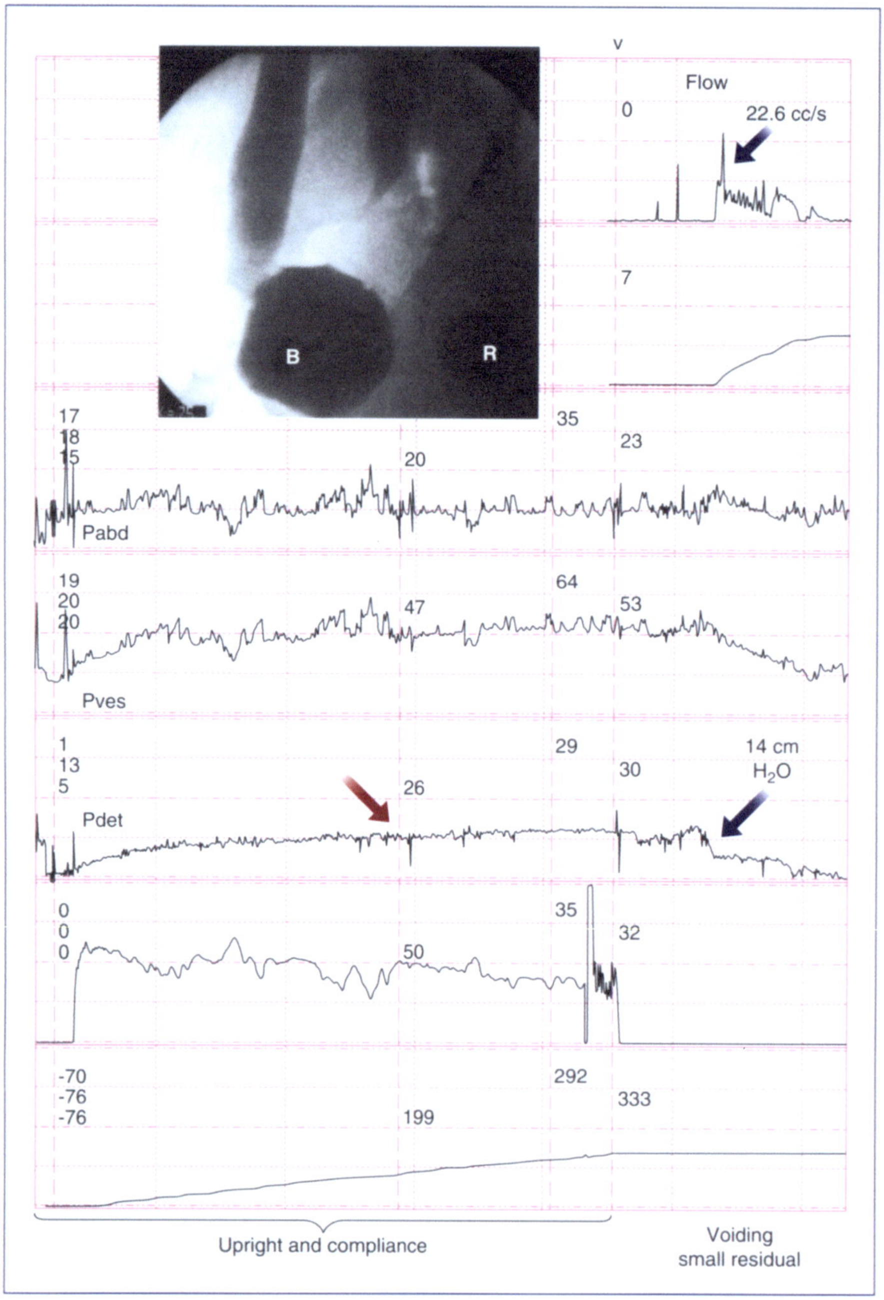

FIGURE 5-35. Videourodynamics in a woman with sacral dysgenesis. This 25-year-old woman was born with sacral dysgenesis. She had an artificial sphincter inserted for urinary incontinence at age 14 years and then developed bilateral vesicoureteral reflux that was unresponsive to multiple ureteral reimplantations. Her renal function deteriorated and she had recurrent febrile urinary tract infections. Ultrasound showed bilateral moderate to marked hydroureteronephrosis. She had no urinary incontinence and was able to void normally with the artificial sphincter.

On bladder filling, she has a first sensation at 76 cc and first desire to void at 199 cc. There is a steep rise in pressure up to 26 cm H_2O, consistent with decreased bladder compliance on filling (*red arrow*). The fluoroscopic image (*inset*) shows grade 4–5 bilateral reflux. This image also shows a small-capacity bladder (*white B*) despite the infusion of 300 cc. A large amount of the infused volume is refluxing. The reflux also most likely dampens the poor compliance measurement. This image shows the reservoir of the artificial sphincter (*white R*). She voids by opening the artificial sphincter with a Pdet of 14 cm H_2O and Qmax of 22.6 cc/s (*blue arrows*). She subsequently underwent augmentation ileocystoplasty and bilateral reimplants.

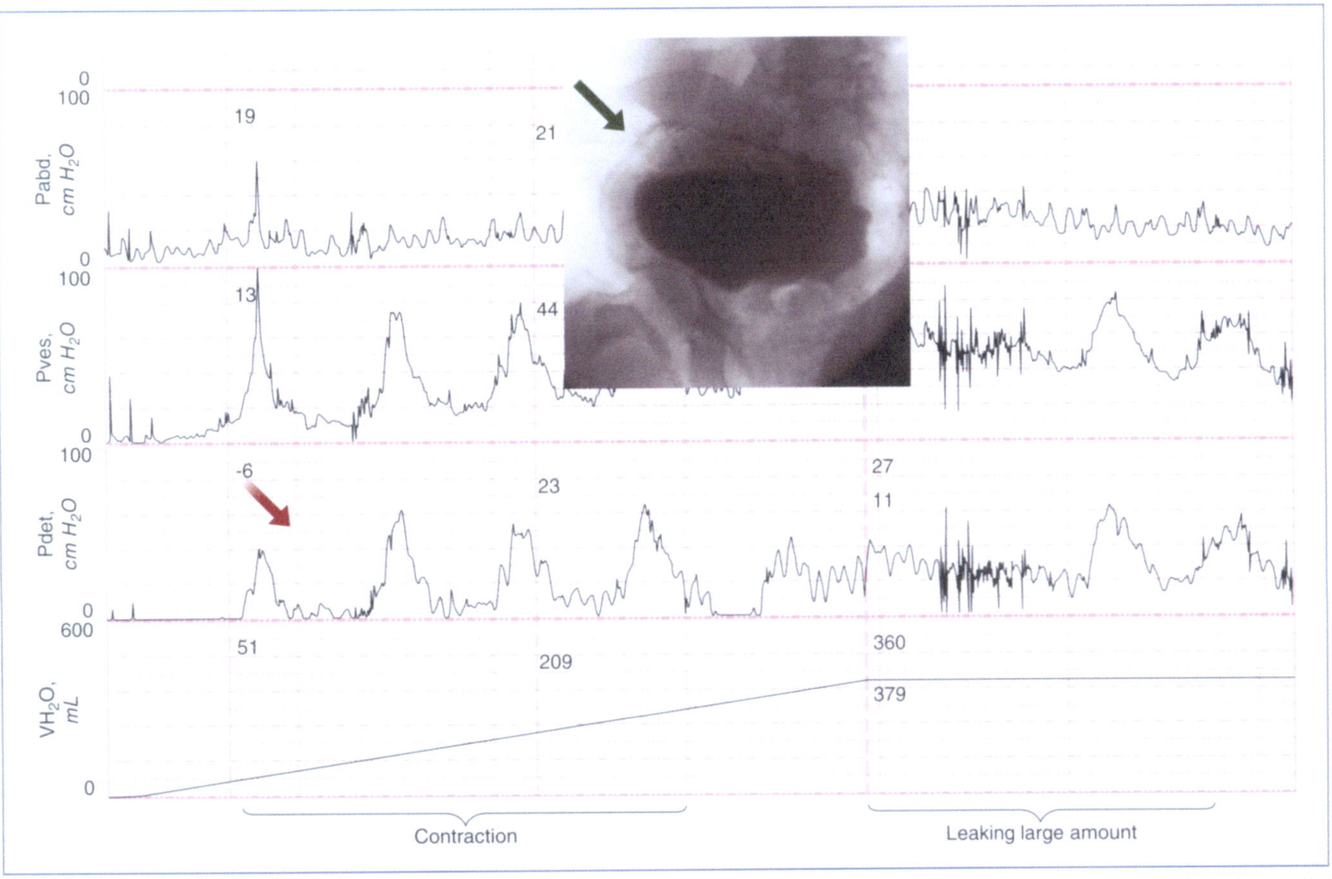

FIGURE 5-36. Videourodynamics of a woman with an Indiana pouch. This 44-year-old woman underwent pelvic exenterations for uterine cancer. She had an Indiana pouch urinary diversion at the time. She performs clean intermittent catheterization every 1 to 2 hours and has volumes of 50 to 250 cc. She wears a stoma bag at night to prevent any leakage. She denies any leakage associated with stress urinary incontinence, but feels the pressure of the pouch when it is full, which leads to leakage. She also wakes up every 1 to 2 hours to catheterize to prevent leakage.

On pouch filling, she has a first sensation at 51 cc, desire to empty the pouch at 209 cc, and the capacity was 380 cc. There are multiple uninhibited contractions elicited (*red arrow*) with pressure up to 61 cm H_2O. Urinary leakage is seen at the stoma (*inset; green arrow*). No reflux is demonstrated. The study showed that the capacity was good, but the pouch was not quiescent.

References

1. Abrams P, Andersson KE, Birder L, *et al.*: Recommendations of the International Scientific Committee. In *Incontinence*. Edited by Abrams P, Cardozo L, Khoury S, Wein A. 4th International Consultation. Paris, France: Health Publications; 2009:1767–1820.
2. Peterson AC, Webster GD: Urodynamic and videourodynamic evaluation of voiding dysfunction. In *Campbell-Walsh Urology*, vol 3. Edited by Wein A, Kavoussi LR, Novick AC, Partin AW, Peters CA. Philadelphia, PA: Saunders Elseveir; 2007:1986–2010.
3. Abrams P, Blaivas JG, Stanton SL, Andersen JT: The standardisation of terminology of lower urinary tract function. The International Continence Society Committee on Standardisation of Terminology. *Scand J Urol Nephrol Suppl* 1988, 114:5–19.
4. Abrams P, Cardozo L, Fall M, *et al.*: The standardisation of terminology of lower urinary tract function: report from the Standardisation Sub-committee of the International Continence Society. *Neurourol Urodyn* 2002, 21:167–178.
5. Hosker G, Rosier P, Gajewski J, *et al.*: *Incontinence*. Edited by Abrams P, Cardozo L, Khoury S, Wein A. 4th International Consultation. Paris, France: Health Publications; 2009:413–540.
6. Schafer W, Abrams P, Liao L, *et al.*: Good urodynamic practices: uroflowmetry, filling cystometry, and pressure-flow studies. *Neurourol Urodyn* 2002, 21:261–274.
7. Jorgensen JB, Jensen KM, Bille-Brahe NE, Morgensen P: Uroflowmetry in asymptomatic elderly males. *Br J Urol* 1986, 58:390–395.
8. Bottaccini MR, Gleason DM: Urodynamic norms in women. I. Normal versus stress incontinents. *J Urol* 1980, 124:659–662.
9. McGuire EJ, Cespedes RD, Cross CA, O'Connell HE: Videourodynamic studies. *Urol Clin North Am* 1996, 23:309–321.
10. Chancellor MB, Rivas DA, Bourgeois IM: Laplace's law and the risks and prevention of bladder rupture after enterocystoplasty and bladder autoaugmentation. *Neurourol Urodyn* 1996, 15:223–233.
11. Landau EH, Jayanthi VR, Churchill BM, *et al.*: Loss of elasticity in dysfunctional bladders: urodynamic and histochemical correlation. *J Urol* 1994, 152:702–705.
12. Toppercer A, Tetreault JP: Compliance of the bladder: an attempt to establish normal values. *Urology* 1979, 14:204–205.
13. McGuire EJ, Woodside JR, Borden TA, Weiss RM: Prognostic value of urodynamic testing in myelodysplastic patients. *J Urol* 1981, 126:205–209.
14. Lose G, Griffiths D, Hosker G, *et al.*: Standardisation of urethral pressure measurement: report from the Standardisation Sub-Committee of the International Continence Society. *Neurourol Urodyn* 2002, 21:258–260.

15. Wyndaele JJ, Kovindha A, Madersbacher H, *et al.*: Neurologic urinary and faecal incontinence. In *Incontinence*. Edited by Abrams P, Cardozo L, Khoury AE, Wein A. 4th International Consultation. Paris, France: Health Publications; 2009:793–960.

16. Chancellor MB, Blaivas JG, Kaplan SA, Axelrod S: Bladder outlet obstruction versus impaired detrusor contractility: the role of outflow. *J Urol* 1991, 145:810–812.

17. Chapple C, Herschorn S, Abrams P, *et al.*: Tolterodine treatment improves storage symptoms suggestive of overactive bladder in men treated with alpha-blockers. *Eur Urol* 2008 [epub ahead of print].

18. Griffiths D, Hofner K, van Mastrigt R, *et al.*: Standardization of terminology of lower urinary tract function: pressure-flow studies of voiding, urethral resistance, and urethral obstruction. International Continence Society Subcommittee on Standardization of Terminology of Pressure-Flow Studies. *Neurourol Urodyn* 1997, 16:1–18.

19. Schafer W: Analysis of bladder-outlet function with the linearized passive urethral resistance relation, linPURR, and a disease-specific approach for grading obstruction: from complex to simple. *World J Urol* 1995, 13:47–58.

6 Bladder Ultrasound in Voiding Dysfunction

Andrea Tubaro and Mario De Gennaro

Bladder ultrasonography is part of the primary evaluation of patients with voiding dysfunction and is often performed in conjunction with a physical examination. Neurogenic and non-neurogenic voiding dysfunctions often result in similar lower urinary tract symptoms and the diagnosis of the underlying condition is important to plan proper management of the condition and, whenever possible, to cure it.

Suprapubic evaluation of the urinary bladder does not require sophisticated technology; a simple abdominal probe (3.5–5.0-MHz convex) and standard two-dimensional ultrasound (US) equipment suffice. The examination is performed with the patient lying in a supine position on the examination bed. Imaging is usually performed using a suprapubic window and a comfortably full bladder is required for morphological imaging for a proper evaluation of bladder morphology (*eg*, bladder symmetry, bladder wall conditions such as neoplasms or diverticula, bladder wall thickness, intravesical prostatic protrusion, middle lobes of the prostate) and the presence of urinary stones or foreign bodies. Evaluation of the postvoiding residual is carried out immediately following voiding and can be performed using standard US equipment or dedicated instruments. Although there are no standardization documents in the peer-reviewed literature regarding the orientation of bladder US pictures, they are usually oriented assuming that the patient is lying down on his or her back, so that the abdominal wall is at the top of the picture, the posterior wall of the bladder is on the bottom, the bladder neck is shown on the right side, and the cranial part of the bladder is on the left side. The urinary bladder is generally scanned in different planes, including sagittal and axial. A measurement of bladder volume can be performed with standard ultrasonography; generally, the craniocaudal and anteroposterior diameters are taken in a picture of the median sagittal plane and the laterolateral diameter is shown in an axial picture obtained at the largest transverse diameter of the bladder. Diameters must be orthogonal among themselves.

The pathophysiology of voiding dysfunction differs according to the patient's gender (*eg*, acute urinary retention due to benign prostate obstruction in men versus urinary retention in sexually abused women) and age (*eg*, chronic retention in newborns with urethral valves or in children with myodysplasia, bladder outlet obstruction in men with bladder stones secondary to benign prostatic obstruction).

Bladder US is an ideal tool to rule out possible comorbidities that may be responsible for the observed dysfunction (*eg*, bladder neoplasms, stones, foreign bodies); it may allow the diagnosis of the underlying cause (*eg*, enlarged prostate protruding into the urinary bladder, valve-like middle lobe of the prostate) and show the consequences of the voiding dysfunction on the urinary bladder and the upper urinary tract (*eg*, bladder diverticula, bladder hernia, dilatation of the ureter secondary to vesicourethral reflux).

Interestingly, the term *bladder ultrasound* is frequently used in the urological world, but radiologists use the term *lower abdomen ultrasonography*. The difference is not semantic, as while the former concentrates on the urinary bladder, the latter includes pelvic organs that may be involved in several types of comorbidities, particularly in women.

The aim of this chapter is to provide an example of the different conditions that may be observed in outpatient practice when managing patients with voiding dysfunction.

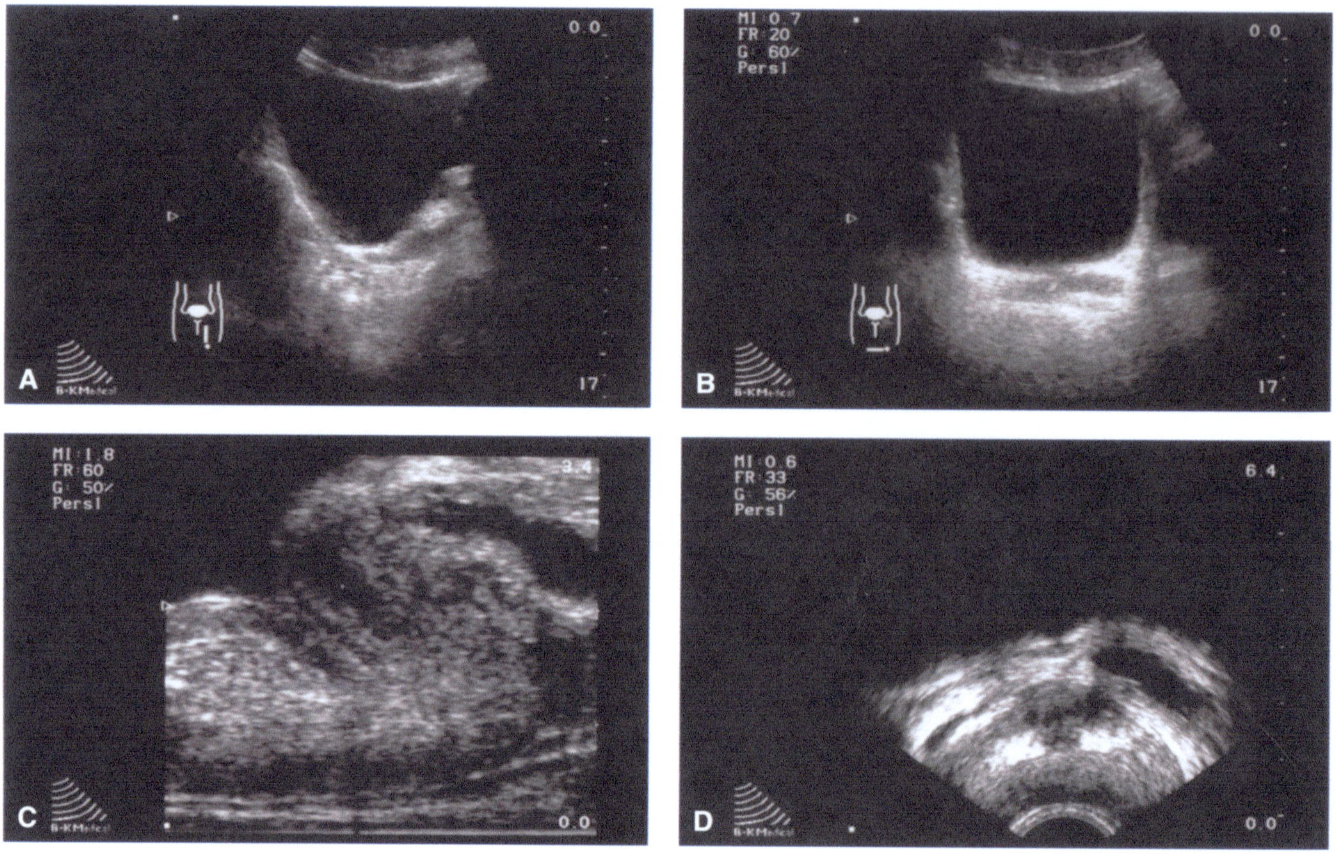

FIGURE 6-1. Suprapubic ultrasound imaging in a young adult male. **A,** On a midline, sagittal section, the bladder neck shape depends on the morphology of the prostate gland. In this case, it appears as a lower echogenic area with minimal funneling. **B,** In a transverse view, the bladder has a typical "square box" shape; the small prostate gland never appears on the largest transverse bladder section. **C,** Anatomic details of the bladder neck are better appreciated on transrectal imaging showing normal bladder neck funneling. The hypoechogenic muscle fibers of the genital sphincter can be observed on either side of the prostatic urethra. **D,** On a transrectal transverse section, a normal transitional zone of the prostate can be observed.

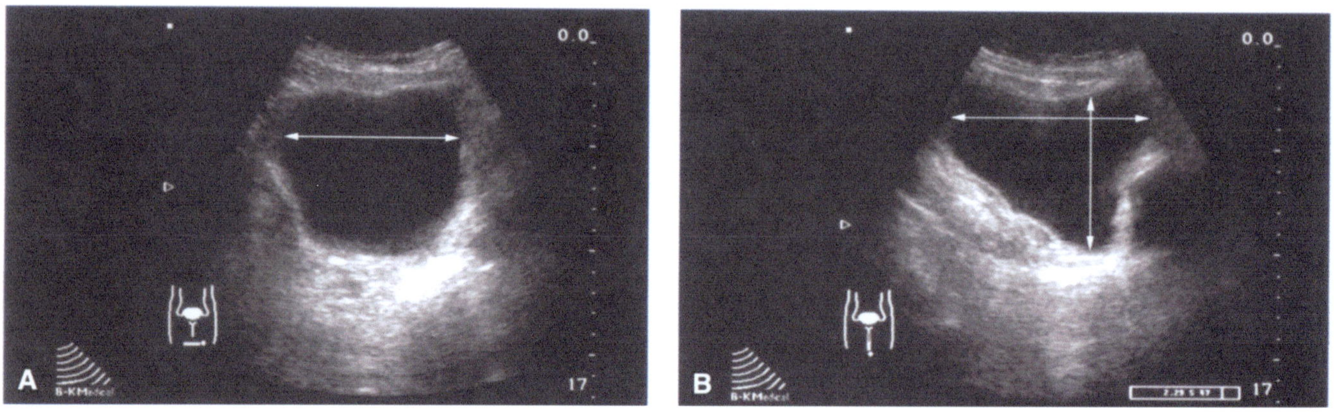

FIGURE 6-2. Bladder volume measurement. Bladder volume can be measured on the midline sagittal (**A**) and largest transverse (**B**) sections of the bladder obtained from a suprapubic window. Craniocaudal and anteroposterior diameters are measured on the sagittal picture, while the laterolateral diameter is derived from the transverse section. A measurement of the anteroposterior diameter on the transverse section is associated with a higher degree of error, because this section is rarely orthogonal with the sagittal section. The *arrows* in **A** show the transverse diameter and in **B** they show the craniocaudal and anteroposterior diameters.

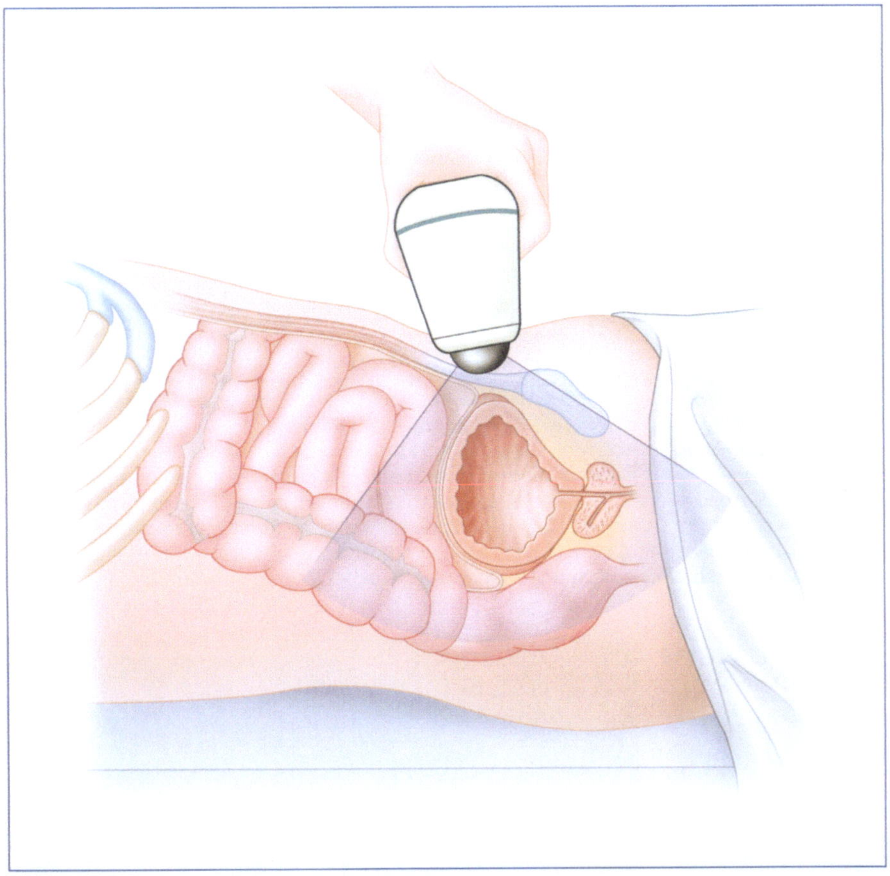

FIGURE 6-3. Automated measurement of bladder volume. An automated ultrasound (US) system has been developed to allow medical personnel who are not trained in ultrasonography to measure bladder volume, avoiding the need for full-range US equipment for measuring postvoid residual and to increase the accuracy of a bladder-volume measurement. Measurement is carried out with the patient lying on his or her back and a standalone US probe is placed on the suprapubic region aiming at the urinary bladder. A gender option is available to adjust for the presence of the uterus in women (this is not required in women who have had their uterus removed). When activated, the probe performs a series of isocentric scans on the bladder to compensate for deviations of the bladder shape from a perfect sphere (in this case, a single image would suffice). Although bladder scanning is performed blindly (there is no real-time image available), a proper position of the probe with respect to the bladder is controlled; in case the bladder perimeter is found to be close to the image borders or if the image borders cut through the bladder perimeter, the software suggests that the user repeats bladder scanning and it provides information about how the probe should be repositioned. Automated US scanning is an accurate alternative to in-and-out catheterization for the measurement of bladder volume [1]. (*Adapted from* Verathon Inc.; Bothel, WA).

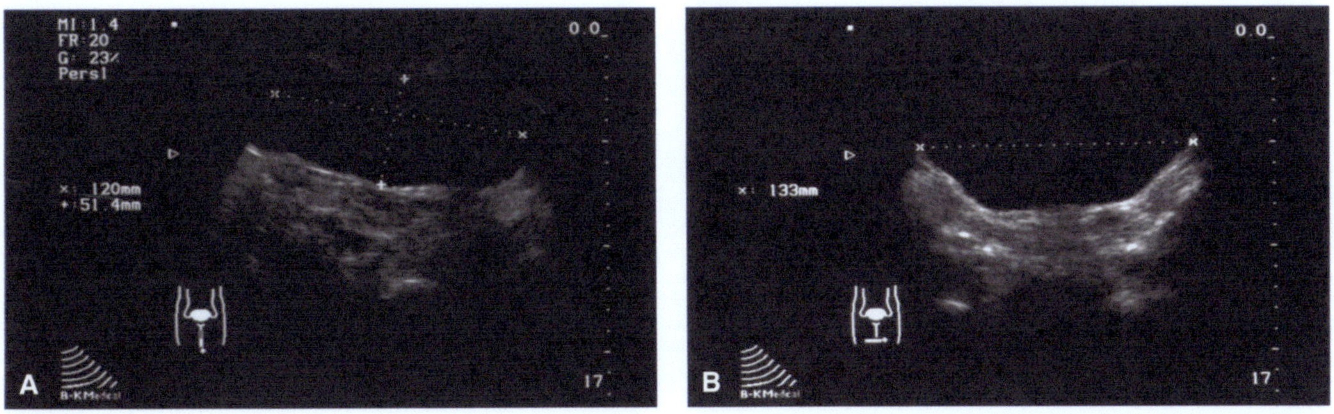

FIGURE 6-4. Acute urinary retention. Bladder volume is measured for a number of different reasons, including calculation of voiding efficiency (the bladder volume before and after voiding is measured) and evaluation of chronic or acute urinary retention. Although the evidence of an overdistended bladder is usually sufficient to diagnose acute retention, the measurement of bladder volume can be sometimes inaccurate, particularly in the case of large volumes.

Suprapubic imaging of the bladder in a male patient with acute urinary retention (3.5-MHz convex probe) is shown. Sagittal (**A**) and transverse (**B**) imaging reveals an overdistended bladder that does not fit (in the sagittal view) in the acoustic window; consequently, the estimated bladder volume of 410 mL is quite inaccurate compared to the real volume of drained urine (905 mL). **A**, x—120 mm; +—51.4 mm. **B**, x—133 mm.

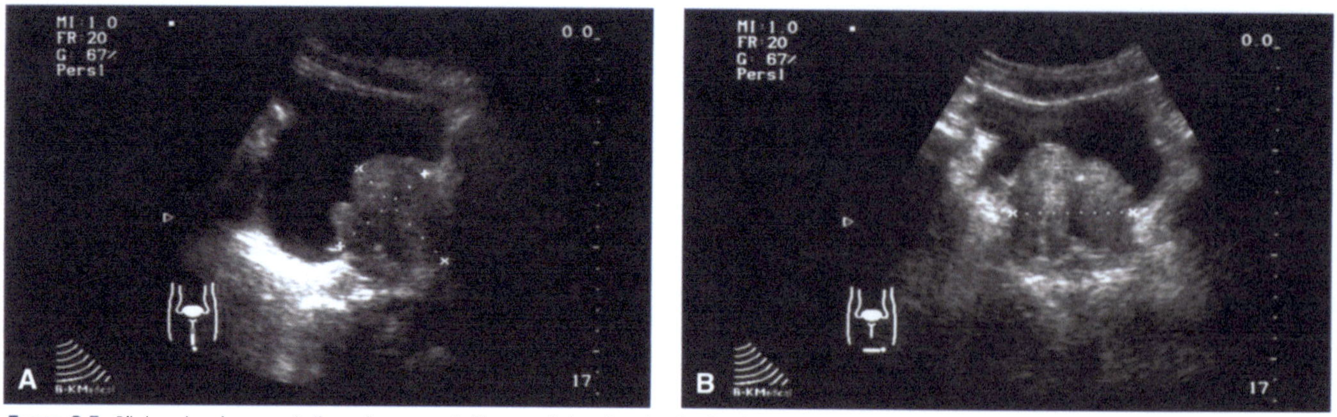

Figure 6-5. Bilobar benign prostatic enlargement. The prostate gland can be imaged easily from a suprapubic window during bladder imaging. Nonetheless, benign enlargement is appreciated and proper quantification of the prostate volume may be hampered by the acoustic shadow of the pubic bone that makes imaging of the lowermost part of the gland difficult. Anteroposterior and craniocaudal diameters are measured in a midline sagittal plane (**A**) while the laterolateral diameter is obtained from a transverse section (**B**). In this patient, the longitudinal diameter of the prostate was underestimated because of the pubic bone and only the craniocaudal diameter of the prostate could be measured. The estimated prostate volume is 92 mL on sovrapubic imaging and 122 mL on transrectal ultrasonography; the latter value proved to be comparable with MRI imaging of the lower abdomen that was performed for other reasons. **A**, x—60.4 mm; +—53.0 mm. **B**, x—57.9 mm.

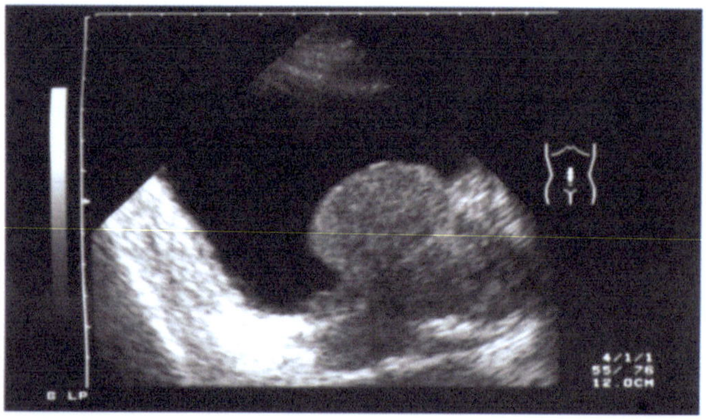

Figure 6-6. Trilobar hypertrophy with intravesical protrusion. In male patients, benign prostatic enlargement is the leading cause of voiding dysfunction and suprapubic ultrasound (US) is frequently used to identify enlarged prostates. US imaging of the bladder not only provides information about prostate volume, but also about the gland morphology. Evaluation of the bladder neck area requires a comfortably distended bladder to allow separation of the posterior bladder wall from the trigone. A large middle lobe protruding into the bladder is clearly shown, suggesting the possibility of bladder outlet obstruction.

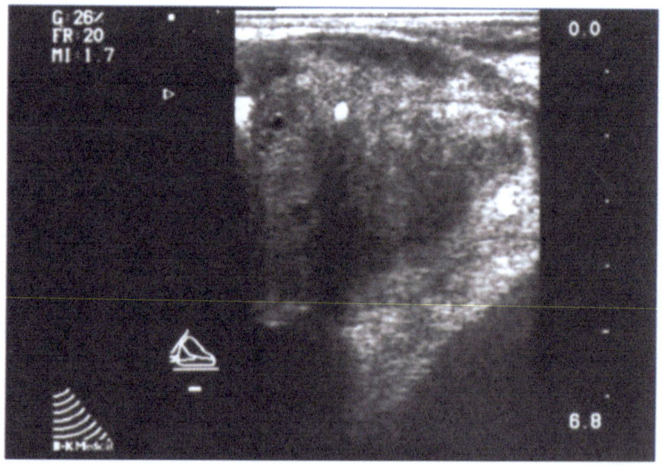

Figure 6-7. Trilobar benign prostatic enlargement without intraprostatic protrusion. Whenever an elevated bladder neck is suspected on bladder ultrasound (US) because the internal urethral orifice is elevated from the trigone, additional transrectal imaging is often required to confirm the diagnosis. There is consensus about the criteria used to distinguish an isolated middle lobe of the prostate from an elevated bladder neck on US; both conditions are usually considered to be trilobar hypertrophy. This figure, obtained using a linear probe through a midline sagittal plane, shows an elevated bladder neck (a white spot is visible when the bladder neck is imaged along a midline sagittal plane) positioned nearly 6 cm above the US probe while the verumontanum is positioned 15 mm away from the rectal probe. The severe curvature of the prostatic urethra is responsible for the observed voiding dysfunction.

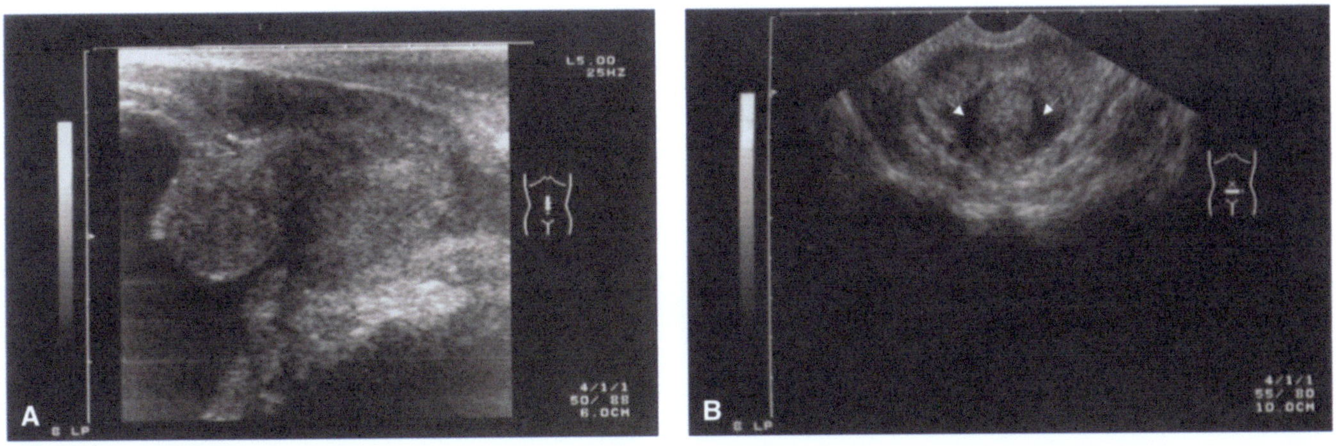

FIGURE 6-8. Isolated middle lobe of the prostate. The suspicion of middle lobe hypertrophy of the prostate on suprapubic ultrasound (US) often requires additional transrectal imaging that may help in obtaining a definitive diagnosis, as in this figure showing an isolated middle lobe in a 58-year-old man. Transurethral resection of the middle lobe without touching the lateral lobes allows proper resolution of bladder outlet obstruction and maintenance of anterograde ejaculation in this patient. The use of a linear US is preferable to transrectal imaging of the benign prostate to avoid distortion of the anatomical structures and to better understand the modifications on the bladder neck and urethra that are caused by enlarged prostates (**A**). On the transverse view (**B**), the hypoechogenic signal of the genital sphincter (*arrows*) is clearly visible and help with diagnosing an isolated middle lobe from an elevated bladder neck is associated with prostatic enlargement.

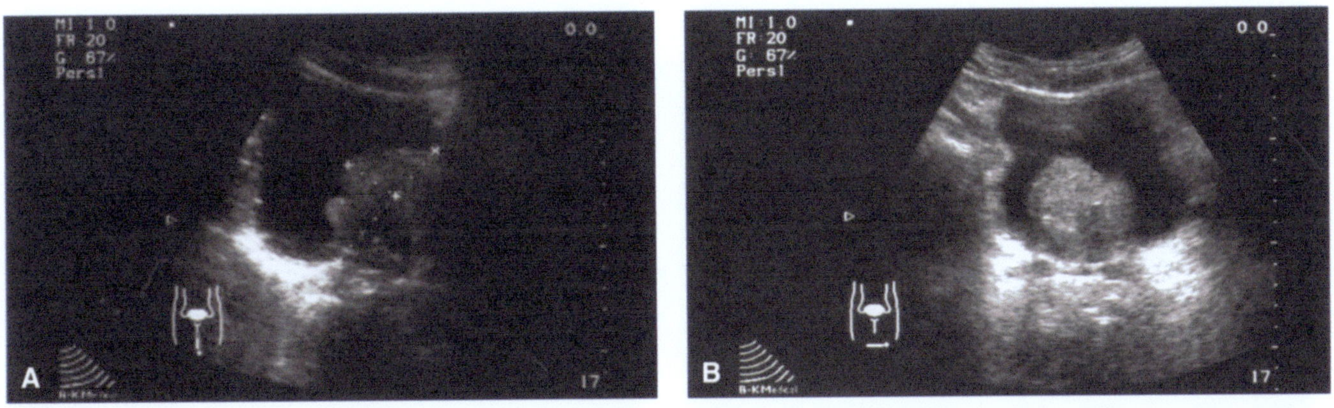

FIGURE 6-9. Intraprostatic protrusion (IPP). IPP, a concept first proposed by Ohnishi *et al.* [2] and subsequently popularized by Chia *et al.* [3], has been used as a proxy for benign prostatic obstruction (BPO). **A,** Protrusion of the prostate gland on a midline sagittal plane with respect to a plane passing for the bladder neck level is measured (27 mm in this case). Protrusion grades (grade 1: ≤ 5 mm, grade 2: 5–10 mm, grade 3: > 10 mm) are associated with an increasing risk of obstruction. IPP is an independent predictor of BPO in multivariate analysis and IPP grade 3 has a sensitivity and specificity of 76% and 92%, respectively, for the diagnosis of bladder outlet obstruction. **B,** Prostate protrusion also is clearly visible on a transverse section, although no quantitative data are available for such a projection. **A,** x—70.4 mm; +—27.0 mm.

Complications of Benign Prostatic Hyperplasia

Although rare, complications of bladder outlet obstruction can still result in irreversible damage and are responsible for the ominous reputation of prostatic hypertrophy in previous centuries. Most benign prostatic hyperplasia complications can be easily diagnosed by bladder ultrasonography.

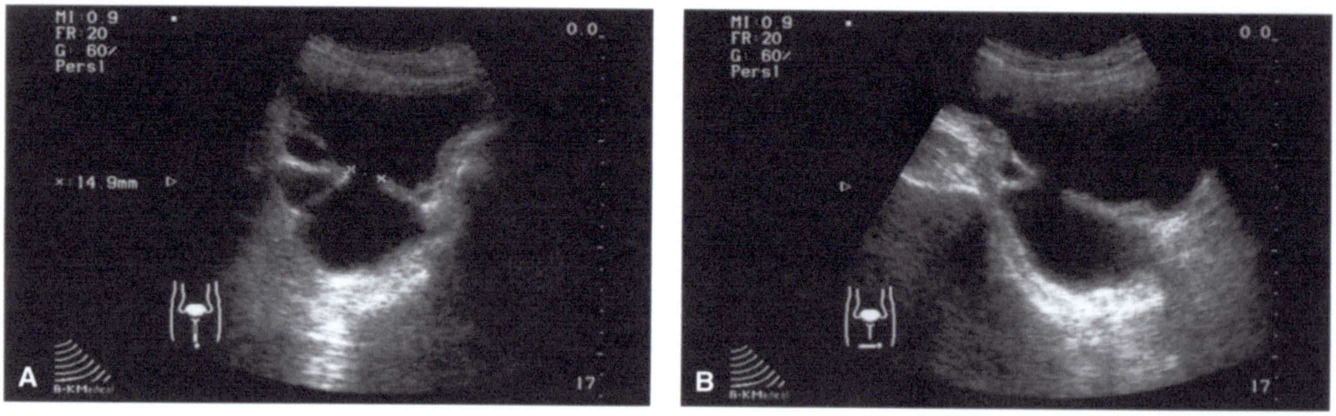

Figure 6-10. Bladder diverticula. Shown is bladder diverticula in a male subject with urethral stenosis following transurethral resection of the prostate (3.5-MHz convex probe). A suprapubic drain was placed to relieve chronic urinary retention. The diverticulum neck of the largest diverticulum is clearly visible in both sagittal (**A**) and transverse (**B**) views. **A**, x—14.9 mm.

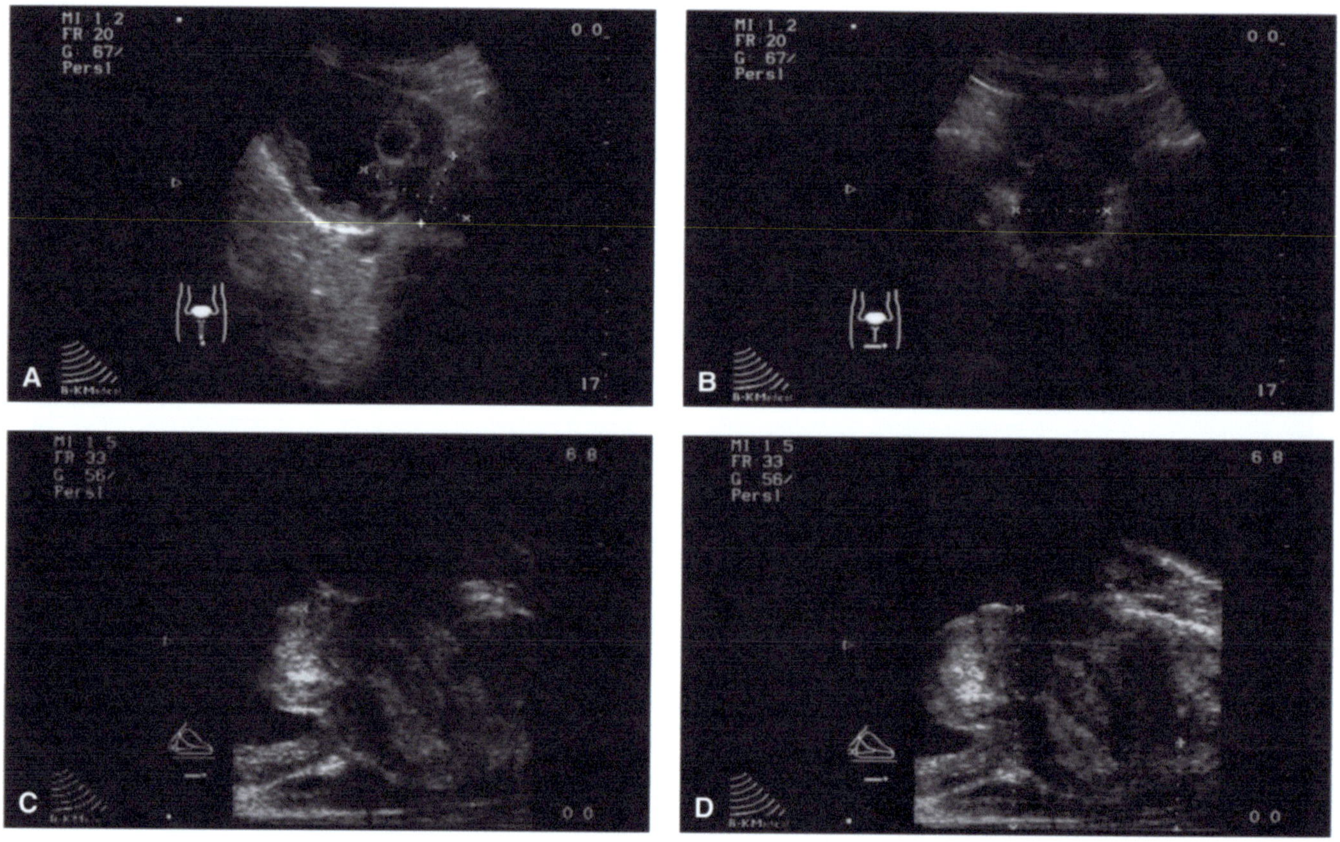

Figure 6-11. Acute and chronic renal failure due to benign prostatic hyperplasia (BPH). Although the Medical Therapy of Prostatic Symptoms trial suggested that renal failure is a rare occurrence in the progression of BPH, occasionally patients with acute and chronic renal failure can be observed in emergency rooms or outpatient clinics for acute renal failure due to acute urinary retention [4]. Renal failure may occur following long-lasting obstruction of the upper urinary tract due to chronic urinary retention associated with benign prostatic enlargement. In this case, a relatively small prostate (44 mL) caused acute renal failure (serum creatinine: 16.2 mg/dL) and chronic renal failure (serum creatinine: 9.5 mg/dL) because of its particular shape, which is characterized by the presence of a valve-like middle lobe that is visible on a sovrapubic midline sagittal picture (**A**) underneath the balloon of a Foley catheter, but it is better appreciated in transrectal midline sagittal views with (**C**) and without (**D**) the catheter. In the absence of a Foley catheter, the middle lobe causes a severe curvature of the prostatic urethra that is 15 mm away from the probe rectum at the verumontanum level and 38 mm from the rectum at the bladder neck level.

Continued on the next page

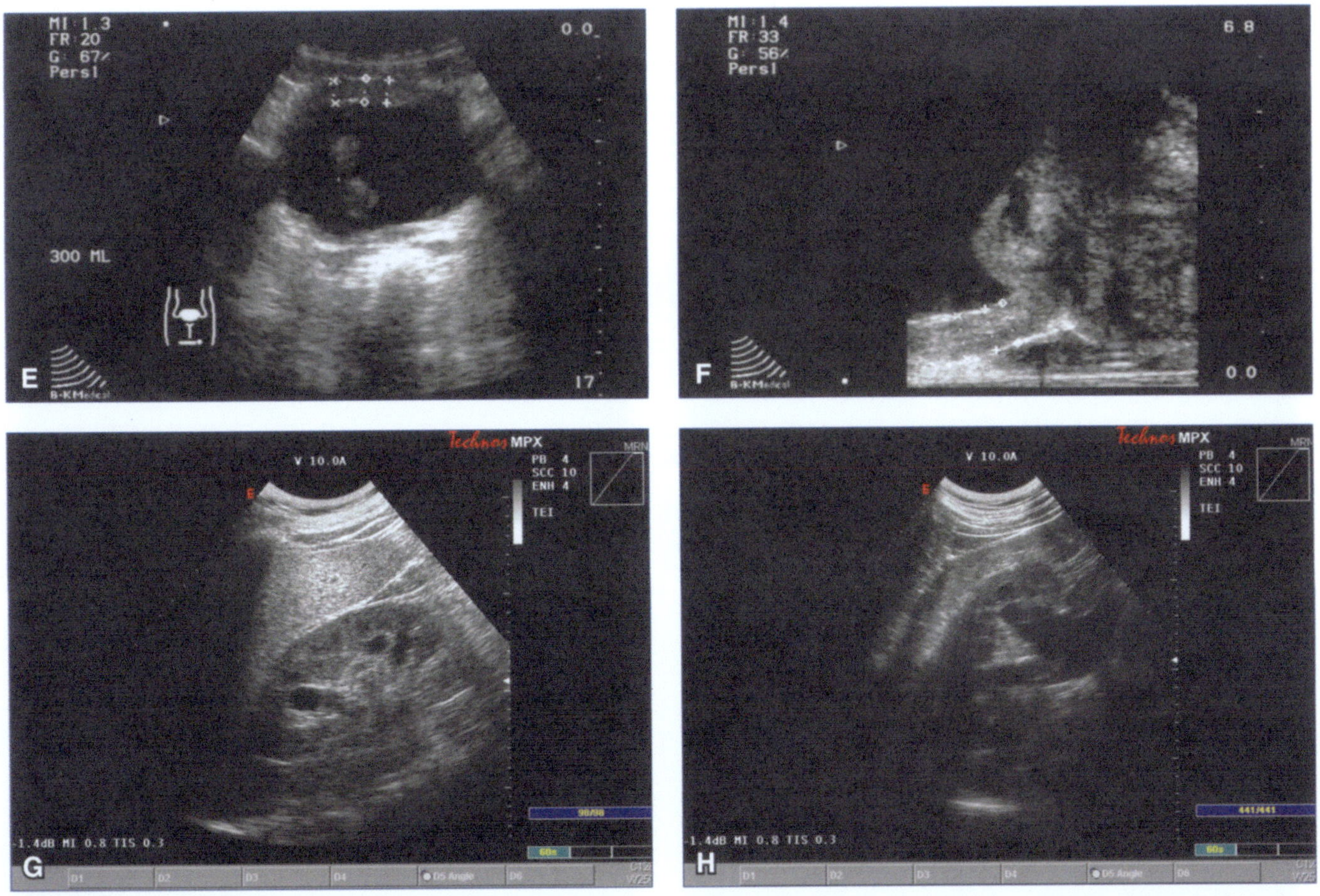

Figure 6-11. *(Continued)* Severe benign prostatic obstruction can result in significant hypertrophy of the detrusor with increased bladder wall thickness (BWT). A 10-mm thickness was observed at the anterior bladder wall with suprapubic ultrasonography and a 7.8-mm mean value of thickness was measure at the trigone level from transrectal sonography. (In male subjects, the relationship between BWT at the trigone and anterior or later bladder walls is still unknown.) Mild hydronephrosis (**G**, **H**) is still evident after 1 week of bladder drainage with an indwelling catheter. **A**, x—54.6 mm; +—35.5 mm. **B**, x—43.5 mm. **C**, x—17.9 mm. **D**, x—38.5 mm; +—15.2 mm. **E**, x—10.3 mm; +—10.8 mm; ◊—11.1 mm. **F**, x—7.88 mm; +—7.66 mm; ◊—7.75 mm.

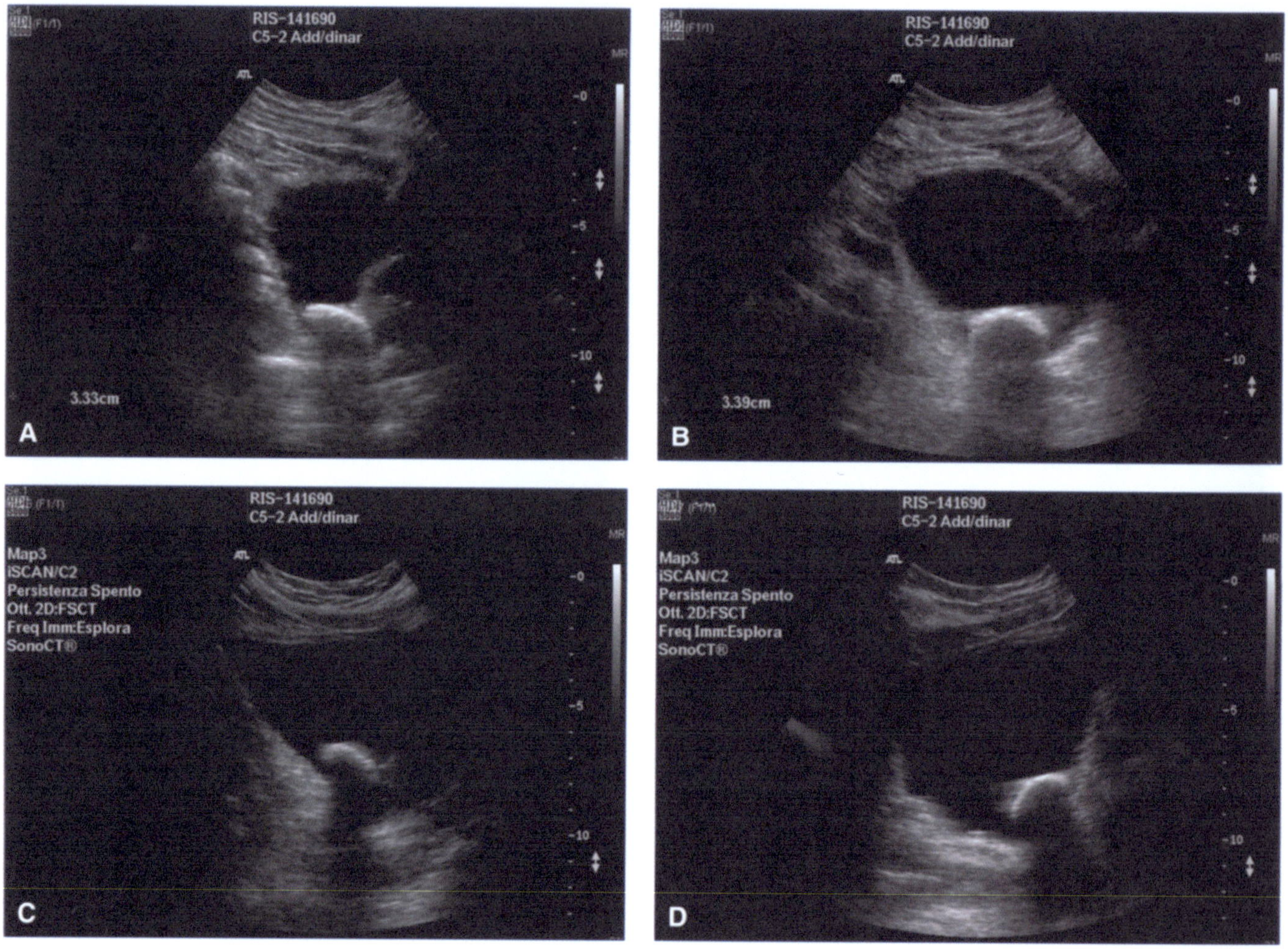

FIGURE 6-12. Bladder stones. Bladder stones appear as a strongly echogenic curved line resembling the curved surface of a sea pebble with a clear back shadow. The stone is usually located in the lowest part of the bladder that is either the trigone or retrotrigonal area on the midline sagittal (**A**) and transverse (**B**) sections. Differential diagnoses with calcified urothelial tumors depend on the stone mobility when the patient is in either the right (**C**) or left (**D**) lateral decubitus. When multiple stones are present in the urinary bladder, identification of the exact stone number can be difficult on ultrasound and a plain x-ray film of the lower abdomen is recommended.

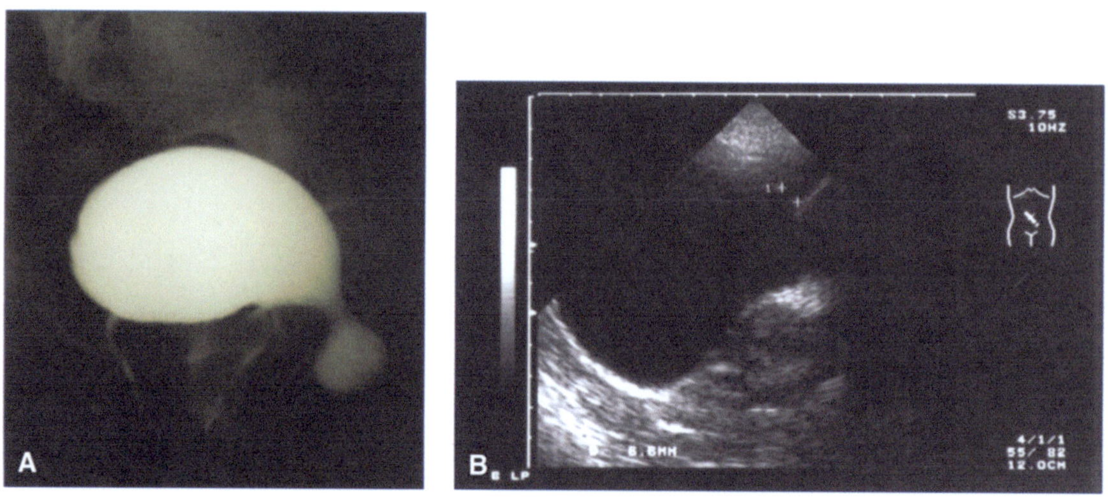

FIGURE 6-13. Bladder hernia. Bladder hernia (**A**) is a rare form of diverticulum that finds its way into the inguinal canal. The diagnosis of bladder hernia on ultrasonography is difficult; the differential diagnosis with a simple diverticulum is based on the long neck of the herniated cul de sac. As is shown in **B**, the distal part of the hernia is usually not visible on the same ultrasound picture. In simple bladder diverticulum, the diverticulum neck is always short and the diverticulum itself is adjacent to the bladder cavity. Voiding cystography (**B**) helps in understanding the anatomical details of the condition. Bladder diverticulum and hernia are more commonly seen in male patients and represent possible complications of benign prostatic obstruction, suggesting the need for deobstructive surgery. *Arrows* in **B** indicate the neck of the diverticulum.

Bladder Neoplasm

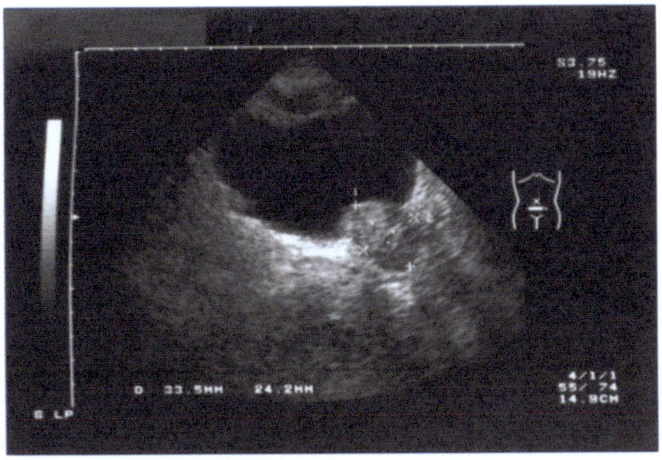

Figure 6-14. Bladder ultrasound may sometimes reveal unexpected comorbidities that impact patient management. Bladder neoplasm is one of the disorders possibly associated with voiding dysfunction that may be responsible for storage symptoms and hematuria. Suprapubic ultrasonography requires a comfortably distended bladder to avoid mucosal infolds and help identify intrinsic bladder wall disorders like the neoplasm shown here. Occasionally, storage symptoms may reduce bladder compliance and a patient's ability to maintain a distended bladder. The tumor mass clearly invades the perivesical fat. Bladder imaging should always be carried out through multiple imaging planes, not only through the midsagittal and transverse planes. *Lines* and x's indicate the diameters of the bladder tumor.

Acute Prostatitis

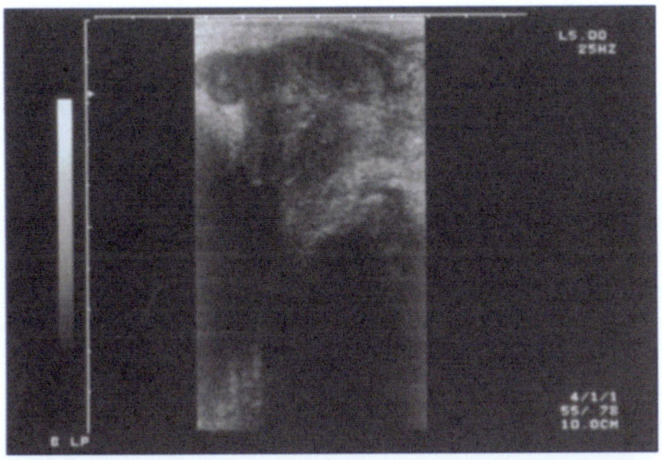

Figure 6-15. Acute inflammatory disorders of the prostate (*ie*, acute prostatitis) may be responsible for voiding dysfunctions of various severities, including acute urinary retention. The diagnosis is mainly clinical (sudden onset of perineal pain, dysuria, and fever; severe pain on digital rectal exploration) and suprapubic ultrasonography is of little help. On transrectal sonography, the ultrasound texture of the prostate is characterized by multiple hypoechogenic areas, as in renal ultrasonography of acute pyelonephritis.

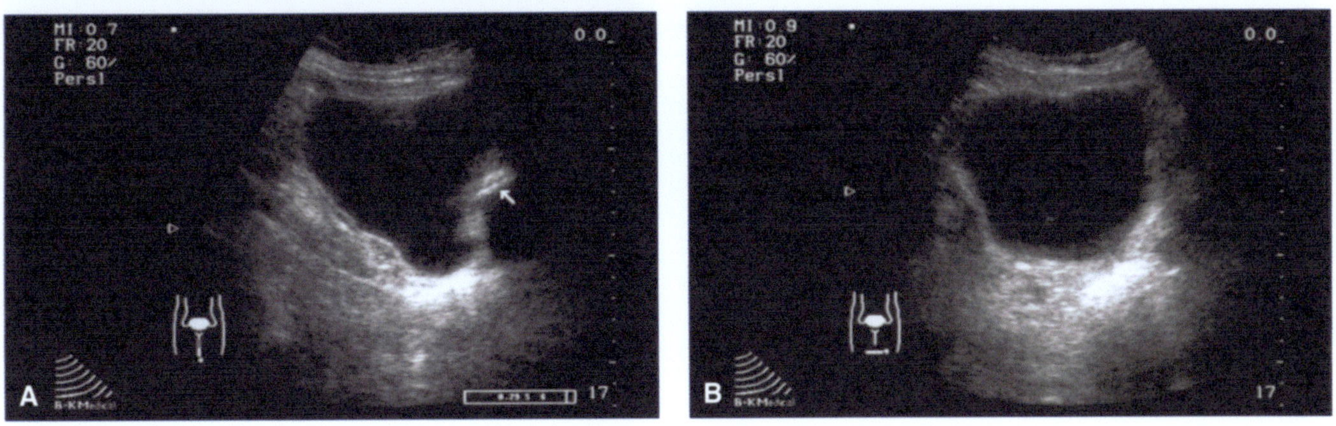

Figure 6-16. Voiding dysfunction in orthotopic neobladders. Orthotopic neobladders are not immune to voiding dysfunction and knowledge gained from the ultrasound (US) appearance of ileal and colon pouches is of importance. A case of voiding dysfunction in a 62-year-old man with orthotopic neobladder for a pT3 neoplasm of the bladder is shown. A Studer orthotopic ileal pouch was performed in 1998, but stenosis of the urethral anastomosis developed. The stricture recurred following cold knife incision of the stenosis and a wall stent was positioned. These US pictures provide a 10-year followup. The wall stent (*arrow*) is visible in the longitudinal scan (**A**). An ingrowth of fibrous tissue inside the lumen of the wall stent requires yearly endoscopic resection. **B**, On a transverse section, the orthotopic ileal neobladder looks very much like a normal urinary bladder.

Bladder Wall Thickness

Ultrasound (US) measurement of detrusor hypertrophy was first proposed in pediatric urology as a marker of bladder outlet obstruction and was then applied to adult urology, as a possible proxy of voiding dysfunction and bladder decompensation [5]. The pioneering work of Kojima *et al.* [6] provided the first evidence of a relationship between bladder wall thickness/bladder mass and bladder outlet obstruction. Further research conducted in Europe confirmed the validity of this approach and showed rapid recovery of detrusor hypertrophy following deobstructive surgery [7–9]. However, technical limitations of current US technique limit the use of such a parameter to clinical research. In women, detrusor hypertrophy was associated with the urodynamic diagnosis of detrusor overactivity [10].

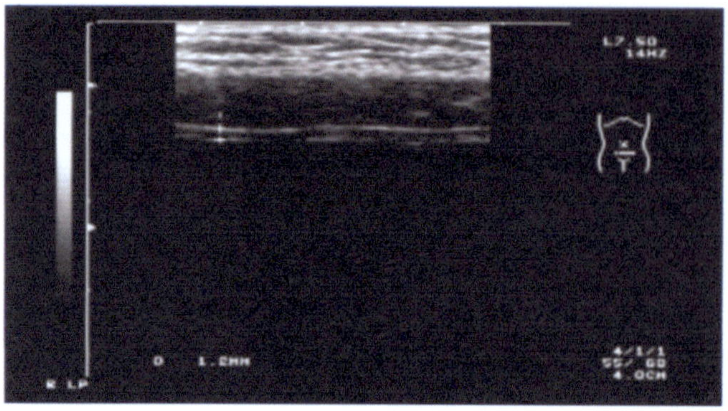

FIGURE 6-17. Normal bladder wall in a child. Bladder wall imaging in children has been applied to diagnose bladder outlet obstruction. This image, taken in a 7-year-old boy using a 7.50-MHz small-parts ultrasound probe, shows how the measurement of bladder wall thickness can be straightforward in children. The hyperechogenic subcutaneous fat tissue is visible on top of a more hypoechogenic muscle layer (abdominus rectus muscles). Two hyperechogenic lines (*markers*), separated by a hypoechogenic layer, define the inner and outer layers of the detrusor muscle. Urine appears as a black transonic area in the lower two-thirds of this image.

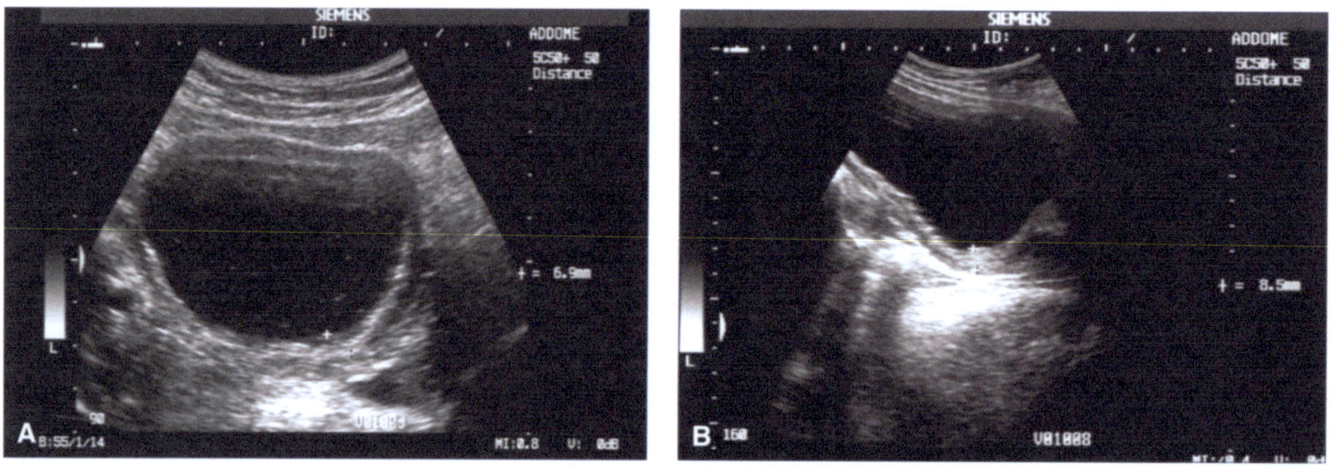

FIGURE 6-18. Detrusor hypertrophy in children. Ultrasound (US) measurement of bladder wall thickness was first introduced in the pediatric population as a proxy for bladder outlet obstruction. An 11-year-old girl with dysfunctional voiding presented with a recurrent urinary tract infection that was resistant to conventional antibacterial therapy. She voided no more than three times a day with interrupted (staccato) flow and significant postvoid residual (PVR). At US, the bladder shows a thickened wall (6, 9 mm) (**A**), particularly at the posterior site (8.5 mm) (**B**) and a diffuse echogenicity of the bladder content. No dilatation of the ureters can be observed. After proper treatment with biofeedback and pelvic floor exercises, the urinary tract infection was cured and PVR and flow curves ameliorated in 3 months.

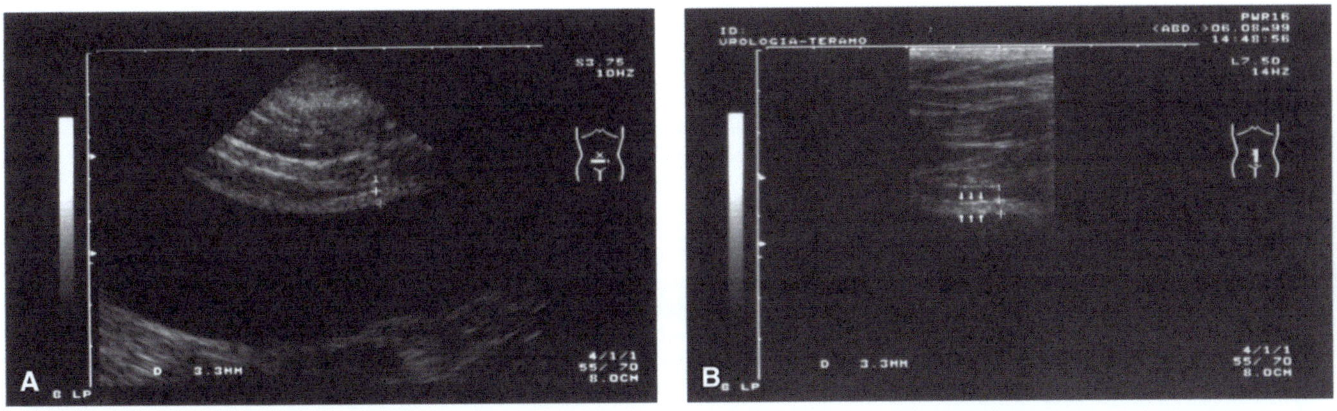

FIGURE 6-19. Normal bladder wall in an adult male. Ultrasound imaging of the bladder wall in a 67-year-old man using a 3.75-MHz electronic sector probe and a 7.5-MHz linear scanner is shown. Aging causes the bladder wall to become hyperechogenic. The bladder wall and a homogeneous hyperechogenic layer on top of the transonic urine content of the bladder are visible. The echogenicity of the bladder wall in the elderly population does not depend on the use of medium- or high-resolution probes (**A** and **B**, respectively). According to our standard reference values, a 3.3-mm bladder wall thickness is considered to be normal and not associated with bladder outlet obstruction. The + signs indicate callipers that measure bladder wall thickness and *arrows* indicate the outer and inner margin of the bladder wall.

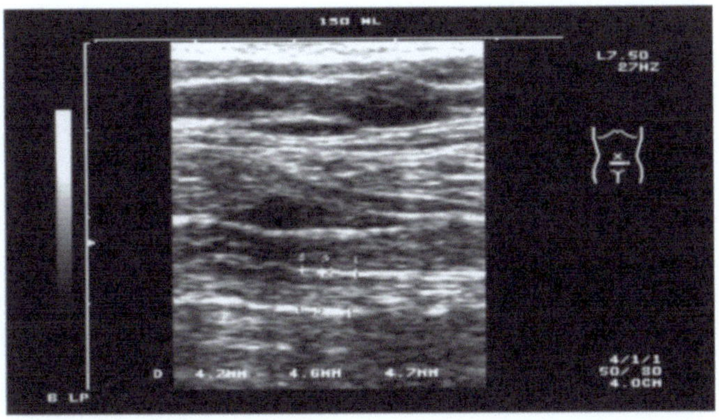

FIGURE 6-20. Detrusor hypertrophy in an elderly man. Ultrasound imaging of the bladder wall can be tricky in elderly patients, particularly in the case of elevated body mass index. In this image, obtained using a 7.5-MHz linear probe, the bladder wall is identified by two hyperechogenic lines delineating the outer and inner layers of the detrusor muscle, which appears to be hyperechogenic. Confounding reflections are seen underneath the bladder wall inside the urine volume that is not transonic because of reflections from the bladder wall. Values of 4.6 to 4.7 mm are borderline for bladder outlet obstruction. The + signs indicate callipers measuring bladder wall thickness in triplicate. Bladder wall thickness measurements are 4.6 to 4.7 mm.

FIGURE 6-21. Normal bladder wall thickness (BWT) in a young woman. The measurement of BWT on transvaginal ultrasound has been proposed by Khullar *et al.* [10] for the diagnosis of detrusor overactivity. To avoid the effect of bladder volume on bladder thickness, a measurement is taken with a volume of 50 mL or lower. BWT is measured in the trigone, anterior, and posterior walls and values are then averaged. Values of 5 mm or higher were found to be highly predictive of detrusor overactivity. In this case, a BWT of 2.3 mm was measured at the trigone level. ×—2.31 mm; +—2.31 mm; ◊—2.37 mm.

FIGURE 6-22. Automated measurement of bladder wall thickness (BWT) and bladder mass. A conventional measurement of BWT and bladder mass in male subjects by suprapubic ultrasound (US) has a number of limitations and problems in standardizing the technique. BWT is inversely related to bladder volume, but imaging of the bladder wall is poor for volumes below 100 mL and the variation of BWT for increasing bladder volumes is lower than the US probe resolution for volumes over 400 mL. Therefore, measurements are usually obtained with bladder volumes of 150 to 300 mL. The bladder wall includes adventitia, detrusor muscle, and urothelium. A distinction of the three layers can be straightforward in some patients and impossible in others, making a comparison among measurements from different centers difficult. Consequently, normative data for different gender and age groups are not available and no consensus has been reached for the threshold BWT/bladder mass values for the diagnosis of bladder outlet obstruction. Research into the development of an automated system to measure BWT/bladder mass is ongoing.

Continued on the next page

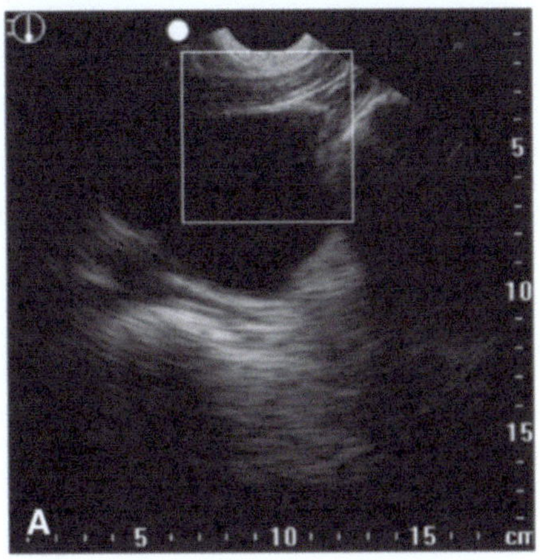

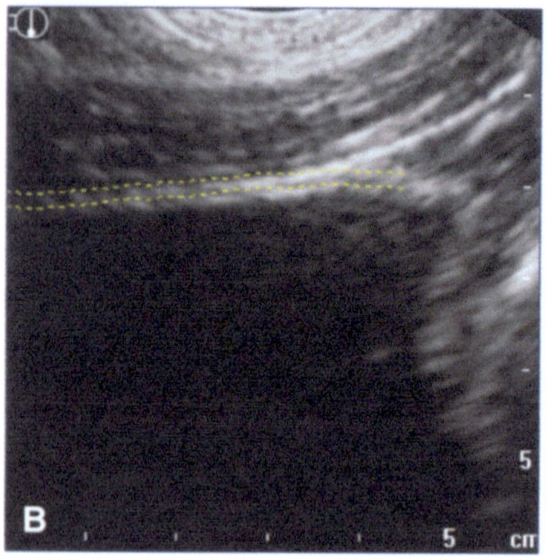

Figure 6-22. *(Continued)* An automated measurement of bladder volume can be obtained by using dedicated devices that provide an accurate estimation of urine volume and can be operated by caregivers with minimal training. The handheld device, the BladderScan BVM 9500 (Verathon Inc.; Bothell, WA), is blindly pointed at the urinary bladder and proper scanning is confirmed by the device when the entire profile of the bladder is contained within the scanner window. The bladder volume is calculated by sophisticated three-dimensional rendering methods. A recent technical development of this device allows automated recognition of the bladder wall. The detrusor wall thickness and bladder volume are used to calculate bladder mass. **A** shows the area of interest for measuring bladder wall thickness. Automated image patter–recognition software identifies the inner and outer margin of the bladder wall as highlighted by the two *dotted lines* in **B**. Validation of this new device is ongoing and preliminary results are encouraging.

Female Bladder

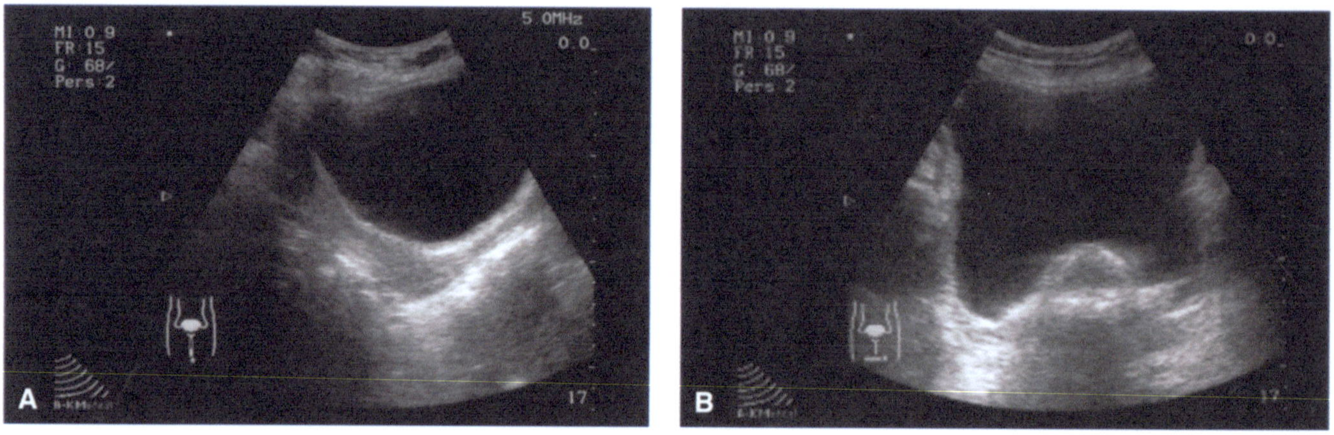

Figure 6-23. Female urinary bladder with uterus. The urinary bladder is often used as an acoustic window to scan female pelvic organs, but it also is imaged in patients with voiding dysfunction who are looking for intrinsic disorders of the bladder and for genital prolapse [11]. The morphology of female urinary bladder depends on the presence of the uterus and a calculation of bladder volume may be affected by a strong deviation of the bladder shape from a perfect sphere.

Bladder ultrasonography in a female subject (5.0-MHz convex probe) is shown. The shape of the female bladder also depends on the presence or absence of the uterus. In this case, the uterus, which is clearly visible in the midline sagittal plane (**A**), does not seem to modify the bladder shape in this section while its impact on the posterior bladder wall is clearly evident in a transverse image (**B**).

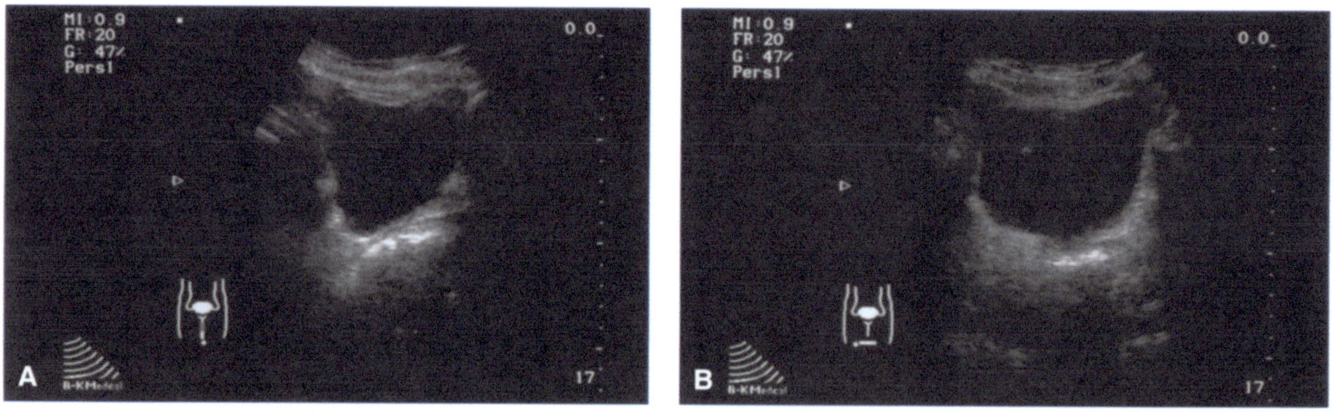

Figure 6-24. Urinary bladder in a female subject who underwent hysterectomy. In the absence of the uterus, the female urinary bladder has a morphology similar to that of the young male bladder in both longitudinal (**A**) and transverse (**B**) sections.

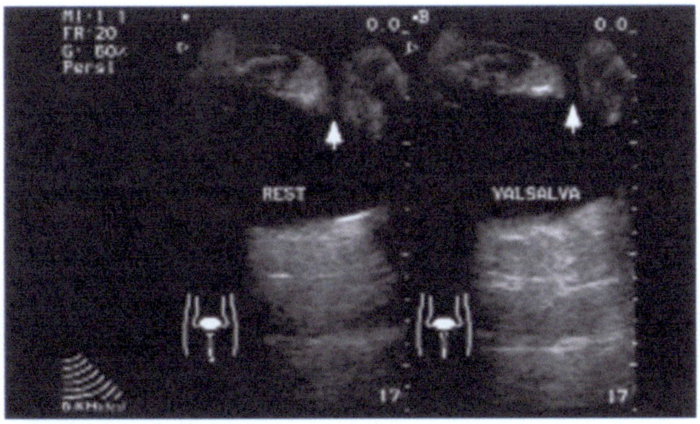

Figure 6-25. Bladder imaging in female stress urinary incontinence. Perineal (translabial) imaging of the urinary bladder is used to explore the anatomy of the urinary bladder and pelvic floor organs. The urethra, bladder neck (*arrows*), and urinary bladder of a 56-year-old woman who has stress urinary incontinence is shown. Straining (Valsalva) causes a 17-mm descent of the bladder neck compared to baseline (rest) without any significant rotation of the urethral axis [11].

Bladder Imaging in Pediatric Urology

Ultrasound (US) imaging of the bladder is ideal in the pediatric population, which benefits the most from the lack of radiation hazard and the noninvasive nature of the technique. Voiding dysfunction is not an uncommon diagnosis in young patients of both genders. In general, the use of US imaging in children has been very inventive and successful in a continuous search to avoid x-ray exposure and invasive imaging techniques.

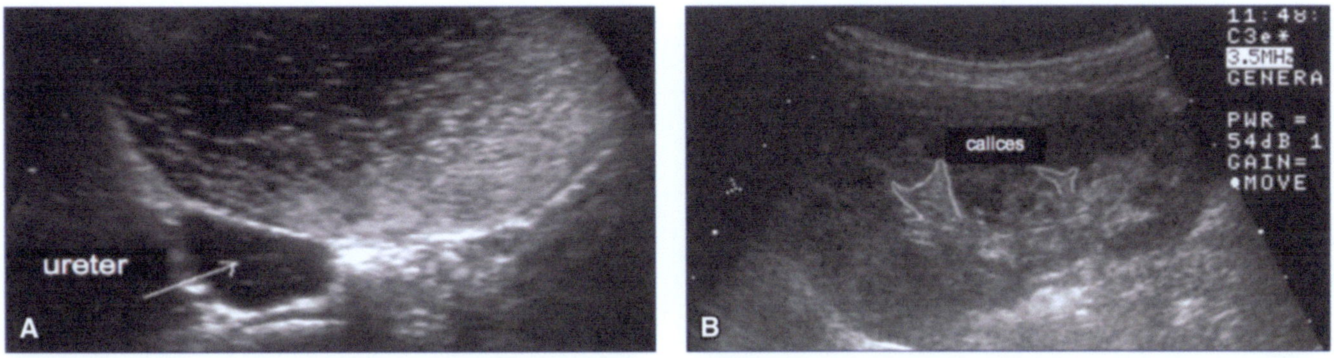

Figure 6-26. Secondary vesicoureteral reflux in children. Severe bladder outlet obstruction can result in failure of the antireflux mechanism, posing a severe threat to the upper urinary tract. Ultrasound cystography can be performed to confirm vesicoureteral reflux. A contrast agent instilled in the urinary bladder can be observed in the dilated ureter (**A**; *arrow*) and in the upper urinary tract (**B**).

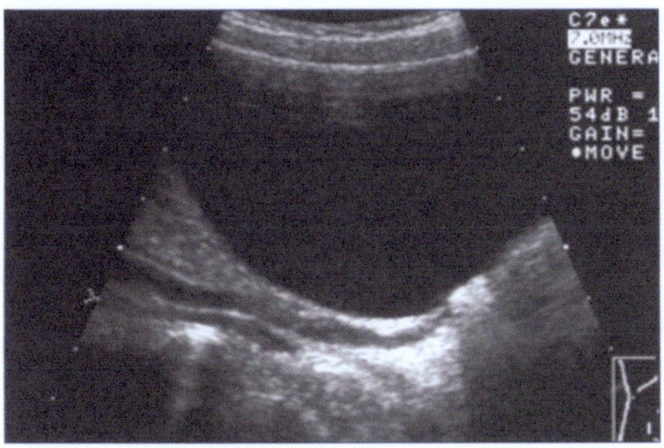

Figure 6-27. Collagen injection for reflux. Adolescent patients are often treated by adult urologists, who are often unaware of procedures previously performed in these young patients or who may not be familiar with the modifications produced in the lower urinary tract morphology. Dysfunctional voiding is certainly prevalent in the male adult population, but is not at all infrequent in the female pediatric subjects.

Suprapubic ultrasonography reveals hyperechogenic material at the intramural ureter level in a child who was injected for grade 2 vesicoureteral reflux. Mild dilatation of the pelvic ureter is visible.

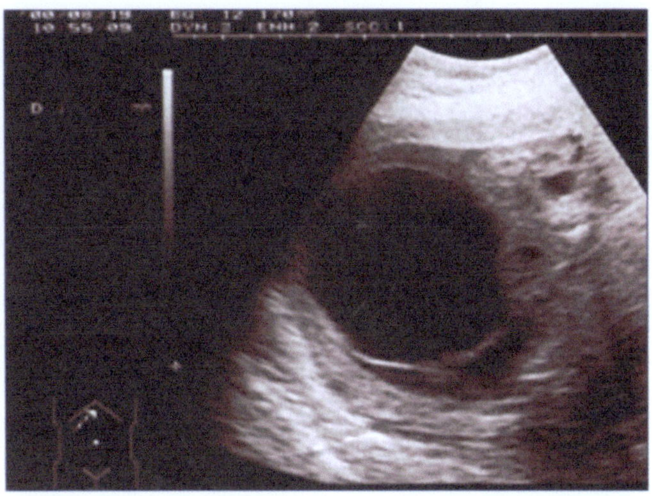

Figure 6-28. Fetal bladder imaging. Antenatal ultrasound of a male fetus: the abdomen is completely occupied by an enormous bladder, which presents as a unique cavity. The kidneys are hyperechogenic and very small and the oligohydramnios is severe, with a substantial absence of fluid. The newborn died in the first 2 days of life.

Urethral Valves

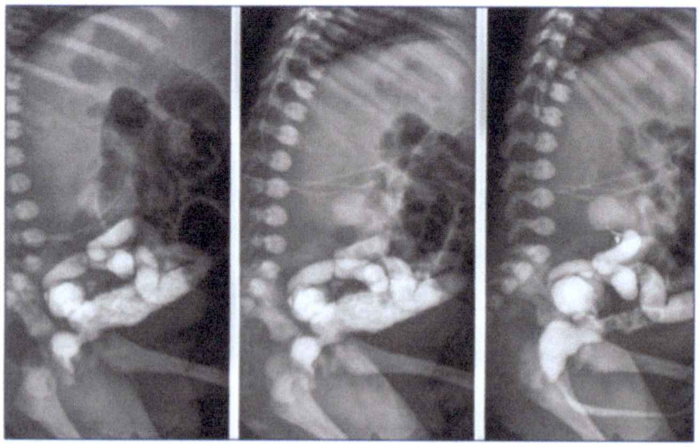

FIGURE 6-29. Newborn (2 days old) with severe posterior urethral valves, diagnosed prenatally. There is evidence of posterior urethra dilatation and narrowing under the sphincteric area; gross bilateral reflux is observed.

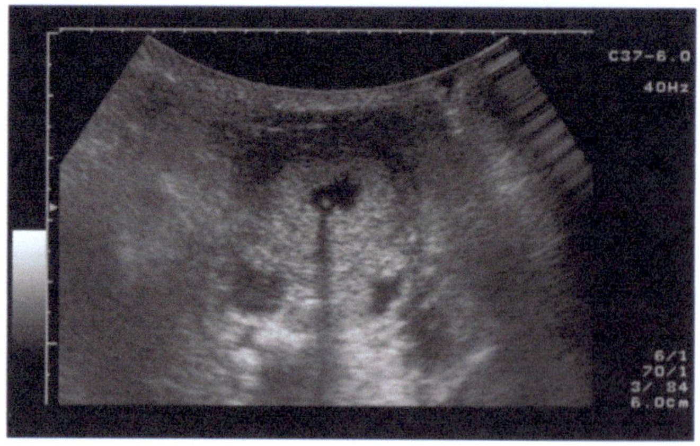

FIGURE 6-30. Urethral valves. Ultrasound at 2 days: very small bladder with severely thickened bladder walls and widely dilated ureters.

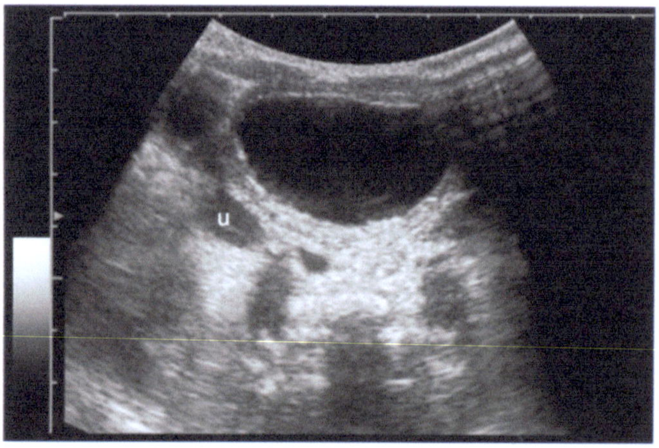

FIGURE 6-31. Ultrasound at 15 days, after the endoscopic section of the posterior urethral valve: the bladder is wide and dilated, and the bladder wall remains thickened but only one ureter (*u*) is dilated.

Nonneurogenic–Neurogenic Bladder

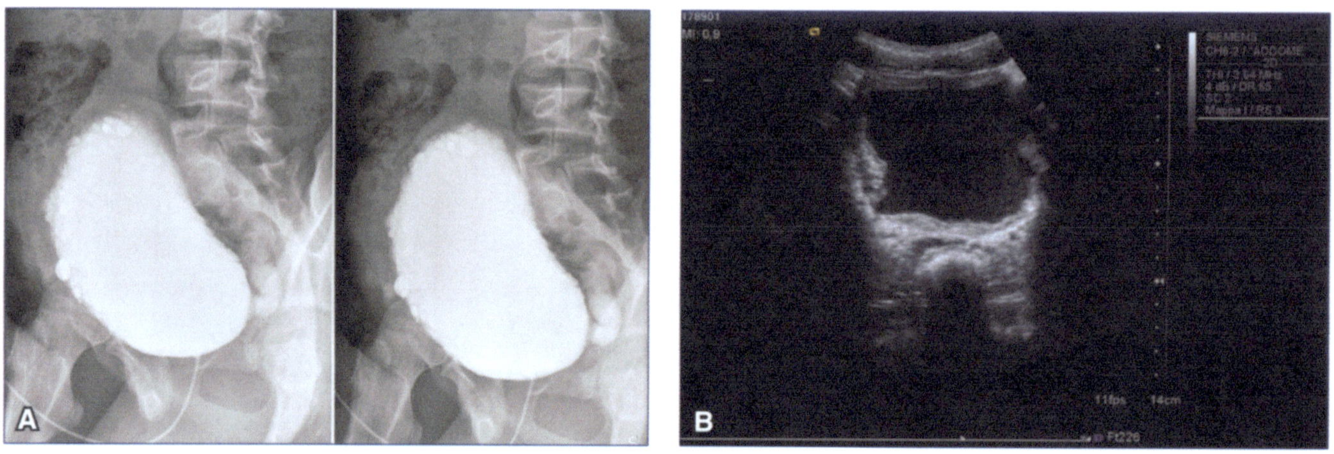

FIGURE 6-32. Nonneurogenic–neurogenic bladder (Hinman syndrome) in a 16-year-old boy. The patient presented with urinary retention, febrile urinary tract infections, severe constipation, and voiding difficulties. A cystogram (**A**) revealed a severely trabeculated bladder with pseudodiverticula, left distal reflux in the dilated ureter, and no micturition at cystoureterography. Signs of fecal impaction are evident over the bladder and at plain film. Cystometry and pressure-flow studies showed an underactive bladder, with low-pressure detrusor contraction and subtotal postvoid residual urine. At flowmetry, an interrupted curve is observed.

Ultrasound (US) of the upper urinary tract shows no dilation, but does show hyperechogenic echostructure and scarce corticomedullary differentiation with hypoplasia of the right kidney. Bladder US (**B**) shows a wide bladder with diffusely irregular and thickened walls (average 7–8 mm); inside the bladder is corpuscolated content. An MRI shows no spinal lesions. **B**, +—6.2 mm.

Conclusions

This selection of ultrasound (US) images is just an example of how complex the subject of US bladder imaging in voiding dysfunction can be. There is an absolute need to develop, maintain, and possibly improve our understanding of US bladder imaging in this area, regardless of who is the specialist involved in the management of voiding dysfunction. Those who believe voiding dysfunction is mainly due to benign prostatic hyperplasia will be surprised by the variety of challenging conditions that urologists may face in their daily practice. Voiding dysfunction in children, adolescents, and women certainly are not trivial issues and deserve proper knowledge of their pathophysiology and imaging. There is a clear call for specialists who are active in the area of voiding dysfunction to develop knowledge in and research this fascinating area.

References

1. Brouwer TA, Eindhoven BG, Epema AH, Henning RH: Validation of an ultrasound scanner for determining urinary volumes in surgical patients and volunteers. *J Clin Monit Comput* 1999, 15:379–385.
2. Ohnishi K, Watanabe H, Ohe H, Saitoh M: Development and clinical significance of protrusion of hypertrophic prostate into the bladder observed by transrectal ultrasonotomography. *Nippon Hinyokika Gakkai Zasshi* 1985, 76:1194–1200.
3. Chia SJ, Heng CT, Chan SP, Foo KT: Correlation of intravesical prostatic protrusion with bladder outlet obstruction. *BJU Int* 2003, 91:371–374.
4. McConnell JD, Roehrborn CG, Bautista OM, *et al.*: The long-term effect of doxazosin, finasteride, and combination therapy on the clinical progression of benign prostatic hyperplasia. *N Engl J Med* 2003, 349:2387–2398.
5. Kaefer M, Barnewolt C, Retik AB, Peters CA: The sonographic diagnosis of infravesical obstruction in children: evaluation of bladder wall thickness indexed to bladder filling. *J Urol* 1997, 157:989–991.
6. Kojima M, Inui E, Ochiai A, *et al.*: Noninvasive quantitative estimation of infravesical obstruction using ultrasonic measurement of bladder weight. *J Urol* 1997, 157:476–479.
7. Manieri C, Carter SS, Romano G, *et al.*: The diagnosis of bladder outlet obstruction in men by ultrasound measurement of bladder wall thickness. *J Urol* 1998, 159:761–765.
8. Tubaro A, Carter S, Hind A, *et al.*: A prospective study of the safety and efficacy of suprapubic transvesical prostatectomy in patients with benign prostatic hyperplasia. *J Urol* 2001, 166:172–176.
9. Oelke M, Hofner K, Jonas U, *et al.*: Diagnostic accuracy of noninvasive tests to evaluate bladder outlet obstruction in men: detrusor wall thickness, uroflowmetry, postvoid residual urine, and prostate volume. *Eur Urol* 2007, 52:827–834.
10. Khullar V, Salvatore S, Cardozo L, *et al.*: A novel technique for measuring bladder wall thickness in women using transvaginal ultrasound. *Ultrasound Med Biol* 1994, 4:220–223.
11. Tubaro A, Artibani W, Bartram C, *et al.*: Imaging and other investigations. In *3rd International Consultation on Incontinence*. Edited by Abrams P, Cardozo L, Khoury S, Wein A. Plymouth, UK: Health Publication; 2005:707–797.

7

Pelvic Floor Rehabilitation

Bary Berghmans, Maura Seleme, Erik Hendriks, Nol Bernards, and Marijke Van Kampen

Pelvic floor rehabilitation, namely pelvic physical therapy, is one of the management mainstays of pelvic floor dysfunctions. The pelvic floor does not act on its own; it works in synergy with other parts of the human body. As such, pelvic floor dysfunctions may lead not only to impairments of local organs and tissues, such as weakness of the pelvic floor muscles (PFMs), or to activity limitations, such as coughing with involuntary loss of urine, but also to restriction in the person's participation in social, physical, and psychological activities, such as withdrawal from regular sport activity or theater visits.

Considering each person to be a sociopsychosomatic entity, pelvic physical therapy may need to focus on behavioral and physical activities for increasing general function, well being, and fitness. Life-long regular adequate physical activity is warranted for prevention of many health problems and diseases, and also to prevent a dysfunctional pelvic floor. Physical activity is also important during pregnancy and after delivery. Effective peri- and postnatal interventions to prevent or treat incontinence, especially for women who are at risk, are deemed important.

Pelvic floor rehabilitation focuses on the prevention and treatment of all kinds of functional disorders of the abdominal, pelvis, and lower back region, such as urinary incontinence and overactive bladder, that are considered to be highly prevalent health problems in both genders but predominantly women. Other important pelvic floor dysfunctions are pelvic organ prolapse (POP) and micturition disorders; in men, they are related to benign hypertrophy of the prostate (BPH) or prostate cancer.

Pelvic physical therapy is often considered to be the first-choice treatment due to its noninvasive character, results in terms of symptom relief, the possibility of combining physical therapy with other treatments, low risk of side effects, and moderate to low costs. Important restrictions for success might be a lack of motivation, the adherence and perseverance of both the patient and therapist, and the time needed for physical therapy.

Pelvic physical therapy modalities contain interventions such as physical therapeutic diagnostics, education and information for patients, behavioral treatment, PFM training, bladder training, training with vaginal cones, electrical and magnetic stimulation, and biofeedback.

In stress urinary incontinence, which is one of the most prevalent health problems related to the pelvic floor, a focus is on improving the extrinsic closing mechanism of the urethra. Physical therapy is focused on strength improvement and coordination of the peri- and paraurethral and PFMs. PFM training is especially effective.

For bladder overactivity, physical therapy aims to reduce or eliminate involuntary detrusor contractions through reflex inhibition. Here, electrical therapy appears to be an effective intervention. In mixed urinary incontinence, the physical therapeutic diagnostic and therapeutic process focuses on the predominant factors. With respect to POP, there is substantial evidence that perioperative physical therapy is an intervention that reduces the risk in the presence of pelvic floor symptoms after prolapse surgery.

Radical prostatectomy and BPH are the most important causes of incontinence and micturition disorders in men. Adequate programs of PFM training, after transurethral radical prostatectomy, decrease the duration and extent of urinary incontinence, improving adequate micturition and quality of life.

This chapter will focus on the prevention, diagnosis, analysis, evaluation, and treatment of pelvic floor and bladder dysfunctions. With pelvic physical therapy, most patients can be treated to a satisfactory level. Clinical practice guidelines have been published in several countries. For the time being, little is known about the implementation of these guidelines and their use in daily pelvic floor rehabilitation.

The physical therapeutic processes, algorithms, and flowcharts described in this chapter are based on these guidelines. To assess the indication for and the effects of pelvic floor rehabilitation, high methodological quality diagnostic tools, outcome measures, and performance indicators must be used.

This field will have its permanent role in the multidisciplinary approach of the pelvic floor, but only if the clinical practice of pelvic physical therapy, performed with adequate skills and experience, is based on high-quality scientific evidence and if the development of new concepts will continuously be stimulated.

Physical Therapy Prediagnostic Phase

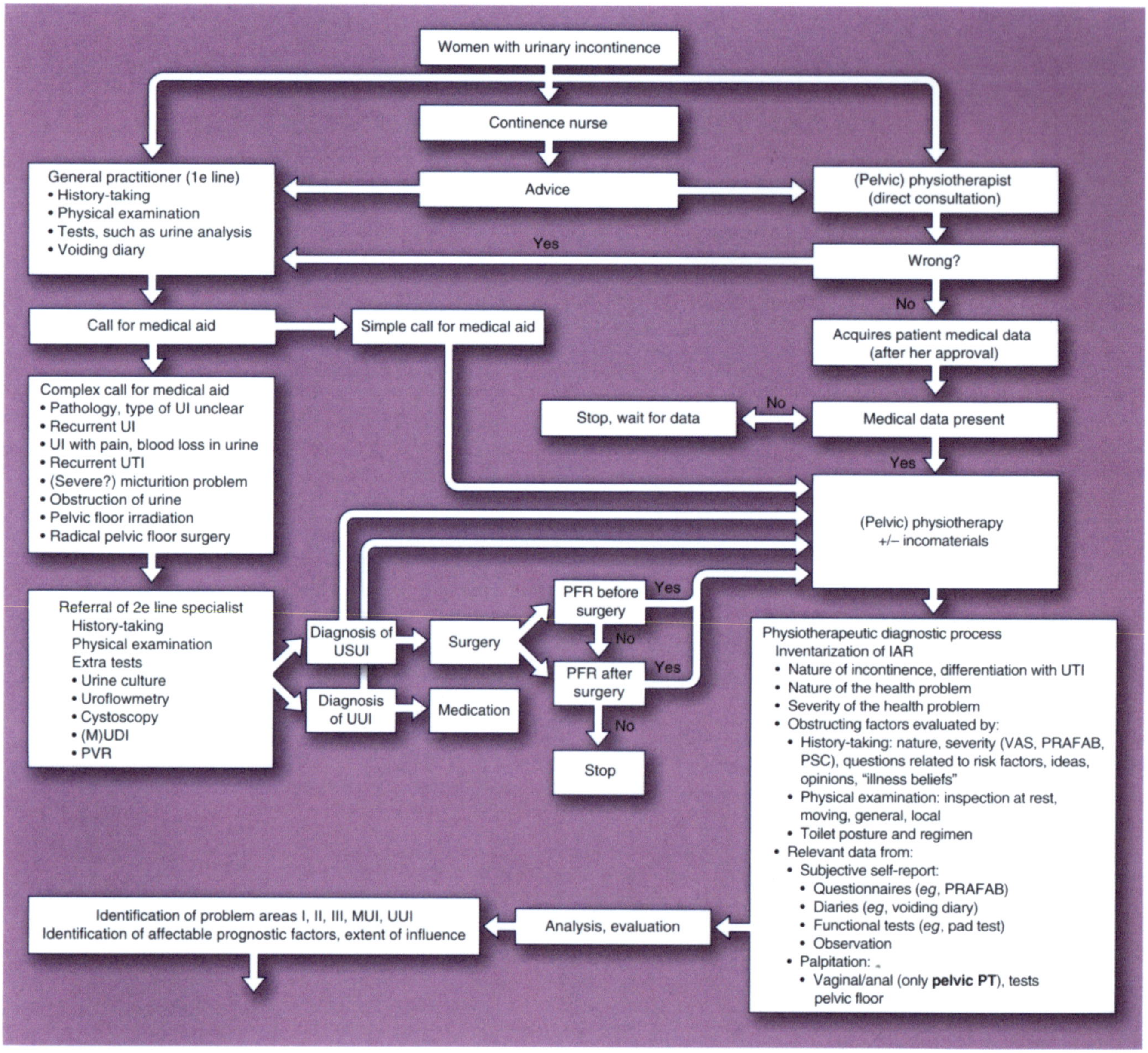

FIGURE 7-1. Flowchart showing treatment procedures for women with urinary incontinence (UI). IAR—impairments, activity limitations, restrictions in participation; (M)UDI—(mobile) urodynamic investigation; PFR—pelvic floor rehabilitation; PRAFAB—protection, amount, frequency, adjustment, body image assessment tool; PSC—patient-specific complaint; PVR—postvoid residual; USUI—urodynamic stress urinary incontinence; UTI—urinary tract infection; UUI—urgency urinary incontinence; VAS—visual analogue scale.

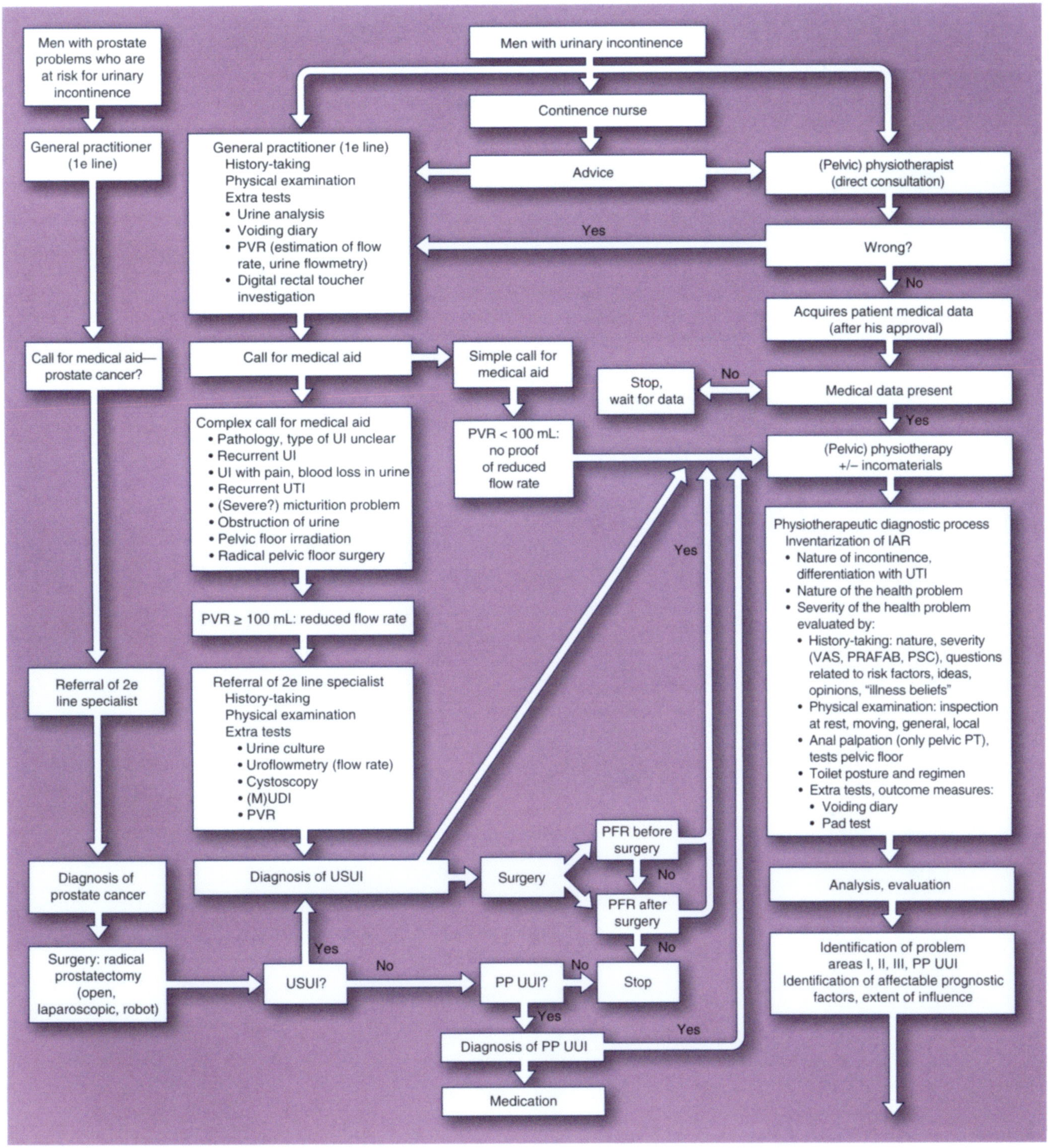

FIGURE 7-2. Flowchart showing treatment procedures for men with urinary incontinence (UI). IAR—impairments, activity limitations, restrictions in participation; (M)UDI—(mobile) urodynamic investigation; PFR—pelvic floor rehabilitation; PP UUI—postprostatectomy urgency urinary incontinence; PRAFAB—protection, amount, frequency, adjustment, body image assessment tool; PSC—patient-specific complaint; PVR—postvoid residual; USUI—urodynamic stress urinary incontinence; UTI—urinary tract infection; UUI—urgency urinary incontinence; VAS—visual analogue scale.

Referral for Pelvic Physical Therapy: Details That Are Needed
Possible causal factors leading to the development of the health problem; *eg*, labor
Local factors that may inhibit recovery and adjustment; *eg*, prolapse of the uterus
General factors that may inhibit recovery and adjustment; *eg*, hormonal disturbances
Diagnostic data of the referrer, such as the patient's capability of a conscious contraction and relaxation of the pelvic floor muscles

FIGURE 7-3. Referral and medical data. In many countries, the pelvic physical therapist must receive a written referral from a medical doctor before treatment begins. Sometimes referrals can also be made indirectly on the advice of a midwife or obstetrician.

In addition to routine patient data, the referral documentation must include, at least, the nature of the intervention requested and an estimate of the relevant health problem severity. Details such as those given in this table are also needed [1].

In case medical data are missing, the physical therapist (after having discussed this with the patient) should contact the referrer to get these data. In the case of a direct consultation of the physical therapist (without referral), medical data such as medication use, other pathologies, or surgery in the past are needed. The patient is asked to provide this information. If there is doubt, the physical therapist has the responsibility to obtain these data before starting the physical therapeutic diagnostic process.

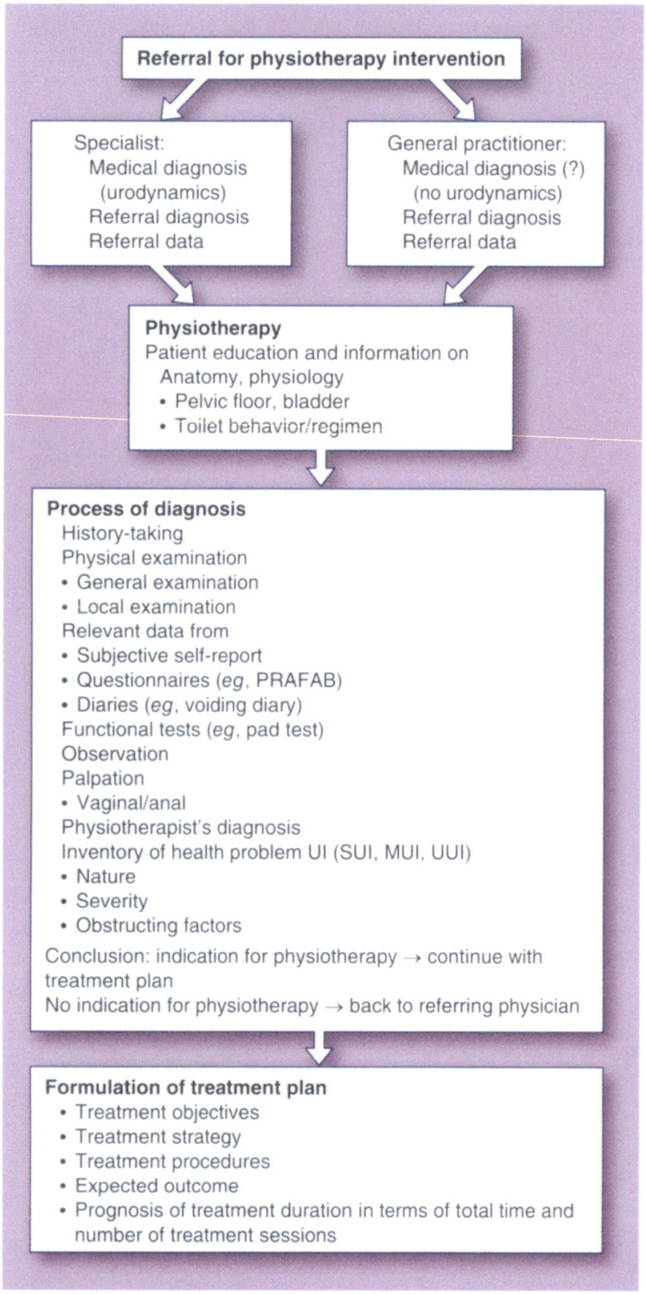

FIGURE 7-4. Flowchart of referral and physical therapeutic diagnostic processes [1].

Urine Voiding Diary

Date	Time	Amount Voided	Activity	Leakage*, 0–3 scale	Reason for accident	Fluid intake (amount/type)
10/23	6:30 AM	300 mL	Getting up/ breakfast	0	Getting to bathroom	16 oz coffee, 6 oz juice
	9:15	300 mL				8 oz water
	9:45	100 mL	Working	1	Urge	10 oz water
	11:00	150 mL				
	12:45 PM	200 mL	Working/ at lunch	0		8 oz water
	2:15	300 mL	Bending	1	Sitting	4 oz water
	3:30	100 mL			Urge	
	5:00	150 mL	Leaving work	0		—
	6:30	125 mL	Exercise class	2		12 oz water
	8:00	—	Dinner	0	Eating	4 oz wine, 8 oz water
	10:45	100 mL	Getting ready for bed	0		—

Leakage: 0 = no leakage; 1 = drops; 2 = wet underwear or light pad; 3 = soaked pad or clothing

Figure 7-5. Voiding diary. A (mostly 3-day) voiding diary, filled out adequately by the patient, provides important and easy way to get symptomatic information and indications about the type and severity of urinary incontinence; it should be part of every physical therapeutic diagnostic process.

A patient who has stress urinary incontinence (SUI) usually has a normal voiding frequency (8 times in 24 hours) and bladder volume (350–500 mL) and has mean voiding volumes between 200 and 400 cc/void, but with neither urgency nor nycturia. The patient reports losing small amounts of urine (drops, spurts) during physical exertion. A patient with urgency urinary incontinence (UUI) has a voiding frequency that often is much higher than 8 voids/24 hours and usually loses more urine (up to the complete contents of the bladder) compared to a patient with SUI. The patient may void less than 150 mL urine per each void, suggesting a reduced functional bladder capacity. Combinations of the aforementioned symptoms of SUI and UUI are considered to reflect mixed urinary incontinence (MUI) [2]. UI—urinary incontinence.

Assessment of the Pelvic Floor

Visual observation: first impression of the patient's ability to contract by visual observation; no quantification of inward movement
PFM palpation intravaginally (or intrarectally): registration squeeze pressure and inward/upward lift PFM: so far it is the recommended technique; often the modified Oxford grading scale is used for quantification of strength (*see* Fig. 7-10)
Surface EMG: registration of motor unit activity of pudendal nerve fibers: extrapolation from EMG data to PFM strength, power, and endurance with caution
Vaginal squeeze pressure measurement, pressure manometry, dynamometric force: always together with the simultaneous observation of inward movement of the perineum
PFM ultrasound: assess the correctness of a PFM contraction, its anatomical position, and muscle volume, no quantification of PFM strength possible: in the future it may be more widely available for physical therapists
Pelvic organ prolapse quantification measures and quantifies the position of all segments of the vagina and perineum [4]

Figure 7-6. Assessment of the pelvic floor. Assessment of the function and strength of the pelvic floor is an important part of the physical therapeutic diagnostic process. Suggested assessment of the measurement pelvic floor muscle (PFM) function and strength and the position of pelvic organs before and after treatment is provided [3]. EMG—electromyogram.

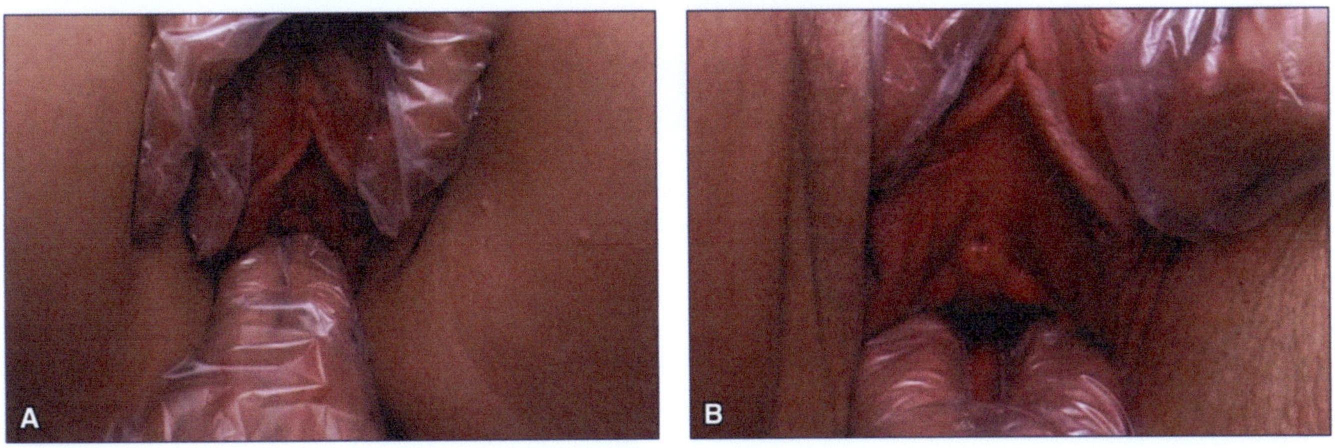

Figure 7-7. Digital palpation of the superficial bulbospongiosus muscle. **A**, First, the index and middle finger must be inserted until the second phalanx. **B**, Next, the fingers spread out and the patient tries to tighten the vagina by squeezing the fingers of the physical therapist with the bulbospongiosus muscle. This muscle can be more superficial than the pubovaginal muscles. Its principal function is closing of the vulva. Indications for this technique might be a lack of coordination, vaginal flatus, or sexual problems.

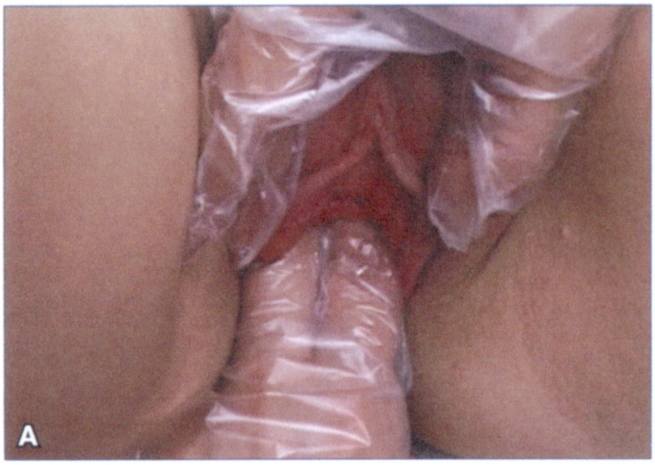

Modified Oxford Scale

0 = No contraction

1 = Flicker

2 = Weak

3 = Moderate contraction (pelvic floor lift is checked)

4 = Good contraction (pelvic floor lift is checked)

B

FIGURE 7-8. Assessment of the pelvic floor, contraction of the levator ani muscles. Pelvic floor muscle (PFM) palpation can be done intravaginally or intrarectally; with this technique, squeeze pressure and inward/upward lift of the PFM can be registered. **A,** For an assessment of the contraction of the levator ani muscles, the pelvic physical therapist inserts fingers from below inside the vagina until the levator ani muscles can be felt. The patient is instructed to contract the PFM ("withhold a flatus, contract the anus inwards, stop the urine"). A correct contraction is a simultaneous squeezing around the physical therapist's index and middle finger and inward/upward movement or elevation of the levator ani muscles. **B,** To quantify the strength of the contraction, the modified Oxford grading scale is often used [5]. PFM relaxation should be tested after a contraction. Therefore, the investigator should always start with a contraction and then ask for relaxation.

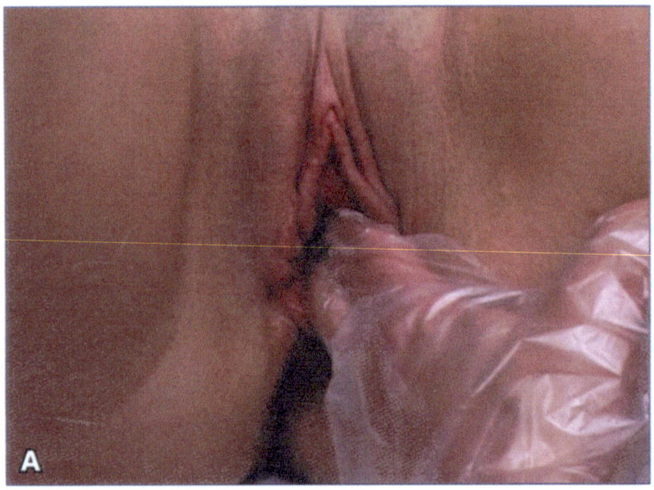

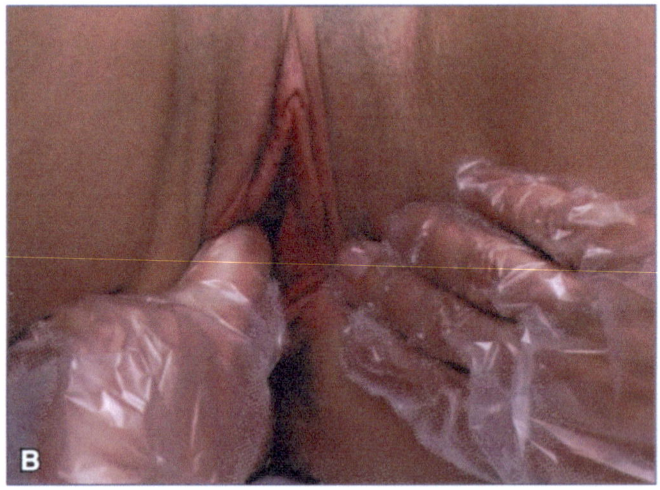

FIGURE 7-9. Pelvic floor muscle (PFM) contraction against the lateral vaginal wall. The patient contracts the PFM as a reaction to the resistance of the physical therapist's fingers against the left (**A**) and right (**B**) vaginal wall. This technique stimulates the propriocepsis (sometimes the strength of the contraction of one side is superior to the other).

Suggested Outcome Measures to Assess the Severity of Urinary Leakage and QOL

3 days of leakage episodes

Leakage index

Pad test (48, 24, and 1 h; short tests with standardized bladder volume)

PRAFAB-Q [7]

Incontinence Impact Questionnaire (short form)

General and disease-specific QOL questionnaires (SF-36, ICIQ UI SF, BFLUTS)

Global perceived effect

A

FIGURE 7-10. Assessment of the severity of urinary leakage, quality of life (QOL), and global perceived effect. **A,** Suggested outcome measures for the assessment of severity of urinary leakage and QOL, before and after treatment [3].

Continued on the next page

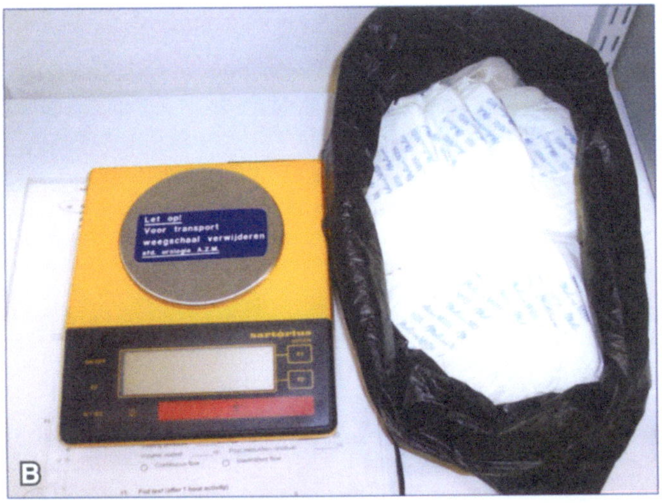

FIGURE 7-10. *(Continued)* **B,** Balanced, preweighed pads and a registration form for the pad test. In clinical practice, a 24-hour pad test seems to be preferable. This test correlates well with symptoms of incontinence and has good reproducibility, but on the other hand it also has poorer compliance than the 1-hour International Continence Society (ICS) pad test. Unless applied with a fixed bladder volume, the 1-hour ICS pad test is not very accurate. A pad weight gain greater than 1 gram suggests a positive 1-hour test and greater than 1.3 grams is a positive 24-hour test. A pad test lasting longer than 24 hours has little advantage [8]. In stress urinary incontinence and mixed urinary incontinence (MUI) with predominant stress factor, the pad test can be used for an assessment of severity. In overactive bladder, this test is less useful because the preweighed pads might not be big enough to measure the loss of urine accurately. BFLUTS—Bristol Female Lower Urinary Tract Symptoms; ICIQ UI SF—International Consultation on Incontinence Modular Questionnaire Urinary Incontinence short form; PRAFAB-Q—Protection, Amount, Frequency, Adjustment, Body Image Assessment Tool Questionnaire; SF-36—SF-36® Health Survey.

Score

Protection

1. I never use protection for urine loss
2. I sometimes use protection or I have to change my underwear because of urine loss
3. I normally use protection or change my underwear several times a day because of urine loss
4. I always have to use protection because of urinary incontinence ☐

Amount

1. The amount of urine loss is just a drop or less
2. Sometimes I lose a trickle
3. The loss of urine is so much that it wets my protection or clothes noticeably
4. The loss of urine is so much that my protection is soaked or leaks ☐

Frequency Involuntary loss of urine occurs:

1. Once a week or less
2. More than once but less than three times a week
3. More than three times a week, but not every day
4. Every day ☐

Subscore "urine loss" = PR + A + F ☐

Adjustment Implications of urine loss:

1. I am not hampered in my daily activities
2. I have stopped some activities, such as some sports and physically demanding activities
3. I have stopped most physical activities that caused an involuntary loss of urine
4. I almost never go out ☐

Body (or self) image

1. I am not bothered by my urine loss
2. I think urine loss is annoying and troublesome, but I am not greatly bothered by it
3. Urine loss makes me feel dirty
4. I am disgusted by myself because of my urinary incontinence ☐

Subscore "impact" = A + B ☐

Total score PRAFAB ☐

FIGURE 7-11. The Protection, Amount, Frequency, Adjustment, Body Image Assessment Tool Questionnaire (PRAFAB-Q) Score [7]. The PRAFAB-Q has been validated in Dutch. Psychometric testing of the English version was not performed. Nevertheless, this questionnaire is provided in English to give readers insight into the items and scoring system (minimum–maximum 5–20 points; range 16 points).

The PRAFAB-Q score is quick and easy to administer compared to a pad test with a standardized bladder volume or quality of life questionnaires and has the additional value of including the subjective aspects of urinary incontinence (UI) [7,9]. The brief and simple PRAFAB-Q demonstrated good psychometric properties to justify its use in clinical practice as well as research to evaluate the treatment effects for UI in women [6].

Minimally important difference (MID) refers to "the smallest score difference which patients perceive as beneficial and which would mandate, in the absence of troublesome side effects and excessive cost, a change in the patient's management" [10]. Taking into account the influence of PRAFAB baseline scores on the magnitude of the MIC, the MIC was in a range of two to three points for nonsevere SUI and four to five points for severe stress urinary incontinence for nonsevere urgency urinary incontinence (UUI) in a range of three to four points and four to five points for severe UUI.

Physical Therapy Therapeutic Phase

Formulation of the Treatment Plan	
Treatment objectives	Explicit formulation of a reduction of impairments, activity limitations, and participation restrictions on organ, personal, and societal levels [11] or improvement, *ie*, full restoration of functions, activities, and participation. Objectives also depend on prognostic factors and the extent of influence of physical therapy on those factors.
Treatment strategy	Information, instruction, and education of the patient. Patient-centered, active, and professional care. Treatment according to an individual optimal dose–response relation. Motivational support, positive feedback, and reinforcement. Provision of home BF/ES devices if they are needed and available. Stimulation execution of a home-training program in line with the level of an office-bound program. Regular tests of therapy progress.
Treatment procedures	Each session starts with a regular assessment of the results so far, the patient's experiences, feedback of the physical therapist, and the formulation of expectations, as well as the choice of treatment modality, tools, parameters, duration and intensity of the session according to guidelines, (individual) protocol and patient's status, reaction, and acceptance.
Expected outcome	Stabilization, improvement, total recovery, cure to be discussed beforehand and during treatment with the patient, adaptation if necessary.
Prognosis of treatment duration	In terms of the total time and number of treatment sessions, to be discussed beforehand, adaptation if relevant.

FIGURE 7-12. Treatment plan. After the evaluation and analysis of all medical and physical therapeutic data, based on the nature and the severity of the health problem, the pelvic physical therapist will formulate a treatment plan. BF/ES—biofeedback/electrical stimulation.

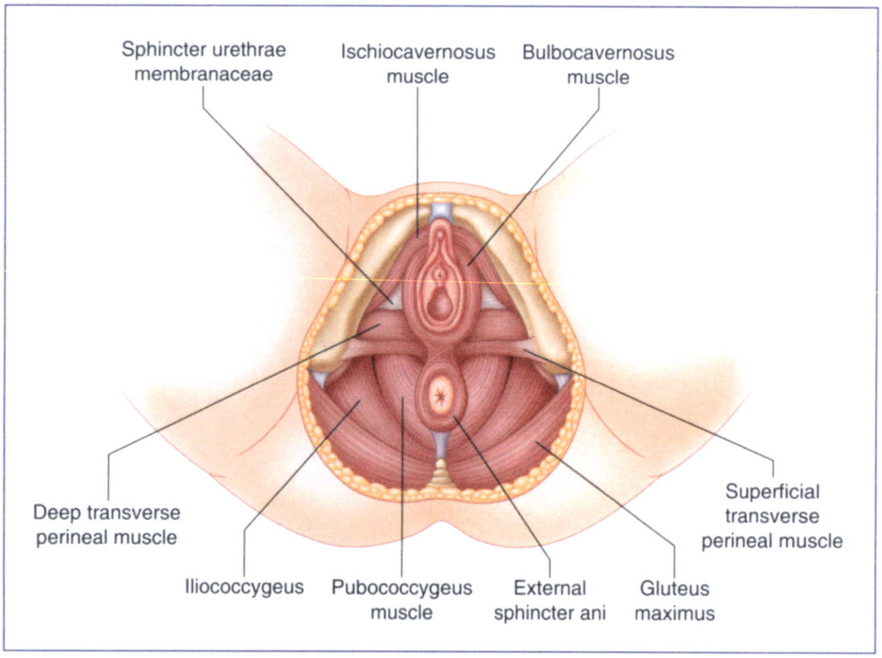

FIGURE 7-13. Information and education. Physical treatment starts with informing and educating the patient about the underlying health problem, its cause and prognosis, the influence of negative and positive factors, and expectations of both the patient and the health care provider. Also, the function and relationship of the pelvic floor muscles and organs with lower urinary tract function will be explained with the use of diagrams, anatomical models, and drawings like the one shown here [1].

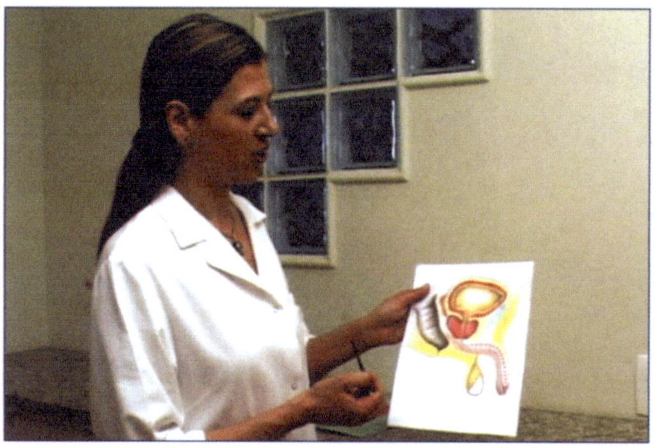

FIGURE 7-14. Information and education of the patient using anatomical drafts. Instructing the patient also motivates the patient and invites him or her to actively participate during treatment [1]. Building up confidence and providing a safe, professional atmosphere is an important first step toward the success of treatment. Visualization with the help of anatomical models or drafts gives insight and knowledge about the normal and pathological situation.

Therapy for Stress Urinary Incontinence in Women

Therapeutic training/management for distinguished problem areas

I. SUI + dysfunction pelvic floor + no awareness of pelvic floor:

Digital palpation by patient or physical therapist

Manual techniques such as tapping, stretching, intravaginal massage

Electrical stimulation (intravaginal/extravaginal) + PFMT

Biofeedback + PFMT

Objective: restoration of awareness of the pelvic floor

If awareness is restored → the next section

Unsatisfactory results → back to the referring physician

II. SUI + dysfunction of the pelvic floor + awareness of the pelvic floor:

PFMT + home exercises; isolated contractions of the pelvic floor → awareness of the pelvic floor; single tasks → double tasks → multiple tasks → automatic controlled tasks; optional: vaginal cones

Objective: total recovery of the functionality of the pelvic floor

Unsatisfactory results → back to the referring physician

III. SUI + dysfunction pelvic floor + function pelvic floor malinfluenced by disorders of the tractus respiratorius, other parts of the tractus motorius, or the toilet regimen or behavior

PFMT + home exercises

Exercises to achieve adequate respiration, postural exercises, relaxation exercises, and lift instruction

Objective: the reduction or elimination of malinfluence disorders, improved functionality of the pelvic floor

Unsatisfactory results → back to the referring physician

IV. SUI + no dysfunction of the pelvic floor

PFMT + home exercises; optional: vaginal cones

Objective: compensation. Expectation: total recovery is not likely

Unsatisfactory results → back to the referring physician

V. SUI + general obstructing factors

Objective: maximal possible reduction of these negative factors

Unsatisfactory results → back to the referring physician

Evaluation

Treatment results, changes in the patient's health status, course of action of the physical therapist

Concluding treatment period and reporting to referring physician

FIGURE 7-15. Algorithm of the process of therapy for stress incontinence in women [1]. PFMT—pelvic floor muscle training; SUI—stress urinary incontinence.

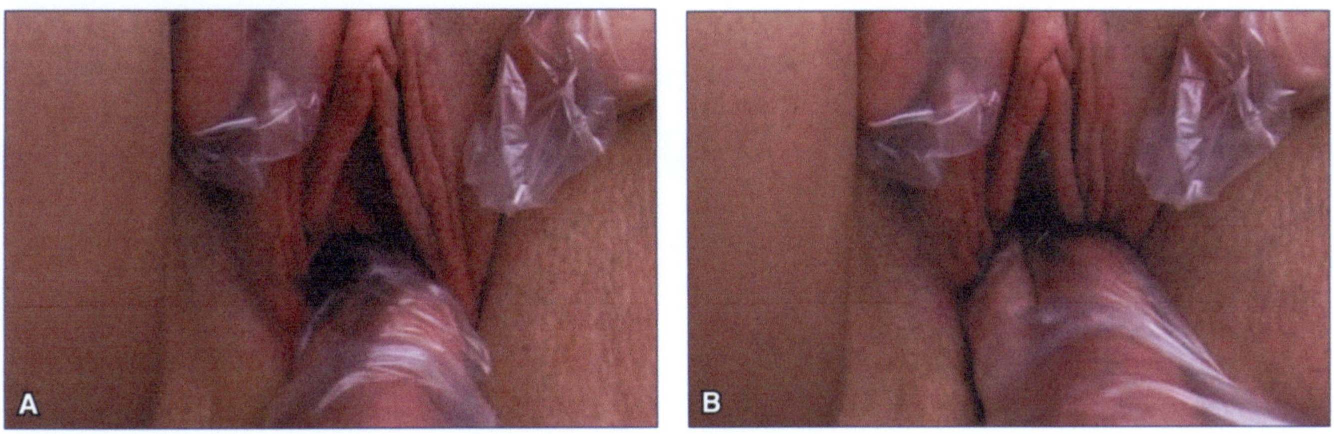

FIGURE 7-16. Perineal or intravaginal massage. **A**, Perineal massage is used to stimulate the propriocepsis and for relaxation if there is overactivity of the perineal muscles, a painful scar, or dyspareunia. **B**, This technique is also used as a preventive antenatal technique to prepare for the descent of the baby during the second stage of labor. The hypothesis is that as a result the pelvic floor muscles (PFMs) will be more flexible and better prepared to let the head of the baby pass without overstretching the PFMs and damaging the perineum. According to Kalichman [12], perineal massage in the last weeks of gestation reduces the likelihood of perineal trauma (mainly episiotomies) and ongoing perineal pain. Moreover, this massage is generally well accepted by women. Therefore, women should be made aware of the likely benefit and should be provided with information on how to massage [12]. Perineal massage during the second stage of labor is not recommended [12].

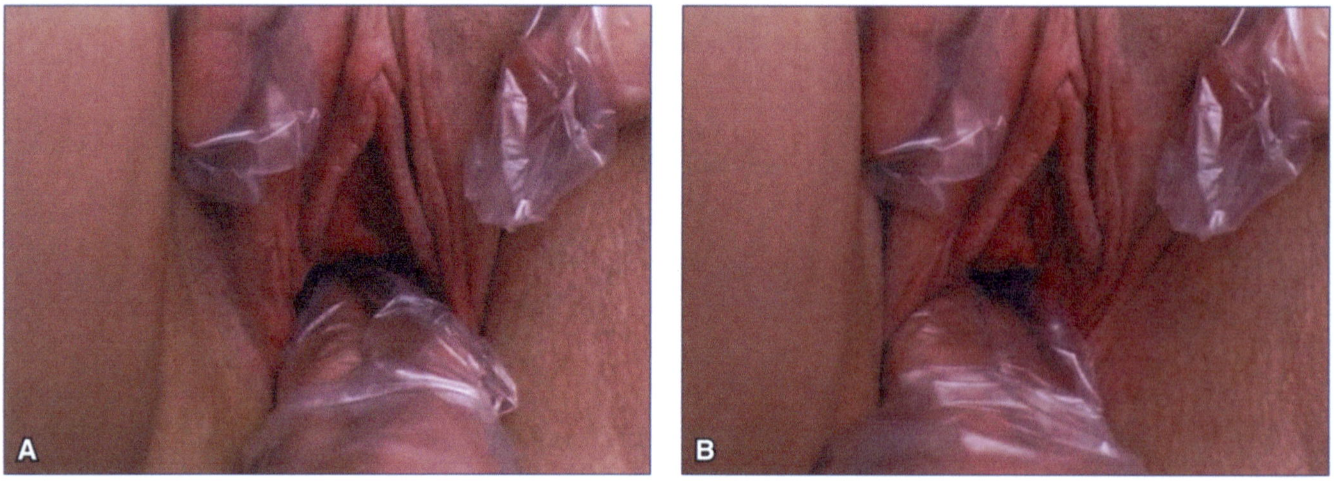

Figure 7-17. Manual techniques in women who are not able to contract the pelvic floor correctly. Over 30% of women do not contract the pelvic floor muscles correctly at the first consultation [13,14]. If they are not able to contract, manual techniques such as touch (**A**), tapping, massage, fast stretching (**B**), or electrical stimulation can be used. Most patients learn to contract if they are given some time by themselves at home to practice.

PFMT Treatment Plan

Stress urinary incontinence or mixed urinary incontinence with a predominant stress factor [3]

- Aim for close to the maximum contractions
- Building up to 8–12 contractions 3 times per day, first hold for 1–3 s, then 6–8 s; hold and relax
- Add 3–4 fast contractions
- In addition to the strength-training regimen, precontract and hold the contraction before and during coughing, laughing, sneezing, and lifting (conscious precontraction/"the Knack") to avoid any involuntary loss of urine
- Ask the patient to suggest where and when exercises should be performed
- Supply an exercise diary or use a computerized biofeedback adherence measurement
- If available, discuss whether the use of biofeedback motivates the patient to exercise

Urgency urinary incontinence or mixed urinary incontinence with a predominant urgency factor

- Aim to inhibit detrusor contractions by intentionally using (sub)maximal PFM contractions
- Hold the contraction as long as needed to stop the urgency to void [15]

Figure 7-18. Treatment plan with pelvic floor muscle (PFM) training for women with urinary incontinence. Integrate the acquired skills and abilities into regular daily activities to reach permanent therapy success.

The treatment duration and frequency may be different in each patient. In general, the total treatment duration will take 6 weeks to 3 months. The treatment duration and frequency depend on specific treatment targets and problems, as well as the apprenticeship and training skills of the patient.

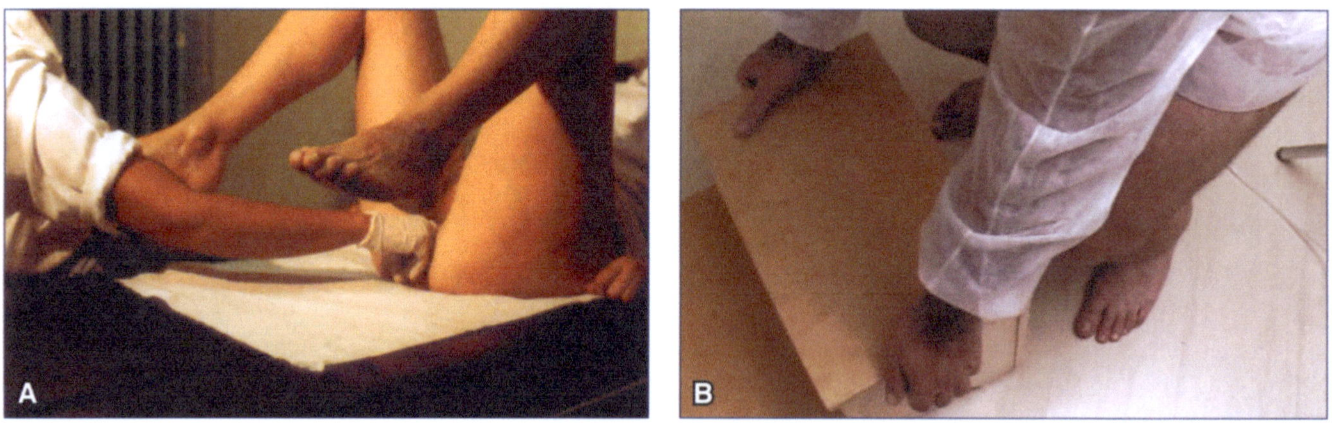

Figure 7-19. Pelvic floor muscle training (PFMT) for stress urinary incontinence (and mixed urinary incontinence with predominant stress factor). Explain the correct pelvic floor muscle (PFM) contraction and practice before checking the ability to contract. First have intensive in-office guidance to perform conscious and selective PFM contractions and then PFMT at home. Set up an individual home-training program and then follow up with weekly or more frequent supervised training [3].

The first part of PFMT can involve digital palpation to support and control PFM contractions during coughing. Lift one or two legs, as seen in **A,** followed by more functional exercises such as lifting weights (**B**), sitting down, or standing up.

Continued on the next page

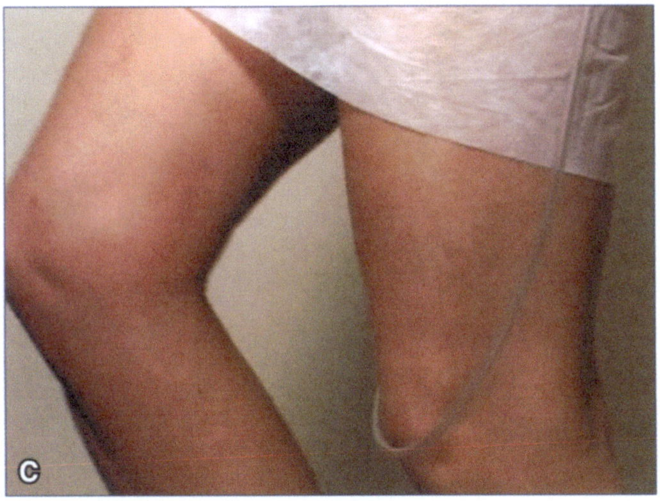

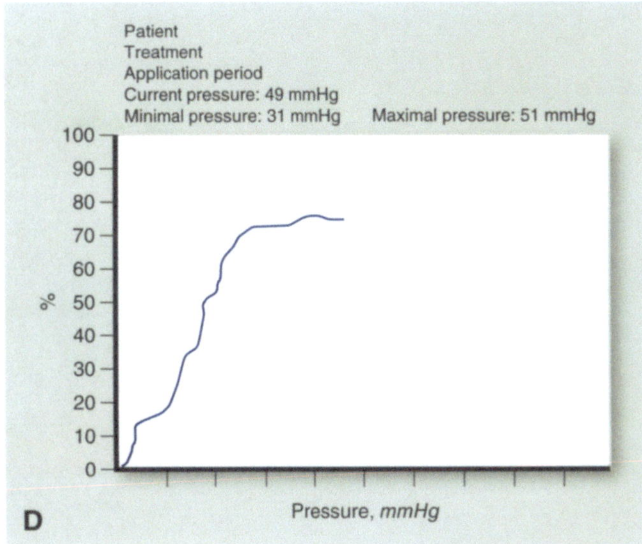

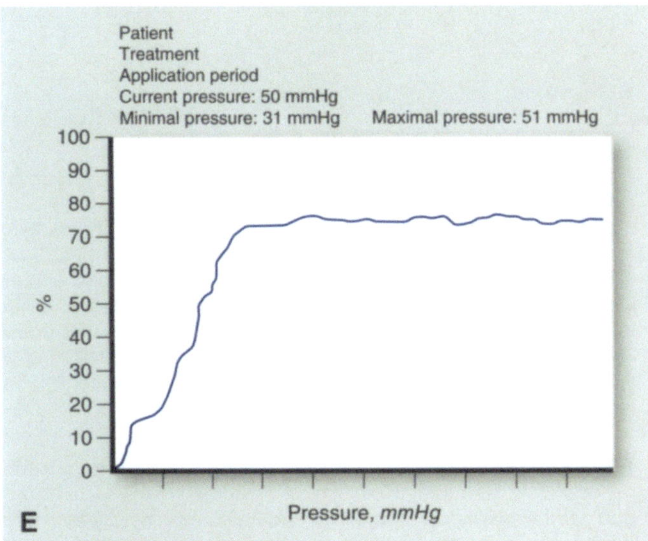

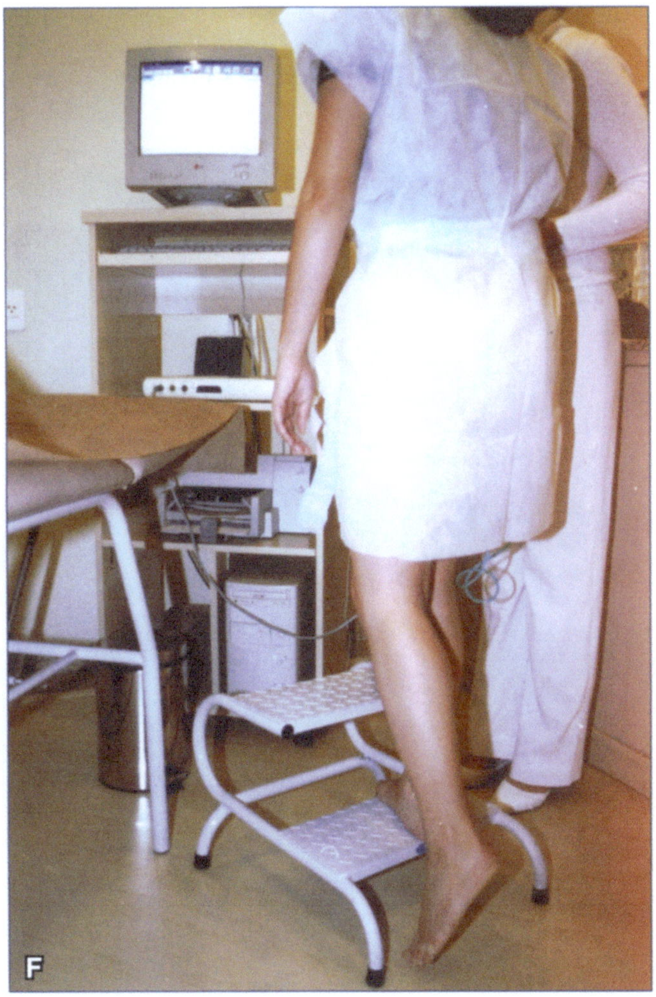

FIGURE 7-19. *(Continued)* **C–E,** PFMT supported by electromyogram (EMG) or pressure biofeedback.

F, Climbing up and going down stairs might be a difficult task for some patients, and biofeedback might be helpful in guiding the execution of correct PFM contractions.

Before beginning to climb up or go down the stairs, the PFM contraction must start and should be held during the whole effort. For training in these positions, the physical therapist can choose between the use of EMG or pressure biofeedback. Some professionals prefer EMG biofeedback for strength training because the PFM signal with this technique undergoes less interference of the abdominal muscles than with pressure biofeedback. (**A** and **B** *courtesy of* IRPP; Lille, France. **C–F** *courtesy of* Ibramed; Rio de Janeiro, Brazil.)

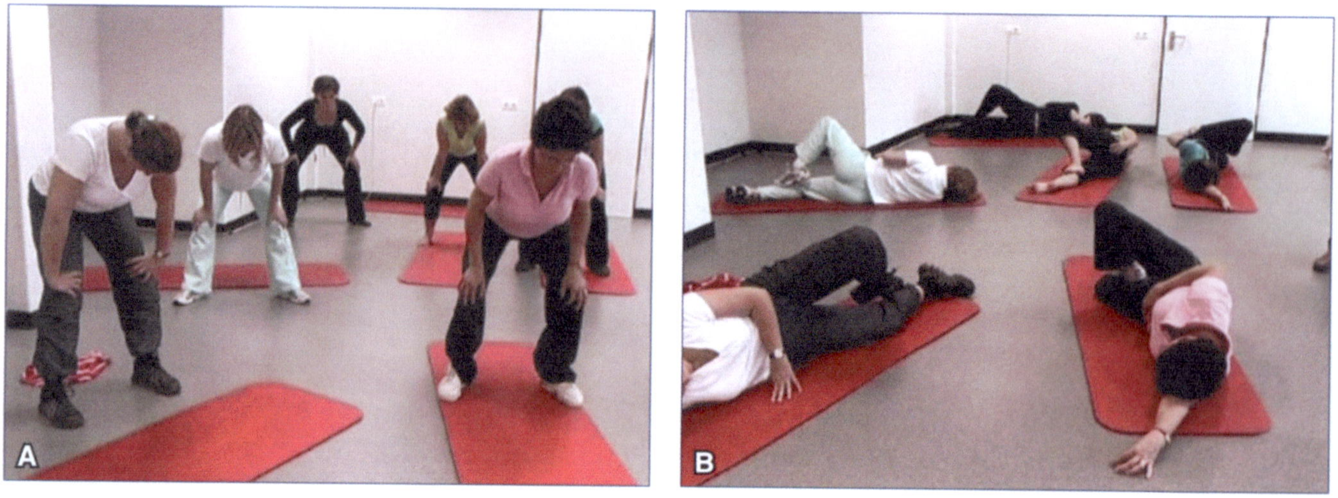

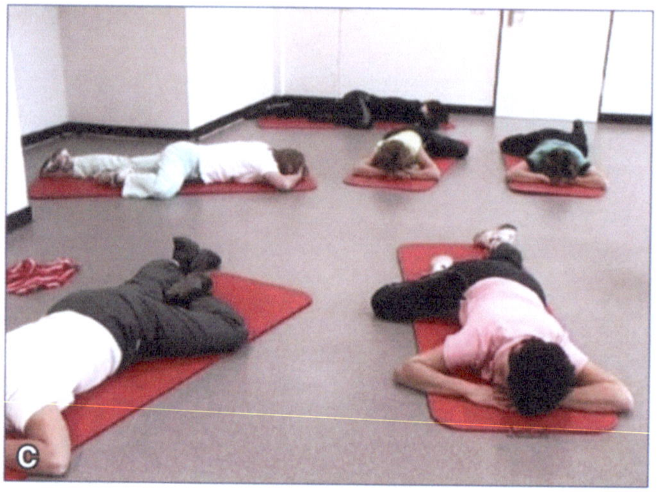

FIGURE 7-20. Group training for the pelvic floor muscles (PFMs) and postpartum. After individual tests of the ability to contract PFMs correctly, an option for continued PFM training (PFMT) might be group training (**A**). Combined with general fitness exercises (with music), such a protocol can be attractive, motivating participation and enhancing adherence, especially of those women who find exercises difficult to conduct regularly. Individual and group training might be equally effective [16]. The lateral position (**B**) facilitates the perception of the PFM contraction. Also, lying on the stomach (**C**) simplifies feeling how to contract the PFMs.

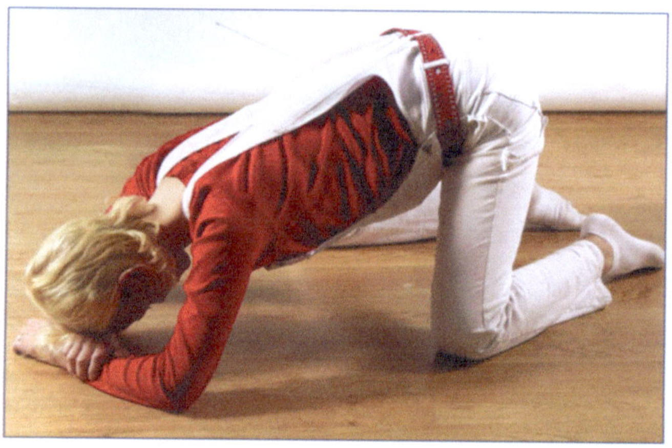

FIGURE 7-21. Peripartum exercises to prevent or treat urinary incontinence. Results from epidemiological studies show that women who have had a baby are at an increased risk of developing urinary incontinence (UI); it seems that both pregnancy and delivery are risk factors [17].

Pelvic floor muscle training (PFMT), either individually or in groups, is commonly used to prevent and treat UI related to pregnancy and childbirth, and the effect has been documented in several randomized clinical trials (RCTs). Following a Cochrane review of RCTs [18], pregnant women without prior incontinence who did "intensive" antenatal PFMT were less likely to report UI in late pregnancy and up to 6 months postpartum than were women who did not or had not received PFMT advice as part of usual antenatal care. Postnatal women with persistent incontinence symptoms 3 months after delivery were less likely to report UI 12 months after delivery than women who did no PFMT or received no PFMT advice as part of usual postnatal care [18]. It seems that the more intensive the program, the greater the treatment effect [18] .

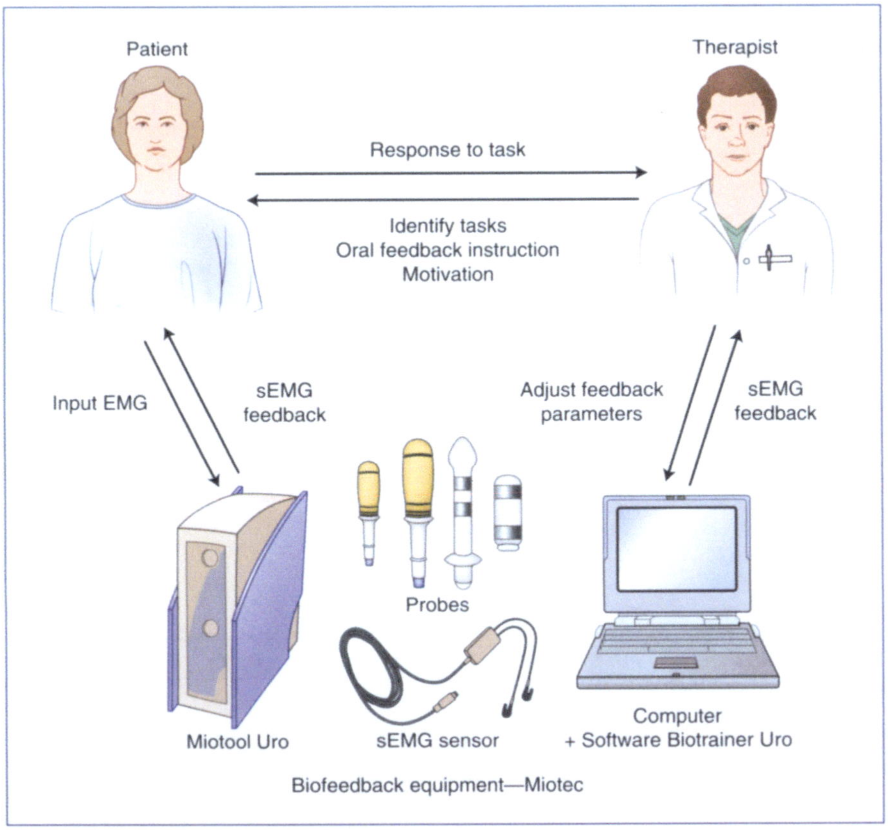

FIGURE 7-22. Electromyogram (EMG) biofeedback as an adjunct to pelvic floor muscle (PFM) exercises. The interaction between a patient and the physical therapist using biofeedback together with PFM exercises or bladder training requires knowledge, experience, and insight into cognitive strategies of the physical therapist, as well as the understanding, sufficient cognitive capacity, and motivation of the patient. The physical therapist must be familiar with the equipment and materials used. Also, all biofeedback equipment and devices for use at home must be easy to handle, safe, and clean. (*Courtesy of* Miotec Equipamentos Biomédicos Ltda; Porto Alegre, Brazil.) sEMG—surface EMG.

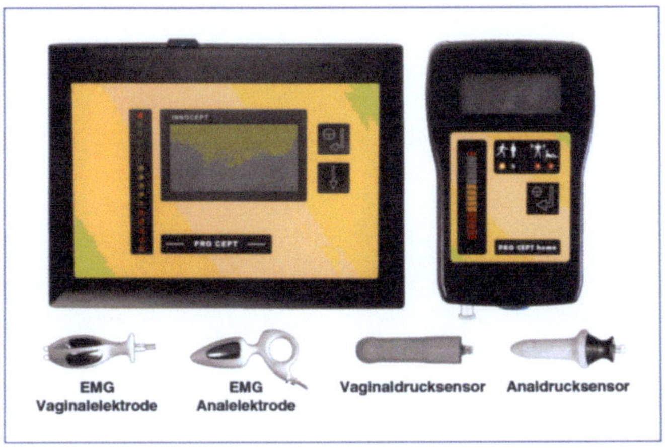

FIGURE 7-23. Practice pelvic floor muscle (PFM) training and biofeedback (BF) in women with stress urinary incontinence or mixed urinary incontinence with a predominant stress factor. BF is no therapy in and of itself; it is only an adjunct to PFM exercises [19]. BF involves the use of equipment to provide visual or auditory feedback about PFM function, which enables a patient to train, strengthen, and increase their endurance and to coordinate PFM contractions. Simple auditory BF can also be provided by the physical therapist, informing the patient when a contraction is felt through digital intravaginal or intrarectal examination during the PFM contraction. EMG—electromyogram. (*Adapted from* Biobedded Medizintechnik, Inc.; Gladbeck, Germany.)

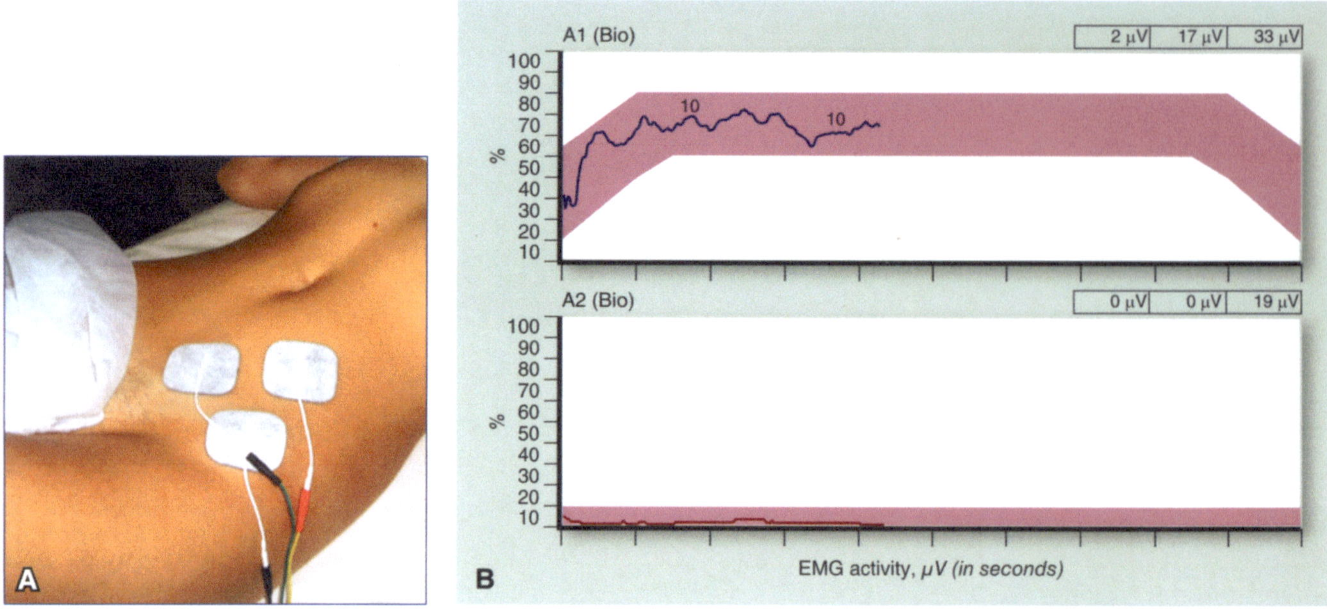

FIGURE 7-24. Electromyogram (EMG) biofeedback (BF). EMG BF, here shown as registered by surface electrodes (**A**), can be used to visualize onscreen (**B**) selective pelvic floor muscle activity (*blue line*) together with the control of any synergistic abdominal muscle activity (*red line*) [1]. (*Courtesy of* VIVALTIS; Montpellier, France.)

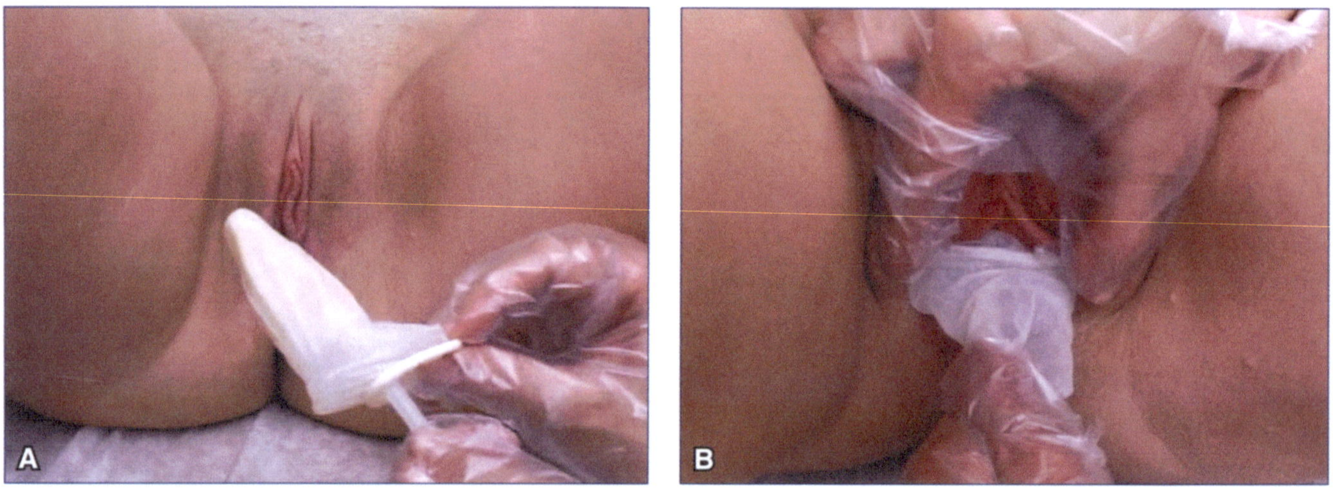

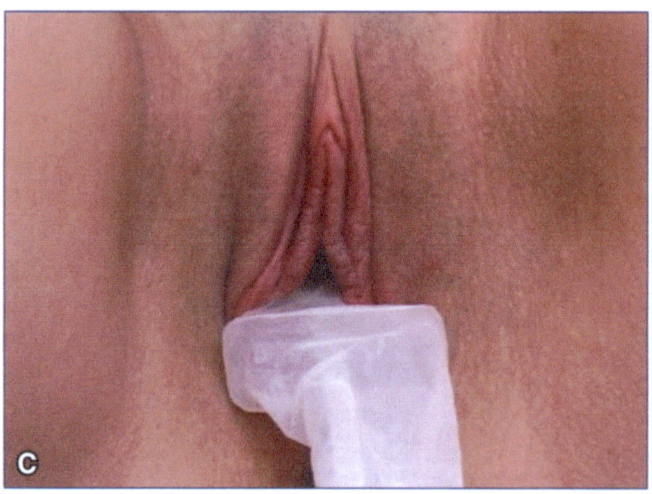

FIGURE 7-25. Biofeedback (BF) with vaginal squeeze pressure measurement. Besides electromyogram BF, manometric BF using pressure devices as shown in **A** can be used.

Technique: first cover the probe with a condom. Put a little gel on top of the probe to avoid any pain or discomfort. **B,** Insert the probe intravaginally about 3.5 cm. Inflate the probe slowly with air and continuously control the already inserted volume to avoid any side effects.

C, The probe should completely link up to the distal part of the vagina without any pain. Wait for 1 or 2 minutes before starting any measurement or training, because the intravaginal temperature will first modify the air inside the probe, changing the outcome of the pressure measurement.

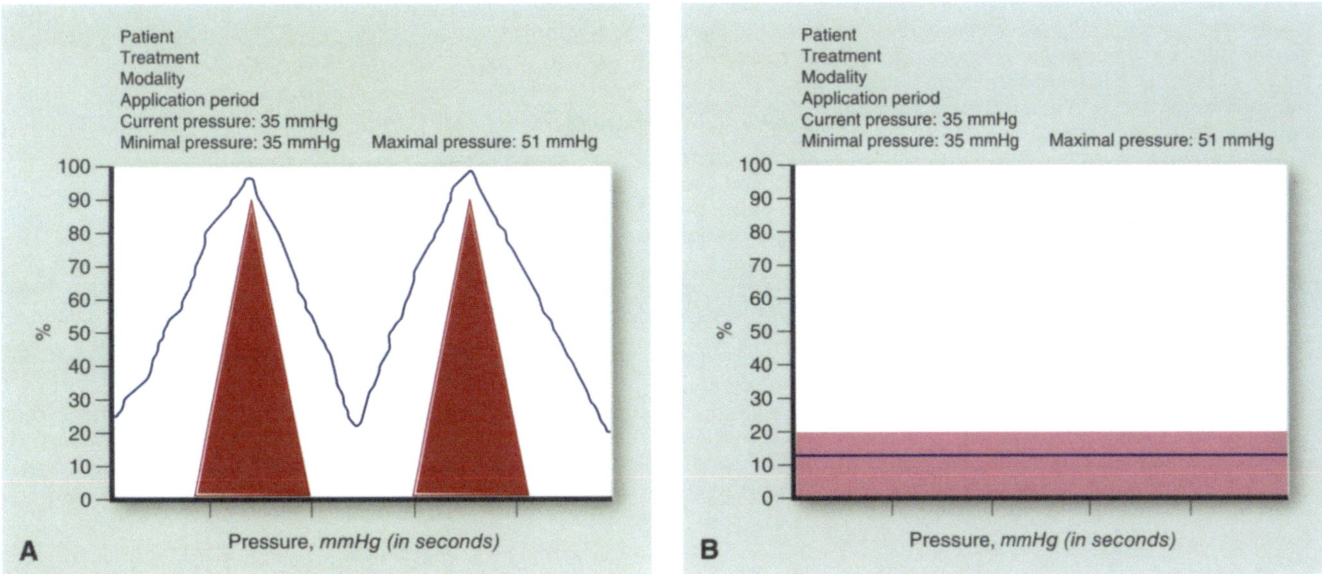

FIGURE 7-26. Quick pelvic floor muscle (PFM) contractions with manometric biofeedback (BF) registration. Both quick and slow PFM contractions should be part of the PFM training program. BF might help to motivate patients to adhere to the program [19].

Quick PFM contractions usually have a maximum duration of 1 to 3 seconds. The patient is instructed to contract the PFM in such a way that the *blue line* will not touch or cross the *red target area*. Between two contractions, the patient is asked to completely relax the PFM. Especially during the first sessions this might be difficult, as can be seen in **A**, where the *blue line* does not reach the lowest possible level, which corresponds with complete PFM relaxation.

Immediately after the training session, a rest period of at least twice the training period is needed, to allow the fast twitch fibers to recover. Because complete relaxation has been shown to be difficult, during this session the target for relaxation (*red*) was set on maximal 20%. **B,** The patient succeeded to stay within this target (*blue line*). (*Courtesy of* Ibramed; Rio de Janeiro, Brazil.)

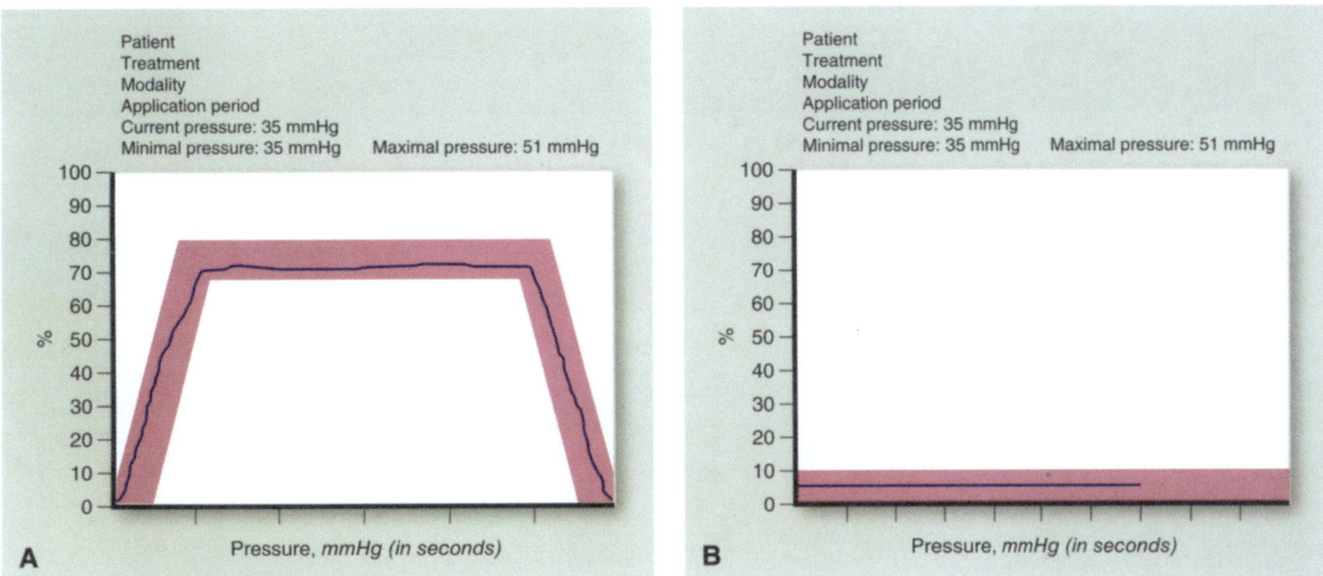

FIGURE 7-27. **A** and **B,** Slow pelvic floor muscle (PFM) contractions with manometric biofeedback registration. Slow PFM contractions have an ideal duration of up to 10 seconds. The patient must try to contract the PFM in such a way that the *blue line* is kept within the *red area*.

After a slow contraction, a rest period of at least the same working time is required. In case the screen shows that the patient cannot relax sufficiently, in the beginning the objective might be 20% with a gradual decrease to less than 10%. (*Courtesy of* Ibramed; Rio de Janeiro, Brazil.)

Figure 7-28. Clinical practical case of woman with stress urinary incontinence (SUI). A 33-year-old woman, diagnosed as having urodynamic SUI 7 months after a traumatic first vaginal delivery and no relevant surgery, was referred to a pelvic physical therapist. The details of her case are given in this figure.

First, treatment instruction and the education of selective pelvic floor muscle (PFM) using contraction and relaxation is performed, using digital palpation (*see* Fig. 7-8), tapping and stretching techniques (*see* Fig. 7-17), or instrumental BF (*see* Fig. 7-23), which is aimed at restoring PFM awareness.

If available, use a home biofeedback (BF) device (*see* Fig. 7-23) with the registration of exercise data and adherence to a home exercise program. Every week, perform one 30-minute physical therapy session and then discuss BF results, PFM training (PFMT), and further instruction. After three in-office PFMT + BF sessions using different activities such as coughing and different positions (*see* Fig. 7-19) and home PFMT for 3 weeks, full restoration of PFM awareness was achieved. Continue with only PFMT and more functional exercises (*see* Fig. 7-19). After another six sessions during the next 2 months, there was a total recovery of PFM functionality. Another 3 months of home PFMT led to total recovery, which was maintained for 2 years as of publication. Outcome measures after 6 months showed: 0 pads; 24-h pad test results of 2 g/24 h; 0 incontinence episodes; visual analogue scale (VAS) 1/10; and strength 5/5.

SUI Clinical Practice Case

Physical examination, observation, intravaginal digital palpation: no awareness of how to contract PFM

Number of pads/24 h: 11

24-h pad test: 84 g/24 h

1-h pad test: 21 g

Incontinence episodes: every increase in intra-abdominal pressure (lifting, sneezing, coughing, laughing, standing up)

VAS 10/10

Strength PFM (modified Oxford scale): 3/5

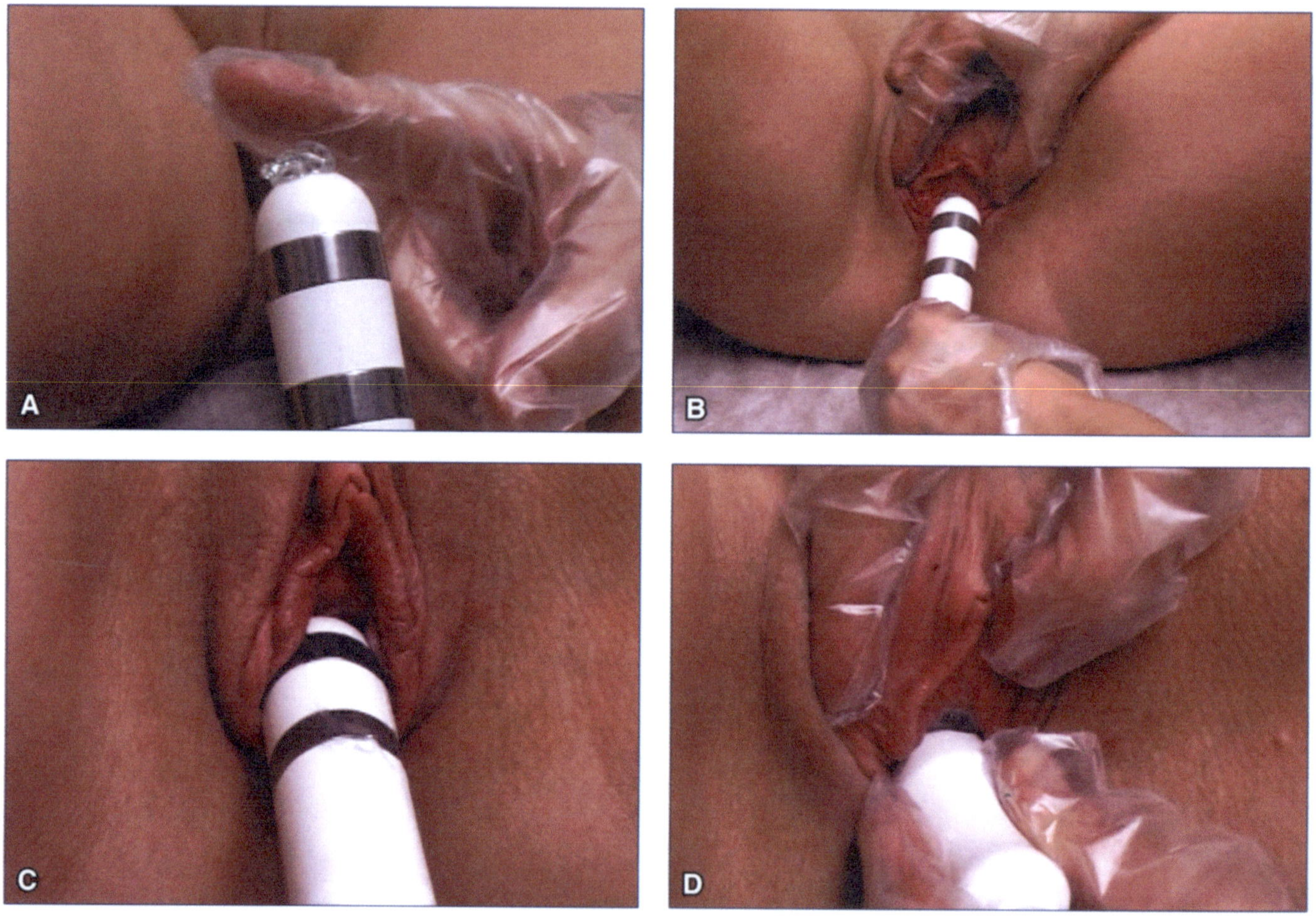

Figure 7-29. Pelvic floor muscle (PFM) training + electrical stimulation (ES) in women with stress urinary incontinence (SUI) or with mixed urinary incontinence in the case of predominant stress factor. Until now, there was no convincing evidence that ES has any additional effect on PFM exercises or is useful as a standalone therapy in women with SUI. It is hypothesized that ES might help those women who are unaware of how to contract the PFM and are not able to do so voluntarily to regain awareness of the PFM by creating an artificial PFM contraction. This hypothesis is still to be tested in a high-quality randomized clinical trial [20].

Parameters for the creation of artificial PFM contractions are frequency 50 Hz, frequency modulation 0.1 second, maximum pulse duration 200 milliseconds, biphasic duty circle 13 seconds 5/8, rectangular at home 20 min/d, and office 1 to 3 times 30 min/wk for 3 months [21]. **A,** It is necessary to put gel on top of the electrical stimulation probe to assure an adequate transmission of the electrical current to the PFM.

After spreading the external vaginal lips (**B**), the physical therapist inserts the probe gently from below. For proper transmission of the electrical current, the metal rings of the probe must be positioned as close as possible to the PFM (**C** and **D**). In the case of the mal position, the patient might experience pain provocation and unpleasant sensations.

In case the patient herself cannot hold the probe inside the vagina (for instance, she strains the PFM instead of contracting inward, pushing the probe outside), the pelvic physical therapist should support the probe during electrical stimulation (**D**).

Continued on the next page

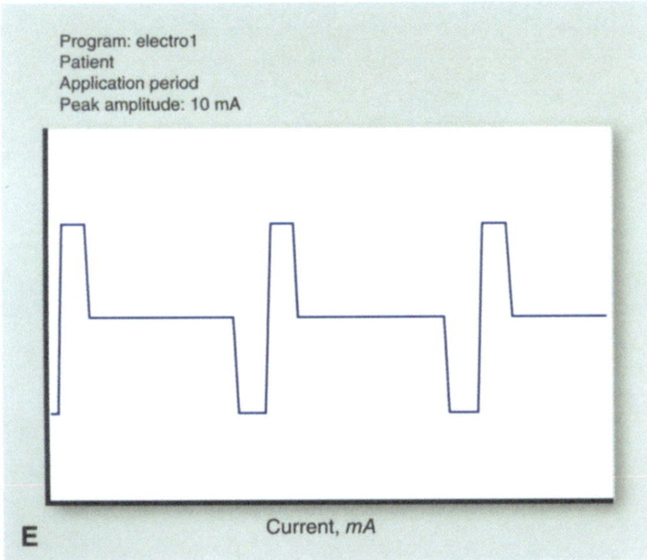

FIGURE 7-29. *(Continued)* During the active electrical stimulation period, the patient contracts the PFM simultaneously (**E**). (**A–D** *courtesy of* ABAFI; Curitiba, Brazil; **E** *courtesy of* Ibramed; Rio de Janeiro, Brazil.)

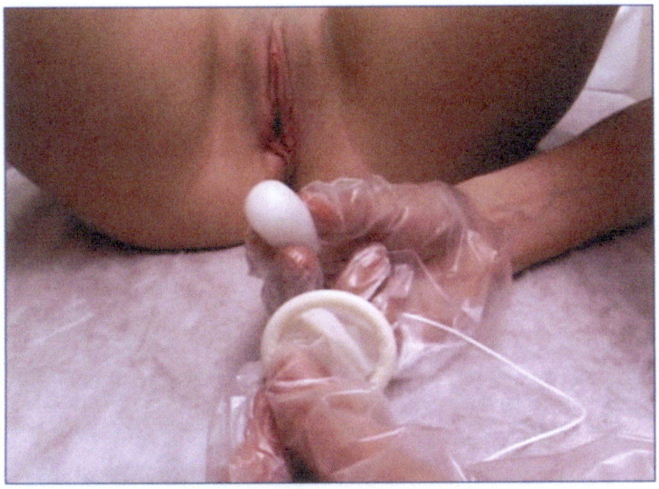

FIGURE 7-30. Vaginal cones. Training the pelvic floor muscle (PFM) with vaginal cones (VCs) is another treatment modality used in women with stress urinary incontinence. Before training, VCs should first be covered with a condom. VCs are inserted intravaginally just above the levator plate. One set consists of cones with different weights (mostly between about 28 and 110 g) but with the same shape. The hypothesis behind this treatment modality is that, in order to strengthen the pelvic floor, the woman holds cones with progressive weights within the vagina by reflexive PFM contractions. Although VC training seems to be superior to no treatment [22], there are doubts about its efficacy and side effects. Holding VC for as long as 15 to 20 minutes, as recommended, may result in unwanted PFM reactions, such as muscle fatigue, pain, or decreased blood supply or oxygen consumption [3]. On the other hand, home VC training with PFM contractions around the cone while simultaneously trying to pull it out in different positions might be useful but needs to be tested in a high-quality randomized clinical trial [3].

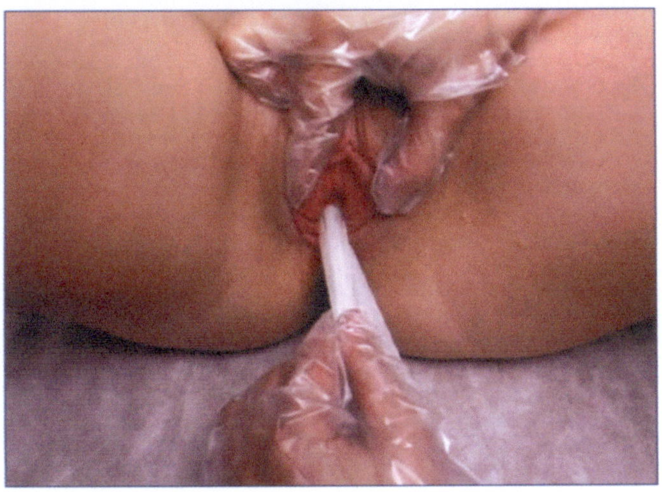

FIGURE 7-31. Stretch reflex using vaginal cones (VCs). The stretch reflex offers good training for propriocepsis. This can be performed by inserting a finger intravaginally or with a VC. The patient is instructed to react immediately to a pull outward as shown here. In this way, both quick pelvic floor muscle contractions and the propriocepsis of the perineum are stimulated.

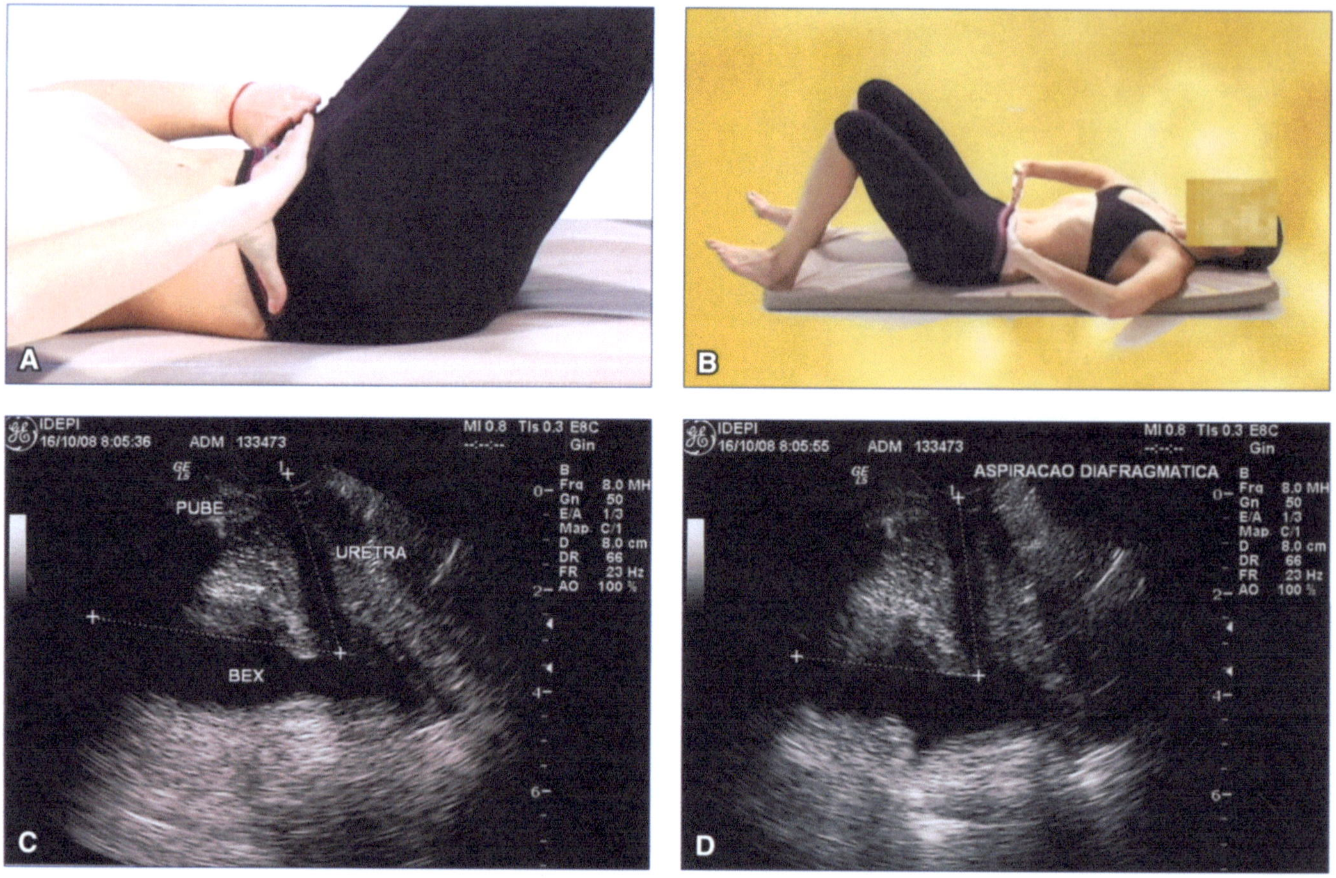

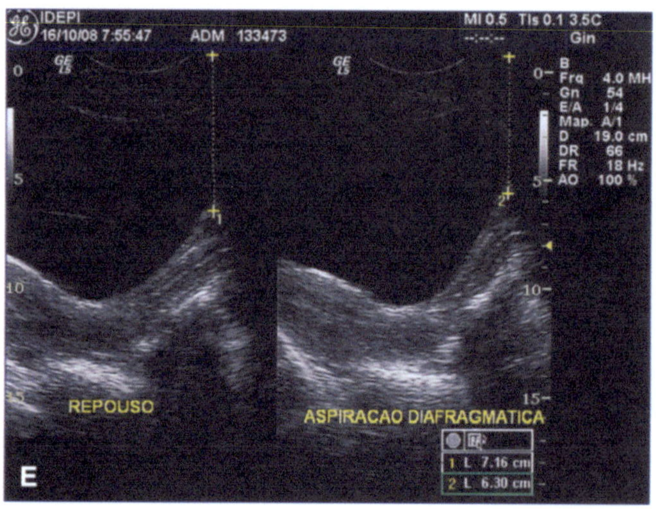

Figure 7-32. Abdominal hypopressive gymnastics for the pelvic floor. Another approach for pelvic floor rehabilitation is the use of hypopressive gymnastics, which are postural techniques that promote lifting the pelvic organs toward the diaphragm, reducing the intra-abdominal pressure and inducing a pelvic floor muscle (PFM) reflex contraction [23]. The original aim was abdominal toning in order to prevent pelvic floor dysfunctions in postpartum women [24].

Although this hypothesis needs to be confirmed in a high-quality study, hypopressive techniques might be a useful strategy for women who are unable to or unaware of how to contract their PFM. Indications for this technique might be postpartum pelvic floor dysfunctions, such as prolapse or urinary incontinence (UI).

The hypopressive technique (**A** and **B**) follows four steps: 1) slow and deep diaphragm inspiration; 2) full expirations (exhale); 3) diaphragm aspiration (progressive contraction of transversus abdominalis and intercostalis muscle); and 4) hold for 10 to 20 seconds (or more) in apnoe.

Hypopressive techniques consist of holding different static positions during a diaphragmatic inspiration, each between 30 seconds and 1 minute long, repeated during 10-minute, twice-daily intervals for a minimum of 3 months.

Sonographic study. **C–I** are from a 30-year-old nulliparous woman without UI and without any former experience in exercising the PFM.

This sonographic study has been realized with a LOGIQ 5 (GE; Amersham, UK) device, abdominal routing with a convex 4-mHz probe, and endovaginally with an 8-mHz probe, during rest and during a diaphragmatic aspiration.

C shows a 65-degree angle between the urethra and the vaginal wall during rest, observed with endovaginal sonography with the bladder minimally filled.

D, The angle between the urethra and the vaginal wall increases by 12 degrees, from 65 degrees during rest to 77 degrees, caused by the diaphragmatic aspiration maneuver, observed with endovaginal sonography with the bladder minimally filled.

E, Measures realized by Goedert A.V. Instituto de Diagnósticos Especiais: based on abdominal sonography with a full bladder, there is a 1.4-cm elevation of the bladder neck during the diaphragmatic aspiration maneuver.

MRI analysis. A comparison **F** during rest with **G** during a diaphragmatic aspiration shows an abdominal wall contraction, elevation of the pelvic organs such as the uterus and the bladder, and the contraction and elevation of the levator ani muscles.

Continued on the next page

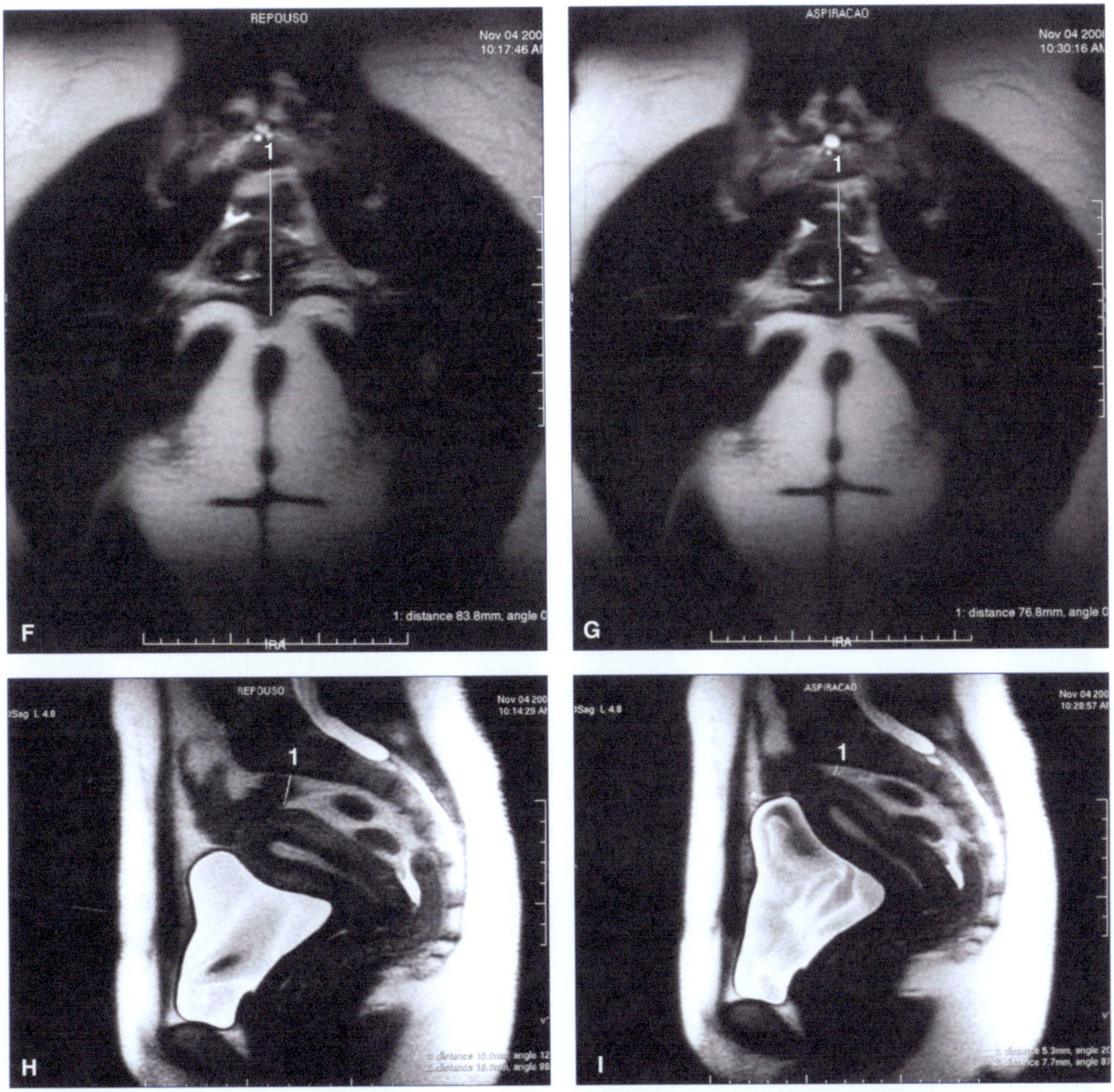

FIGURE 7-32. *(Continued)* **F** and **G** show a distance between the levator ani muscles and the sacrum of 83.8 mm during rest (**F**) and of 76.8 mm during a diaphragmatic aspiration (**G**).

H demonstrates the abdominal muscles during rest and **I** after an abdominal muscle contraction. The angle between the uterus and vagina changes from 31 degrees at rest (**H**) to 45 degrees after diaphragmatic aspiration (**I**). The technique of diaphragmatic aspiration might be useful in patients with voiding problems caused by a descent of the uterus, because lifting the uterus might give space to the formerly oppressed urethra and consequently facilitate the passing of urine. So far this hypothesis has been based only on clinical experience.

Therapeutic Training/Management for Distinguished Problem Areas

Process of therapy

I. PP SUI + dysfunction pelvic floor + no awareness of pelvic floor:

- Digital palpation by patient and/or physical therapist
- Biofeedback + PFMT
- Only in the case of the inability or incapacity of contraction: electrostimulation (intravaginal/extravaginal) + PFMT

Objective: restoration of awareness of the pelvic floor

- If awareness is restored → see next section
- Unsatisfactory results during pilot treatment → back to referring physician

II. PP SUI + dysfunction pelvic floor + awareness of the pelvic floor:

- PFMT + home exercises; isolated contractions of the pelvic floor → with awareness of pelvic floor, single tasks → double tasks → multiple tasks → automatic controlled tasks

Objective:

- Total recovery of the functionality of the pelvic floor
- Duration and extent of urinary incontinence after PPI
- Improvement of the adequate micturition and quality of life
- Improvement of the strength external urethral sphincter during periods of increased abdominal pressure
- Hypertrophy striated muscles increasing the external mechanical pressure on the urethra
- Unsatisfactory results after 3 months → back to referring physician

III. PP SUI + dysfunction pelvic floor + function pelvic floor malinfluenced by disorders tractus respiratorius, other parts tractus motorius, toilet regimen, toilet behavior

- PFMT + home exercises
- Exercises to achieve adequate respiration, postural exercises, relaxation exercises, and lift and squeeze instruction

Objective: reduction or elimination mal-influence disorders, improvement functionality pelvic floor

- Unsatisfactory results after 3 months → back to referring physician

IV. PP SUI + no dysfunction of the pelvic floor (most likely intrinsic sphincter deficiency)

- PFMT + home exercises

Objective: compensation. Expectation: total recovery is not likely

- Unsatisfactory results → back to referring physician

V. PP SUI + general obstructing factors

Objective: maximal possible reduction of these negative factors

- Unsatisfactory results? Back to referring physician

In limited cases of PP UUI:

A) + PP SUI (= MUI) related to:

- Dysfunction of the pelvic floor with or without awareness
- No dysfunction of the pelvic floor
- General obstruction factors

All objectives and treatment modalities mentioned above

B) − PP SUI (stress-induced urgency?) related to:

- Dysfunction (weakness) of the pelvic floor
- PFMT + home exercises
- Relaxation exercises

Objective: total recovery of the functionality of the pelvic floor

- Duration and extent of urinary incontinence after PPI
- Improvement of adequate micturition and quality of life
- Improvement of the strength of the external urethral sphincter during periods of increased abdominal pressure
- Hypertrophy of striated muscles, increasing external mechanical pressure on urethra
- Inhibition of nonphysiological urgency sensations

Related to bladder overactivity

- Electrical stimulation (office and home bound, if available) only
- Electrical stimulation (office and home bound, if available) + PFMT + home exercises
- Electrical stimulation (office and home bound, if available) + bladder training + home exercises
- Bladder training + home exercises
- Bladder training + PFMT + home exercises
- PFMT + home exercises
- PFMT + biofeedback + home exercises
- Relaxation exercises

Objective: inhibition of involuntary detrusor contractions

Evaluation

Treatment results: changes in incontinence and the quality of life

Concluding treatment period and reporting to referring physician

Figure 7-33. Algorithm of the process of therapy for post-prostatectomy incontinence (PPI) in men. PPI mostly leads to stress urinary incontinence (SUI) and in some cases urgency urinary incontinence (UUI). MUI—mixed urinary incontinence; PFMT—pelvic floor muscle training; PP—post-prostatectomy.

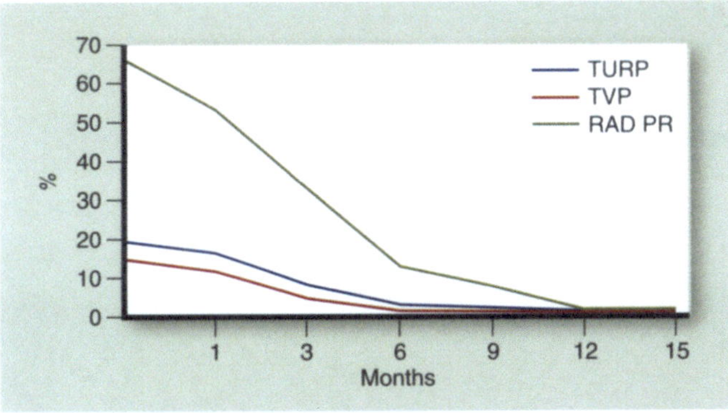

FIGURE 7-34. Incidence of incontinence after transurethral and radical prostatectomy. Urinary incontinence is a significant problem in many men who are undergoing prostate surgery. Symptoms of incontinence after prostatectomy tend to improve over time without intervention [40]. RAD PR—radical prostatectomy; TURP—transurethral radical prostatectomy; TVP—transvesical prostatectomy.

Treatment Modalities for PPI

Pelvic floor muscle training, biofeedback, and electrical stimulation [26]

Number of pelvic floor exercises varied from 36 to 100 exercises per day

Most programs used strength and endurance exercises

Home exercises were divided into three sessions every day: in the morning, in the afternoon, and in the evening

Some therapists instructed their patients to practice interruption of the urinary stream during voiding

Biofeedback involves the use of a device to provide visual or auditory feedback

Electrical stimulation involves any type of stimulation by using transcutaneous electrodes or a rectal probe

FIGURE 7-35. Post-prostatectomy treatment modalities.

Therapeutic Training/Management of Postvoid Dribbling

Absent postvoid urethral milking, residual unexpelled urine in the bulbar urethra

Digital palpation by patient or physical therapist

PFMT

Additional: bulbar urethral massage is performed with the finger behind the scrotum and moving forward and upward

Objective:

- Eliminate the urine left in the bulbar urethra after voiding
- Restoration of awareness of the pelvic floor

FIGURE 7-36. Definition of dribble and the algorithm of the process of physical therapy for postvoid dribble in men. "Terminal dribbling" is the prolonged final part of micturition when the flow has slowed to a dribble. Postvoiding dribble is the involuntary loss of urine immediately after a man has finished passing urine, usually after leaving the toilet. PFMT—pelvic floor muscle training.

Outcome Measures for PPI, LUTS, and Postvoid Dribble

- Outcome measures of PPI
  - Different pad tests
    - 20-min, 40-min, or 1-h ICS and 24- and 48-h pad tests [25]
    - Total volume: amount of urine loss: at home the patient must note the amount of urine loss using a balance with an accuracy of 1 g. 24-h pad test: 2/8/100 g, 1-h ICS pad test: .5 g
    - Total number of pads: 0 and 1 pad is defined as continent
  - Voiding diaries
    - Number of incontinent episodes/24 h, voiding patterns and fluid intake (type and amount)
  - PFM strength test by intrarectal digital palpation
    - Modified Oxford scale: 0–5
  - Subjective severity
    - Visual analogue scale: 0–10
  - Quality of life questionnaires
    - ICS-Male Q
    - IIQ-7
    - EORTC QLQ C30
- Outcome measures for lower urinary tract symptoms
  - American Urological Association Symptom Score
  - International Prostate Symptom Score
- Outcome measures of postvoid dribble
  - Total volume/void: amount of urine loss in grams, usually a small amount of 2–4 g

FIGURE 7-37. Outcome measures in post-prostatectomy incontinence, lower urinary tract symptoms, and postvoid dribble. EORTC QLQ C30—European Organisation for Research and Treatment of Cancer Quality of Life Questionnaire; ICS—International Continence Society; IIQ-7—Incontinence Impact Questionnaire; PFM—pelvic floor muscle.

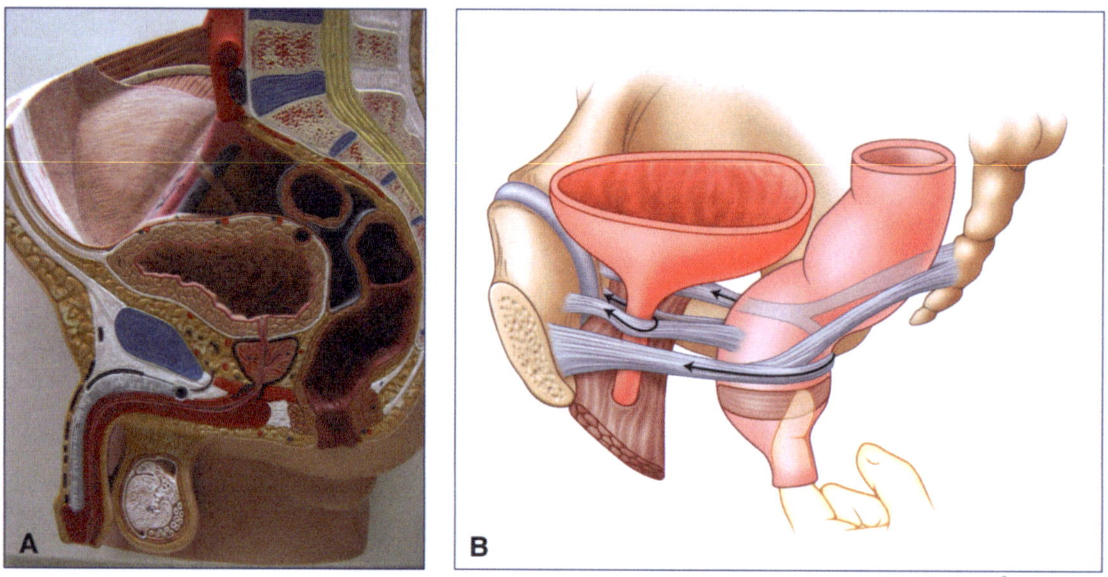

FIGURE 7-38. Pelvic floor muscle training (PFMT) for postprostatectomy incontinence; practice. PFMT was started before prostatectomy or immediately after catheter withdrawal: scheme of treatment.

For the first treatment, the anatomy, pelvic floor, and bladder function were explained using anatomical models (**A**).

Patients were educated in pelvic floor muscle (PFM) awareness and learned how to contract and relax PFM while in a supine position (**B**).

PFM exercises (PFMEs) are manually controlled by a therapist including a verbal explanation and palpation. Contractions can be visualized by using a mirror.

Second and followup treatments include PFMEs in different positions. Patients were invited to practice PFMEs before any activity that might induce incontinence, such as sneezing, coughing, lifting, transferring, or rapid movements. PFMEs should be recommended to all cooperative incontinent patients after transurethral prostatectomy (TURP) or radical prostatectomy [25,26].

Incontinence treatment after TURP took mostly a few weeks [27]. Patients with PPI were treated for as long as any degree of incontinence persisted with a time frame of 1 year.

PFMT guided by a physical therapist enhanced regular PFMT and reduced PPI significantly when it was compared to patients training on their own [28].

Adverse effects of PFM training after prostatectomy are rarely described [29]. Every patient receives individual treatment from once a week to once a month.

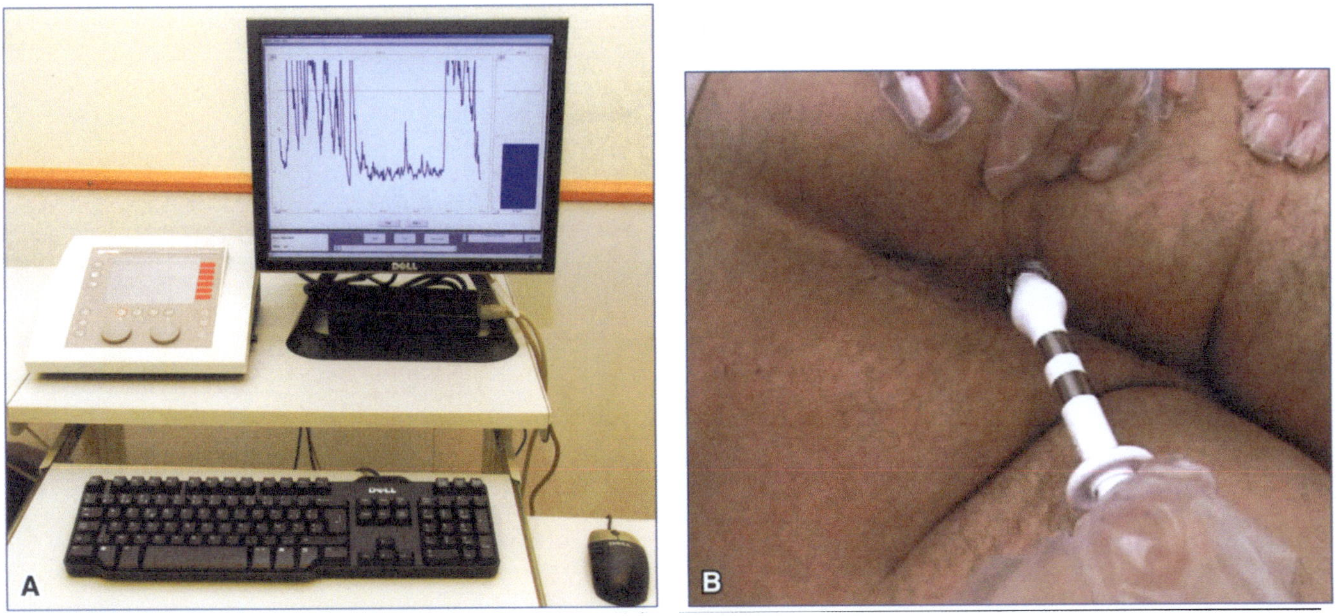

FIGURE 7-39. **A,** Pelvic floor muscle (PFM) training, biofeedback, and electrical stimulation after post-prostatectomy incontinence. Biofeedback can be used as a learning tool to show men how to contract the PFM using visual or auditory feedback. Although no additional effect could be proved by adding biofeedback to exercises alone or verbal instructions, most patients choose this method because it registers their PFM contractions in a clear way.

Also, the use of electrical stimulation (ES) could not add any proven additional effect to exercises performed alone or with instructions only [29,30]. ES after prostatectomy is mostly used in patients with weak PFMs. The parameters for this study were a pulse duration between 200 and 600 microseconds and a frequency of 50 Hz for stress urinary incontinence and between 5 and 10 Hz for overactive bladder.

B, Biofeedback and electrical stimulation of the pelvic floor with an anal probe.

The anal probe should be inserted gently and with the use of gel. In the case of the use of electrical stimulation, ideally the patient tries to contract the PFMs or the external sphincter ani simultaneously with the artificial contraction that is provoked by the electrical current without using the gluteal, abdominal, or adductor muscles.

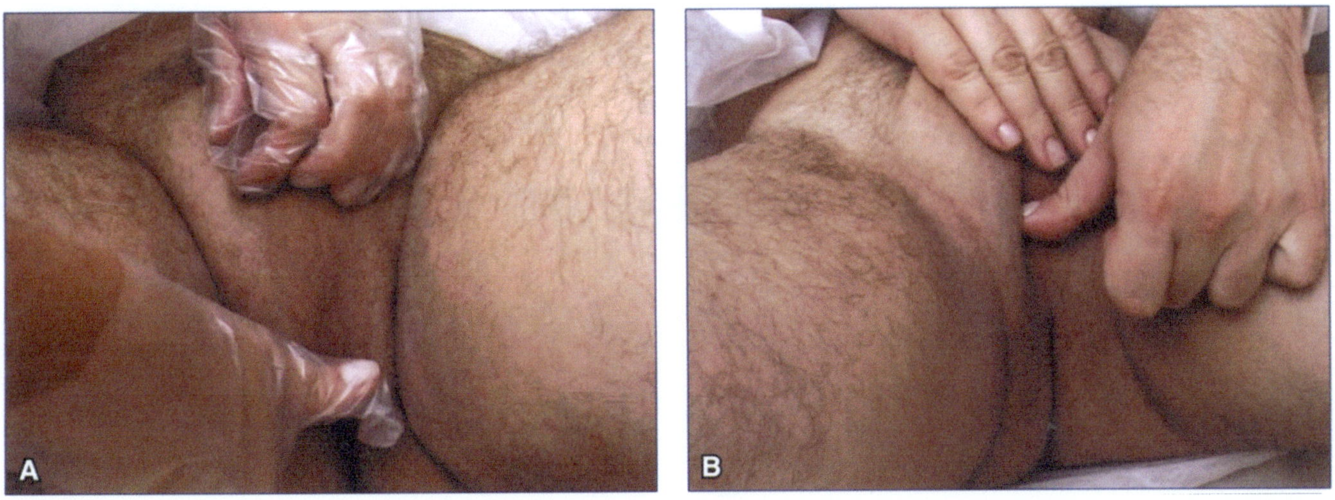

FIGURE 7-40. Postvoid dribble in men. Terminal dribbling is the prolonged final part of micturition when the flow has slowed to a dribble while postvoiding dribble is the involuntary loss of urine immediately after a man has finished passing urine, usually after leaving the toilet.

Therapeutic training/management for distinguished problem areas include: 1) absent postvoid urethral milking, residual unexpelled urine in the bulbar urethra; 2) digital palpation by the patient or physical therapist; 3) pelvic floor muscle training; 4) and bulbar urethral massage (**A** and **B**). The objective is to eliminate the urine left in the bulbar urethra after voiding [31] and to restore awareness of the pelvic floor.

In the case of a male patient who has postvoid dribble, bulbar massage can be performed. The first time, the physical therapist does the procedure while explaining the technique and teaching the patient how to execute this treatment modality. The thumb should be moved from behind the scrotum in a forward and upward direction. The next time the patient himself will do the bulbar massage and will be instructed to perform this at home after every void to avoid any postvoid dribble.

Process of UUI Therapy

Therapeutic training/management for distinguished problem areas

I. UUI related to idiopathic bladder overactivity
- Electrical stimulation (office and home bound, if available) only
- Electrical stimulation (office and home bound, if available) + PFMT + home exercises
- Electrical stimulation (office and home bound, if available) + bladder training + home exercises
- Bladder training + home exercises
- Bladder training + PFMT + home exercises
- PFMT + home exercises
- PFMT + biofeedback + home exercises
- In the case of concurrent hypertone PFM, local relaxation exercises

Objective: inhibition of involuntary detrusor contractions
- Unsatisfactory results→back to referring physician

II. UUI related to neurogenic bladder overactivity
- PFMT + home exercises
- PFMT + biofeedback + home exercises
- Electrical stimulation (office and home bound, if available) only
- Electrical stimulation (office and home bound, if available) + PFMT + home exercises
- Bladder training + home exercises
- Bladder training + PFMT + home exercises
- Behavioral therapy

Objective: maximal possible reduction urgency incontinence, compensation, adaptation

III. UUI related to no dysfunction of the pelvic floor (intrinsic closing mechanism failure)
- PFMT + home exercises
- PFMT + biofeedback + home exercises
- Relaxation exercises

Objective: compensation, total recovery not likely
- Unsatisfactory results →back to referring physician
- Unsatisfactory results → back to referring physician

IV. UUI related to disregulation bladder (central and/or peripheral sensitization)
- Local relaxation exercises
- General relaxation exercises
- Electrical stimulation (office and home bound, if available) only
- Electrical stimulation (office and home bound, if available) + home relaxation exercises
- Modified activity program
- Behavioral therapy

Objective: desensitization, maximal possible reduction urgency, compensation, adaptation
- Unsatisfactory results → back to referring physician

V. UUI related to dysfunction pelvic floor + no awareness of pelvic floor (extrinsic closing mechanism failure)
- Digital palpation by patient or physical therapist
- Electrical stimulation + PFMT
- Biofeedback + PFMT

Objective: restore awareness of the pelvic floor
- If awareness restored → see next section
- Unsatisfactory results → back to referring physician

VI. UUI related to dysfunctional pelvic floor + awareness of the pelvic floor
- If hypotone pelvic floor muscles → PFMT + home exercises; isolated contractions of the pelvic floor → with awareness of pelvic floor, single tasks → double tasks → multiple tasks → automatic controlled tasks
- If hypertone, PFM relaxation exercises

Objective: total recovery (of the functionality of the pelvic floor) → elimination of urgency incontinence
- Unsatisfactory results → back to referring physician

Evaluation

Treatment results: changes in incontinence and quality of life

Concluding treatment period and reporting to referring physician

FIGURE 7-41. Algorithm of the process of therapy for urgency urinary incontinence (UUI). PFM—pelvic floor muscle; PFMT—pelvic floor muscle training.

9-Point Global Rating Scale

- ☐ 1. Very much improved
- ☐ 2. Much improved
- ☐ 3. Moderately improved
- ☐ 4. Slightly improved
- ☐ 5. Unchanged
- ☐ 6. Slightly worse
- ☐ 7. Moderately worse
- ☐ 8. Much worse
- ☐ 9. Very much worse

Figure 7-42. Global perceived effect. As for stress urinary incontinence, for the assessment of urgency urinary incontinence both objective and subjective outcome measures are used, such as quantification of bladder overactivity (*eg*, the detrusor activity index (*see* Fig. 7-43), bladder diaries, quality of life questionnaires (*eg*, I-QOL), and questionnaires to assess severity (*eg*, Protection, Amount, Frequency, Adjustment, Body Image Assessment Tool Questionnaire) or impact (*eg*, IIQ-7).

Besides these outcome measures, a rating of the global perceived effect at each assessment is important because it gives an impression about meaningful change or a benefit caused by the physical therapeutic intervention. The patient is asked to rate his or her overall status change from baseline using the global rating scale, a nine-point global rating scale, as shown here, or on an 11-point scale with the addition of "completely recovered" or "worse than ever," by using the following question: "How is your current condition compared to how it was before you started physical therapy treatment?" Ratings of 4 to 6 are considered to be no meaningful change (minimal clinical important change or benefit).

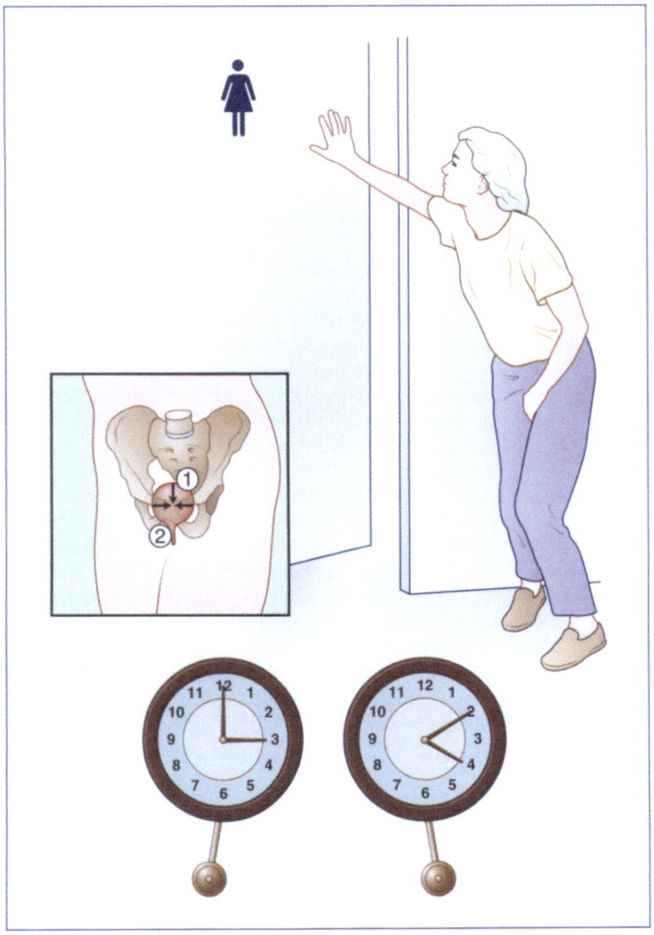

Figure 7-43. Bladder training (BLT) in patients with overactive bladder or mixed urinary incontinence (in the case of predominant urgency factor). BLT is a rather simple, usually not costly, and safe treatment modality without side effects [20].

The objective of BLT is to restore normal bladder function through a process of patient education along with a mandatory or self-adjustable voiding regimen that gradually increases the time interval between consecutive voids.

BLT is especially attractive for use in elderly patients who refrain from other therapies such as medication. It can be used as solid treatment or combined with drug therapy or pelvic floor muscle training (PFMT); the combination is sometimes called LUTE (lower urinary tract exercises = BLT + PFMT). The BLT effect might be augmented with caffeine reduction if the patient's intake is greater than 100 mg/d.

To practice BLT, use the following steps: 1) determine the initial voiding interval, based on the baseline voiding frequency; 2) set a 1-hour interval during waking hours, but make an individual adjustment if this time period is initially too long; 3) if there are fewer leakage episodes than the week before, urgency can be controlled by the individual by smoothly adhering to the scheme and increasing the schedule by 15 to 30 minutes each week; 4) inform and educate patients on normal bladder function and control; 5) teach patients distraction and relaxation techniques, pelvic floor muscle contraction, and relaxation; 6) follow supervised self-monitoring using voiding diaries; 7) the clinician will offer feedback and evaluate progress, provide positive reinforcement, and change the schedule if necessary. If there is no improvement after 3 weeks of BLT, reevaluate and reconsider the therapy.

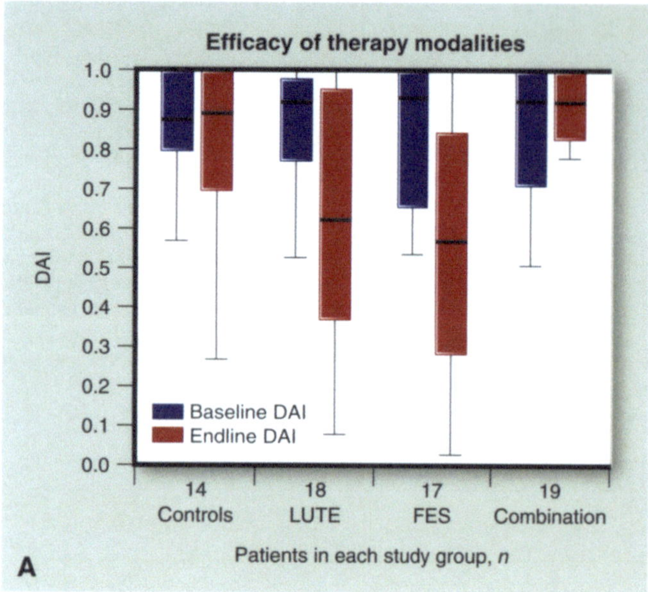

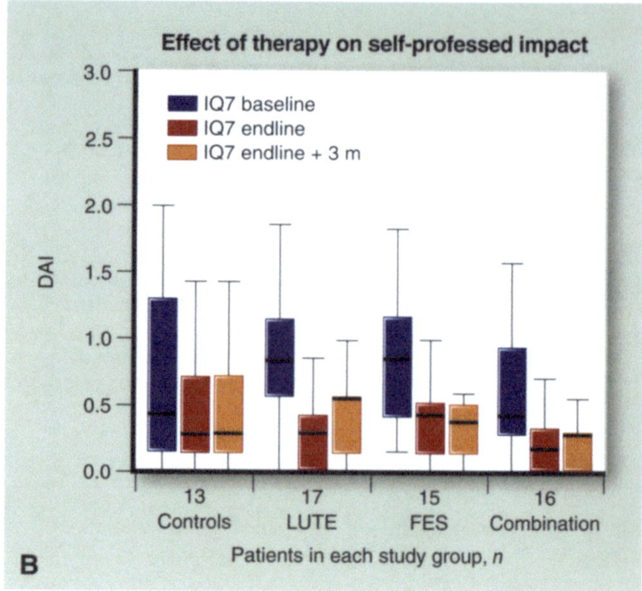

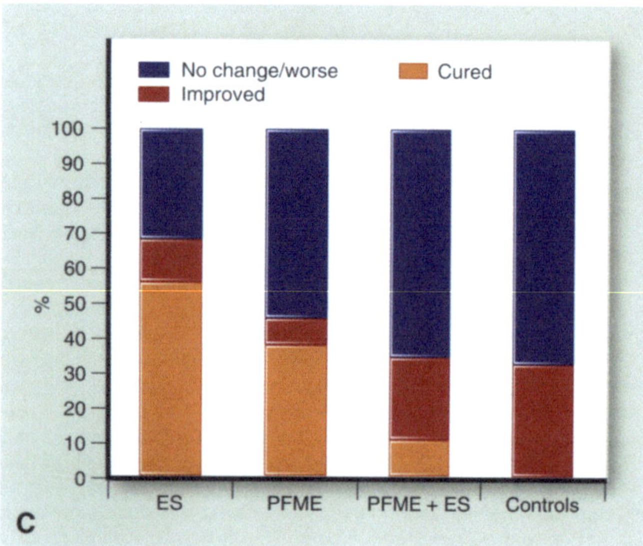

FIGURE 7-44. Efficacy of functional electrical stimulation in women with proven overactive bladder (OAB). Of the different treatment modalities used for women with OAB, functional electrical stimulation (FES) might be the treatment of first choice [20].

This figure shows (**A**) the Detrusor Activity Index (DAI) and (**B**) the Impact Incontinence Questionnaire (IIQ-7) outcomes and (**C**) percentages of cured, improved, and no change/worse of a randomized clinical trial in women with OAB comparing FES, pelvic floor muscle exercises, and bladder training (lower urinary tract exercises), a combination of the former treatment modalities and no treatment (controls). Women with symptomatic OAB received ambulatory urodynamics (ACM). Based on both urodynamic variables of ACM and the micturition diary, the DAI for each patient was calculated. The DAI model quantifies detrusor activity during consecutive filling phases during extramural ambulatory cystometry [32]. A DAI score of 0 represents no OAB, DAI greater than 0.50 defines proven OAB, and 1 represents severe OAB. OAB patients received nine treatment sessions, once weekly, of office-bound and daily home-based FES (*see* Fig. 7-44). DAI and IIQ-7 were measured before starting and after FES, and 3 months after treatment. The only decrease in DAI scores in the FES group was statistically significant (P = 0.032) in comparison with no treatment. FES seems to be effective [15]. PFME—pelvic floor muscle exercise.

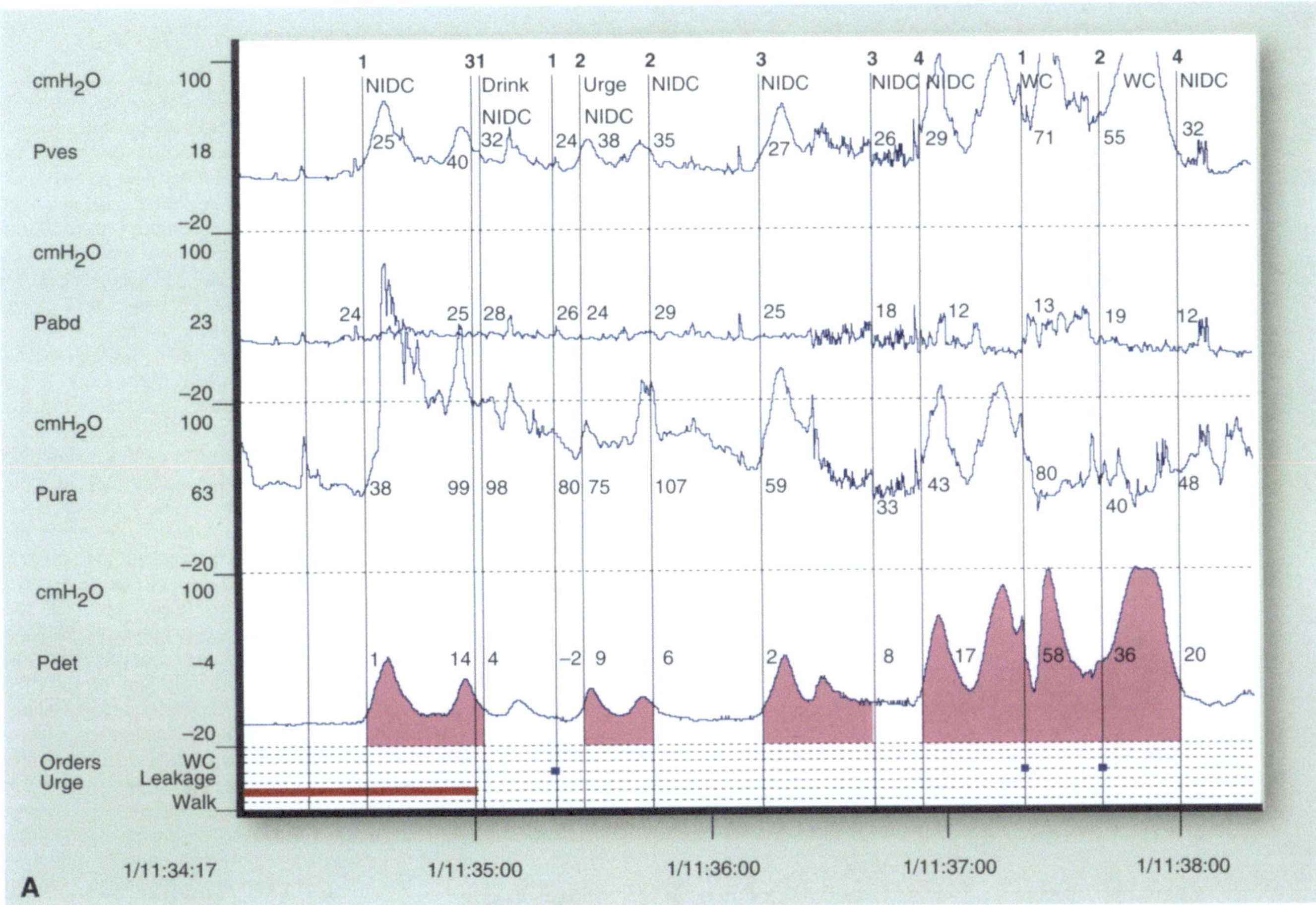

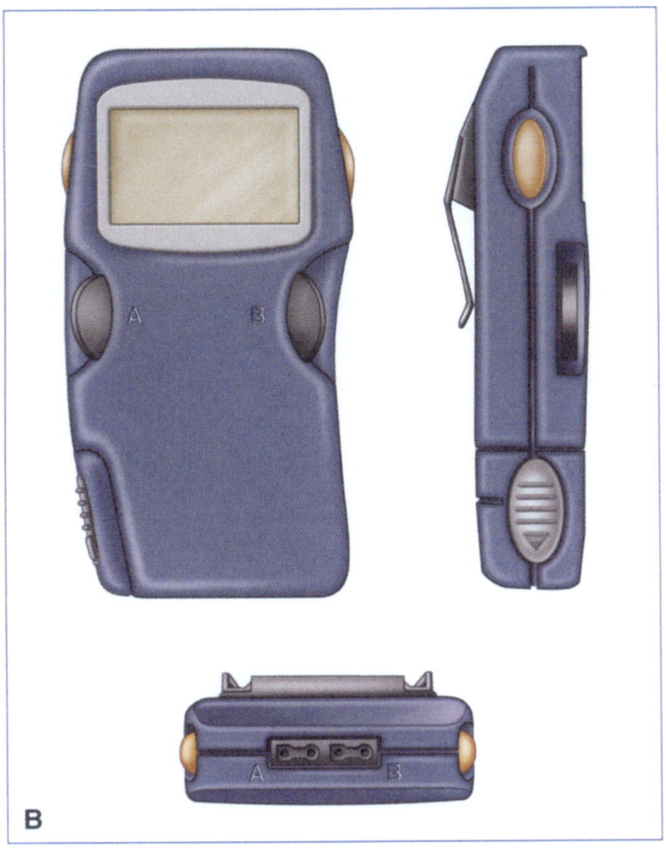

Figure 7-45. Practical case of overactive bladder (OAB) using the ProUrge system (Biobedded Medizintechnik, Inc.; Gladbeck, Germany) (**A**). Details of the registration of ambulatory urodynamic investigation in a 59-year-old woman with proven OAB are given. Involuntary detrusor contractions can be seen during the filling phase of the bladder.

The patient underwent ambulatory urodynamics using the Detrusor Activity Index (DAI) model [31], resulting in a pretreatment DAI of 0.68 (proven OAB) and 0.03 posttreatment (nonoveractive). Treatment consisted of nine 30-minute office-based functional electrostimulation (FES) sessions (**B**), once weekly, and home-based FES of two 20-minute sessions per day with an interval of more than 6 hours. FES was applied vaginally through a plug-mounted electrode. The maximum level of current stimulation was 100 mA (I_{eff} = 6 mA). The current characteristics were maximal tolerable stimulation, a frequency modulation of 0.1-second trains of rectangular biphasic 200-µsec-long pulses that varied stochastically between 4 and 10 Hz. Besides the DAI, the Incontinence Impact Questionnaire-7 was used to measure the self-professed impact of incontinence. In this patient, the objective cure and no more impact of incontinence were realized. All sessions were realized according to protocol. There were no side effects or adverse events and the results were maintained at least for 24 weeks after the end of treatment. (**B** *adapted from* Biobedded Medizintechnik, Inc.; Gladbeck, Germany.)

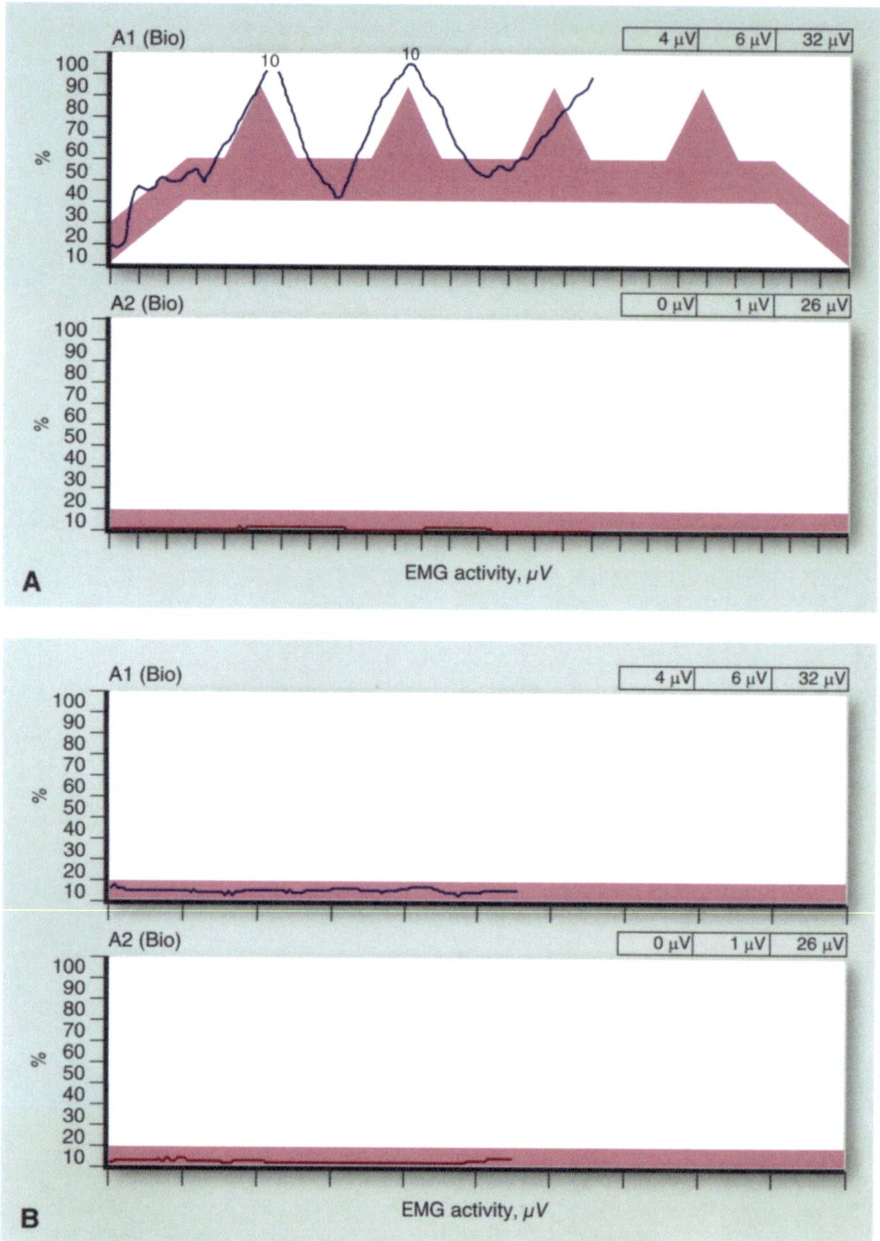

FIGURE 7-46. Pelvic floor muscle training (PFMT) with or without biofeedback (BF) for overactive bladder (OAB) or mixed urinary incontinence (in the case of predominant urgency factor). Until now, the role of PFMT with or without BF for OAB was yet to be established. Limited randomized clinical trial evidence [15, 33,34] and clinical experience show that PFMT aim at the inhibition of overactivity of the bladder. The patient is taught specific pelvic floor muscle exercises (PFMEs) to likely facilitate and restore the detrusor inhibition reflex (DIR) by selective pelvic floor muscle (PFM) contraction [35]. In many patients with OAB, the level of activation is so high that selective PFM contraction in order to achieve reciprocal bladder inhibition is very difficult if not impossible [36]. Teaching selective PFM contraction and relaxation is an important first step. Although the additional benefit has not been shown yet [34], BF as an adjunct to PFMT may help to achieve selective contraction and relaxation (discussed earlier). **A,** Once this is achieved, a selective PFM contraction focuses on facilitating the DIR. After using digital palpation by the physical therapist to test a patient's ability to hold contractions for at least 20 seconds, patients are instructed to do so, followed by a relaxation period of 10 seconds. More functional training (PFME during daily living activities) completes the exercise program. The treatment duration is between 3 and 6 months and the treatment frequency is once per week in the office and daily at home.

A shows a continuous PFM submaximal contraction with some rapid peaks to inhibit sudden sensations of urgency. The PFM contractions must be strong enough to realize a depolarization of the afferent pudendal nerve fibers, ultimately leading to a stimulation of the DIR [15]. During the PFM contraction(s), the abdominal muscles stay relaxed.

B, During the training session the patient gets time to rest, but during daily life the patient must continue the PFM contraction until inhibition of the detrusor is realized or the toilet is reached. (*Courtesy of* VIVALTIS; Montpellier, France.)

PFMT Training Protocol: Neurogenic OAB With or Without BF

4-8 × 6-contractions, 6-s rest; 3-s contractions, 3-s rest; 30-s contractions, 30-s rest in different positions can be considered if without BF

Group training (6–8 patients)

1 h/wk during outpatient treatment; home exercises 1–2 times per day can be considered if without BF

FIGURE 7-47. Neurogenic overactive bladder practices pelvic floor muscle training (PFMT) with or without biofeedback (BF). The role of pelvic floor physical therapy for bladder problems in specific neurological diseases is minimally investigated; for PFMT, only stroke is investigated. PFMT for stroke patients provided a significant improvement of frequency of voiding, 24-hour home pad test, and pelvic floor muscle endurance. No data are available on the use of BF as an adjunct to PFMT.

PFMT Training Protocol: Neurogenic OAB Practice (PFMT + ES)

ES

Interferential currents carrier frequency of 2000-Hz treatment with a frequency of 5–10 Hz, 10–50 Hz, and 50 Hz, 10 min of each frequency, 3 min rest in between

PFMT

10 3-s PFM contractions, 3-s rest, 5 5-s PFM contractions, 10-s rest, 5 15-s PFM contractions, 30-s rest; others: 5 times in different positions

Home exercises: 20 PFM contractions 3–5 times per week; 6 months in the sitting and standing positions, respectively

6 sessions during 21 d on an outpatient basis

Figure 7-48. Neurogenic overactive bladder practice (pelvic floor muscle training [PFMT] + electrical stimulation [ES]). The role of pelvic floor physical therapy for bladder problems in specific neurological diseases is minimally investigated. So far, PFMT combined with ES is only investigated in multiple sclerosis (MS) patients with urinary incontinence [37]. PFMT + ES decreased the urgency, frequency, incontinence, and nocturia and improved the bladder emptying and pelvic floor muscle (PFM) activity compared with patients who received only mobilizations. The prognosis of PFMT effect in MS patients might be higher in those without pelvic floor spasticity or detrusor external sphincter dyssynergia [38].

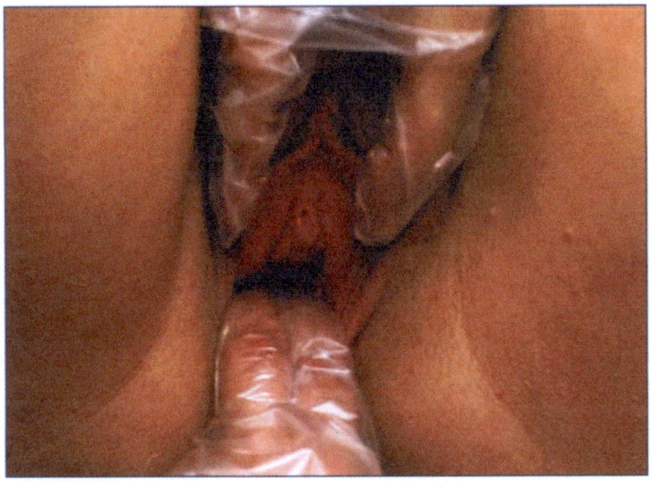

Figure 7-49. Inspection of an anterior vaginal wall prolapse. During the digital palpation, the investigator asks the patient for a maximal push down to demonstrate any existence of anterior vaginal wall prolapse. If so, the nature and severity (degree) must be assessed. The pelvic organ prolapse quantification examination (POP-Q) [13] is used to quantify the degree of the pelvic organ prolapse. In this image, an anterior vaginal wall prolapse, grade I, can be identified.

DeLancey *et al.* [39] showed, in a randomized clinical trial comparing 151 women with prolapse and 135 controls with normal support determined by POP-Q, that women with prolapse have reduced muscle strength and generated less vaginal closure force during pelvic floor muscle (PFM) contraction than controls.

Physical therapeutic interventions for prolapse include PFM assessment, PFM exercise, and PFM bracing against increased intra-abdominal pressure (*eg*, lifting, coughing). The working mechanisms of the PFM training (PFMT) for the aid of prolapse are morphological changes ("stiffness" of the pelvic floor, *ie*, a rigid but still flexible adequate layer of pelvic floor components such as muscles and collagen tissue) occurring after strength training and the use of a conscious contraction during the increase in abdominal pressure in daily activities [40]. There is urgent need to clarify the importance and place of PFMT in the prevention and management of prolapse [41].

References

1. Berghmans LCM, Bernards ATM, Bø K, Grupping MHM: Guidelines for the physiotherapeutic management of genuine stress incontinence. *Phys Ther Rev* 1998, 3:133–147.
2. ICS Pelvic Floor Clinical Assessment Group: Terminology of pelvic floor function and dysfunction. *ICS Report*, 2001.
3. Bø K, Berghmans B, Mørkved S, Kampen M Van, eds: *Evidence-Based Physiotherapy for the Pelvic Floor: Bridging Science and Clinical Practice*, edn 1. Philadelphia: Elsevier; 2007.
4. Bump RC, Mattiasson A, Bø K, *et al.*: The standardisation of terminology of female pelvic organ prolapse and pelvic floor dysfunction. *Amer J Obstet Gynecol* 1996, 175:10–17.
5. Laycock J: Clinical evaluation of the pelvic floor. In *Pelvic Floor Re-education*. New York: Springer-Verlag; 2003:42–48.
6. Hendriks E, Bernards A, Berghmans B, Bie R: The psychometric properties of the PRAFAB-questionnaire: a brief assessment questionnaire to evaluate severity of urinary incontinence in women. *Neurourol Urodyn* 2007, 26:998–1007.
7. Vierhout ME: Meting van ongewenst urineverlies bij de vrouw. [Measurement of unvoluntary urine loss in women]. *Nederlands Tijdschrift voor de Geneeskunde* 1990, 134:1837–1840.
8. Donovan J, Bosch R, Gotoh M, *et al.*: Symptoms and quality of life assessment. In *Incontinence*, vol 1, edn 3. Paris: Health Publication; 2005:519–585.
9. Berghmans LCM, Hendriks HJM, Bø K, *et al.*: Conservative treatment of stress urinary incontinence in women: a systematic review of randomized clinical trials. *Br J Urol* 1998, 82:181–191.
10. Jaeschke R, Singer J, Guyatt GH: Measurement of health status. Ascertaining the minimal clinically important difference. *Control Clin Trials* 1989, 10:407–415.
11. World Health Organization: International classification of functioning, disability and health. Available at www.who.int/classifications/icf/en/
12. Kalichman L: Perineal massage to prevent perineal trauma in childbirth. *J Isr Med Assoc* 2008, 10:531–533.
13. Bump R, Hurt WG, Fantl JA, *et al.*: Assessment of Kegel exercise performance after brief verbal instruction. *Am J Obstet Gynecol* 1991, 165:322–329.
14. Bø K, Larsen S, Oseid S, *et al.*: Knowledge about and ability to correct pelvic floor muscle exercise in women with urinary stress incontinence. *Neurourol Urodynam* 1988, 7:261–262.
15. Berghmans LCM, Van Waalwijk van Doorn ESC, *et al.*: Efficacy of physical therapeutic modalities in women with proven bladder overactivity. *Eur Urol* 2002, 41:581–588.
16. Janssen CC, Lagro-Janssen AL, Felling AJ: The effects of physiotherapy for female urinary incontinence: individual compared with group treatment. *Br J Urol Int* 2001, 87:201–206.
17. Viktrup L, Rortveit B, Lose G: Risk of stress urinary incontinence twelve years after the first pregnancy and delivery. *Obstet Gynecol* 2006,108:248–254.
18. Hay-Smith EJC, Fairbrother KA, Morkved S, Herbison P: Pelvic floor muscle training for prevention and treatment of urinary and faecal incontinence in antenatal and postnatal women. *Cochrane Database Syst Rev* 2008, CD007471 (online).

19. Berghmans LCM, Frederiks CMA, Bie RA de, *et al.*: Efficacy of biofeedback, when included with pelvic floor muscle exercise treatment, for genuine stress incontinence. *Neurourol Urodynam* 1996, 15:37–52.

20. Wilson D, Hay-Smith J, Berghmans B, *et al.*: Adult conservative management. In *Incontinence*, vol 2, edn 3. Paris: Health Publication; 2005:857–964.

21. Fall M, Madersbacher H: Peripheral electrical stimulation. In *Urodynamics: Principles, Practice and Application*, edn 2. Edinburgh, UK: Churchill Livingstone; 1994:495–520.

22. Herbison GP, Dean N: Weighted vaginal cones for urinary incontinence. *Cochrane Database Syst Rev* 2002, DOI: 10.1002/14651858.CD002114.

23. Caufriez M: *Thérapies Manuelles et Instrumentales en Uro-gynécologie*, vol 2. Brussels, Belgium: Maite; 1989.

24. Caufriez M: *Gymnastique Abdominale Hypopressive*. Brussels, Belgium: 1997.

25. Hunter KF, Moore KN, Glazener CMA: Conservative management for postprostatectomy urinary incontinence. *Cochrane Database Syst Rev* 2007, 2:1–43.

26. Van Kampen M, De Weerdt W, Van Poppel H, *et al.*: Effect of pelvic-floor reeducation on duration and degree of incontinence after radical prostatectomy: a randomized controlled trial. *Lancet* 2000, 355:98–102.

27. Chang PL, Tsai TH, Huang ST, *et al.*: The early effect of pelvic floor muscle exercise after transurethral prostatectomy. *J Urol* 1998, 160:402–405.

28. Overgård M, Angelsen A, Lydersen S, Mørkved S: Does physiotherapist-guided pelvic floor muscle training reduce urinary incontinence after radical prostatectomy? A randomised clinical trial. *Eur Urol* 2008, 54:438–448.

29. Moore KN, Griffiths D, Hughton A: Urinary incontinence after radical prostatectomy: a randomized controlled trial comparing pelvic muscle exercises with or without electrical stimulation. *Br J Urol Int* 1999, 83:57–65.

30. Wille S, Sobottka A, Heidenreich A, *et al.*: Pelvic floor exercises, electrical stimulation and biofeedback after radical prostatectomy: results of a prospective randomized trial. *J Urol* 2003, 170:490–493.

31. Paterson J, Pinnock CB, Marshall VR: Pelvic floor exercises as a treatment for post-micturition dribble. *Br J Urol* 1997, 79:892–897.

32. Van Waalwijk-van Doorn ESC, Ambergen AW: Diagnostic assessment of the overactive bladder during the filling phase: the Detrusor Activity Index. *Br J Urol* 1999, 83(Suppl 2):16–21.

33. Millard R: Clinical efficacy of tolterodine with or without a simplified pelvic floor exercise regimen. *Neurourol Urodynam* 2004, 23:48–53.

34. Wang A, Wang Y, Chen M: Single-blind, randomized trial of pelvic floor muscle training, biofeedback-assisted pelvic floor muscle training, and electrical stimulation in the management of overactive bladder. *Urology* 2004, 63:61–66.

35. Houston KA: Incontinence and the older woman. *Clin Geriatr Med* 1993, 9:157–171.

36. Messelink EJ: The overactive bladder and the role of the pelvic floor muscles. *Br J Urol* 1999, 83(Suppl 2):31–35.

37. Vahtera T, Haaranen Oskela AL: Pelvic floor rehabilitation is effective in patients with multiple sclerosis. *Clin Rehab* 1997, 11:211–219.

38. De Ridder D, Vermeulen C, Ketelaer P, *et al.*: Pelvic floor rehabilitation in multiple sclerosis. *Acta Neurologica Belgica* 1999, 99: 61–64.

39. DeLancey JO, Morgan DM, Fenner DE, *et al.*: Comparison of levator ani muscle defects and function in women with and without pelvic organ prolapse. *Obstetrica Gynecologia* 2007, 109:295–302.

40. Bø K: Can pelvic floor muscle training prevent and treat pelvic organ prolapse? *Acta Obstetrica Gynecologia Scand* 2006, 85:263–268.

41. Thakar R, Stanton S: Management of genital prolapse. *BMJ* 2002, 324:1258–1262.

8

Pharmacology and Pharmacologic Treatment of the Male Bladder Outlet

Doreen E. Chung and Alexis E. Te

The male bladder outlet includes the bladder trigone, bladder neck, prostate, urethra, and external sphincter. One of the most prevalent pathologic conditions affecting the male bladder outlet is benign prostatic hyperplasia (BPH), which is a benign histologic process of hyperplasia that contributes to, but is not solely responsible for, lower urinary tract symptoms (LUTS) in the aging male. Previously, LUTS in older men were considered to be completely a result of increased prostate mass and elevated urethral resistance. These symptoms were known as "prostatism." However, we now understand that LUTS in the aging male are only partially due to BPH and are also caused by age-related detrusor dysfunction as well as bladder outlet obstruction-related detrusor dysfunction and overactivity [1].

Historically, the only options for the treatment of LUTS in the aging male were surgery and watchful waiting. Transurethral resection of the prostate (TURP) was developed in the 1920s and became the new gold standard of treatment. TURP is less invasive and morbid than is open prostatectomy; however, it does have some disadvantages. Immediate complications include bleeding, transurethral syndrome, and sepsis [2]. Long-term complications, such as bladder neck contracture, urethral stricture, erectile dysfunction, retrograde ejaculation, and incontinence, may also occur. Both procedures have a small but real mortality risk. With the advent of new drugs to treat BPH-related symptoms, in the last 20 years medical therapy has become the most prevalent form of treatment for BPH-related LUTS [3]. This has also led to a better understanding of the complex pharmacologic basis of the male bladder outlet and related pathophysiologies. This chapter focuses on the pharmacology and pharmacologic treatment of the male bladder outlet.

This chapter is divided into two parts. The first half discusses the pharmacology of the bladder outlet, knowledge that is essential to understand the pharmacologic treatment of LUTS in the aging male. In order to fully appreciate the pharmacology of the bladder outlet, we have also included figures of relevant anatomy, neuroanatomy, and the pathophysiology of BPH.

The second half of this chapter illustrates the pharmacologic treatment of the male bladder outlet, specifically the treatment of BPH-related symptoms. The symptoms of BPH can be treated through various mechanisms including urethral smooth muscle relaxation, the inhibition of prostate growth, and anticholinergic activity. We describe the major drug classes and their mechanism of action, efficacy, side effects, and key studies. As well, we discuss combination therapies. At the end of the chapter, we discuss phytotherapy and newer therapies that are currently being introduced for the treatment of BPH-related symptoms. A better understanding of the pharmacology and pharmacologic treatment of the male bladder outlet will aid the physician in clinical decision-making for the treatment of LUTS in the aging male.

Background Information

Relevant Anatomy of the Male Bladder Outlet

Components of the Male Bladder Outlet
Bladder trigone
Bladder neck
Prostate
Urethra
External sphincter

Figure 8-1. Components of the male bladder outlet.

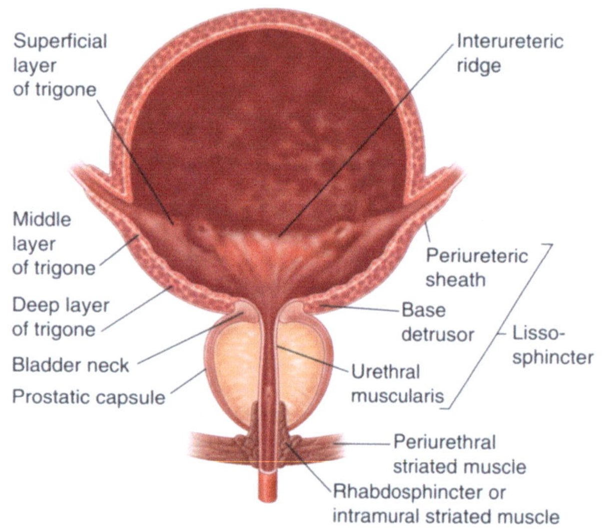

Figure 8-2. Male bladder outlet. At the trigone, three distinct layers of smooth muscle are present: a superficial longitudinal layer, a middle circular layer, and an inner longitudinal layer. The middle circular layer of smooth muscle contracts at the level of the bladder neck and contributes to continence. This layer has adrenergic innervation and contracts in response to adrenergic stimulation. The inner longitudinal layer of smooth muscle runs continuously from the bladder base to the prostatic urethra. Histologic studies show that the smooth muscle fibers in the prostatic urethra interdigitate with the prostatic capsule [4]. In addition to smooth muscle, the male urethra is also composed of striated muscle. There are two striated muscle components, the periurethral striated muscle of the pelvic floor and the rhabdosphincter. The periurethral striated muscle extends from the base of the bladder, through the prostatic capsule, and across the membranous urethra. The rhabdosphincter is located at the prostatic apex and is composed of circular fibers. It is located medial to the periurethral striated muscle.

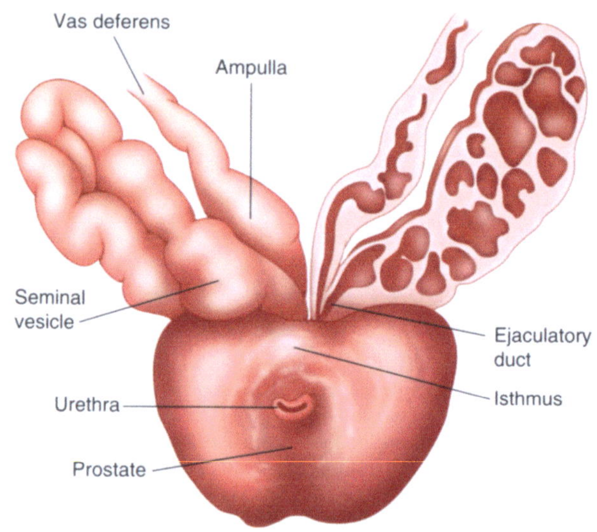

Figure 8-3. Anatomic relationships of the prostate: view from above. The prostate has a broad base superiorly and a narrow apex inferiorly. The base lies adjacent to the inferior surface of the bladder. The apex of the prostate is continuous with the rhabdosphincter and the prostatic urethra runs through the entire length of the prostate. The major glandular elements of the prostate empty into the prostatic urethra. The seminal vesicles and vas deferens lie posterior to the prostate, between the rectum and the prostate. The ejaculatory ducts are located at the junction between the vas deferens and seminal vesicles and enter the prostate base where it fuses with the bladder. They then follow a course through the prostate for nearly 2 cm parallel to the distal prostatic urethra before reaching the verumontanum.

Prostate Compartments and Cell Types

Compartment	Cell types
Prostatic epithelium	Stem cells
	Basal epithelial cells
	Transit-amplifying cells
	Neuroendocrine cells
	Terminally differentiated luminal secretory epithelial cells [1]
Prostatic stroma	Smooth muscle cells
	Fibroblasts
	Endothelial cells

FIGURE 8-4. The prostate. The main function of the prostate gland is to secrete seminal fluid. The two major functional compartments of the prostate gland are the prostatic epithelium (70% of the gland) and the prostatic stroma (30% of the gland). The prostatic epithelium is responsible for the secretion of hormones and enzymes and the prostatic stroma provides structural support.

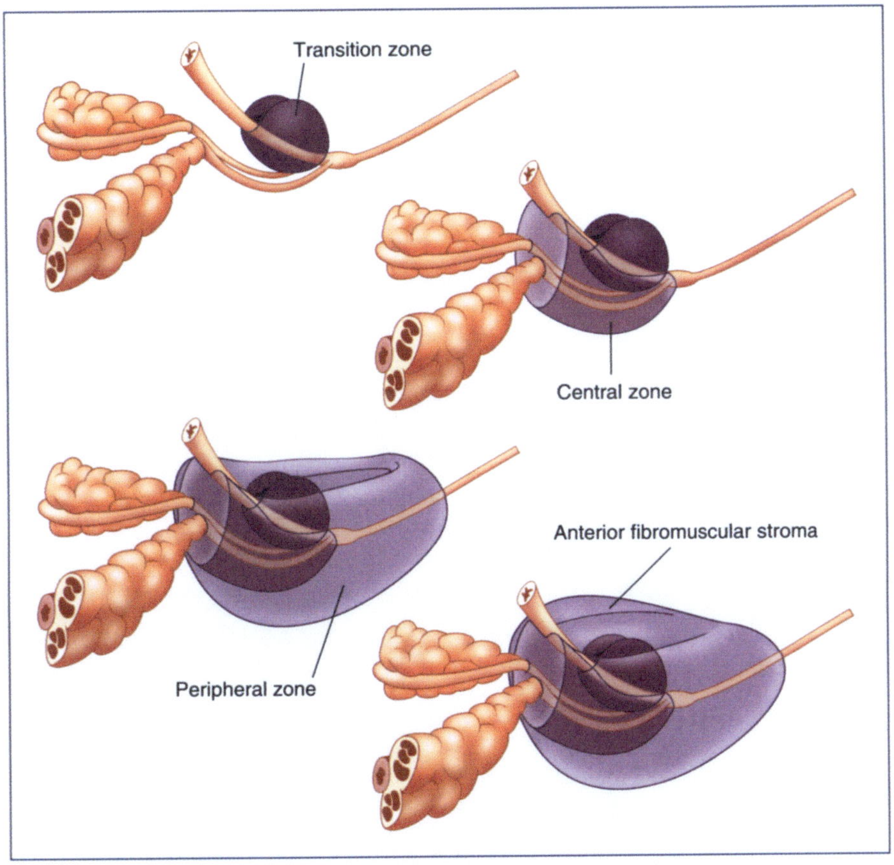

FIGURE 8-5. Zones of the prostate. The transition zone surrounds the urethra proximal to the ejaculatory ducts. The central zone surrounds the ejaculatory ducts and extends under the bladder base. The peripheral zone encompasses the apical, lateral, and posterior aspects of the prostate. The anterior fibromuscular stroma extends from the bladder neck to the striated urethral sphincter.The anterior fibromuscular stoma of the prostate is continuous with the bladder wall posterior to the urethra. (*Adapted from* McNeal [4].)

Peripheral Nerves

Three sets of peripheral nerves control the male bladder outlet:

1. The parasympathetic nervous system (S2–S4)
2. The sympathetic nervous system (T10–L2)
3. The somatic nervous system

FIGURE 8-6. Nervous control of the male bladder outlet.

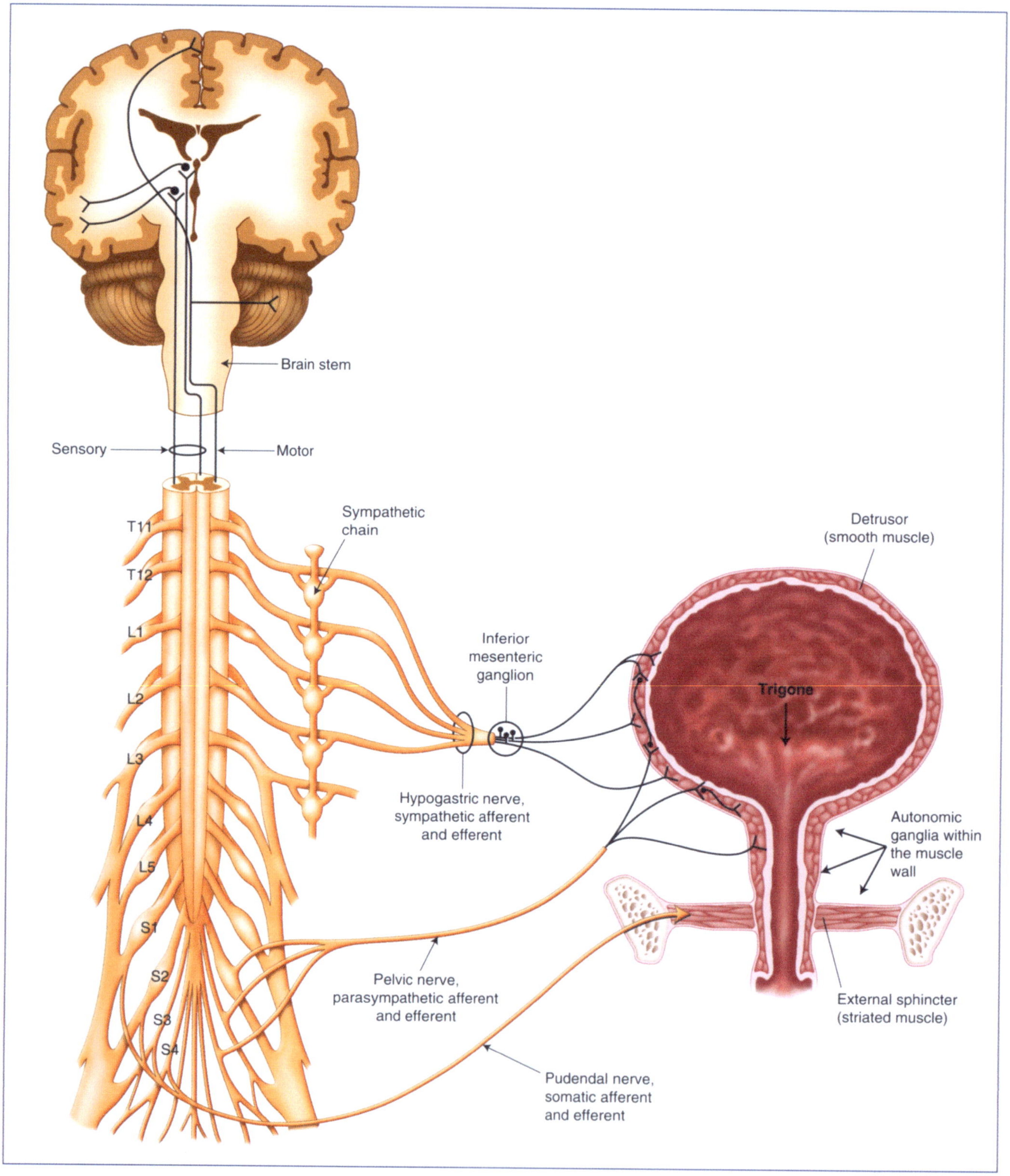

FIGURE 8-7. Innervation of the male bladder outlet. The pelvic parasympathetic (cholinergic) nerves originate from the sacral spinal cord (S2–4) and release the excitatory neurotransmitter acetylcholine. They cause a contraction of the bladder and relaxation of the urethra. Peripheral sympathetic (noradrenergic) nerves originate from the lumbar spinal cord (T10–L2). They inhibit the bladder body and excite the bladder base and urethra to promote urine storage. The pudendal nerve contains both afferent (sensory) and efferent (motor) neurons. Excitation results in contraction of the external urethral sphincter. The external urethral sphincter neurons are located in Onuf's nucleus, along the lateral border of the ventral horn.

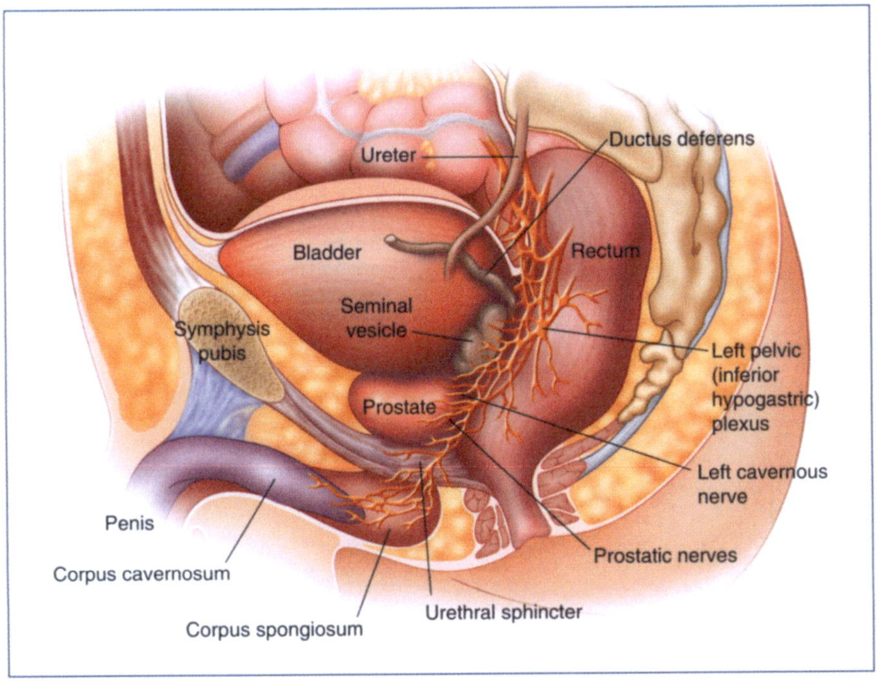

FIGURE 8-8. The pelvic (prostatic) plexus: basic anatomy, lateral view. The pelvic plexus (which includes the prostatic nerves) receives parasympathetic fibers from the sacral spinal cord as well as sympathetic fibers from the hypogastric nerves. Both cholinergic and noradrenergic nerves innervate the smooth muscle bundles of the prostatic stroma [5]. The smooth muscle of the prostatic capsule is innervated only by cholinergic (parasympathetic) nerves. During ejaculation, sympathetic stimulation causes the expulsion of prostatic fluid into the urethra.

Pathophysiology of Benign Prostatic Hyperplasia

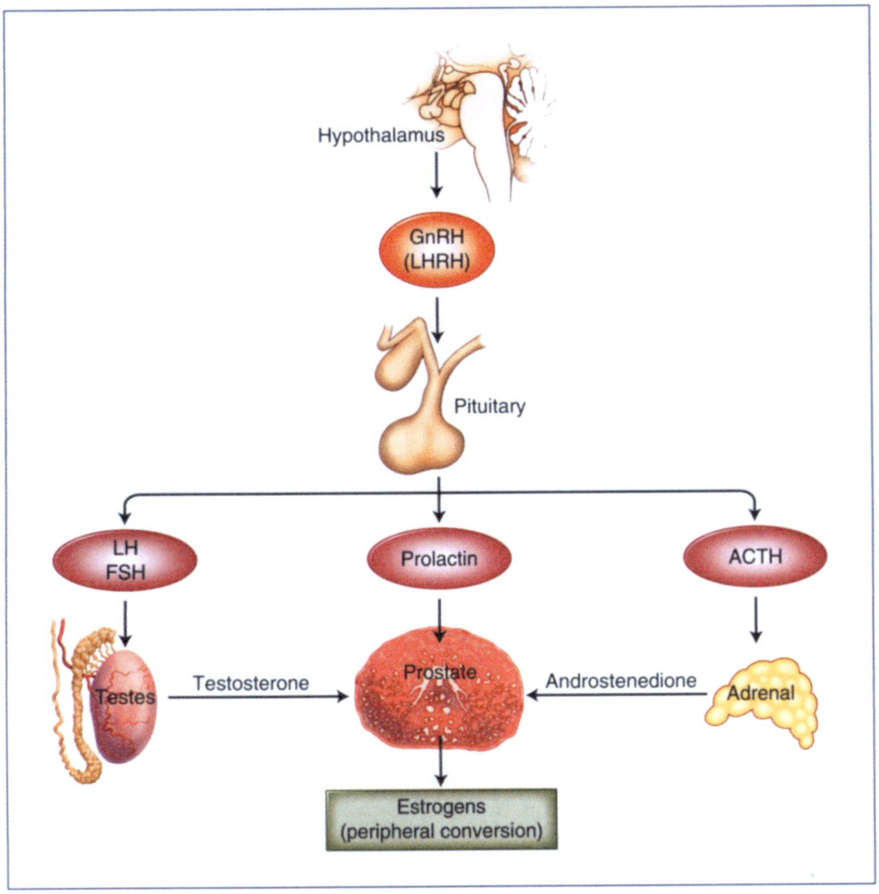

FIGURE 8-9. Endocrine control of prostatic growth. Testosterone, dihydrotestosterone, and estrogens are responsible for the growth, differentiation, and biologic functions of the prostate [6]. Luteinizing hormone–releasing hormone (LHRH), also known as gonadotropin-releasing hormone (GnRH), stimulates the pituitary to secrete the gonadotropin luteinizing hormone (LH) and follicle-stimulating hormone (FSH), which stimulate the Leydig cells of the testes to synthesize testosterone. Adrenocorticotropic hormone (ACTH) released from the pituitary stimulates the adrenal gland to secrete minor androgens, such as androstenedione. Estrogens in the male are formed through the peripheral conversion of testosterone and adrenal androgens. Prolactin is also thought to play a role in prostate growth.

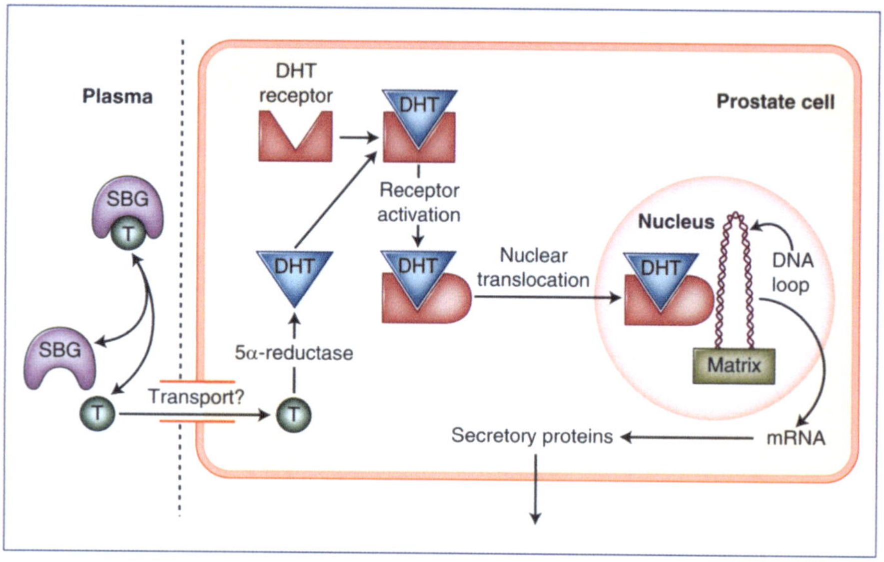

FIGURE 8-10. How testosterone causes prostate cell growth. Testosterone (T) in the serum is bound to serum-binding globulins (SBGs). Unbound testosterone enters the prostate cell, where it is converted by 5α-reductase (type II) to dihydrotestosterone (DHT). DHT binds to a cytosolic (androgen receptor) and is translocated to the nucleus. Inside the nucleus the androgen receptor localizes in matrix acceptor sites and subsequently activates or represses certain target genes by regulating production of their mRNA. The RNA is then transported to the cytoplasm, where it is translated into a variety of proteins (*eg*, secretory proteins such as prostate-specific antigen). Ultimately, cell growth occurs.

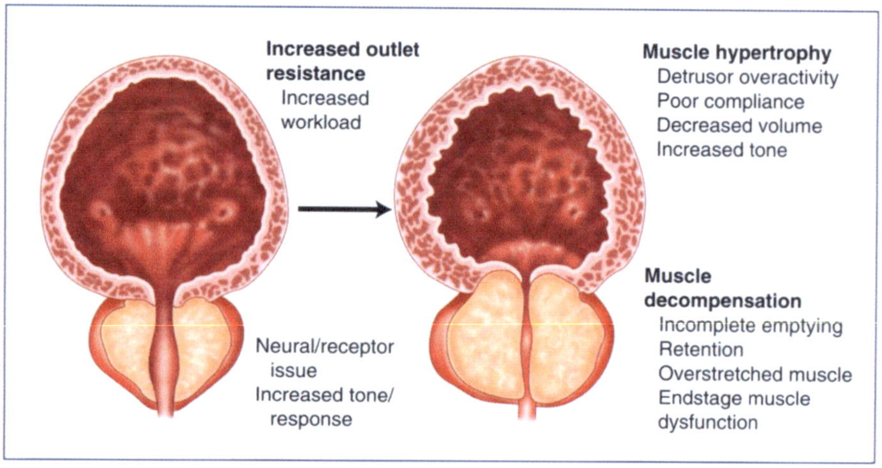

FIGURE 8-11. Pathophysiology of lower urinary tract symptoms in the aging male. Aging and neurogenic factors lead to overactive bladder (OAB). Bladder outlet obstruction leads to OAB.

Pharmacology of the Male Bladder Outlet

Receptor Pathways in the Male Bladder Outlet
Muscarinic mechanisms
Purinergic mechanisms
Adrenergic mechanisms
α-Adrenergic mechanisms
β-Adrenergic mechanisms
Nitric oxide
Peptidergic innervation
Tachykinins
Neuropeptide Y
Vasoactive intestinal polypeptide
Opiods
Calcitonin-gene-related peptide

FIGURE 8-12. Receptor pathways in the male bladder outlet.

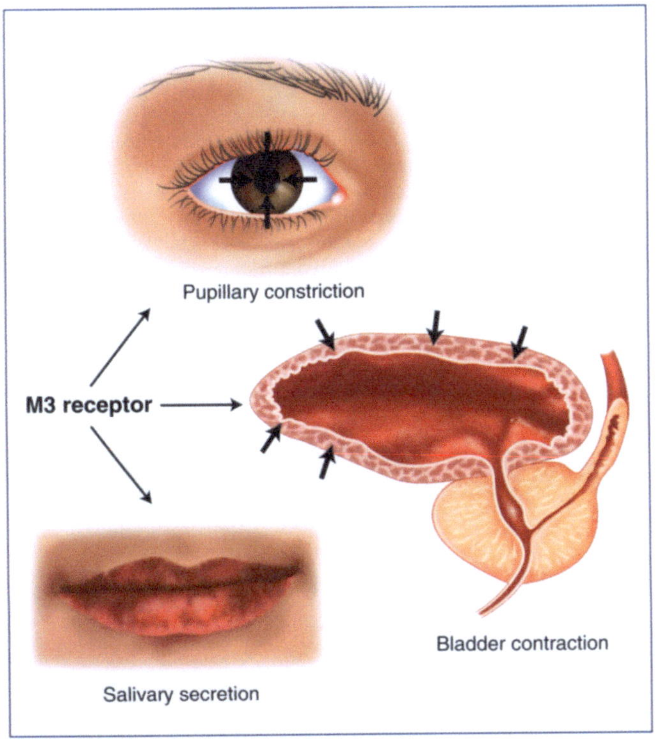

FIGURE 8-13. Muscarinic mechanisms. Humans have at least five different muscarinic receptors subtypes according to molecular cloning, M1–M5 [7–9]. Pharmacologically, three different receptors have been found: M1, M2, and M3 [10]. Studies show that in the bladder M2 receptors are the most prevalent, but M3 receptors are responsible for cholinergic contractions [11]. Other actions of the M3 receptor subtype include salivary secretion and papillary constriction [12].

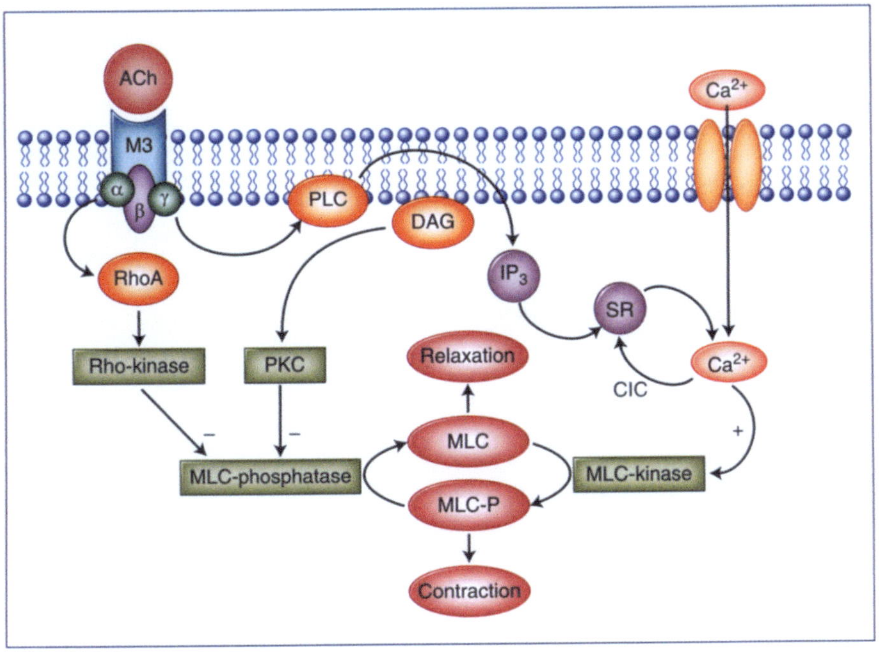

FIGURE 8-14. Muscarinic receptor activation. Acetylcholine binds to the M3 receptor. Phospholipase C (PLC) is activated and catalyzes a reaction that forms inositol triphosphate (IP_3) and diacylglycerol (DAG). IP_3 stimulates the release of intracellular calcium stores from the sarcoplasmic reticulum (SR). Calcium binds to calmodulin and activates myosin light-chain kinase (MLC-kinase), which phosphorylates myosin light chains (MLCs). The phosphorylation of an MLC leads to crossbridge formation between myosin and actin, which causes a smooth muscle contraction. In addition to intracellular calcium release, a transmembrane flux of calcium ions through L-type Ca^{2+} channels may also be involved in detrusor smooth muscle contraction [6]. It has also been proposed [13] that the coactivation of M2 receptors could enhance the response to M3 stimulation. There is also evidence for cholinergic innervation to the urethra. In vivo [14,15] and in vitro [14], external cholinergic agonists contract urethral smooth muscle. CIC—calcium-induced calcium release; MLC-P—myosin light chain phosphorylated; MLC-phosphatase—myosin light-chain phosphatase; PKC—protein kinase C.

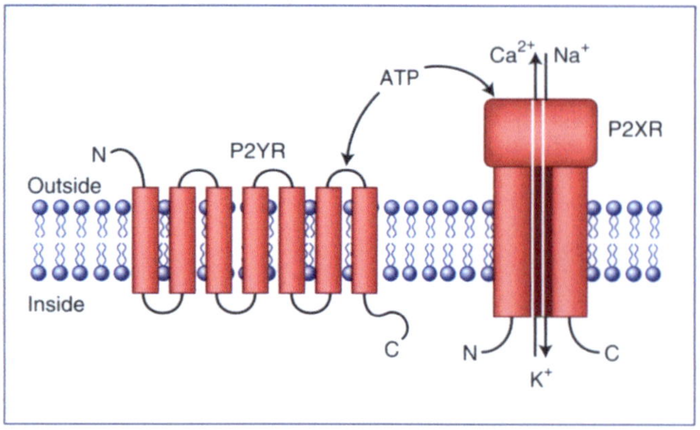

FIGURE 8-15. Purinergic mechanisms. ATP acts on two families of purinergic receptors. The P2X receptor (P2XR) is a part of the ion channel family and the P2Y receptor (P2YR) is a G-protein–coupled receptor [15,16]. In many animal species, such as the rat, guinea pig, and rabbit, there is a significant purinergic contribution to detrusor parasympathetic innervation [15]. In humans, no evidence has been found so far for significant purinergic neurotransmission in the normal response to stimulation; however, there may be a role in pathologic states such as bladder outlet obstruction and overactive bladder [10,11,17,18]. P2X1 is the predominant type of P2XR in the human bladder [18] and its expression is upregulated in the obstructed bladder compared to controls [18]. P2X3 receptors are also present in the human bladder.

Pharmacologic Properties of α-Adrenergic Mechanisms

	α_1 Receptor subtype		
	α_{1A}	α_{1B}	α_{1D}
Tissue where mRNA is found	Prostate, blood vessels, liver, heart, cerebral cortex, lung	Blood vessels, spleen, lung	Bladder, blood vessels, cerebral cortex, prostate
Structure	466 amino acids	515 amino acids	560 amino acids
Human chromosome location	Chromosome 8	Chromosome 5	Chromosome 20
Function	Human: prostate smooth muscle contraction	Human: vascular smooth muscle contraction	Human: vascular smooth muscle contraction
	Rat: kidney, vasoconstriction, vas deferens contraction	Rat: spleen contraction	Rat: aorta contraction

FIGURE 8-16. Pharmacologic properties of α-adrenergic mechanisms [12]. In the male prostate and urethra, the α_{1A} subtype is most prevalent. The α-adrenoreceptor subtypes α_{1A}, α_{1B}, and α_{1D} are present in blood vessels. In humans, α_{1D} receptors predominate in the bladder. Although α-adrenergic stimulation is not significant to bladder function, α-adrenergic stimulation leads to increased urethral tone and intraurethral pressure. α-Antagonists are used to treat symptoms of increased functional urethral resistance, such as benign prostatic hyperplasia. However, blocking α-receptors in vascular smooth muscle can lead to side effects such as postural hypotension. Pharmacologic and electrophysiologic studies demonstrate that adrenergic activity may modulate cholinergic activity in the pelvic ganglia. In the cat, the activation of α_2-adrenergic receptors inhibits excitatory cholinergic ganglia [19]. In contrast, β-adrenergic agonists promote transmission in vesical ganglia.

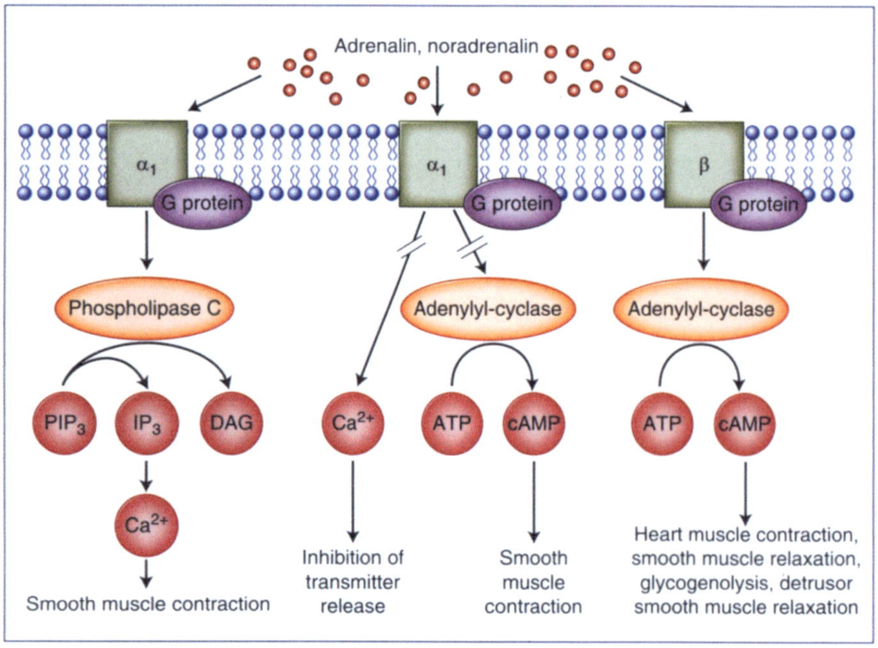

FIGURE 8-17. Adrenergic mechanisms: β-adrenergic mechanisms. The stimulation of β2 and β3 receptors leads to relaxation of the detrusor smooth muscle. Adrenergic stimulation results in detrusor smooth muscle relaxation through β3 adrenoreceptor activation. It follows that β3-adrenoreceptor agonists have been proposed as a potential treatment for overactive bladder [20]. β-adrenergic stimulation is mediated through the stimulation of adenylate cyclase and elevation in cAMP levels. DAG—diacylglycerol; IP_3—inositol triphosphate; PIP_3—phosphatidylinositol triphosphate.

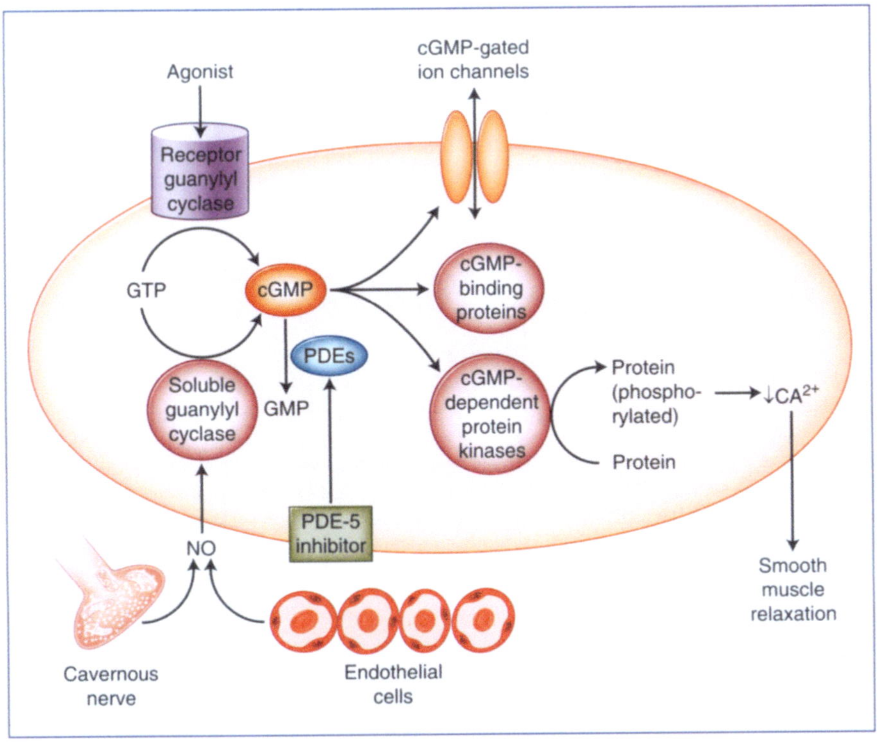

Figure 8-18. Nitric oxide (NO). NO causes relaxation of smooth muscle. NO synthase (NOS) synthesizes NO. The release of NO stimulates guanylyl cyclase to produce cyclic guanosine monophosphate(cGMP). The second messenger cGMP activates cGMP-dependent protein kinases and binding proteins. The phosphorylation of ion channels and proteins leads to the inhibition of voltage-dependent calcium channels and the sequestration of intracellular calcium by the endoplasmic reticulum, blocking calcium influx. This leads to smooth muscle relaxation. GTP—guanosine triphosphate; PDE 5—phosphodiesterase 5; PDEs— phosphodiesterases.

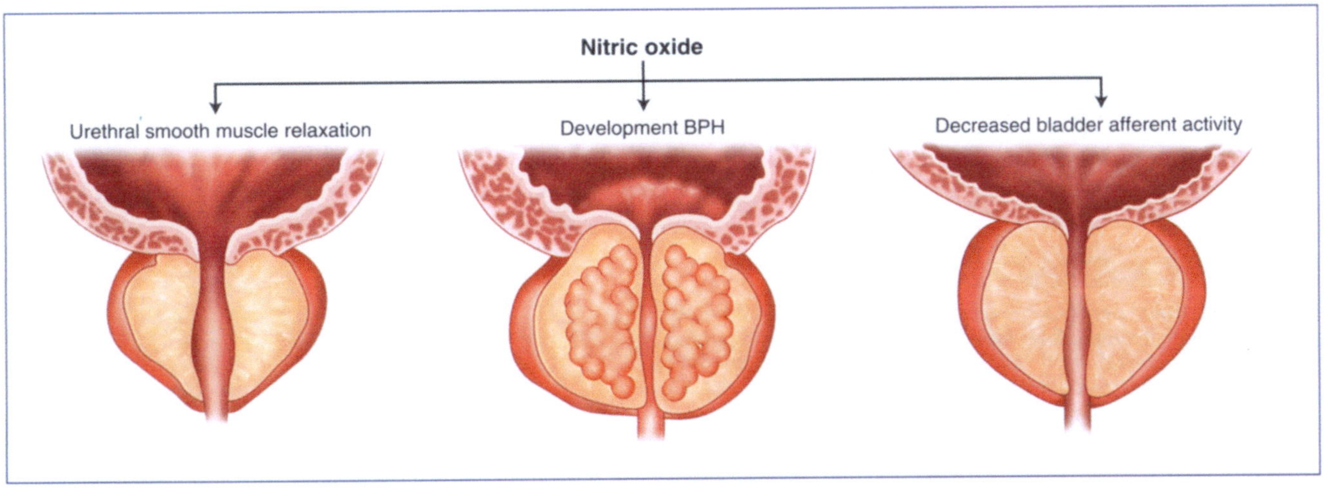

Figure 8-19. Role of nitric oxide (NO) in the male lower urinary tract. NO synthase has been found in the human prostate by immunohistochemical and biochemical means [21,22] and has been identified as the main inhibitory neurotransmitter responsible for urethral smooth muscle relaxation during micturition [23,24]. NO levels are reduced in benign prostatic hyperplasia (BPH) [25] and it is thought that NO may play a role in the development of BPH. NO also plays a role in mediating bladder afferent activity [26]. Phosphodiesterases (PDEs) 1 to 5 have been found in human detrusor smooth muscle [27]. Vinpocetine, a PDE 1 selective inhibitor, has been tested in patients who have refractory detrusor overactivity that is unresponsive to conventional anticholinergic drugs with encouraging but preliminary results [28].

Peptidergic Innervation

Neuropeptides in the Bladder
Substance P
Neurokinin A
Neurokinin Y
CGRP
VIP
PACAP
Enkephalins

Figure 8-20. Neuropeptides in the bladder. Bladder and afferents contain many neuropeptides, according to immunohistological studies. These include substance P, neurokinin A, neuropeptide Y, calcitonin gene-related peptide (CGRP), vasoactive intestinal polypeptide (VIP), pituitary adenylate cyclase-activating peptide (PACAP), and enkephalins [29,30]. Many of these peptides have been localized to the capsaicin-sensitive C fibers in the bladder. In response to noxious stimulation, they contribute to inflammatory responses by triggering plasma extravasation, vasodilation, and alterations in bladder smooth muscle activity [30]. In addition, these peptides are involved in signal transmission at the afferent terminals in the spinal cord.

Tachykinin Peptide Family

Tachykinin	Receptor
Substance P	NK1
Neurokinin A	NK2
Neurokinin B	NK3

Figure 8-21. The tachykinin peptide family. The tachykinin peptide family is characterized by a common C-terminal sequence Phe-Xaa-Gly-Leu-Met-NH2. The main members of this family are substance P, neurokinin A, and neurokinin B. Tachykinins are present in both the central and peripheral nervous systems. In the peripheral nerves, tachykinins are predominantly localized to the terminals of unmyelinated sensory C fibers. The principal tachykinin receptors belong to a superfamily of seven transmembrane-spanning G protein-coupled receptors [31]. All three receptor subtypes in humans—NK1, NK2, and NK3—have been identified in the bladder [32].

Neuropeptides in the Prostate
NPY
VIP
Opioids
Met-enkephalin
Leu-enkephalin
Tachykinins
CGRP

Figure 8-22. Neuropeptides in the prostate. The human prostate also contains many neuropeptides that are involved in afferent signaling, including neuropeptide Y (NPY), vasoactive intestinal polypeptide (VIP), opioids, tachykinins, and calcitonin-gene-related peptide (CGRP). The role of these peptides has not yet been clearly elucidated [33].

Pharmacology Treatment of the Male Bladder Outlet

Pharmacologic Agents for BPH Therapy
Alpha blockers
Androgen suppression
Combination therapy
Phytotherapy
Botulinum toxin

Figure 8-23. Pharmacologic agents for benign prostatic hyperplasia (BPH) therapy. Advances in pharmacologic agents for BPH have radically altered the nature of treatment, which used to be primarily surgical. Over the past two decades, medical therapy has become the most common way to treat BPH. Therapy may be targeted at either the treatment of symptoms or at preventing the progression of disease. The main categories of pharmacologic agents include α-adrenergic blockers, androgen suppression agents, anticholinergic agents, phytotherapeutic agents, and botulinum toxin. These agents can be used alone or in combination.

Outcomes of Medical Therapies: Estimates of Change in Efficacy Scores/Rates

	AUA/IPSS			Peak flow rate (Qmax)			QOL question score		BPH impact index	
	3–9 mo	10–16 mo	> 16 mo	3–9 mo	10–16 mo	> 16 mo	3–9 mo	10–16 mo	3–9 mo	10–16 mo
Alpha blockers										
Alfuzosin	-4.44			2.05			-1.10			
Doxazosin	-5.10	-5.63		3.11	2.98	1.90*	-1.25	-1.47	-2.00	-2.47
Tamsulosin	-4.63	-7.53*		1.85	1.86*		-1.43			
Terazosin	-6.22	-5.99		2.51	1.94	2.61*	-1.70*	-1.37	-1.45*	-2.09
Hormonal										
Finasteride	-3.44	-3.40	-2.37	2.11	1.66	1.95	-0.75	-0.87	-1.50	-1.21
Combinations										
Alfuzosin/finasteride	-6.10*			2.30*						
Doxazosin/finasteride	-5.64	-6.53		3.96	3.38		-1.15	-1.57	-2.20	-2.57
Terazosin/finasteride	-5.90*	-6.21*		3.50*	2.63				-1.55*	-2.03
Placebo	-2.44*	-2.33*	-1.03*	0.86*	0.48*	0.48*	-0.65*	-0.67*	1.00*	-0.97*

FIGURE 8-24. Comparison of outcomes of medical therapies for benign prostatic hyperplasia (BPH). *Asterisks* indicate numbers based on single-arm analyses. AUA—American Urological Association; IPSS—International Prostate Symptom Score; QOL—quality of life. (*From* Roehrborn *et al.* [34]; with permission.)

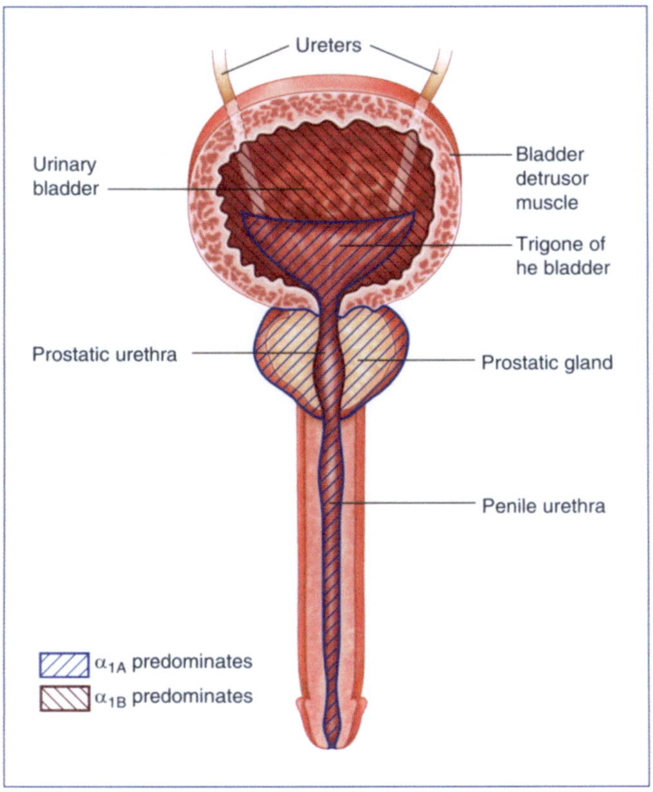

FIGURE 8-25. Distribution of α_1-adrenergic receptors in the lower urinary tract. In the male prostate and urethra, the α_{1A}-adrenergic receptor subtype is most prevalent. In humans, α_{1D} receptors predominate in the bladder. Smooth muscle is one of the dominant components of benign prostatic hyperplasia. (*Adapted from* Roehrborn and Schwinn [35].)

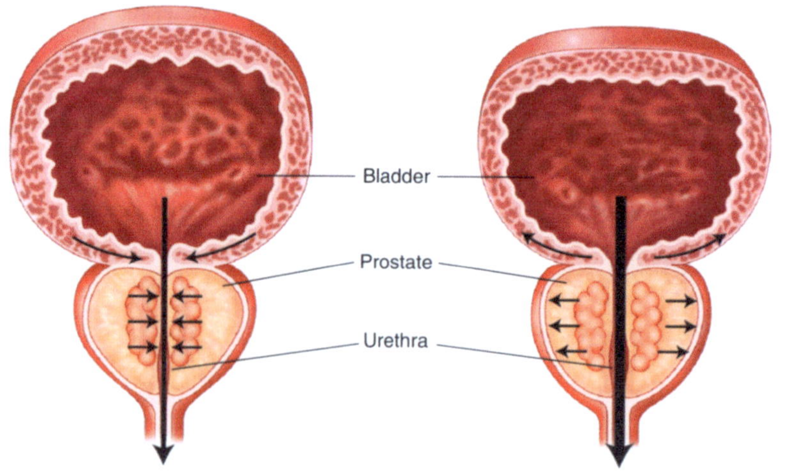

Figure 8-26. Mechanism of action of α-adrenergic blockers. It has been hypothesized that benign prostatic hyperplasia (BPH) causes bladder outlet obstruction and symptoms partially through increased smooth muscle tone. α-Adrenergic stimulation leads to increased urethral smooth muscle tone and intraurethral pressure, although α-adrenergic stimulation is not significant to bladder function. It follows that α-adrenergic blockers are useful in treating BPH symptoms.

Classification of α-Adrenergic Blockers

	Nonselective	α_1-Selective	α_{1A}-Selective
Short-acting	Phenoxybenzamine 10 mg twice a day	Prazosin 2 mg twice a day	
		IR alfuzosin 2.5 mg three times per day	
		Indoramin 20 mg twice a day	
Long-acting		Terazosin 5–10 mg once a day	Tamsulosin 0.4 mg once a day
		Doxazosin 4–8 mg once a day	
		Alfuzosin SR 10 mg once a day	

Figure 8-27. Classification of α-adrenergic blockers. Phenoxybenzamine is rarely used anymore for the treatment of benign prostatic hyperplasia due to side effects such as postural hypotension. Tamsulosin is the only α_{1A}-selective α-adrenergic blocker.

No single agent has proven to be significantly more efficacious than the others. Although tamsulosin is subtype selective for the α_{1A}-adrenoreceptor, it can induce some hypotension, although significantly less than what is observed with terazosin [36]. IR—immediate release; SR—sustained release.

Side Effects of α-Adrenergic Blockers
Dizziness
Postural hypotension
Asthenia
Rhinitis
Sexual dysfunction

Figure 8-28. Side effects of α-adrenergic blockers. Side effects are reported in approximately 5% to 9% of patient populations who take α-adrenergic blockers [37]. These side effects include dizziness, postural hypotension, asthenia, rhinitis, and sexual dysfunction including abnormal ejaculation.

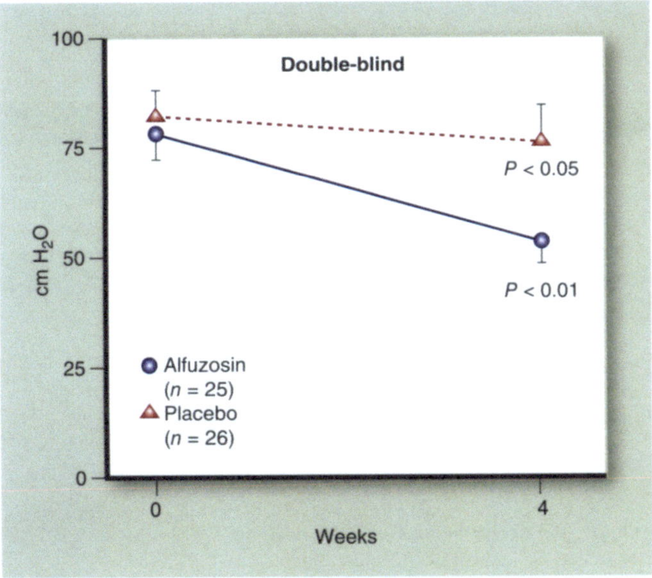

FIGURE 8-29. Effects of α-adrenergic blockers on bladder outlet obstruction [19]. Martorana *et al.* [38] published a randomized, double-blind, placebo-controlled study examining the effect of a 1-month treatment of alfuzosin, at a dose of 2.5 mg three times per day, on pressure-flow urodynamic parameters. In the alfuzosin-treatment group compared with the placebo group, changes in detrusor pressure at maximal flow, detrusor opening pressure, and maximal detrusor pressure were significantly greater. (From Martorana *et al.* [38]; with permission.)

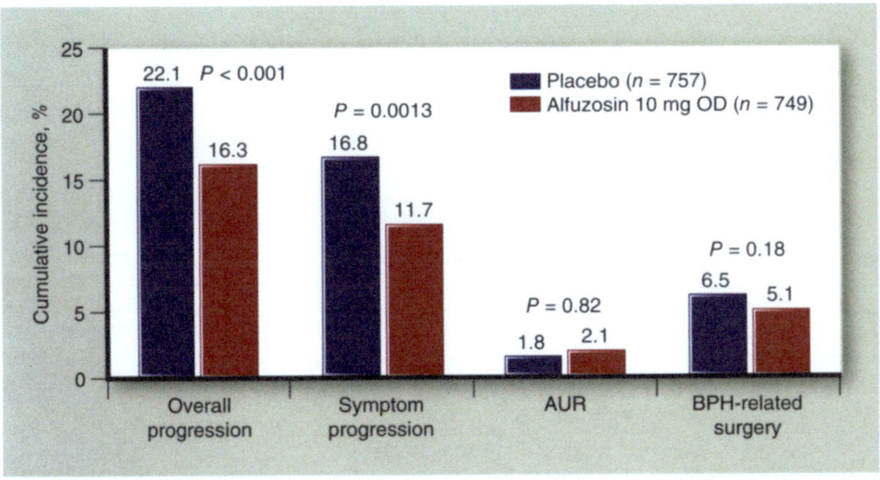

FIGURE 8-30. Cumulative incidence of lower urinary tract symptoms/benign prostatic hyperplasia (BPH) progression events over 2 years in the Alfuzosin Long-Term Efficacy and Safety Study (ALTESS) [39].

The ALTESS researched the impact of alfuzosin on BPH progression [40]. Compared with placebo, alfuzosin did not reduce the risk of acute urinary retention (AUR) (2.1% vs 1.8% for alfuzosin and placebo, respectively, $P = 0.82$) but tended to reduce the risk for BPH-related surgery (5.1% vs 6.5%, $P = 0.18$; RR, 22%; 95% CI, −18, 48%). OD—every day. (From Roerhborn [39]; with permission.)

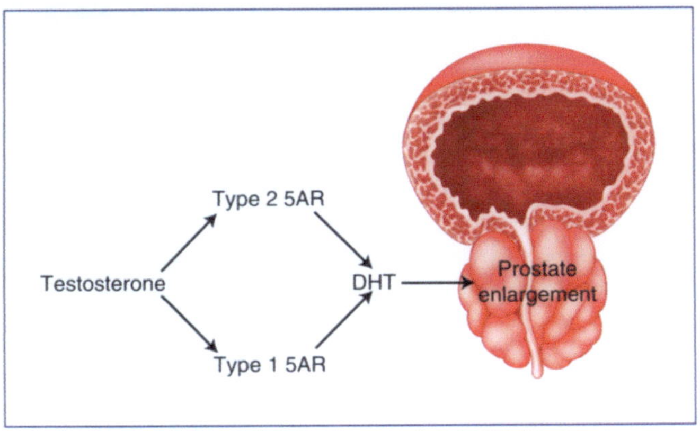

FIGURE 8-31. Role of androgens in benign prostatic hyperplasia (BPH). In the embryo, prostate development requires dihydrotestosterone (DHT). The enzyme 5α-reductase (5AR) converts testosterone to DHT. Castration and pharmacologic agents that suppress testosterone or DHT secretion have been shown to reduce the prostate's size in men with BPH [41]. Reducing prostate volume is hypothesized to decrease the static component of bladder outlet obstruction caused by BPH. The 5AR inhibitors finasteride and dutasteride are safe and efficacious in the treatment of BPH. Studies of antiandrogens such as flutamide and cetrorelix have failed to show treatment-related efficacy [42].

Androgen Suppression
LHRH analogues
Leuprolide
Nafarelin
Goserelin
Buserelin
LHRH antagonists
Cetrorelix
Estrogens
Diethylstilbestrol
Progestational agents
17α-Hydroxycortisone
Megestrol
Anti-androgens
Steroidal
Cyproterone acetate
Zanoterone
Nonsteroidal
Flutamide
Biclutamide
Nilutamide
5α-Reductase inhibitors
Finasteride
Dutasteride

FIGURE 8-32. Classification of androgen suppression. The classification of androgen suppression agents is illustrated. The only pharmacologic agents effective against benign prostatic hyperplasia with minimal side effects are the 5α-reductase inhibitors. LHRH—luteinizing hormone–releasing hormone.

5AR Inhibitors

5AR inhibitor	5AR isoenzyme(s) inhibited	Dosage
Finasteride	Type 2	5 mg daily
Dutasteride	Types 1 and 2	0.5 mg daily

FIGURE 8-33.

Clinical Effects of 5AR Inhibitors
Reduction in serum DHT
Reduction in prostate volume
Decreased risk in the symptomatic progression of BPH (defined as an increase in the AUA symptom score > 4 points) [44]
Reduction in the risk of acute urinary retention
Reduction in the need for surgery for BPH
Decrease in the risk of prostate cancer [45]
Prevention of gross hematuria due to BPH [46]

FIGURE 8-34. Clinical effects of 5α-reductase (5AR) inhibitors. This figure outlines the main clinical effects of 5AR inhibitors. Most of these effects were observed in two major studies, the Medical Therapy of Prostatic Symptoms and Proscar Long-Term Efficacy and Safety Study, which observed the natural history of benign prostatic hyperplasia and the effects of 5AR inhibitors on symptoms and progression. AUA—American Urological Association; DHT—dihydrotestosterone.

Adverse Effects of 5α-Reductase Inhibitors
Decreased libido
Impotence
Decreased ejaculate volume
Ejaculation disorders
Breast enlargement
Breast tenderness
Generalized rash

FIGURE 8-35. Adverse effects of 5α-reductase inhibitors. In the Proscar Long-Term Efficacy and Safety Study (PLESS), finasteride was well tolerated [47]. More specifically, the number of withdrawals from treatment due to adverse effects was similar in the placebo and finasteride groups. Studies of the safety and tolerability of dutasteride yielded similar results and demonstrated that, despite additional 5α-reductase blockade, dutasteride does not appear to have decreased tolerability in comparison to finasteride [48]. The adverse events in the PLESS, which occurred in less than 1% of men and were significantly more prevalent in the finasteride group compared to placebo, are shown.

Findings for PLESS
55% risk reduction in the cumulative risk of undergoing BPH-related surgery over 4 y in the finasteride group
57% risk reduction in the cumulative incidence of acute urinary retention at 4 y in the finasteride group
Significant decrease in the AUA symptom score in the finasteride group
Significantly increased flow rate in the finasteride group
Significant decrease in the prostate volume in the finasteride group

FIGURE 8-36. Findings of the Proscar Long-Term Efficacy and Safety Study (PLESS). The PLESS was a large-scale, multicenter, randomized, double-blind, placebo-controlled trial conducted in 3040 men with moderate-to-severe lower urinary tract symptoms, a Qmax of less than 15 mL/s, and an enlarged prostate on digital rectal examination. Patients were randomized to receive either 5 mg of finasteride or placebo daily for 4 years. Mean prostate volume was 55 cm^3, which indicates bias toward men with larger prostates. AUA—American Urological Association; BPH—benign prostatic hyperplasia.

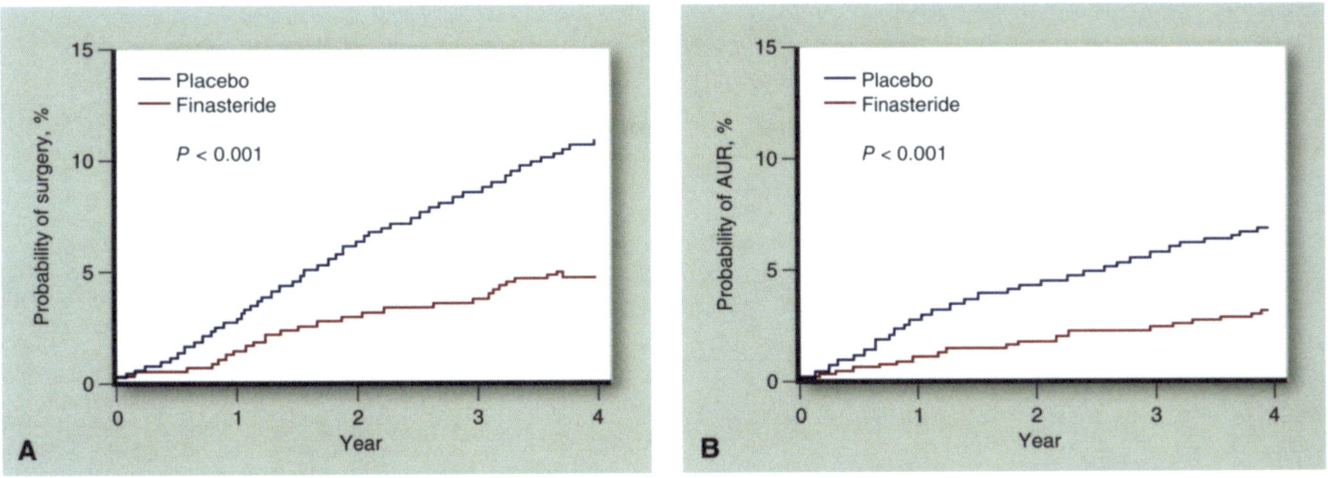

Figure 8-37. Probability of **A**, undergoing surgery for benign prostatic hyperplasia (BPH) or **B**, the development of acute urinary retention (AUR) during the Proscar Long-Term Efficacy and Safety Study. Life-table analyses of the proportion of men with each outcome are shown. In the finasteride group, there was a significant decrease in the probability of BPH-related surgery and the probability of developing AUR. (*Adapted from* McConnell *et al.* [47].)

MTOPS Trial	
Study	MTOPS [44]
Patients, ***number***	3047
Study groups	Placebo
	Doxazosin 8 mg/d
	Finasteride 5 mg/d
	Doxazosin and finasteride
Inclusion criteria	Age ≥ 50
	AUA symptom score 8–30
	Peak flow 4–15 mL/s
Study duration	4.5 y
Risk of AUR	Significantly decreased in combination and finasteride groups ($P < 0.001$)
Risk of BPH surgery	Significantly decreased in combination and finasteride groups ($P < 0.001$)
Symptoms	Significant improvement in the AUA symptom score in all groups
	Combination group is superior to finasteride ($P = 0.006$) and doxazosin ($P < 0.001$)
Other	Risk of overall clinical progression increased with increasing baseline serum PSA levels and baseline prostate volume in placebo ($P \leq 0.001$)
	Maximum urinary flow rate improved in all treatment groups as compared to placebo ($P < 0.001$)
	Median decrease in prostate volume of 19% in the finasteride and combination groups

Figure 8-38. Combination therapy: the Medical Therapy of Prostatic Symptoms (MTOPS) trial. Initial studies of combination therapy assessed finasteride in combination with either terazosin or doxazosin. These studies, the Veterans Affairs and Prospective European Doxazosin and Combination, did not establish benefit for combination therapy over placebo in terms of improving lower urinary tract symptoms or Qmax [49,50]. However, the longer-duration MTOPS has shown a significant benefit of finasteride and doxazosin over monotherapy [44]. AUA—American Urological Association; AUR—acute urinary retention; BPH—benign prostatic hyperplasia; PSA—prostate-specific antigen.

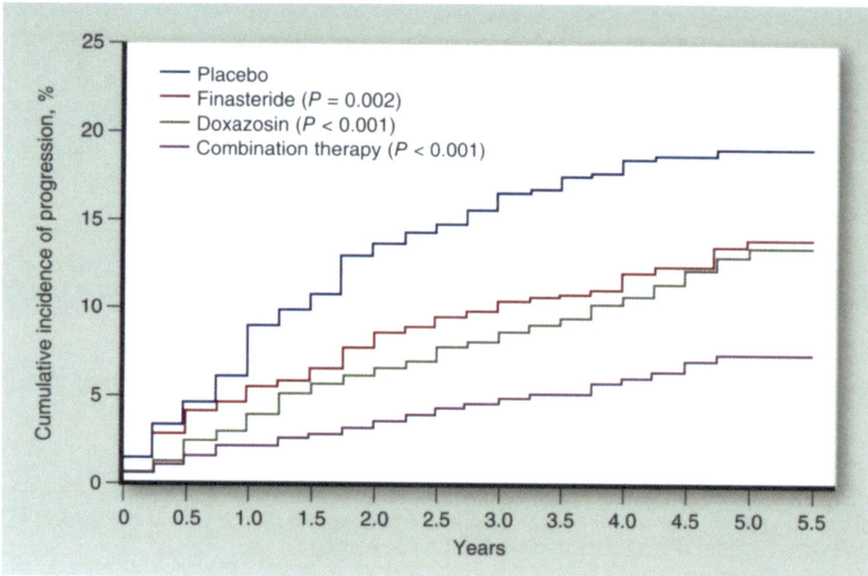

FIGURE 8-39. Cumulative incidence of progression of benign prostatic hyperplasia (BPH) in the Medical Therapy of Prostatic Symptoms (MTOPS) trial. In the MTOPS trial, BPH progression was defined by an increase of at least 4 points over baseline in the American Urological Association symptom score, acute urinary retention, incontinence, renal insufficiency, or recurrent urinary tract infections. In the doxazosin (39% risk reduction, $P < 0.001$) and finasteride (34% risk reduction, $P = 0.002$) groups, as compared with placebo, there was a significant decrease in progression. The reduction in risk associated with combination therapy (66% for the comparison with placebo, $P < 0.001$) was significantly greater than that associated with doxazosin ($P < 0.001$) or finasteride ($P < 0.001$) alone [44]. (*Adapted from* McConnell *et al.* [44].)

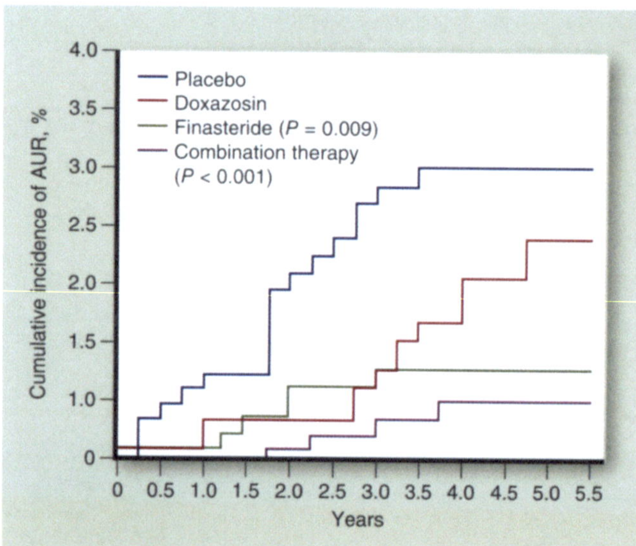

FIGURE 8-40. Cumulative incidence of acute urinary retention (AUR) in the Medical Therapy of Prostatic Symptoms (MTOPS) trial. In MTOPS, the risk of AUR was significantly reduced by combination therapy ($P < 0.001$) and finasteride ($P < 0.009$), but not by doxazosin. (*Adapted from* McConnell *et al.* [44].)

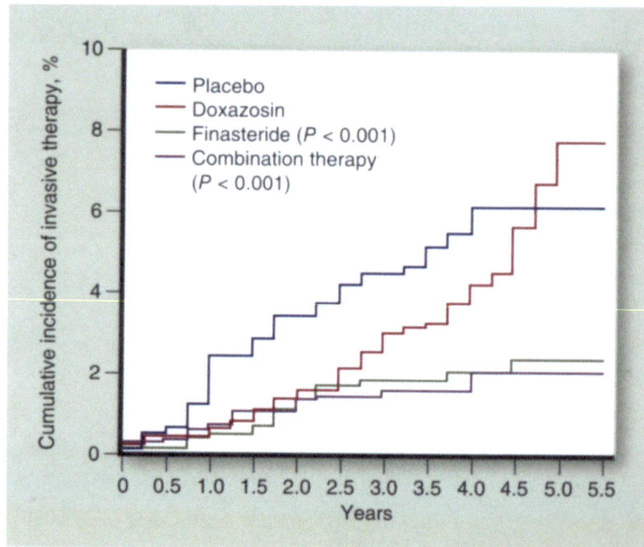

FIGURE 8-41. Cumulative incidence of invasive therapy. The risks of a need for invasive therapy were significantly reduced by combination therapy ($P < 0.001$) and finasteride ($P < 0.001$), but not by doxazosin. (*Adapted from* McConnell *et al.* [44].)

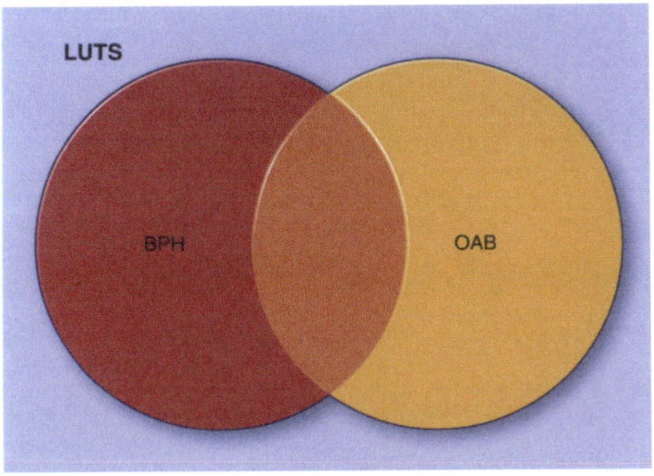

FIGURE 8-42. Anticholinergic therapy for patients with bladder outlet obstruction (BOO) and detrusor overactivity. A significant proportion of men with symptoms of benign prostatic hyperplasia (BPH) also have symptoms of overactive bladder (OAB). The International Continence Society defines OAB as a syndrome characterized by urgency with or without urge incontinence, usually with frequency and nocturia [51]. The link between BPH and OAB symptoms is not well understood [52]. Although many men will have persistent storage symptoms after treatment, urologists have traditionally been reticent to place these men on anticholinergic therapy because of the risk of urinary retention. This issue was specifically addressed by Abrams *et al.* [53] in a randomized, placebo-controlled study with a tolterodine dosage of 2 mg twice daily in men with BOO and detrusor overactivity. Of 221 patients, only one patient in each group suffered from acute urinary retention in the 3-month study period and the tolterodine group had a only a mild mean increase (25 mL) in postvoid residual compared to placebo. At the end of the study, maximum flow rates and maximum detrusor pressure at the maximum flow were essentially identical between the two groups. LUTS—lower urinary tract symptoms.

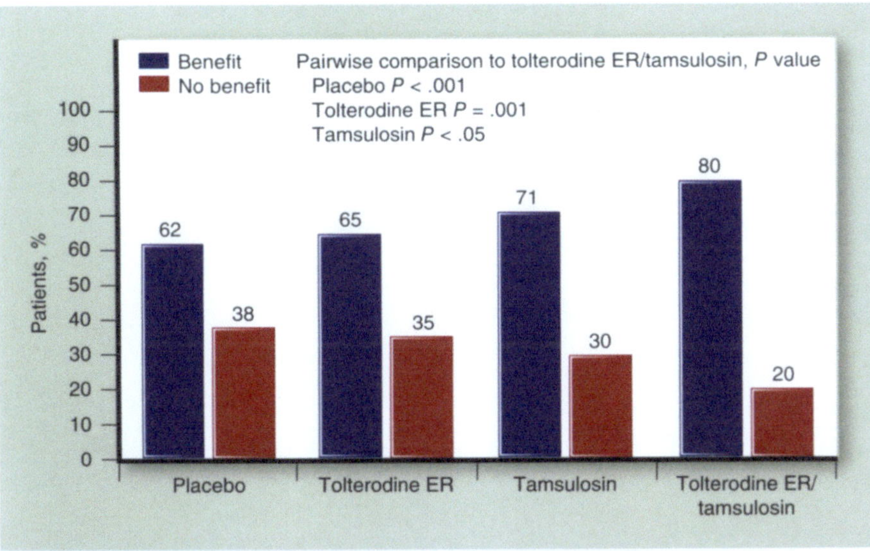

FIGURE 8-43. Tolterodine extended release (ER) plus tamsulosin resulted in a significant benefit at week 12. The results of combination therapy with α-adrenergic blockers and anticholinergics [54] are shown. A total of 172 men (80%) receiving tolterodine ER plus tamsulosin reported a treatment benefit by week 12 compared with 132 patients (62%) receiving placebo ($P < .001$), 146 (71%) receiving tamsulosin ($P = .06$ vs placebo), or 135 (65%) receiving tolterodine ER ($P = .48$ vs placebo). All interventions were well tolerated. The incidence of acute urinary retention requiring catheterization was low (tolterodine ER plus tamsulosin, 0.4%; tolterodine ER, 0.5%; tamsulosin, 0%; and placebo, 0%). (*Adapted from* Kaplan *et al.* [54].)

Phosphodiesterase Inhibitors Currently Available in the United States

	Sildenafil	Vardenafil	Tadalafil
Recommended dosage	25, 50, 100 mg	5, 10, 20 mg	5, 10, 20 mg
Onset of action	15–60 min	15–60 min	15–60 min
Half-life	3–5 h	4–5 h	17.5 h

FIGURE 8-44. Phosphodiesterase inhibitors currently available in the United States. As stated previously, phosphodiesterases have been found throughout the lower urinary tract [55]. In the prostate, phosphodiesterase (PDE) 4 and 5 predominate. PDE 5 has been localized to the urethra and vasculature and PDEs 1 and 4 have been shown to affect detrusor smooth muscle activity. Studies have shown that regular use of sildenafil and tadalafil improves benign prostatic hyperplasia (BPH)-related lower urinary tract symptoms (LUTS), but not the flow rate [56–58]. Kaplan *et al.* [54] conducted a pilot study to compare the efficacy and safety of alfuzosin, sildenafil, or both on LUTS suggestive of BPH and erectile dysfunction [59]. Improvement of the International Prostate Symptom Score was significant with the three treatments, but was greatest with the combination (24.1%) compared with alfuzosin (15.6%) and sildenafil (16.9%) alone ($P < 0.03$). Improvement in the International Index for Erectile Function was slight with alfuzosin (16.7%), marked with sildenafil (49.7%), and greatest with the combination (58.6%).These studies are promising. However, larger and longer-term studies are needed.

Phytotherapeutic Agents to Treat BPH

Scientific name	Common name
Serenoa repens	Saw palmetto berry
Hypoxis rooperi	South African star grass
Pygeum africanum	African plum tree
Urtica dioica	Stinging nettle
Secale cereale	Rye pollen
Cucurbita pepo	Pumpkin seed
Opuntia	Cactus flower
Pinus	Pine flower
Picea	Spruce

Figure 8-45. Origin of phytotherapeutic agents used in the treatment of benign prostatic hyperplasia (BPH). Phytotherapeutic products are extracts derived from fruit, seeds, or the bark of plants. These plant extracts often contain a wide variety of chemical substances including sterols, oils, fatty acids, and phytoestrogens. Which chemical substances in the extracts are clinically important is usually unknown, as is the mechanism of action of these substances. Preparations made by different manufacturers vary widely in terms of the amount of plant extract that they contain.

Action of Plant Extracts

Action of Plant Extracts
Inhibition of 5α-reductase
Anti-inflammatory
Interference with growth factors
Anti-androgen
Inhibition of aromatase
Decrease of sex hormone-binding globulin
Alteration of cholesterol metabolism
α-Adrenergic receptors blockage
Free radical scavenging
Alteration of lipid peroxidation
Modulation of prolactin-induced prostatic growth
Protection of bladder and detrusor function
Placebo effect

Figure 8-46. Action of plant extracts. The potential mechanisms of action of plant extracts are given.

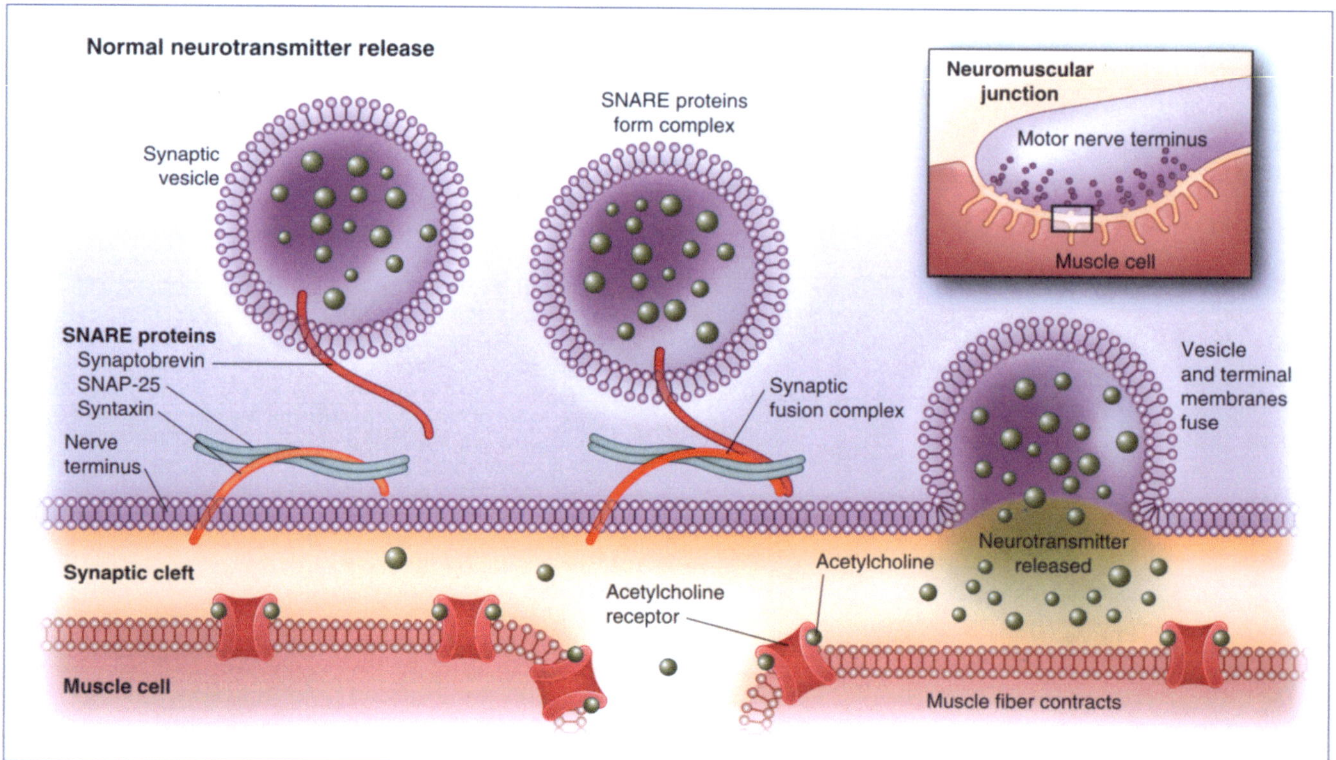

Figure 8-47. Mechanism of action of acetylcholine released from the nerve terminal. Normal fusion and the release of acetylcholine from nerve terminals through interaction of vesicle and membrane-bound (soluble N-ethylmaleimide-sensitive factor attachment protein receptor [SNARE]) proteins are demonstrated. When parasympathetic nerves in the bladder are stimulated, assembly of the SNARE protein complex (*eg*, synaptobrevin, SNAP-25, and syntaxin) occurs, leading to the release of acetylcholine and the activation of postjunctional muscarinic receptors [60]. As a result, the bladder contracts. (*Adapted from* Arnon *et al.* [61].)

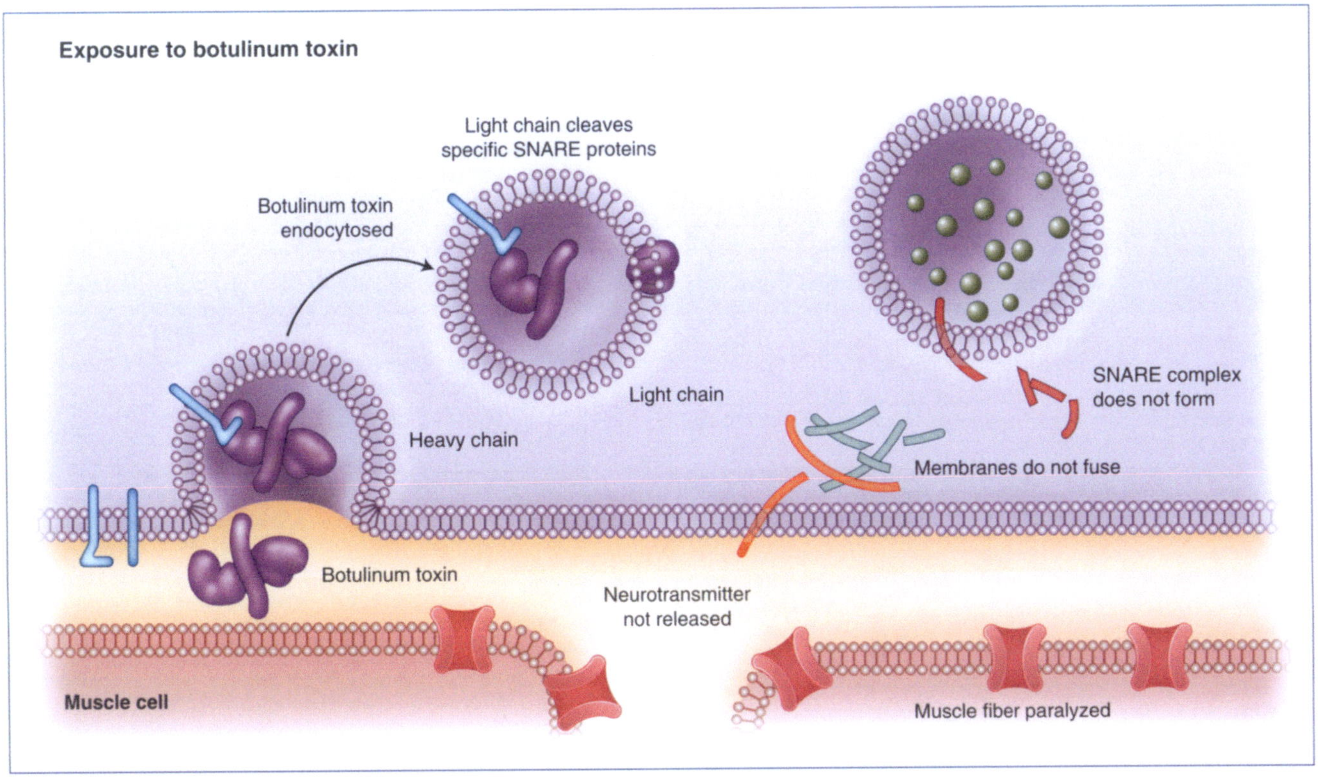

FIGURE 8-48. Mechanism of the action of the botulinum toxin (BTX). BTX preventing acetylcholine release is shown. BTX becomes internalized within the nerve terminal. Next, translocation of the light chain into the cytosol occurs and neurotransmitter release is inhibited by the cleavage of specific soluble N-ethylmaleimide-sensitive factor attachment protein receptor (SNARE) proteins. The muscle fiber is paralyzed. As an investigative medication, BTX injection may be an option for patients who have failed all of the therapies mentioned earlier. There are seven subtypes of BTX and types A and B have been evaluated for lower urinary tract symptoms. Schurch *et al.* [62] found that a BTX-A injection into the detrusor muscle was beneficial in patients with spinal cord injury, detrusor hyperreflexia, and urge incontinence that is resistant to anticholinergic drugs. In a study of 100 patients with non-neurogenic overactive bladder syndrome refractory to anticholinergics, Schmid *et al.* [63] found that 4 and 12 weeks after the injection of 100 U BTX-A toxin into the detrusor muscle, 88% of the patients showed a significant improvement in subjective symptoms, quality of life, and urodynamic parameters. The relief of voiding dysfunction in benign prostatic hyperplasia (BPH) patients after an intraprostatic injection of BTX-A was based on the observation that, in rodents, the prostate undergoes atrophy after a local toxin injection [63]. Maria *et al.* [64] conducted a randomized placebo-controlled study in which BTX-A or saline was injected in 30 consecutive men with BPH [64]. Two months following the injection, 13 patients in the treated group versus three in the control group ($P = 0.0007$ had subjective symptomatic relief). Currently, a multicenter National Institute of Health-sponsored randomized phase II trial is investigating the durability, toxicity, and efficacy of an intraprostatic injection of BTX for the management of BPH.

References

1. Jaffe WI, Te AE: Overactive bladder in the male patient: epidemiology, etiology, evaluation, and treatment. *Curr Urol Rep* 2005, 6:410–418.
2. Roehrborn CG, McConell JD: Benign prostatic hyperplasia: etiology, pathophysiology, epidemiology, and natural history. In *Campbell-Walsh Urology*, edn 9. Edited by Wein AJ, Kavoussi LR, Novick AC, *et al.* Philadephia: Saunders; 2007:2727–2764.
3. Sarma AV, Jacobson DJ, McGree ME, *et al.*: A population based study of incidence and treatment of benign prostatic hyperplasia among residents of Olmsted County, Minnesota: 1987 to 1997. *J Urol* 2005, 173:2048–2053.
4. McNeal JE: The prostate and prostatic urethra: a morphologic synthesis. *J Urol* 1972, 107:1008–1016.
5. Gosling JA: Autonomic innervation of the prostate. In *Benign Prostatic Hypertrophy*. Edited by Hinman F. New York: Springer-Verlag; 1983:349–360.
6. Andersson KE, Wein AJ: Pharmacology of the lower urinary tract: basis for current and future treatments of urinary incontinence. *Pharmacol Rev* 2004, 56: 581–631.
7. Somogyi GT, Tanowitz M, de Groat WC: M1 muscarinic receptor mediated facilitation of acetylcholine release in the rat urinary bladder but not in the heart. *J Physiol* 1994, 480:81–89.
8. Yamaguchi O, Shishido K, Tamura K, *et al.*: Evaluation of mRNAs encoding muscarinic receptor subtypes in human detrusor muscle. *J Urol* 1996 156:1208–1213
9. Wang P, Luthin GR, Ruggieri MR: Muscarinic acetylcholine receptor subtypes mediating urinary bladder contractility and coupling to GTP binding proteins. *J Pharmacol Exp Ther* 1995, 273:959–966.
10. Kondo S, Morita T, Tashima Y: Muscarinic cholinergic receptor subtypes in human detrusor muscle studied by labeled and nonlabeled pirenzepine, AFDX-116, and 4-DAMP. *Urol Int* 1995, 54:150–153.
11. Eglen RM, Reddy H, Watson N, Challiss RA: Muscarinic acetylcholine receptor subtypes in smooth muscle. *Trends Pharmacol Sci* 1994, 15:114–119.
12. Matsui M, Motomura D, Karasawa H, *et al.*: Multiple functional defects in peripheral autonomic organs in mice lacking muscarinic acetylcholine receptor gene for the M3 subtype. *Proc Natl Acad Sci USA* 2000, 97:9579–9584.
13. Hegde SS, Choppin A, Bonhaus D, *et al.*: Functional role of M2 and M3 muscarinic receptors in the urinary bladder of rats in vitro and in vivo. *Br J Pharmacol* 1997, 120:1409–1418.
14. Ek A: Innervation and receptor functions of the human urethra. *Scand J Urol Nephrol Suppl* 1977, 45:1–50.
15. Gosling JA, Dixon JS, Lendon RG: The autonomic innervation of the human male and female bladder neck and proximal urethra. *J Urol* 1977, 118:302–305.
16. Chancellor MB, Kaplan SA, Blaivas JG: The cholinergic and purinergic components of detrusor contractility in a whole rabbit bladder model. *J Urol* 1992, 148:906–909.

17. Palea S, Artibani W, Ostardo E, *et al.*: Evidence for purinergic neurotransmission in human urinary bladder affected by interstitial cystitis. *J Urol* 1993, 150:2007–2012.

18. O'Reilly BA, Kosaka AH, Chang TK, *et al.*: A quantitative analysis of purinoceptor expression in the bladders of patients with symptomatic outlet obstruction. *BJU Int* 2001, 87:617–622.

19. de Groat WC, Booth AM: Inhibition and facilitation in parasympathetic ganglia of the urinary bladder. *Fed Proc* 1980, 39:2990–2996.

20. Furuta A, Thomas CA, Higaki M, *et al.*: The promise of the β3-adrenoreceptor agonists to treat the overactive bladder. *Urol Clin North Am* 2006, 33:539–543.

21. Burnett AL, Maguire MP, Chamness SL, *et al.*: Characterization and localization of nitric oxide synthase in the human prostate. *Urology* 1995, 45:435–439.

22. Dixon JS, Jenn PYP: Development of nerves containing nitric oxide synthase in the human male urogenital organs. *Br J Urol* 1995, 76:719–725.

23. Andersson KE, Persson K: Nitric oxide synthase and the lower urinary tract: possible implications for physiology and pathophysiology. *Scand J Urol Nephrol Suppl* 1995, 175:43–53.

24. Bennett BC, Kruse MN, Roppolo JR, *et al.*: Neural control of urethral outlet activity in vivo: role of nitric oxide. *J Urol* 1995, 153:2004–2009.

25. Bloch W, Klotz T, Loch C, *et al.*: Distribution of nitric oxide synthase implies a regulation of circulation, smooth muscle tone, and secretory function in the human prostate by nitric oxide. *Prostate* 1997, 33:1–8.

26. Kakizaki H, de Groat WC: Role of spinal nitric oxide in the facilitation of the micturition reflex by bladder irritation. *J Urol* 1996, 155:355–360.

27. Truss MC, Uckert S, Stief CG, *et al.*: Effects of various phosphodiesterase inhibitors, forskolin, and sodium nitroprusside on porcine detrusor smooth muscle tonic responses to muscarinergic stimulation and cyclic nucleotide levels in vitro. *Neurourol Urodyn* 1996, 15:59–70.

28. Truss MC, Stief CG, Uckert S, *et al.*: Phosphodiesterase 1 inhibition in the treatment of lower urinary tract dysfunction: from bench to bedside. *World J Urol* 2001, 19:344–350.

29. de Groat WC: Neuropeptides in pelvic afferent pathways. *Experientia* 1989, 43:801–813.

30. Yoshimura N, de Groat WC: Neural control of the lower urinary tract. *Int J Urol* 1997, 4:111–125.

31. Khawaja AM, Rogers DF: Tachykinins: receptor to effector. *Int J Biochem Cell Biol* 1996, 28:721–738.

32. Lecci A, Maggi CA: Tachykinins as modulators of the micturition reflex in the central and peripheral nervous system. *Regul Pept* 2001, 101:1–18.

33. Pennefather JN, Lau WAK, Mitchelson F, Ventura S: The autonomic and sensory innervation of the smooth muscle of the prostate gland: a review of pharmacological and histological studies. *J Auton Pharmacol* 2000, 20:193–206.

34. Roehrborn CG, McConnell JD, Barry MJ, *et al.*: *Guideline on the Management of Benign Prostatic Hyperplasia (BPH)*. American Urological Association Education and Research. Linthicum, MD; 2003. Available online at http://www.auanet.org/content/guidelines-and-quality-care/clinical-guidelines/main-reports/bph-management/preface_toc.pdf

35. Roehrborn CG, Schwinn DA: Alpha-1-adrenergic receptors and their inhibitors in lower urinary tract symptoms and benign prostatic hyperplasia. *J Urol* 2004, 171:1029–1035.

36. De Mey C, Michel MC, JcEwen J, Moreland T: A double-blind comparison of terazosin and tamsulosin on their differential effects on ambulatory blood pressure and nocturnal othostatic stress testing. *Eur Urol* 1998, 33:481–488.

37. Debruyne FM: Alpha blockers: are all created equal? *Urology* 2000, 56(Suppl 1)20–22.

38. Martorana G, Giberti C, Di Silverio F, *et al.*: Effects of short-term treatment with the α1-blocker alfuzosin on urodynamic pressure/flow parameters in patients with benign prostatic hyperplasia. *Eur Urol* 1997, 32:47–53.

39. Roerhborn CG: BPH progression: concept and key learning from MTOPS, ALTESS, COMBAT, and ALF-ONE. *BJU Int* 2008, 101(Suppl 3):17–21.

40. Roehrborn CG for the ALTESS Study Group: alfuzosin 10 mg once daily prevents overall clinical progression of benign prostatic hyperplasia but not acute urinary retention: results of a 2-year placebo-controlled study. *BJU Int* 2006, 97:734–741.

41. McConnell JD: Medical management of benign prostatic hyperplasia with androgen suppression. *Prostate* 1990, 3(Suppl):49–59.

42. Kirby R, Lepor H: Evaluation and nonsurgical management of benign prostatic hyperplasia. In *Campbell-Walsh Urology*, edn 9. Edited by Wein AJ, Kavoussi LR, Novick AC, *et al.* Philadelphia: Saunders; 2007:2760–2801.

43. Evans HC, Goa KL: Dutasteride. *Drugs Aging* 2003, 20:905–916.

44. McConnell JD, Roehrborn CG, Bautista OM, *et al.*: The Medical Therapy of Prostatic Symptoms (MTOPS) Research Group: the long-term effect of doxazosin, finasteride, and combination therapy on the clinical progression of benign prostatic hyperplasia. *N Engl J Med* 2003, 349:2387–2398.

45. Thompson IM, Phyllis MD, Goodman MS, *et al.*: The influence of finasteride on the development of prostate cancer. *N Engl J Med* 2003, 349:215–224.

46. Foley SJ, Soloman LZ, Wedderburn AW, *et al.*: A prospective study of the natural history of hematuria associated with benign prostatic hyperplasia and the effect of finasteride. *J Urol* 2000, 163:496–498.

47. McConnell JD, Bruskewitz R, Walsh P, *et al.*: The effect of finasteride on the risk of acute urinary retention and the need for surgical treatment among men with benign prostatic hyperplasia. *N Engl J Med* 1998, 338:557–563.

48. Roehrborn CG, Boyle P, Nickel JC, *et al.*: Efficacy and safety of a dual inhibitor of 5-alpha-reductase types 1 and 2 (dutasteride) in men with benign prostatic hyperplasia. *Urology* 2002, 60:434–441.

49. Lepor H, Williford WO, Barry MJ, *et al.*: The efficacy of terazosin, finasteride, or both in benign prostatic hyperplasia. *N Engl J Med* 1996, 335:533–539.

50. Kirby RS, Roehrborn C, Boyle P, *et al.*: Efficacy and tolerability of doxazosin and finasteride, alone or in combination, in treatment of symptomatic benign prostatic hyperplasia: the Prospective European Doxazosin and Combination Therapy (PREDICT) trial. *Urology* 2003. 61:119–126.

51. Abrams P: Describing bladder storage function: overactive bladder syndrome and detrusor overactivity. *Urology* 2003, 62(Suppl 2):28–37.

52. Blake-James BT, Rashidian A, Ikeda Y, Emberton M: The role of anticholinergics in men with lower urinary tract symptoms suggestive of benign prostatic hyperplasia: a systematic review and meta-analysis. *BJU Int* 2007, 99:85–96.

53. Abrams P, Kaplan S, Millard R: Tolterodine treatment is safe in men with bladder outlet obstruction and symptomatic detrusor overactivity. *Proceedings of the International Continence Society 32nd Annual Meeting.* Seoul, Korea; September 18–20, 2001:107.

54. Kaplan SA, Roehrborn C, Rovner ES, *et al.*: Tolterodine and tamsulosin for treatment of men with lower urinary tract symptoms and overactive bladder: a randomized controlled trial. *JAMA* 2006, 296:2319–2328.

55. Andersson K-E, Uckert S, Stief C, Hedlund P: Phosphodiesterases (PDEs) and PDE inhibitors for treatment of LUTS. *Neurourol Urodyn* 2007, 26(Suppl):928–933.

56. McVary KT, Roehrborn CG, Kaminetsky JC, *et al.*: Tadalafil relieves lower urinary tract symptoms secondary to benign prostatic hyperplasia. *J Urol* 2007, 177:1401–1047.

57. Mulhall JP, Guhring P, Parker M, *et al.*: Assessment of the impact of sildenafil citrate on lower urinary tract symptoms in men with erectile dysfunction. *J Sex Med* 2006, 3:662–667.

58. Roehrborn CG, McVary KT, Elion-Mboussa A, *et al.*: Tadalafil administered once a day for lower urinary tract symptoms secondary to benign prostatic hyperplasia: a dose finding study. *J Urol* 2008, 180:1228–1234.

59. Kaplan SA, Gonzalex RR, Te AE : Combination of alfuzosin and sildenafil is superior to monotherapy in treating lower urinary tract symptoms and erectile dysfunction. *Eur Urol* 2007, 51:1717–1723.

60. Schiavo G, Santucci A, Dasgupta BR, *et al.*: Botulinum neurotoxins serotypes A and E cleave SNAP-25 at distinct COOH-terminal peptide bonds. *FEBS Lett* 1993, 335:99–103.

61. Arnon SS, Schechter R, Inglesby TV, *et al.*: Botulinum toxin as a biological weapon: medical and public health management. *JAMA* 2001, 285:1059–1070.

62. Schurch B, Stohrer M, Kramer G, *et al.*: Botulinum-A toxin for treating detrusor hyperreflexia in spinal cord injured patients: a new alternative to anticholinergic drugs? Preliminary results. *J Urol* 2000, 164:692–697.

63. Schmid DM, Sauermann P, Werner M, *et al.*: Experience with 100 cases treated with botulinum-A toxin injections in the detrusor muscle for idiopathic overactive bladder syndrome refractory to anticholinergics. *J Urol* 2006, 176:177–185.

64. Maria G, Brisinda G, Civello IM, *et al.*: Relief by botulinum toxin of voiding dysfunction due to benign prostatic hyperplasia: results of a randomized, placebo-controlled study. *Urology* 2003, 62:259–264.

9

Uropharmacology: Botulinum Neurotoxin

David R. Staskin and Christopher P. Smith

This chapter reviews and illustrates the structure and function of botulinum neurotoxin (BoNT). In addition, injection techniques are proposed. Areas for future research are expanding as our knowledge and utilization of the toxin continues to grow. As an example, an improved understanding of toxin deactivation and nerve regeneration would improve our ability to treat the disease as well as target pathways that would prolong the effectiveness of medical interventions. The utilization of BoNT is investigative for lower urinary tract symptoms but holds great promise for modulating efferent and afferent disease as well as symptoms of the bladder and bladder outlet.

Botulinum Neurotoxin: The Disease

BoNT blocks exocytosis of acetylcholine at all peripheral cholinergic sites, including neuromuscular junctions, ganglia of the sympathetic and parasympathetic nervous system, and postganglionic parasympathetic sites. BoNT (Latin *botulus* = "sausage") is produced by the bacterium *Clostridium botulinum*. The toxin is formed by the spores of the bacteria that in an anaerobic environment germinate, grow, and release toxin. Spores (nonheat sensitive) produce bacteria (high Na^+ and acid sensitive), which produce toxin (heat sensitive). An exception is infant intestinal and wound botulism that result from infection with spores that subsequently germinate, resulting in production of toxin and the symptoms of botulism (*see* Fig. 9-1) [1,2].

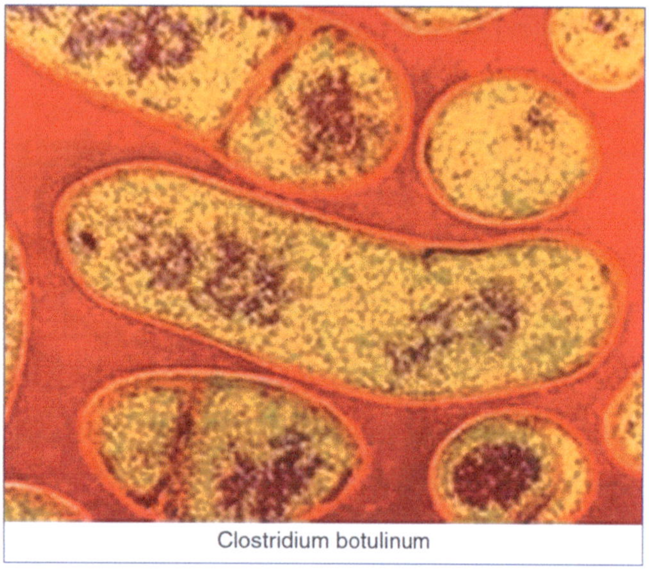

Figure 9-1. Microscopic view of *Clostridium botulinum* bacteria. (*From* Centers for Disease Control and Prevention's Public Health Image Library. http://phil.cdc.gov/phil/home.asp.)

Botulinum Neurotoxin: Measuring Potency

BoNT is the most potent toxin known to man. The median lethal dose (LD_{50}) of BoNT-A for a 70-kg adult male can be calculated to be 35 to 40 U/kg or 1 ng/kg. Of note, because the toxin is a biologic product with inherent variability, variations in potency may occur within a strain and between strains (suBoNTypes). Commercial testing for potency is carried out for each batch of toxin and at several stages of the toxin production process and is standardized by determining the lethal dose in mice. A mouse unit (MU) is equivalent to the amount of toxin constituted in 1 mL that kills 50% (LD_{50}) of a group of 20-g mice within 3 days of intraperitoneal injection (eight to 24 animals/dose, six doses, × four replicates). Toxic doses typically fall within the range of about 0.6 to 2.5 mouse LD_{50} units [3–5]. As local chemodenervation is responsible for the therapeutic effect of BoNT, the potency can also be predicted by directly measuring regional denervation rather than lethality. An aliquot of the toxin can be injected into the gastrocnemius muscle of the hind limb of mice. The amount of toxin activity in a given preparation is assessed by evaluating the fraction of mice that showed complete paralysis of the right hind limb. This method has been primarily used to compare toxins and has demonstrated a significant difference in potency among subtypes. More advanced methods of determining potency are under development [6,7].

Botulinum Neurotoxin: Structure and Subtypes

The BoNT complex and the associated components (where indicated) are illustrated in "ribbon," "surface representation," "amino acid chain," and "graphic" representations (*see* Figs. 9-2 through 9-5). The functions of the individual components are detailed in Figure 9-6.

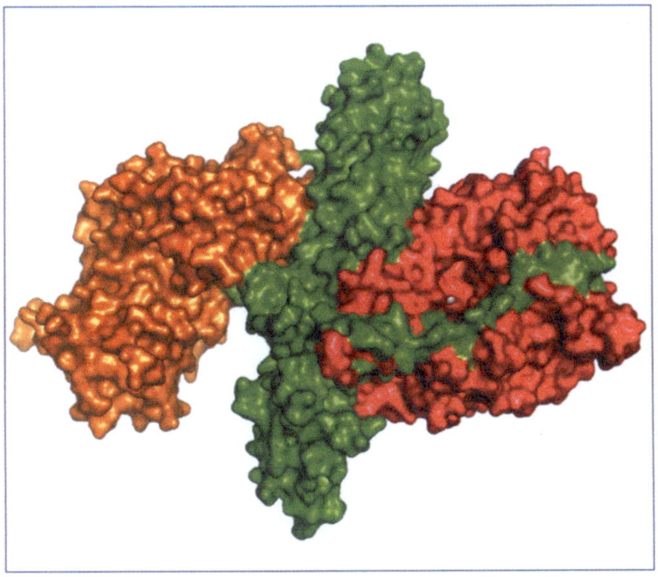

FIGURE 9-2. Botulinum neurotoxin-B "ribbon representation." The catalytic domain is in *red*, the translocation domain is in *green*, and the binding domain is in *orange*. The catalytic zinc is shown as a *sphere in gray* within the catalytic domain. (*Courtesy of* S. Swaminathan, Brookhaven National Laboratory, Upton, NY.)

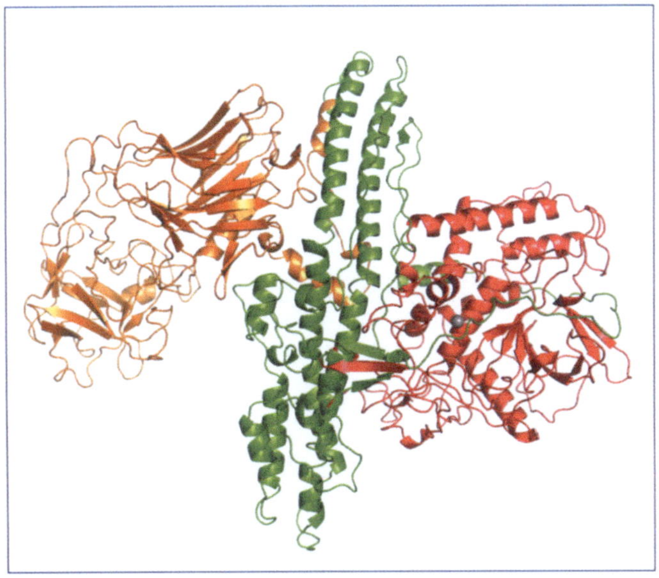

FIGURE 9-3. Botulinum neurotoxin-B "surface representation." The catalytic domain is in *red*, the translocation domain is in *green*, and the binding domain is in *orange*. The catalytic zinc is shown as a *sphere in gray* within the catalytic domain. (*Courtesy of* S. Swaminathan, Brookhaven National Laboratory, Upton, NY.)

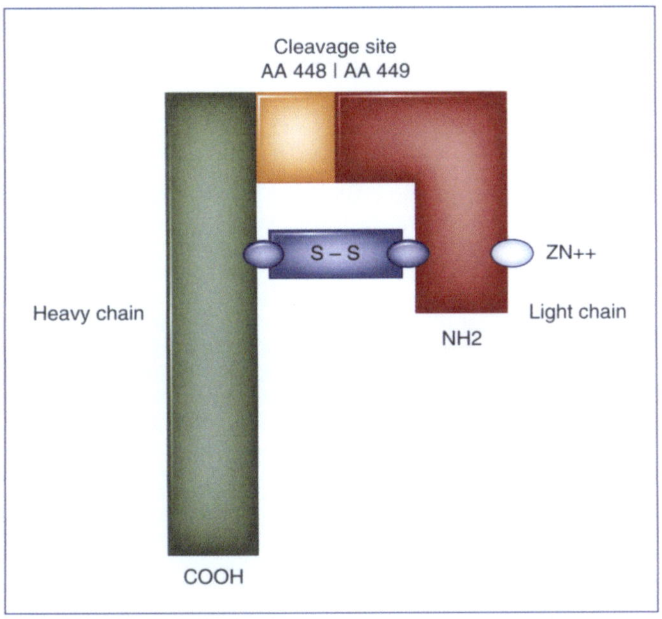

FIGURE 9-4. Botulinum neurotoxin in an "amino-acid chain" representation. The full structure is shown where the proteolytic cleavage (amino acids 448–449) separates the heavy chain (*green–gold*) and light chain (*red*), which after cleavage are still bound by the disulfide (S-S) bond. The zinc (ZN) molecule is noted and is attached to the light chain. (*see* Fig. 9-6 for functional component details.)

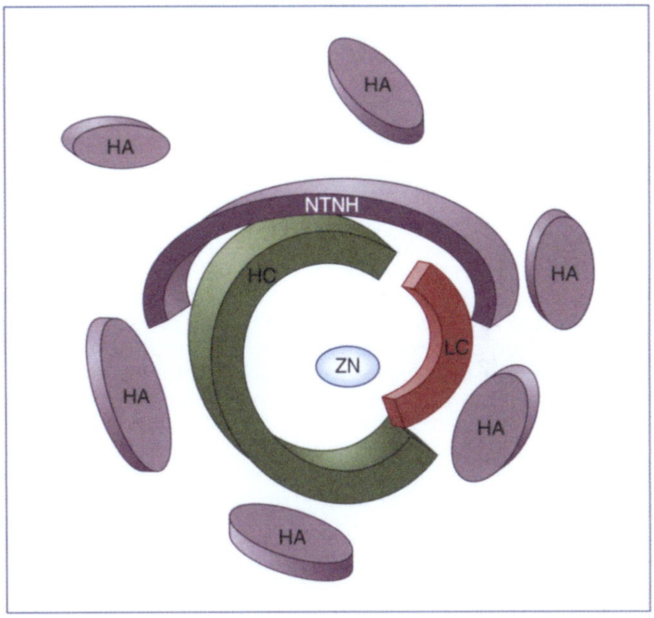

FIGURE 9-5. Botulinum toxin "graphic" representation. The heavy chain (HC) (*green*) and light chain (LC) (*red*) are noted, as well as the zinc (ZN) molecule. In addition, the nonhemagglutinin (NTNH) proteins and hemagglutinin (HA) proteins are illustrated. (*see* Fig. 9-6 for functional component details.)

The Neurotoxin Complex and Associated Components

- Botulinum toxin: di-chain neurotoxin component ($C_{6760}H_{10447}N_{1743}O_{2010}S_{32}$) is149.320 kD
  - Light chain ~50 kD (amino acid #1–#448)
    - Endopeptidase proteolytic activity located at the N-terminal end defunctionalizes one of the proteins (SNAP-25, syntaxin, or synaptobrevin) preventing Ca^{++}-dependent binding of acetylcholine vesicles to the membrane for release
  - Heavy chain ~100 kD (amino acid #449–#1280)
    - Carboxy-terminal half binding to specific receptors
      - Receptors: synaptic vesicle 2 and specific gangliosides
      - Cholinergic specificity and transport into cell
      - Binds to specific transport proteins
        - Transport and formation of endosome
      - Transports light chain out of endosome into cytosol
        - pH-dependent translocation
  - Di-sulfide bond (see Fig. 9-4 only)
    - Binds heavy and light chains together
- Zn^{2+}
  - Important for endopeptidase activity
- NTHN and HA proteins (nontoxic nonhemagglutinin and hemagglutinin) (see Fig. 9-5 only)
  - Protects the molecule that is sensitive to pH and proteolytic enzymes in gut and may not be necessary for lung or blood infection; size of molecule limits penetration of blood-brain barrier

FIGURE 9-6. The neurotoxin complex and associated components.

The term *botulinum neurotoxin* represents seven neurotoxins that are antigenically and serologically distinct but have a similar structure. Human botulism is caused mainly by types A, B, E, and (rarely) F (*see* Fig. 9-7). Types C and D cause toxicity only in animals. Serotypes C and E appeared to be similar to serotype A, whereas serotypes D and F are similar to serotype B. Each serotype cleaves only one peptide bond in its substrate, but the amino acid sequence may be repeated elsewhere in the substrate BoNT-A and BoNT-E cleave synaptosome-associated protein of 25 kD (SNAP-25: Gln197–Arg198 for serotype A; Arg180–Ile181 for serotype E), a presynaptic membrane protein required for fusion of neurotransmitter containing vesicles. BoNT-B, BoNT-D, BoNT-F, and BoNTG cleave a vesicle-associated membrane protein, also known as synaptobrevin. BoNT-C acts by cleaving syntaxin, a target membrane protein, although it can also cleave SNAP-25 [8–11].

The duration of action of the seven toxin serotypes varies, although serotype A is known to have the most sustained action. Whether measured in laboratory animals or in human beings, the duration of serotype A action can be many weeks to many months. This sustained action may be a function of the substrate cleavage product, the intraneuronal half-life of the toxin, or a combination of the two. It is noteworthy that no one has yet determined how the toxin subtypes are metabolized or otherwise eliminated, although nerve sprouting appears to be necessary for nerve reactivation (*see* Fig. 9-7) [9,10].

Seven Known Types of Botulinum Toxin and Their Targets, Representative Agents, and Characteristics		
Type	Target	Available agents and characteristics
A	SNAP-25	Commercial name: Botox (Allergen, Irvine, CA)
		Strain: Hall
		Size: 9000 kD
		Units per vial: 100
		Commercial name: Dysport (Ipsen, Ltd, Slough, UK)
		Strain: NCTC-2916
		Size: 600 kD
		Units per vial: 500
		Commercial name: China Toxin
		Strain: Unknown
		Size: 600–900 kD
		Units per vial: 100
B	VAMP	Commercial name: Myobloc (Elan, Dublin, Ireland)
		Strain: Bean
		Size: 700 kD
		Units per vial: 2500, 5000, 10,000
C1	Syntaxin	
D	VAMP	
E	SNAP-25	
F	VAMP	
G	VAMP	

Figure 9-7. The seven known types of botulinum neurotoxin: targets, representative agents, and characteristics.

Botulinum Neurotoxin: Mechanism of Action (Injection)

The mechanism of action of BoNT injection is outlined in Figures 9-8 through 9-12 [8,10–13]. The toxin is injected into the extracellular space.

Binding/attachment. The heavy chain (carboxy terminus) targets the cell. Subtype toxin binds to receptors on the cell surface (sialic acid/ganglioside/lectin complexes), which are highly specific surface recognition domains for BoNT of cholinergic axon terminals.

Endocytosis. Following the attachment of the heavy chain, the toxin is transported into the neuron. The toxin acquires an intracellular endosomal membrane.

Translocation. The light chain transports the complex out of the endosomal vesicle to reach the cytoplasm: a) an acidic environment is created within the endosome (proton pump) and the pH-induced change in toxin structure results in exposure of previously occult hydrophobic domains; b) insertion of the toxin into the endosome membrane; c) translocation of the light chain–heavy chain complex from the luminal to the cytosolic surface of the membrane; d) reduction and uncoupling of the noncovalent disulfide (S-S) bond that links the heavy chain and light chain with separation; e) restoration of light-chain structure in the more neutral cytoplasmic environment in preparation for proteolysis.

Proteolysis. The light chain of the toxin has endoprotease activity. Proteolysis occurs when the type A toxin degrades the SNAP-25 protein, a type of SNARE protein that mediates fusion of the cellular transport vesicle with the cell membrane or with a target compartment (lysosome). BoNT, depending on the type (see Fig. 9-6), specifically cleaves these SNAREs, and so prevents neurosecretory vesicles from docking/fusing with the nerve synapse plasma membrane and releasing their neurotransmitters.

Sprouting. Sprouting occurs to reestablish function while a functional axonal terminus is formed.

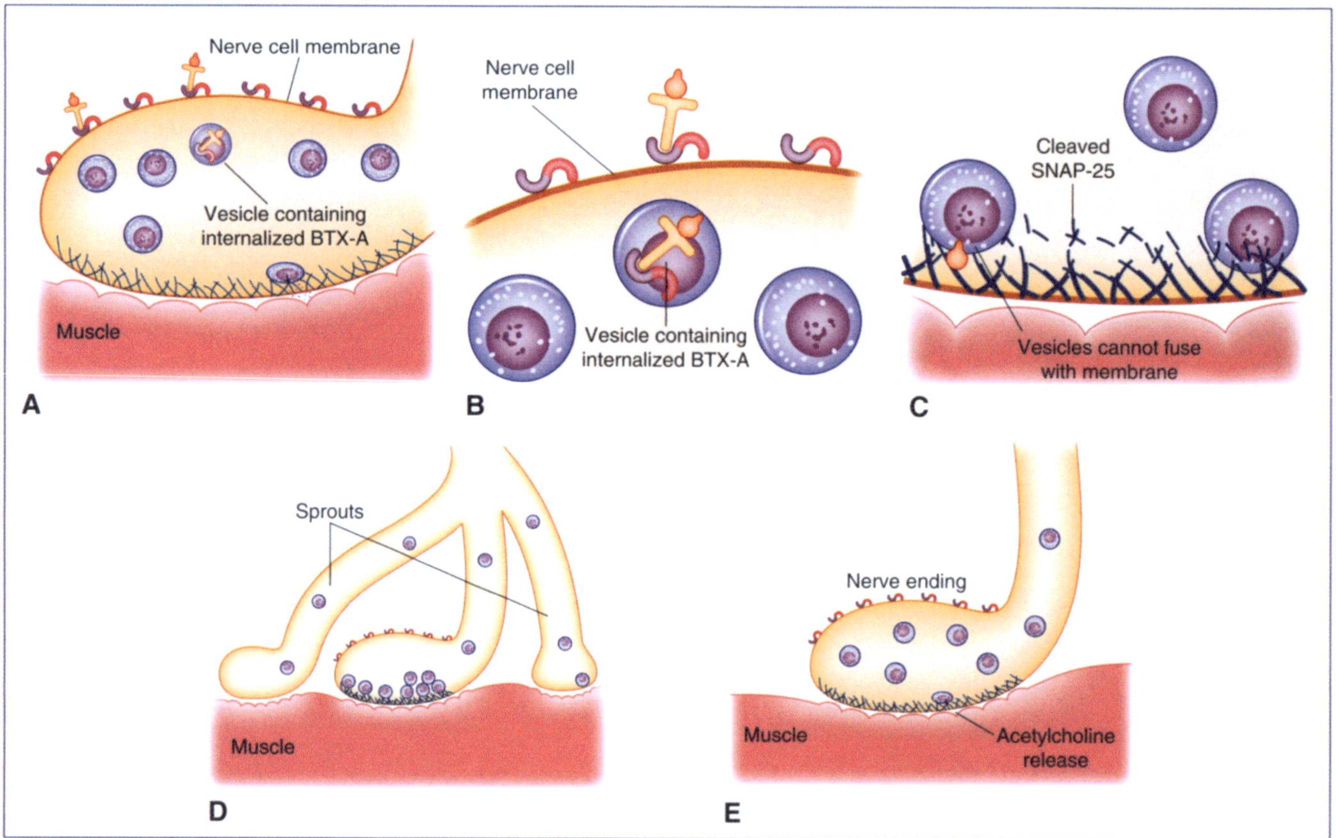

Figure 9-8. **A**, Binding: the heavy chain portion of the active ingredient in botulinum neurotoxin (BoNT) binds to the cell membrane of the parasympathetic motor nerve. **B**, Endocytosis: after binding, the BoNT protein molecule passes through the cell into the cytoplasm. **C**, Proteolysis: cleaving of SNAP-25 elements inhibits acetylcholine release (efferent) and also blocks the release of neuropeptides involved in the transmission of painful sensations including substance P, glutamate, and calcitonin gene–related peptide (afferent). This is illustrated in more detail in Fig. 9-9 and Fig. 9-10. **D**, Nerve sprouting: new nerve endings sprout and connect to the muscle after the original nerve ending is blocked, renewing the ability of the nerve to cause muscle contractions. **E**, Original nerve connection reestablished: new nerve sprouts retract and the original nerve ending regains its function.

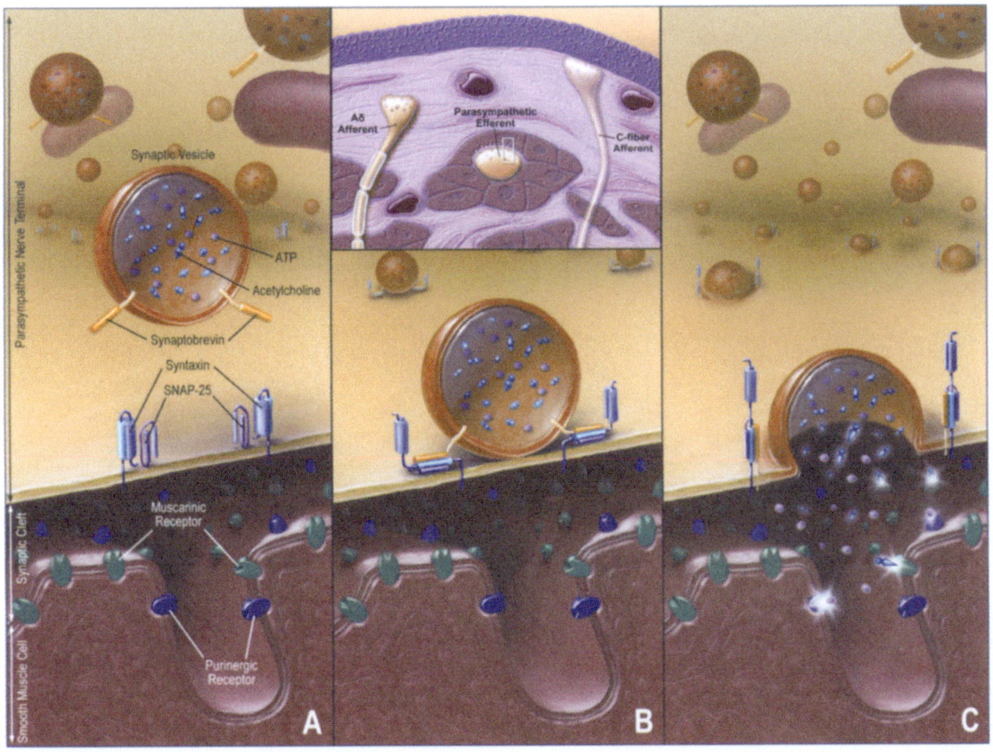

FIGURE 9-9. **A–C**, Normal fusion and release of acetylcholine from parasympathetic nerve terminals via interaction of SNARE proteins. (*Courtesy of* Scott A. Weldon, MA, CMI, Baylor College of Medicine, Houston, TX.)

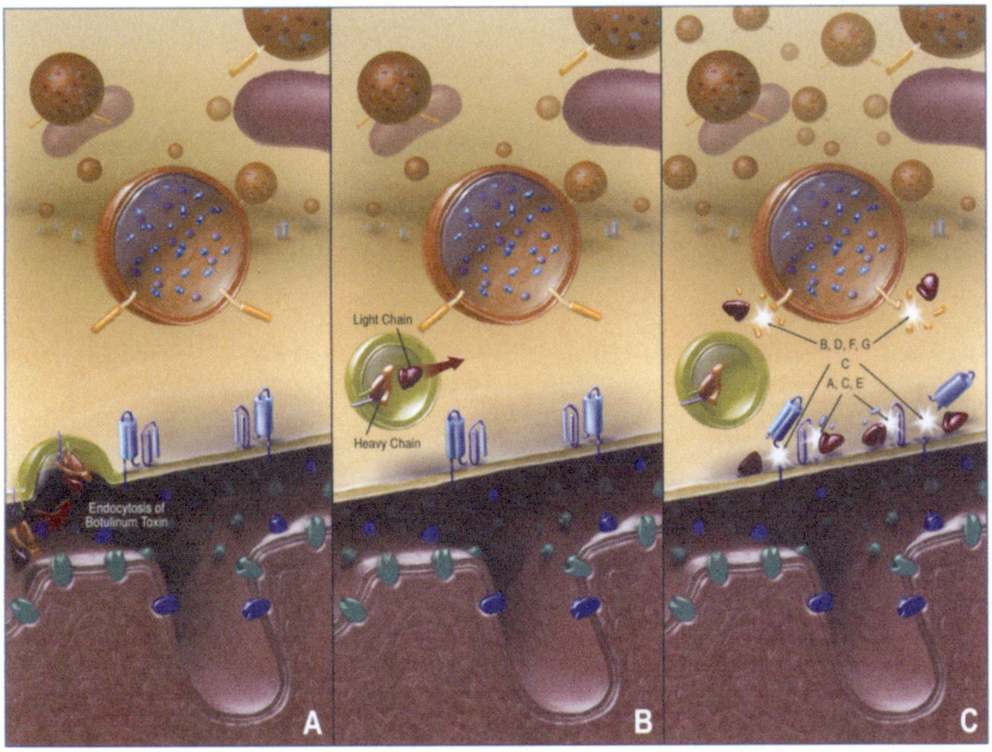

FIGURE 9-10. **A–C**, Binding, internalization, and cleavage of specific SNARE proteins by botulinum neurotoxins resulting in inhibition of transmitter release. (*Courtesy of* Scott A. Weldon, MA, CMI, Baylor College of Medicine, Houston, TX.)

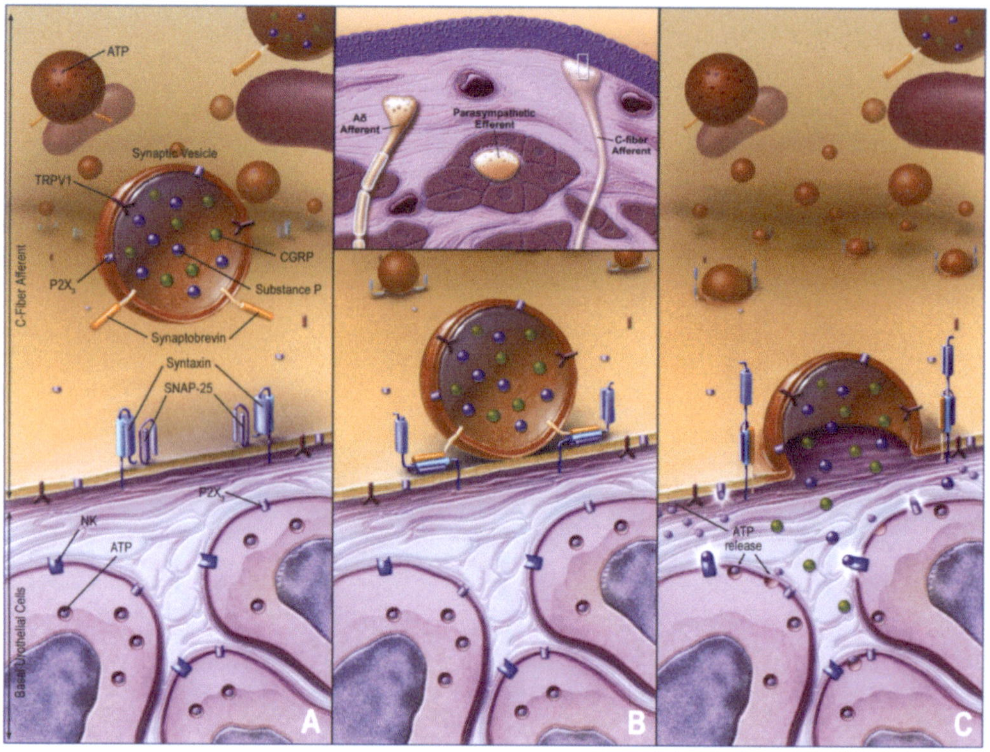

FIGURE 9-11. A–C, Potential action of botulinum toxin on bladder C-fiber afferent terminals. SNARE protein–dependent fusion and release of vesicles containing transmitters (*ie*, calcitonin gene–related peptide [CGRP], substance P) and receptors (*ie*, TRPV1 and P2X3). (*Courtesy of* Scott A. Weldon, MA, CMI, Baylor College of Medicine, Houston, TX.)

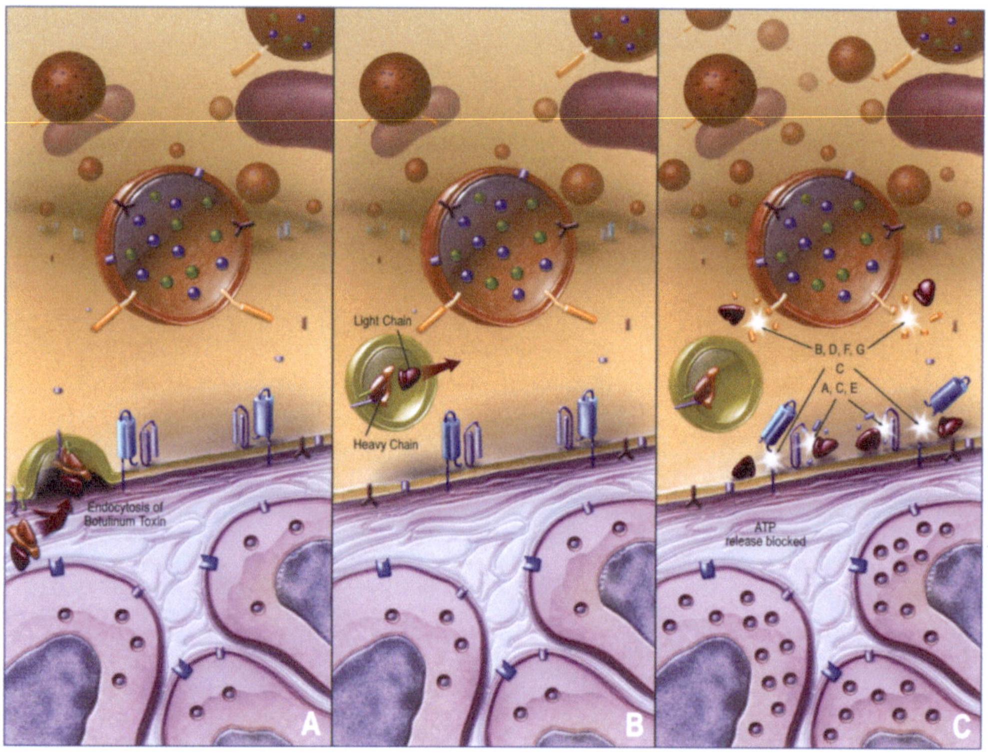

FIGURE 9-12. A–C, Botulinum toxin uptake and cleavage of specific SNARE proteins resulting in inhibition of transmitter release or surface membrane receptor expression. (*Courtesy of* Scott A. Weldon, MA, CMI, Baylor College of Medicine, Houston, TX.)

Botulinum Neurotoxin: Comparison with Tetanus Toxin

The unique mode of action of BoNT can be compared and contrasted with the tetanus toxin (*see* Fig. 9-13). The toxin produced from *Clostridium botulinum* differs from *Clostridium tetani* by inhibiting peripheral acetylcholine release causing flaccid (sagging) paralysis of muscles as opposed to the tetanus toxin blockade of central inhibitory neurotransmitter release resulting in a spastic paralysis. The most significant difference between tetanus toxin and botulinum toxin is the retrograde transmission, discharging, and reuptake by the proximal axon as the tetanus toxin proceeds retrograde along the central nervous system.

Tetanospasmin is transported within the axon and across synaptic junctions until it reaches the central nervous system. There it becomes rapidly fixed to gangliosides at the presynaptic inhibitory motor nerve endings, and is taken up into the axon by endocytosis. The effect of the toxin is to block the release of inhibitory neurotransmitters (glycine and gamma-amino butyric acid) across the synaptic cleft, which is required to check the nervous impulse. If nervous impulses cannot be checked by normal inhibitory mechanisms, it produces the generalized muscular spasms. Tetanospasmin appears to act by selective cleavage of synaptobrevin II, which prevents the release of neurotransmitters by the cells. The A fragment has toxic (enzymatic) activity after the B fragment secures its entry. Binding appears to be an irreversible event. Recovery depends on sprouting a new axon terminal (*see* Fig. 9-8*D*) [13–17].

Differential Toxin Characteristics: *Clostridium botulinum* versus *Clostridium tetani*

Bacteria	*Clostridium botulinum*	*Clostridium tetani*
Toxin	Botulinum toxin	Tetanospasmin (TeTx/TeNT)
Neurotoxin: two-chain metalloendopeptidase	Yes	Yes
Disulphide bridge and zinc	Yes	Yes
Heavy chain: 100 kD	Yes	Yes
Function: entry	Yes	Yes
Endocytosis	Yes	Yes
Light chain: 50 kD	Yes	Yes
Function: enzymatic	Yes	Yes
Vegetative spore	Yes (A, B)	No
Oral poisoning (transcytosis through gut)	No (C)	No
Mehanism of action	Blocks stimulation	Blocks inhibition
Neuortransmitter	Acetylcholine (*see* text for sensory effects)	Glycine/gamma-amino butyric acid
Common steps in neural action	Yes	Yes
Adsorption	Yes	Yes
Binding surface receptors: sialic acid/gangliosides/lectin	Yes	Yes
Endocytosis	Yes	Yes
Cleavage to heavy-light chains	Yes	Yes
Translocation to cytosol (release of light chain by proton pumping and conformational change, insertion, channel formation)	Yes	Yes
Different site of action of light chain	SNAP-25 VAMP Syntaxin	VAMP - synaptobrevin II
Retrograde axon transport	No	Yes
Release	Not permeable to blood-brain barrier (systemically deactivated)	Yes
Repeat of cycle	No	Yes

Figure 9-13. Differential toxin characteristics: *Clostridium botulinum* versus *Clostridium tetani*.

It should be noted that BoNT injection into the bladder is an "off-label" non–US Food and Drug Administration–approved utilization of the substance. Multiple clinical trials are registered and many have been completed (http://clinicaltrials.gov/ct2/results?term=botulinum+toxin+bladder).

It should be emphasized that no standardized injection technique exists for BoNT-A injection in the lower urinary tract. However, no controlled studies have been performed to determine the optimum dose or toxin dilution in neurogenic and OAB patient populations. In addition, the depth optimum depth for injection has also not been studied.

Number of injections: Bladder injections with BoNT-A can be made using either a rigid or flexible cystoscope, under general or local anesthesia. A total of 100 to 300 units of BoNT-A diluted in 10 to 30 mL of preservative saline (*ie*, 10 units/mL, 1 mL/injection) are injected submucosally throughout the bladder using an endoscopic injection needle (see Fig. 9-14A). In our protocol, for idiopathic bladder overactivity, 100 to 200 units are injected, whereas in neurogenic bladder overactivity 200 to 300 units are injected, using the higher dose when complete bladder paralysis is acceptable (*ie*, patient already performing clean intermittent catheterization). Different injection paradigms have been described (*ie*, trigone vs trigone-sparing), although none has been proven to be superior to the other. For patients with interstitial cystitis, 100 units are injected and the template is focused on the bladder trigone, where bladder sensory nerves are most abundant and there is minimal concern about vesico-ureteral reflux (see Fig. 9-14B) [18].

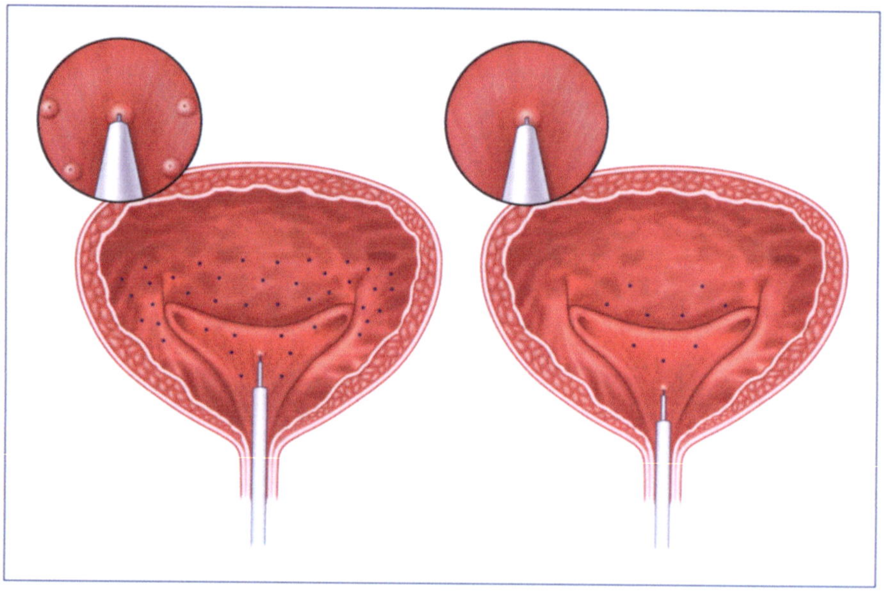

FIGURE 9-14. Diagram depicting botulinum neurotoxin (BoNT) injection sites within the detrusor muscle of the bladder. In contrast to other investigators, we target the trigone because of its rich sensory innervation. **A**, Thirty to 40 injection templates were used for neurogenic or severe idiopathic overactive bladder patients and typically 200 to 300 units of BoNT-A injection. **B**, Ten injection templates were used for moderate idiopathic overactive bladder patients or patients with interstitial cystitis using 100 to 200 units.

Depth of injections: Many questions arise regarding how deep to inject the toxin: intramuscularly, submucosally, or epithelially. Mehnert *et al.* [19] performed a study where neurogenic detrusor overactive patients' bladders were injected intramuscularly with 300 units of BoNT-A mixed with gadolinium. Immediately following injection, patients underwent an MRI study to document the distribution of the gadolinium. The investigators found that almost 18% of injected BoNT-A was localized outside the bladder wall in the extraperitoneal fat. In addition, Kuo [20] demonstrated significant increases in functional bladder capacity, significant reductions in urge episodes, without an increase in postvoid residual in patients with idiopathic overactive bladder undergoing bladder trigone suburothelial injections compared with patients injected intramuscularly outside of the trigonal area. Unfortunately, without the ability to adequately label BoNT, it is impossible to clearly define toxin distribution with different injection paradigms. For this reason we strongly prefer an injection protocol that incorporates the trigone and avoids the posterior wall and dome and places the diluted toxin in a submucosal fashion (see Fig. 9-12). (*Courtesy of* Scott A. Weldon, MA, CMI, Baylor College of Medicine, Houston, TX.)

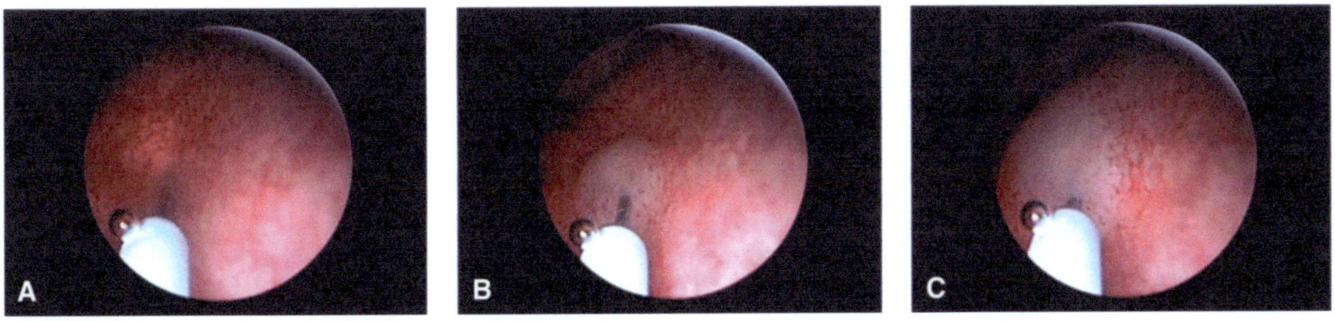

FIGURE 9-15. **A**, Insertion of the needle into the bladder wall. **B**, "Mucosal" injection is shallow, creating a blistering effect of the urothelium with loss of vascular markings and minimal toxin spread. **C**, As the needle is inserted further the injection is then directed submucosally with significant elevation of the mucosal wall in both vertical and horizontal planes and persistence of mucosal vascular markings. Deeper injection may increase the risk of extravesical extravasation.

References

1. Lamanna C: The most poisonous poison. *Science* 1959, 130:763–772.
2. Dickerson JT, Janda KD: The use of small molecules to investigate molecular mechanism and therapeutic targets for treatment of botulinum neurotoxin A intoxication. *ACS Chem Biol* 2006, 1:359–369.
3. Gill DM: Bacterial toxins: a table of lethal amounts. *Microbiol Rev* 1982, 46:86–94.
4. Schantz EJ, Kautter DA: Microbiological methods: standardized assay for clostridium botulinurn toxins. *J AOAC Int* 1977, 61:96–99.
5. Sesardic D, Leung T, Gaines DR: Role of standards in assays of botulinum toxins: international collaborative study of three preparations of botulinum type A toxin. *Biologicals* 2003, 31:265–276.
6. Sugiyama H, Brenner SL, DasGupta BR: Detection of clostridium botulinurn toxin by local paralysis elicited with intramuscular challenge. *Appl Microbial* 1975, 30:420–423.
7. Pearce LB, Borodic GE, Johnson EA, *et al.*: The median paralysis unit: a more pharmacologically relevant unit of biologic activity for botulinum toxin. *Toxicon* 1995, 33:217–227.
8. Foster KA, Bigalke H, Aoki KR: Botulinum neurotoxin—from laboratory to bedside. *Neurotox Res* 2006, 9:133–140.
9. Simpson LL: Identificantio of the major steps in botulinum toxin action. *Ann Rev Pharmacol Toxicol* 2004, 44:167–193.
10. DasGupta BR: Structure and biological activity of botulinum neurotoxin. *J Physiol (Paris)* 1990, 84:220–228.
11. de Paiva A, Meunier FA, Molgo J, *et al.*: Functional repair of motor endplates after botulinum neurotoxin type A poisoning: biphasic switch of synaptic activity between nerve sprouts and their parent terminals. *Proc Natl Acad Sci U S A* 1999, 96:3200–3205.
12. Dong M, Yeh F, Tepp WH, *et al.*: SV2 is the protein receptor for botulinum neurotoxin A. *Science* 2006, 312:592–596.
13. Montecucco C: How do tetanus and botulinum toxins bind to neuronal membranes? *Trends Biochem Sci* 1986, 11:314–317.
14. Schiavo G, Rossetto O, Benfenati F, *et al.*: Tetanus and botulinum neurotoxins are zinc proteases specific for components of the neuroexocytosis apparatus. *Ann N Y Acad Sci* 1994, 710:65–75.
15. Humeau Y, Doussau F, Grant NJ, Poulain B: How botulinum and tetanus neurotoxins block neurotransmitter release. *Biochemie* 2000, 82:427–446.
16. Turton K, Chaddock JA, Acharya KR: Botulinum and tetanus neurotoxins: structure, function and therapeutic utility. *Trends Biochem* 2002, 27:552–558.
17. Schiavo G, Matteoli M, Montecucco C: Neurotoxins affecting neuroexocytosis. *Physiol Rev* 2000, 80:717–766.
18. Karsenty G, Elzayat E, Delapparent T, *et al.*: Botulinum toxin type A injections into the trigone to treat idiopathic overactive bladder do not induce vesicoureteral reflux. *J Urol* 2007, 177:1011–1014.
19. Mehnert U, Boy S, Schmid M, *et al.*: A morphological evaluation of botulinum neurotoxin A injections into the detrusor muscle using magnetic resonance imaging. *World J Urol* 2009, 27:397–403.
20. Kuo HC: Comparison of effectiveness of detrusor, suburothelial and bladder base injections of otulinum toxin a for idiopathic detrusor overactivity. *J Urol* 2007, 178:1359–1363.

10 Urinary Stress Incontinence

Dudley Robinson and Linda Cardozo

The term *urinary stress incontinence* may be used to describe the symptoms or signs of urinary leakage on coughing or exertion, but should not be regarded as a diagnosis. A diagnosis of urodynamic stress incontinence may only be made after urodynamic investigation, which is defined as the involuntary leakage of urine during increased abdominal pressure in the absence of a detrusor contraction [1].

Epidemiology

Stress incontinence is the most commonly reported type of urinary incontinence in women. A large epidemiological study of 27,936 women from Norway has recently been reported [2]. Overall, 25% of women reported urinary incontinence, of which 7% felt it to be significant and the prevalence of incontinence was found to increase with age. When considering the type of incontinence, 50% of women complained of stress, 11% of urge, and 36% of mixed incontinence.

Further analysis has also investigated the effect of age and parity. The prevalence of urinary incontinence among nulliparous women ranged from 8% to 32% and increased with age. In general, parity was associated with incontinence and the first delivery was the most significant. When considering stress incontinence in the age group of 20 to 34 years, the relative risk was 2.7 (95% CI: 2.0–3.5) for primiparous women and 4.0 (95% CI: 2.5–6.4) for multiparous women. There was a similar association for mixed incontinence although not for urge incontinence [3].

Pathophysiology

Causes of Urodynamic Stress Incontinence
Urethral hypermobility
Urogenital prolapse
Pelvic floor damage or denervation
Parturition
Pelvic surgery
Menopause
Urethral scarring
Vaginal (urethral) surgery
Incontinence surgery
Urethral dilation or urethrotomy
Recurrent urinary tract infections
Radiotherapy
Raised intra-abdominal pressure
Pregnancy
Chronic cough (bronchitis)
Abdominal/pelvic mass
Fecal impaction
Ascites
(Obesity)

FIGURE 10-1. There are various different underlying causes that result in weakness of one or more of the components of the urethral sphincter mechanism. The bladder neck and proximal urethra are normally situated in an intra-abdominal position above the pelvic floor and are supported by the pubourethral ligaments. Damage to either the pelvic floor musculature (levator ani) or pubourethral ligaments may result in descent of the proximal urethra such that it is no longer an intra-abdominal organ, resulting in leakage of urine per urethram during stress.

More recently, the "midurethral theory" or "integral theory" has been described by Petros and Ulmsten [4]. This concept is based on earlier studies suggesting that the distal urethra and midurethra play an important role in the continence mechanism [5] and that the maximal urethral closure pressure is at the midurethral point [6]. This theory proposes that damage to the pubourethral ligaments supporting the urethra, impaired support of the anterior vaginal wall to the midurethra, and weakened function of part of the pubococcygeal muscles, which are inserted adjacent to the urethra, are responsible for causing stress incontinence.

Surgery for Urinary Stress Incontinence

Anterior Colporrhaphy

Anterior colporrhaphy is now rarely performed for the treatment of stress urinary incontinence and, due to relatively low short-term success rates, can no longer be recommended. Although it is usually the best operation for a cystourethrocele, the cure rates for urodynamic stress incontinence are poor compared to suprapubic [7] and midurethral tape procedures.

Marshall-Marchetti-Krantz Procedure

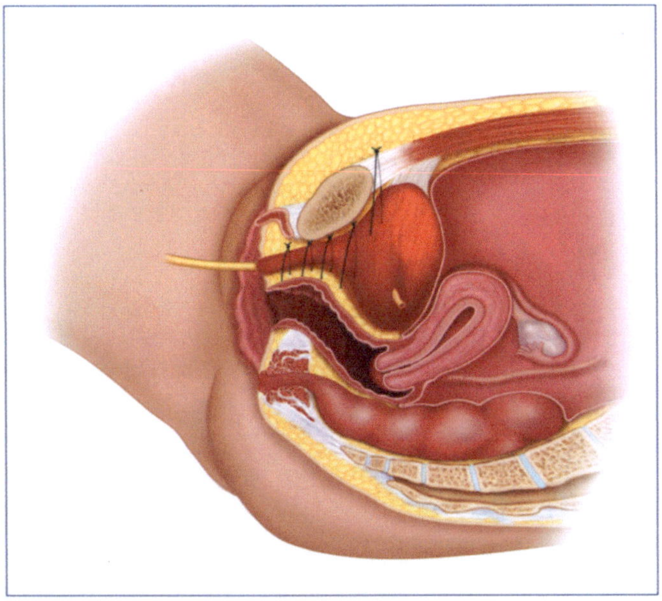

Figure 10-2. The Marshall-Marchetti-Krantz procedure [8] is a suprapubic operation in which the paraurethral tissue at the level of the bladder neck is sutured to the periosteum or perichondrium of the posterior aspect of the pubic symphysis. This procedure elevates the bladder neck but will not correct any concomitant cystocele. It has been largely superseded by the Burch colposuspension because its complications include osteitis pubis in 2% to 7% of cases. (*Adapted from* Cardozo and Staskin [9].)

Bladder Neck Suspension Procedures

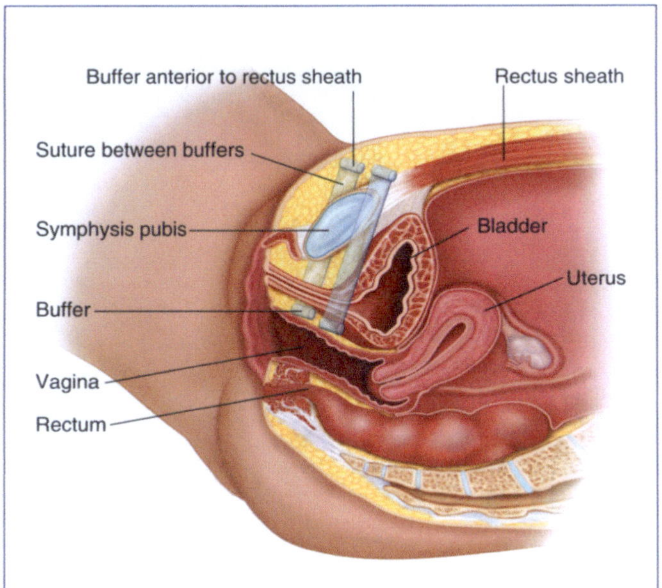

Figure 10-3. Endoscopically guided bladder neck suspensions are simple to perform, but they are less effective than open suprapubic procedures and are now seldom used [10–12]. In each of these operations, a long needle is used to insert a loop of nylon on each side of the bladder neck; this is tied over the rectus sheath to elevate the urethrovesical junction. Cystoscopy is employed to ensure accurate placement of the sutures and to detect any damage to the bladder caused by the needle or the suture. In the Stamey procedure, buffers are used to avoid the sutures cutting through the tissues and, in the Raz procedure, a helical suture of Prolene is inserted deep into the endopelvic fascia lateral to the bladder neck to avoid cutting through. The main problem with each of these operations is that they rely on two sutures, which may break or pull through the tissues. However, endoscopically guided bladder neck suspensions are quick and easy to perform. They can be carried out under regional blockade and postoperative recovery is fast. Temporary voiding difficulties are common after long needle suspensions, but these usually resolve and there are few other complications. (*Adapted from* Cardozo and Staskin [9].)

Colposuspension

The Burch colposuspension has been modified by many authors since its original description [13]. Until relatively recently, colposuspension has been the operation of choice in primary urodynamic stress incontinence as it corrects both stress incontinence and a cystocele. However, it may not be suitable if the vagina is scarred or narrowed by previous surgery.

While the colposuspension is now well recognized as an effective procedure for stress incontinence, it is not without complications. Detrusor overactivity may occur de novo or may be unmasked by the procedure [14], which may lead to long-term urinary symptoms. Voiding difficulties are common postoperatively and, although they usually resolve within a short time after the operation, long-term voiding dysfunction may result. In addition, a rectoenterocele may be exacerbated by repositioning the vagina [15]. However, the colposuspension is the only incontinence operation for which long-term data are available. Alcalay *et al.* [16] have reported a series of 109 women with an overall cure rate of 69% at a mean of 13.8 years.

Technique

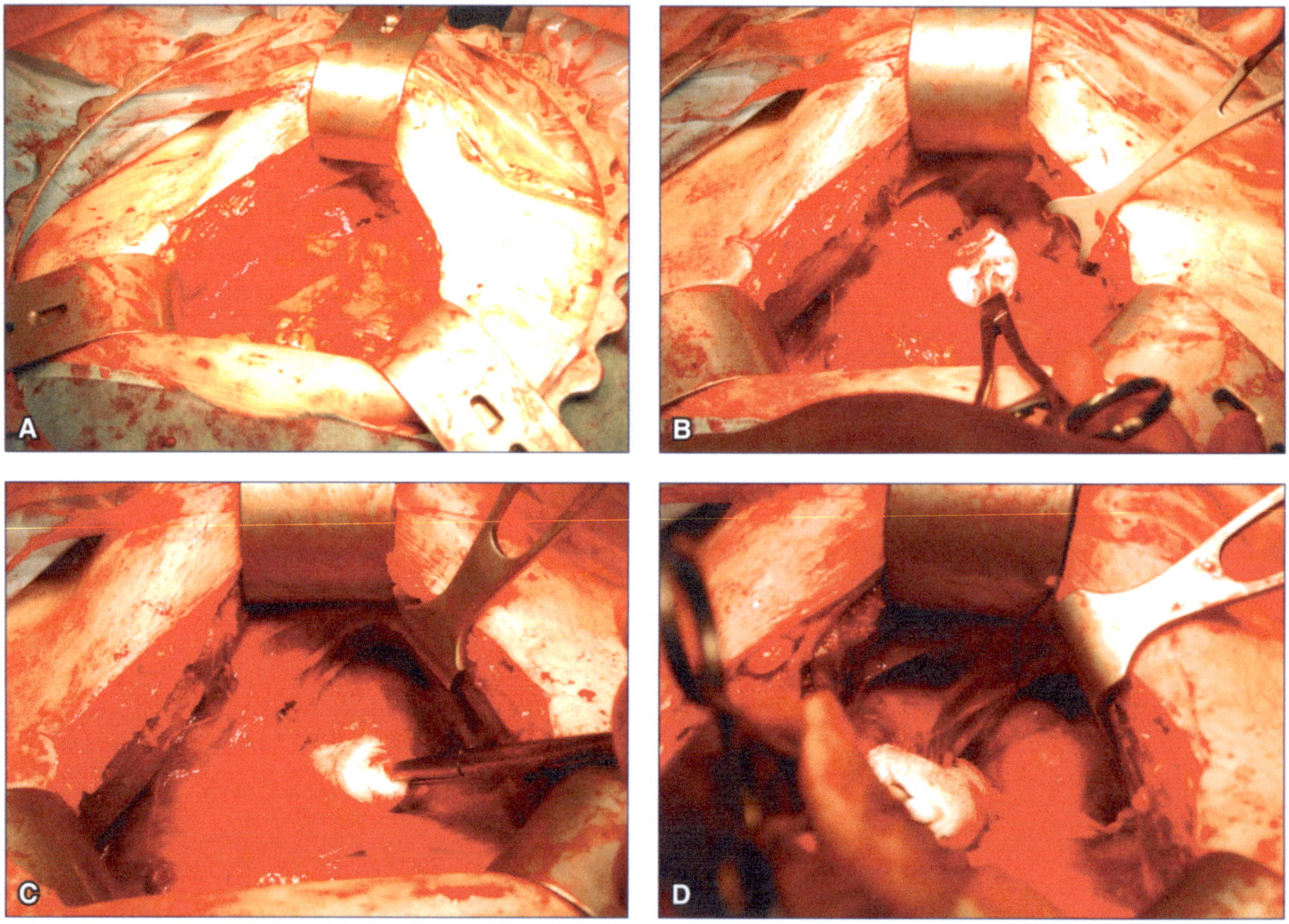

Figure 10-4. The patient is positioned on the operating table in the modified lithotomy position using Lloyd-Davies stirrups. The abdomen and vagina are then prepared as a sterile operating field in order to allow manipulation of the vaginal fornices and bladder neck by the surgeon. An indwelling Foley catheter is then inserted and the balloon is inflated with 6 mL of water to allow identification of the bladder neck.

A low transverse suprapubic incision approximately 1 cm above the pubic symphysis is made and the rectus fascia is incised taking care not to open the peritoneal cavity unless a concomitant intra-abdominal procedure is being performed. **A,** A Turner-Warwick self-retaining retractor may then be inserted and **B,** the retropubic space (Cave of Retzius) is opened using both sharp and blunt dissection until **C,** the white paravaginal tissue lateral to the bladder neck and urethra is identified. Vaginal manipulation is also used to further assist in the elevation of the lateral vaginal fornices while the bladder is swept medially. Two to four delayed absorbable sutures are inserted into the paravaginal fascia on each side and each is tied down onto the vaginal tissue, ensuring hemostasis. **D,** The first suture is at the level of the bladder neck and 1 cm lateral. The suture is then passed vertically through the ipsilateral iliopectineal ligament, taking care not to pull the bladder neck open, and left untied.

Continued on the next page

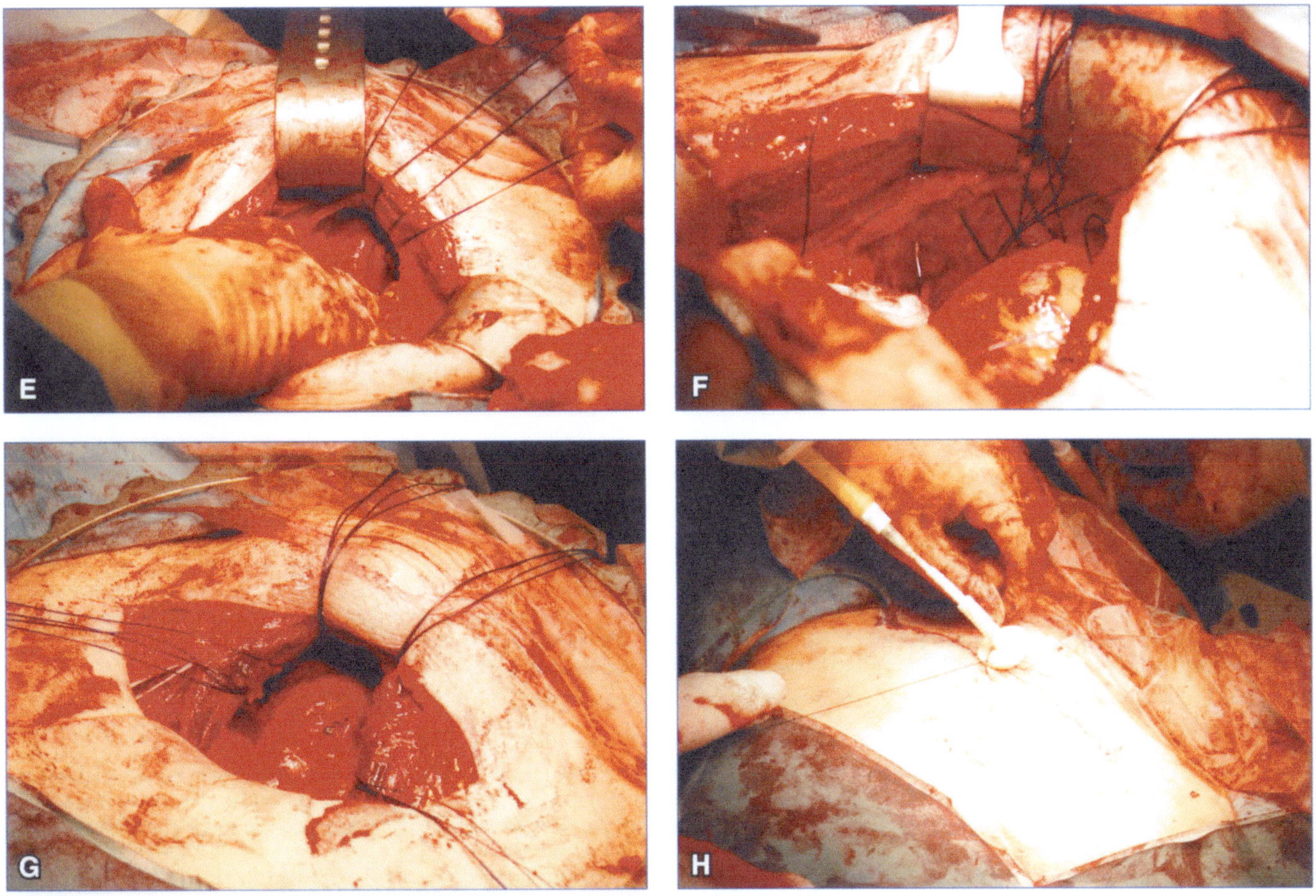

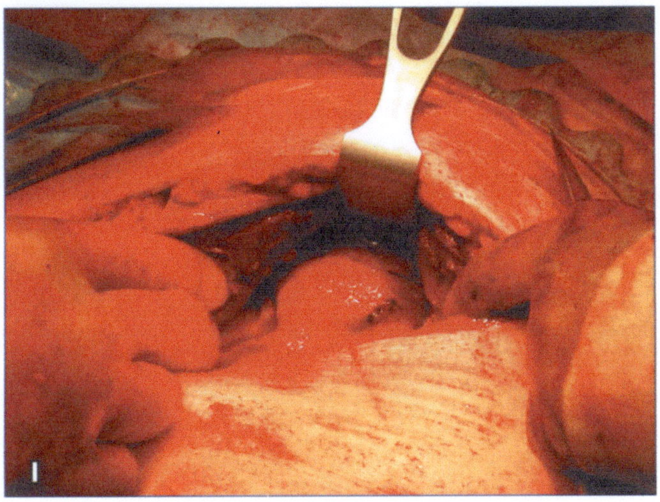

Figure 10-4. *(Continued)* **E,** Each subsequent suture is then placed 1 cm lateral and 1 cm cephalad and **F,** all are left untied before the sutures are placed on the opposite side. **G,** Once all the sutures are positioned correctly, each lateral fornix is elevated by an assistant, allowing the sutures to be tied easily without tension. **H,** The bladder is left on free drainage using a suprapubic catheter for 48 hours prior to starting a clamping regimen. When the urinary residuals are less than 100 mL, the suprapubic catheter may be removed. **I,** After checking for adequate hemostasis, the retropubic space is drained with a Redi-vac suction drain and the abdomen is closed.

Laparoscopic Colposuspension

FIGURE 10-5. Minimally invasive surgery is attractive and its use has extended to surgery for stress incontinence and the development of laparoscopic colposuspension. Although many authors have reported excellent short-term subjective results from laparoscopic colposuspension [17], early studies have shown results that are inferior to the open procedure [18,19].

More recently, two large, prospective, randomized, controlled trials have been reported from Australia and the United Kingdom, comparing laparoscopic and open colposuspension. In the Australian study, 200 women with urodynamic stress incontinence were randomized to either laparoscopic or open colposuspension [20]. Overall, there were no significant differences in the objective and subjective measures of cure or in patient satisfaction at 6 months, 24 months, or 3 to 5 years. While the laparoscopic approach took longer (87 vs 42 min; $P < 0.0001$), it was associated with less blood loss ($P = 0.03$) and a quicker return to normal activities ($P = 0.01$).

These findings are supported by the United Kingdom multicenter, randomized, controlled trial of 291 women with urodynamic stress incontinence, comparing laparoscopic to open colposuspension [21]. At 24 months, the intention-to-treat analysis showed no significant difference in cure rates between the procedures. Objective cure rates for open and laparoscopic colposuspension were 70.1% and 79.7%, respectively, while subjective cure rates were 54.6% and 54.9%, respectively.

These studies have confirmed that the clinical effectiveness of the two operations is comparable, although the cost effectiveness of laparoscopic colposuspension remains unproven. A cost analysis comparing laparoscopic to open colposuspension was also performed alongside the United Kingdom study [22]. Over the first 6-month followup period, the health care resources used translated into costs of £1805 for the laparoscopic group versus £1433 for the open group.

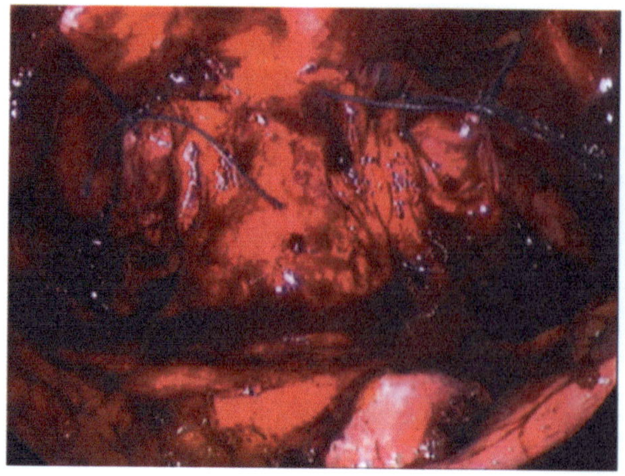

Pubovaginal Sling

Sling procedures are often performed as secondary operations in which there is scarring and narrowing of the vagina. The sling material can either be organic (rectus fascia or porcine dermis) or inorganic (Prolene; Ethicon, Livingston, UK; Mersilene; Ethicon, Livingston, UK; Marlex; or Silastic; Dow Corning, Midland, MI). The sling may be inserted either abdominally, vaginally, or by a combination of both. Normally, the sling is used to elevate and support the bladder neck and proximal urethra, but not intentionally to obstruct it.

Sling procedures may be associated with a high incidence of side effects and complications. It is often difficult to decide how tight to make the sling. If it is too loose, incontinence will persist and if it is too tight, voiding difficulties may be permanent. Women who will be undergoing insertion of a sling must be prepared to perform clean, intermittent self-catheterization postoperatively. In addition, there is a risk of infection, especially if inorganic material is used. The sling may erode into the urethra, bladder, or vagina, in which case it must be removed, which can be exceedingly difficult.

Technique

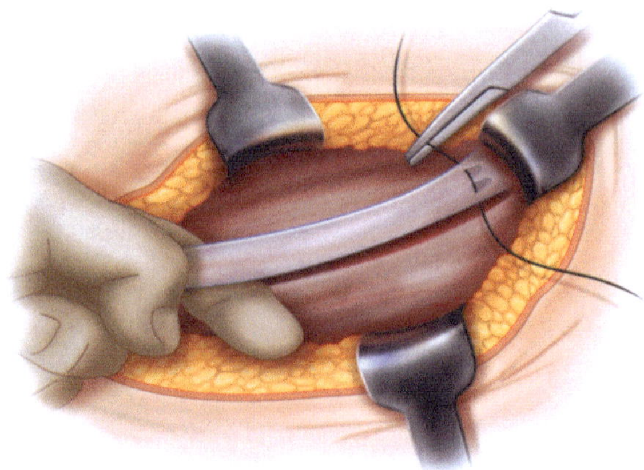

A

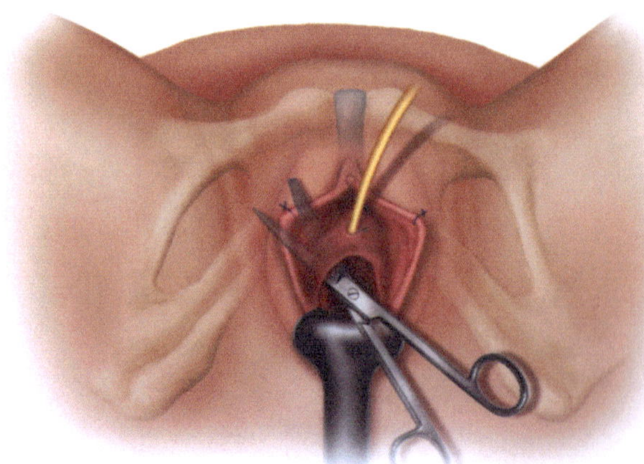

B

FIGURE 10-6. The procedure is performed in the dorsal lithotomy position and utilizes an abdominal and vaginal approach. A transverse suprapubic incision is first made just above the pubic symphysis and the rectus fascia is identified. Two parallel horizontal incisions 2 cm apart are then made in the fascia and a 16-cm sling of rectus fascia is mobilized. Each end of the strip of fascia is then secured with a nonabsorbable suture and the ends left long (**A**).

Following the insertion of an indwelling Foley catheter, a curvilinear vaginal incision is made in the anterior vaginal wall just below the level of the bladder neck. Next, a tunnel is created superficially to the pubocervical fascia using a combination of both sharp and blunt dissection in a plane toward the patient's ipsilateral shoulder until the endopelvic fascia is perforated (**B**).

Continued on the next page

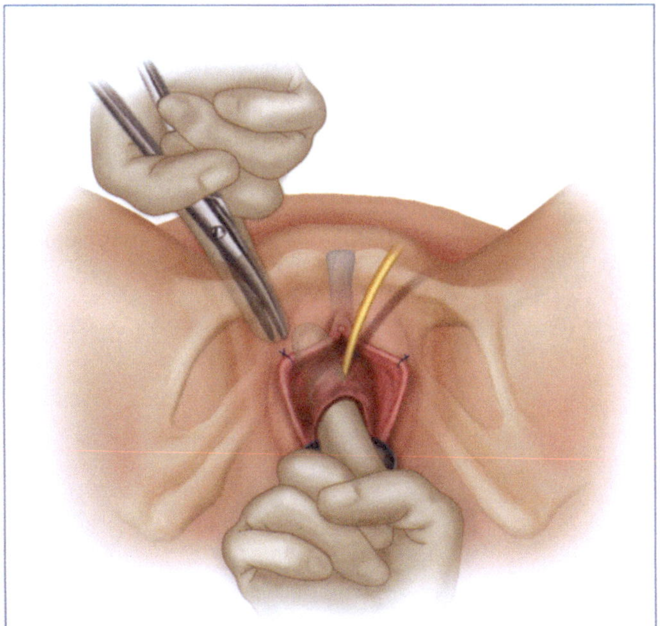

C

FIGURE 10-6. *(Continued)* A long, curved clamp may then be carefully passed downward from the abdominal incision using the vaginal finger as a guide and also to protect the bladder and urethra (**C**). The long sutures attached to the end of the harvested fascial sling may then be pulled through the abdominal incision on each side, allowing placement of the sling under the bladder neck. Two small incisions are then made in the rectus fascia and the suture ends are pulled through prior to tying them over the rectus fascia without tension (**D**). The rectus fascia may then be closed using a delayed absorbable suture prior to closing the abdominal and vaginal incisions. At the end of the procedure, a suprapubic catheter is left in situ and the bladder is left on free drainage for 48 hours before a clamping regimen is instituted. *(Adapted from* Cardozo and Staskin [9].)

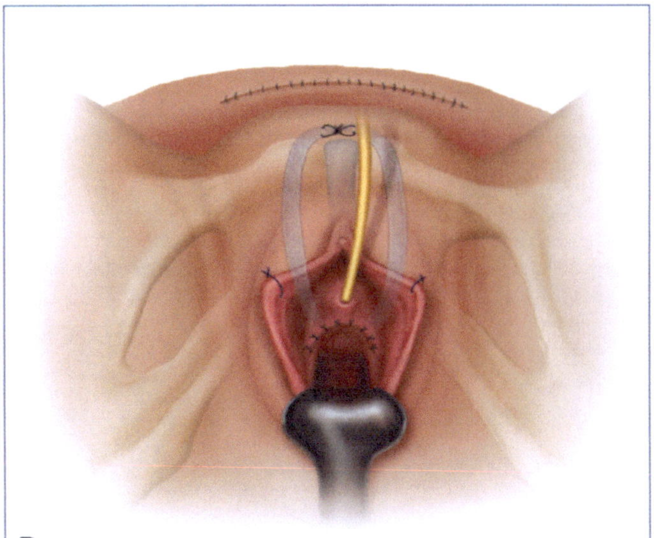

D

The advent of the newer midurethral tape procedures have largely replaced the use of traditional sling procedures and while efficacy rates are comparable, there tends to be fewer complications with the newer synthetic slings. A prospective, randomized study comparing tension-free vaginal tape (TVT), a Pelvicol (Bard Urological; Covington, GA) suburethral sling, and a traditional autologous fascial sling has been reported [23]. Overall, 201 women were randomized in four centers over 6 years and an interim analysis was performed after 50 patients were completed in each arm. Due to high failure and reintervention rates, the Pelvicol arm was closed after this analysis. At the 1-year follow-up, cure rates were 55% and 45% in the TVT and fascial sling arms, respectively, and improvement rates were 93% and 90% in the TVT and fascial sling arms, respectively. In the Pelvicol arm, cure rates were 22% and improvement was 61%. The reintervention rate was 20% in the Pelvicol arm compared to 0% in the other two arms. Consequently, the evidence from this study would suggest that the newer midurethral retropubic tapes are as efficacious as a traditional sling.

Midurethral Tape Procedures: Retropubic Midurethral Tapes

Tension-free Vaginal Tape

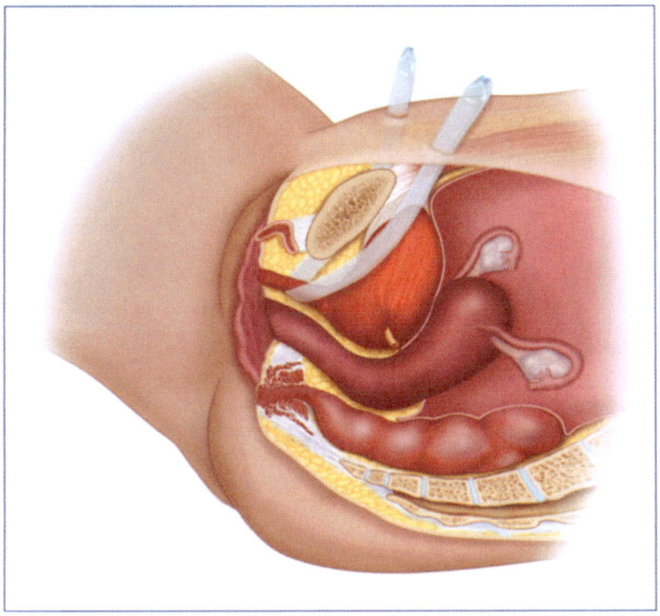

FIGURE 10-7. The tension-free vaginal tape (TVT; Gynecare; Ethicon Women's Health & Urology; Somerville, NJ), first described by Ulmsten in 1996 [24], is now the most commonly performed procedure for stress urinary incontinence in the United Kingdom and more than 2 million have been performed worldwide. A knitted 11-mm by 40-cm polypropylene mesh tape is inserted transvaginally at the midurethra level, using two 5-mm trocars. The procedure may be performed under local, spinal, or general anesthesia. Most women can go home the same day, although some do require catheterization for short-term voiding difficulties (2.5%–19.7%). Other complications include bladder perforation (2.7%–5.8%), de novo urgency (0.2%–15%), and bleeding (0.9%–2.3%) [25].

The initial multicenter study, carried out in six centers in Sweden, reported a 90% cure rate at 1 year in women undergoing their first operation for urodynamic stress incontinence, without any major complications [26]. Long-term results would confirm the durability of the technique with success rates of 86% at 3 years [27], 84.7% at 5 years [28], 81.3% at 7 years [29], and 90% at 11 years [30].

Continued on the next page

Figure 10-7. *(Continued)* The TVT has also been compared to open colposuspension in a multicenter prospective randomized trial of 344 women with urodynamic stress incontinence [31]. Overall, there was no significant difference in terms of objective cure; 66% in the TVT group and 57% in the colposuspension group. However, the operation time, postoperative stay, and return to normal activity were all longer in the colposuspension group. Analysis of the long-term results at 24 months using a pad test, quality of life assessment, and symptom questionnaires showed an objective cure rate of 63% in the TVT arm and 51% in the colposuspension arm [32]. At 5 years, there were no differences in subjective cure (63% in the TVT group and 70% in the colposuspension group), patient satisfaction, and quality of life assessment. However, while there was a significant reduction in cystocele in both groups, there was a higher incidence of enterocele, rectocele, and apical prolapse in the colposuspension group [33]. Furthermore, cost–utility analysis has also shown that at 6 months followup, TVT resulted in a mean cost saving of £243 when compared to colposuspension [34].

A smaller randomized study has also compared TVT to laparoscopic colposuspension in 72 women with urodynamic stress incontinence. At a mean followup of 20 months, objective cure rates were higher in the TVT group when compared to the laparoscopic colposuspension group; 96.8% versus 71.2%, respectively ($P = 0.056$) [35].

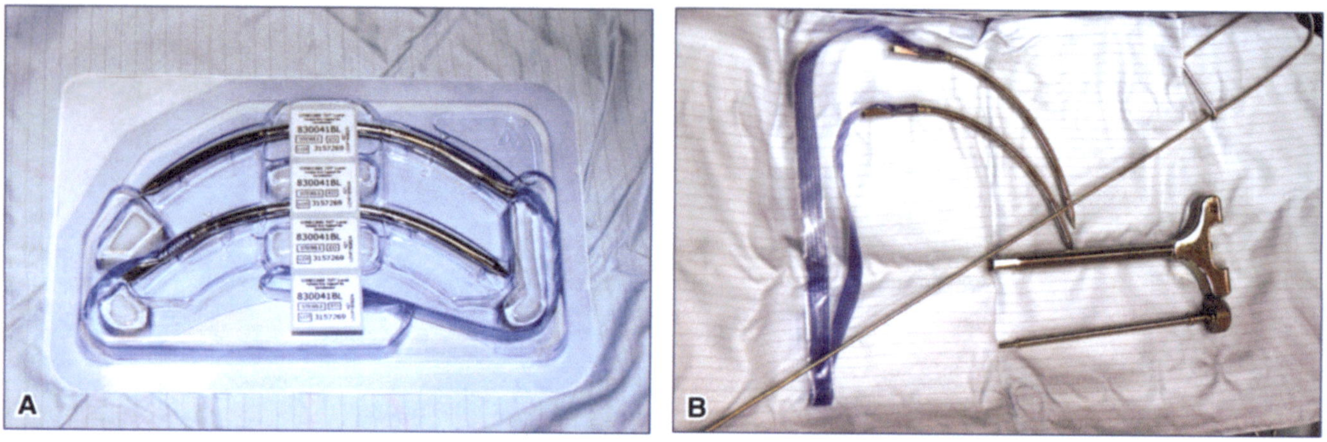

Figure 10-8. The tension-free vaginal tape (Gynecare; Ethicon Women's Health & Urology; Somerville, NJ) device consists of an 11-mm wide by 40-cm long tape of polypropylene mesh, both ends of which are attached to a stainless steel curved 5-mm diameter needle (**A**). The tape is covered by a protective plastic sheath and a reusable stainless steel handle is used to insert the needles (**B**).

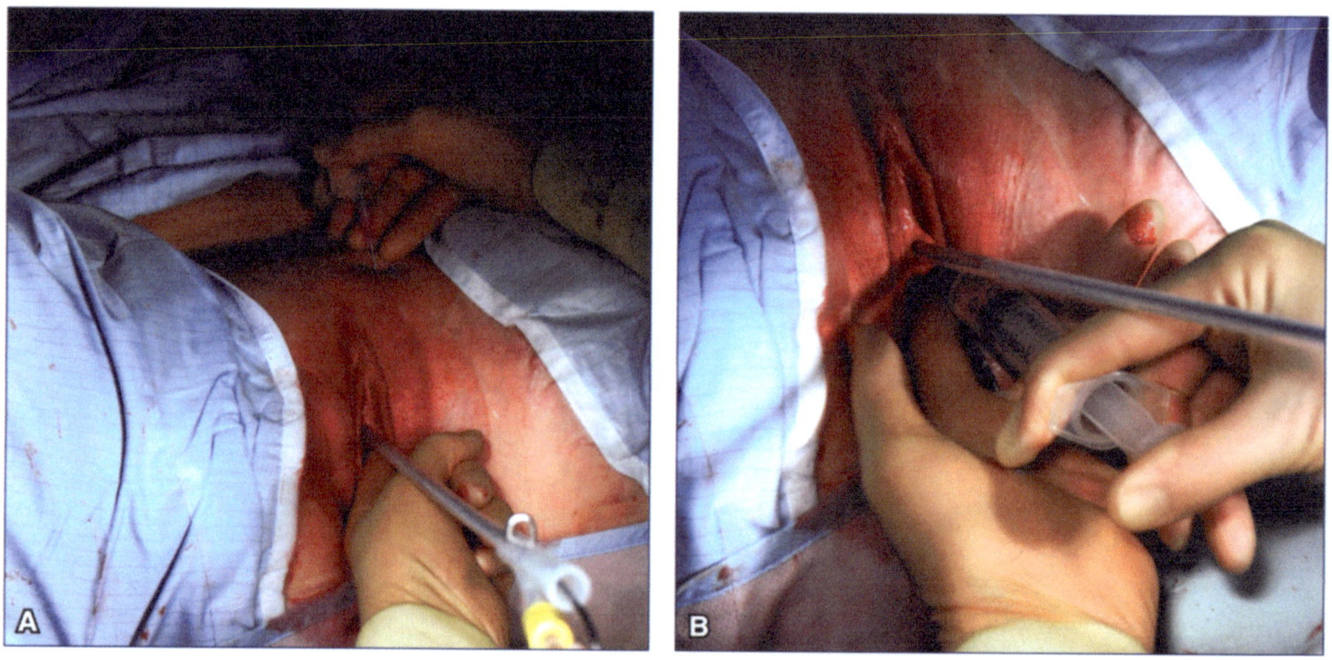

Figure 10-9. The procedure may be performed under local or general anesthesia. The patient is placed in the dorsal lithotomy position and after preparing the vagina and suprapubic area, an indwelling 18-Fr Foley catheter is inserted into the bladder. Once the bladder has been emptied, a rigid catheter guide is then inserted down the catheter in order to deflect the bladder away from the passage of the needle introducers. The use of local anesthesia (20 mL Bupivacaine 0.5% with 1 in 200,000 adrenaline, diluted in 100 mL normal saline) allows effective hydrodissection and vasoconstriction, while at the same time providing effective intra- and postoperative analgesia. Dilute local anaesthetic (20 mL) is injected on each side retropubically, immediately behind the pubic tubercle (**A**). In addition, a further 20 mL are injected paraurethrally on each side up to the level of the urogenital diaphragm (**B**) and 5 mL suburethrally.

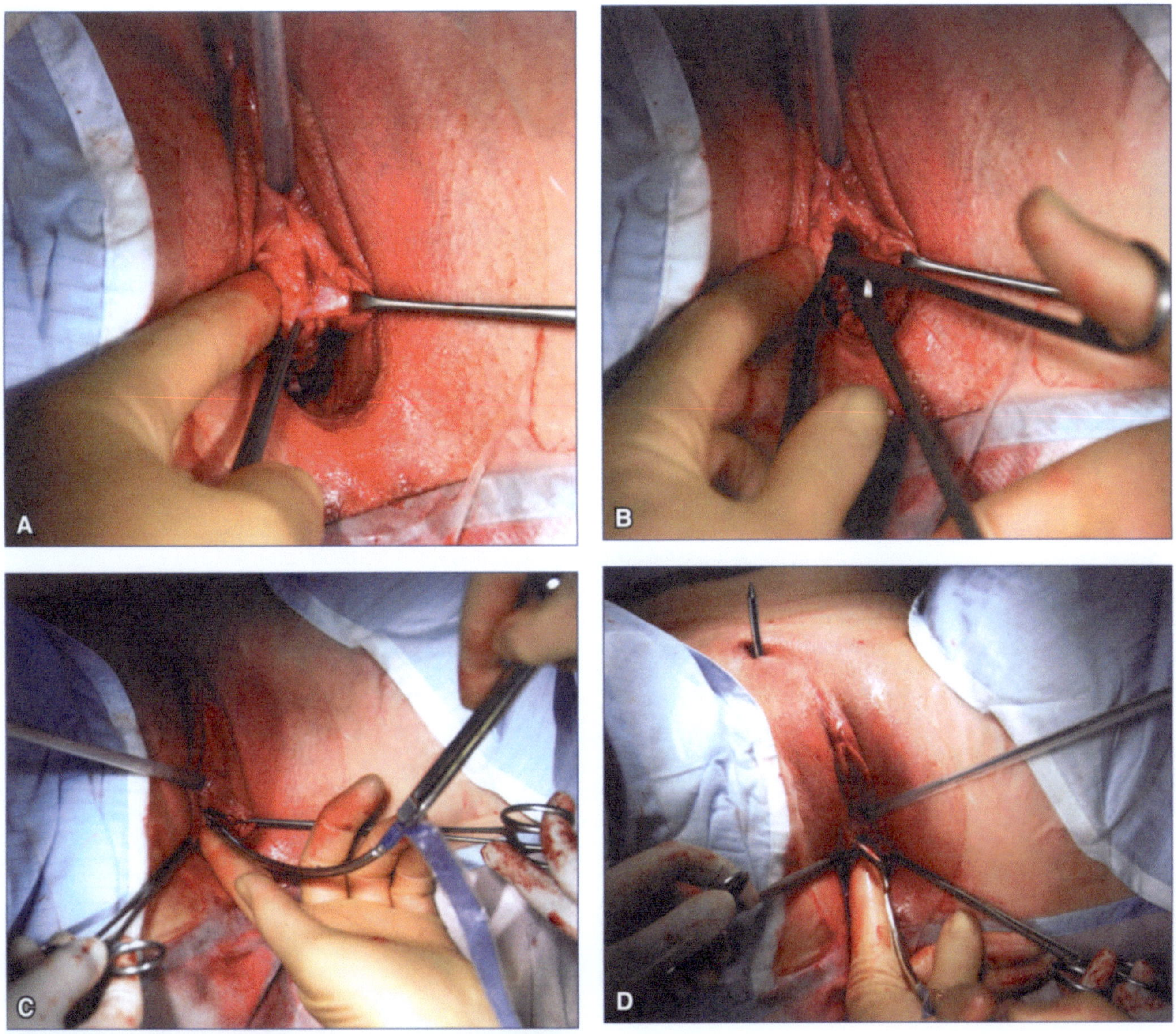

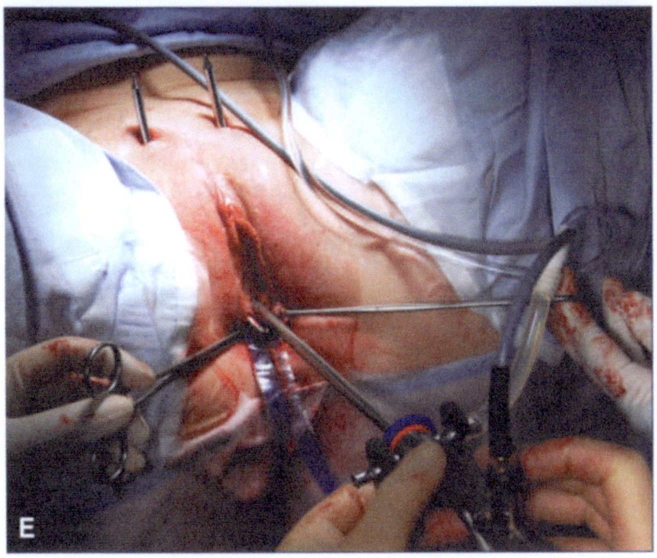

FIGURE 10-10. A 2-cm midline suburethral vaginal incision is made (**A**) and paraurethral dissection is performed using sharp dissection with McIndoe scissors between the vaginal mucosa and pubocervical fascia to the level of the inferior pubic ramus and the urogenital diaphragm (**B**). Two small 0.5-cm suprapubic incisions at the upper border of the pubic tubercle, 2 cm lateral to the midline, may be made to facilitate needle passage through the skin.

The tension-free vaginal tape needle is then placed in the starting position within the dissected paraurethral tunnel with the tip of the needle between the index finger (in the vagina) and the lower border of the pubic ramus (**C**). Prior to the passage of the needle, the bladder is pushed away from the track of the needle using the rigid catheter guide. In a controlled movement, the needle is then pushed through the urogenital diaphragm, the retropubic space, and the rectus fascia, keeping in close contact to the dorsal aspect of the pubic bone. The procedure is then repeated on the contralateral side (**D**).

With the needles still in position, a cystoscopy using a 70° cystoscope is performed to check that there is no bladder injury (**E**). If a bladder perforation is noted the needle is withdrawn, replaced, and passed once again. The cystoscopy is then repeated. Once the integrity of the bladder is confirmed, the bladder is again emptied completely and the tape is pulled through.

Continued on the next page

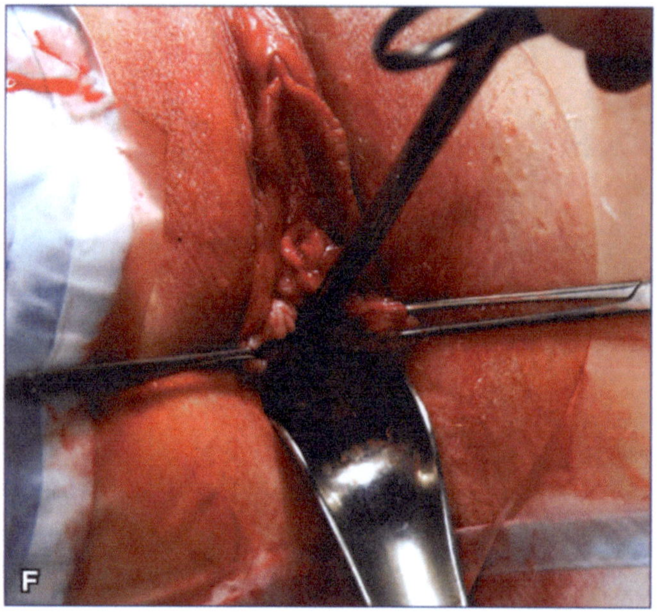
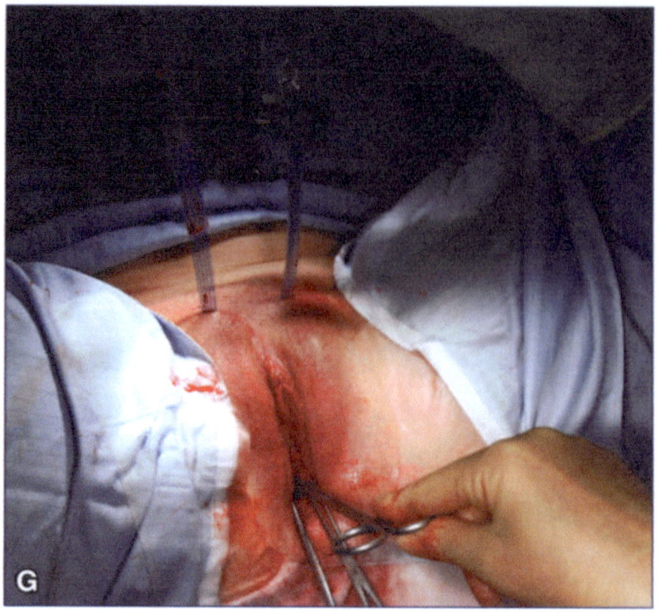

FIGURE 10-10. *(Continued)* In centers that continue to use the cough stress test, the bladder is then refilled with 300 mL normal saline and the patient is asked to cough vigorously. The tape may then be adjusted to a point where there is only a drop of leakage from the urethral meatus. After this final adjustment, the tape is held in position beneath the urethra using a pair of McIndoe scissors (**F**) while the plastic sheaths are removed on each side (**G**).

In centers in which a cough stress test is no longer used, the tape is positioned loosely below the midurethra without tension. Finally, the vaginal incision is closed using an absorbable suture and the suprapubic incisions are closed with Steri-Strips (3M; St. Paul, MN). While an indwelling catheter is not required in all cases, a urethral catheter should be left on free drainage for 48 hours following a bladder injury.

Midurethral Sling Suspension System

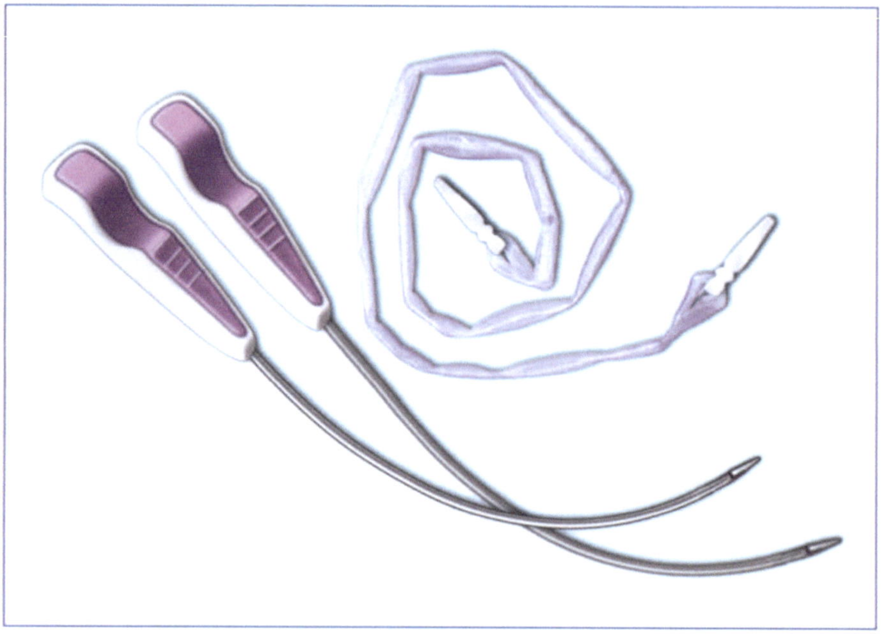

FIGURE 10-11. The SPARC sling system (American Medical Systems; Minnetonka, MN) is a minimally invasive sling using a knit 10-mm wide polypropylene mesh that is placed at the midurethra level by passing the needle via a suprapubic to vaginal approach [36]. The procedure may be performed under local, regional, or general anesthesia. A prospective multicenter study of 104 women with urodynamic stress incontinence has been reported from France [37]. At a mean followup of 11.9 months, the objective cure rate was 90.4% and the subjective cure rate was 72%. There was a 10.5% incidence of bladder perforation and 11.5% of women complained of de novo urgency following the procedure. More recently, SPARC has been compared to tension-free vaginal tape in a prospective randomized trial of 301 women [38]. At short-term followup, there were no significant differences in cure rates, bladder perforation rates, and de novo urgency. There was, however, a higher incidence of voiding difficulties and vaginal erosions in the SPARC group. (*Adapted from* Cardozo and Staskin [9].)

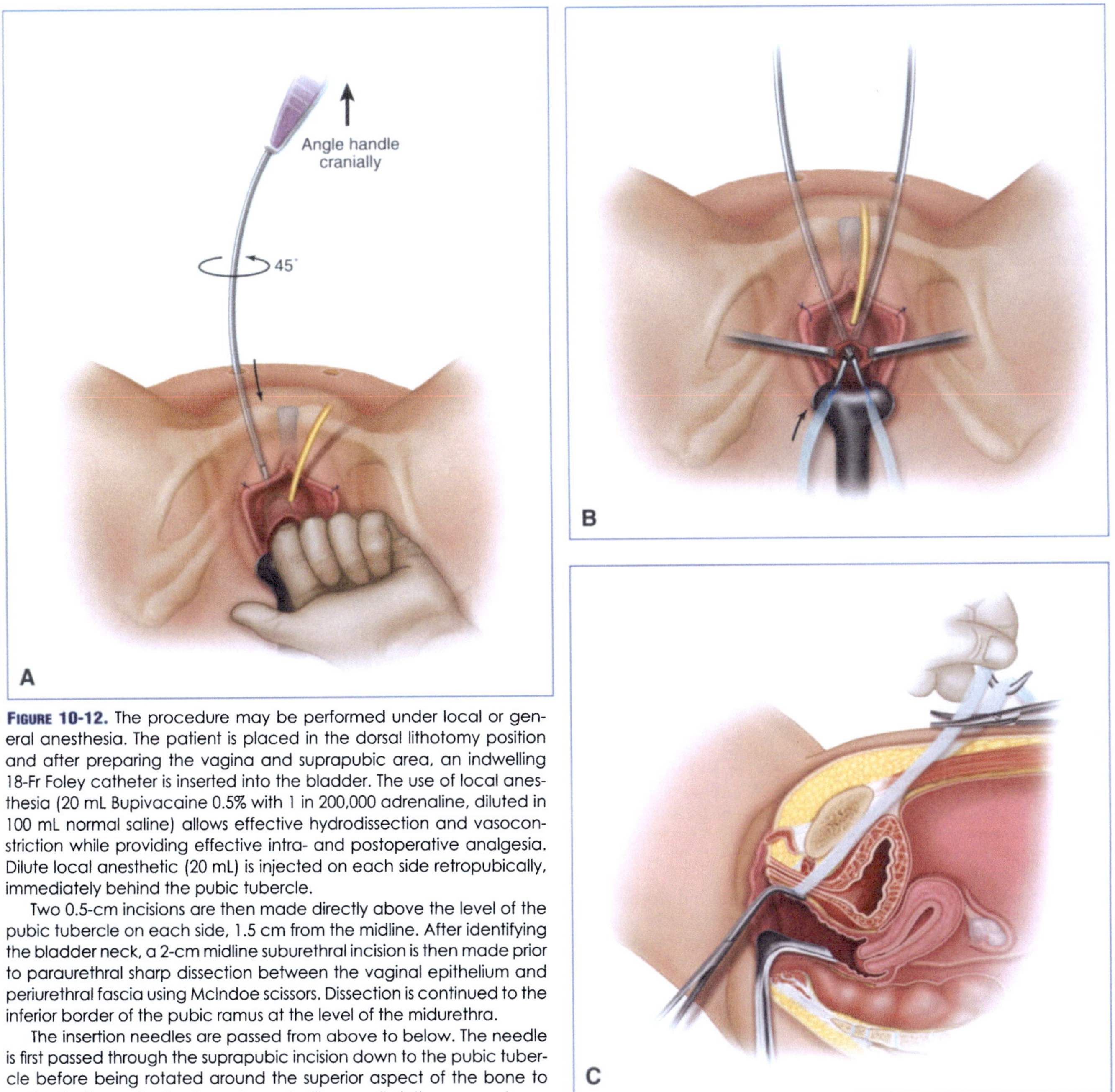

FIGURE 10-12. The procedure may be performed under local or general anesthesia. The patient is placed in the dorsal lithotomy position and after preparing the vagina and suprapubic area, an indwelling 18-Fr Foley catheter is inserted into the bladder. The use of local anesthesia (20 mL Bupivacaine 0.5% with 1 in 200,000 adrenaline, diluted in 100 mL normal saline) allows effective hydrodissection and vasoconstriction while providing effective intra- and postoperative analgesia. Dilute local anesthetic (20 mL) is injected on each side retropubically, immediately behind the pubic tubercle.

Two 0.5-cm incisions are then made directly above the level of the pubic tubercle on each side, 1.5 cm from the midline. After identifying the bladder neck, a 2-cm midline suburethral incision is then made prior to paraurethral sharp dissection between the vaginal epithelium and periurethral fascia using McIndoe scissors. Dissection is continued to the inferior border of the pubic ramus at the level of the midurethra.

The insertion needles are passed from above to below. The needle is first passed through the suprapubic incision down to the pubic tubercle before being rotated around the superior aspect of the bone to perforate the rectus fascia and muscle. The needle is then passed over the posterior aspect of the pubic bone to reach the endopelvic fascia before being guided through the vaginal incision using a finger placed in the vagina or incision itself (**A**). The procedure is then repeated on the opposite side.

Following the passage of both needles, a 70° cystoscope is used to exclude a urethral or bladder injury. Should a perforation be noted, the bladder is emptied, needles repositioned, and a repeat cystoscopy performed.

Next, the connectors on each end of the tape are attached to the needles in the vaginal incision (**B**) and the tape is gently pulled through on each side, taking care to make sure that the tape remains flat under the midurethra. If there is any suspicion of bladder injury, a repeat cystoscopy should be performed. The tape is then held loosely in position beneath the urethra using a pair of McIndoe scissors while the protective plastic sheaths are removed, ensuring that there is no tension on the urethra (**C**). The vaginal incision may then be closed using an absorbable suture and Steri-Strips (3M; St. Paul, MN) are used to close the two small suprapubic incisions. While an indwelling catheter is not required in all cases, a urethral catheter should be left on free drainage for 48 hours following a bladder injury. (*Adapted from* Cardozo and Staskin [9].)

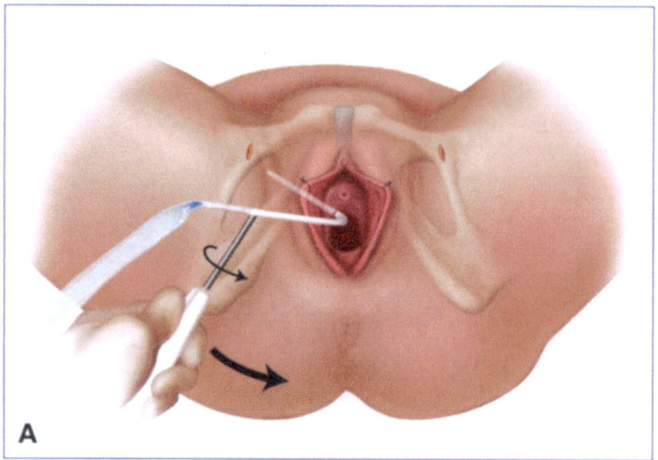

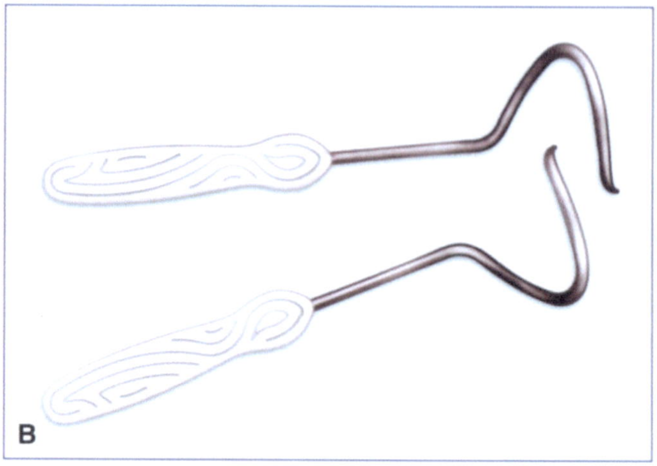

Figure 10-13. The transobturator route for the placement of synthetic midurethral slings was first described in 2001 by Delorme [39]. As with the retropubic sling procedures, transobturator tapes may be performed under local, regional, or general anesthesia and have the theoretical advantage of eliminating some of the complications associated with the retropubic route, such as bladder and urethral perforation. However, the transobturator route may be associated with damage to the obturator nerve and vessels; in an anatomical dissection model, the tape passes 3.4 to 4.8 cm from the anterior and posterior branches of the obturator nerve, respectively, and 1.1 cm from the most medial branch of the obturator vessels [40]. Consequently, nerve and vessel injury, in addition to bladder injury and vaginal erosion, remain potential complications of the procedure.

The transobturator approach may be used as an "inside-out" tension-free vaginal tape obturator approach (TVT-O; Gynecare; Ethicon Women's Health & Urology; Somerville, NJ) (**A**) or, alternatively, an "outside–in" technique (Monarc; American Medical Systems; Minnetonka, MN) (**B**). To date, several studies have documented the short-term efficacy of transobturator procedures. Initial studies have reported cure and improved rates of 80.5% and 7.5%, respectively, at 7 months [41] and 90.6% and 9.4%, respectively, at 17 months [42].

More recently, the TVT-O has been compared to the retropubic tension-free vaginal tape (TVT) approach in an Italian prospective multicenter randomized study of 231 women with urodynamic stress incontinence [43]. At a mean of 9 months, subjectively 92% of women in the TVT group were cured compared to 87% in the TVT-O group. Objectively, on pad testing, cure rates were 92% and 89%, respectively. There were no differences in voiding difficulties and the length of stay, although there were more bladder perforations in the TVT group; 4% versus none in the TVT-O group. A further multicenter prospective randomized trial comparing TVT and TVT-O has also recently been reported from Finland, in which 267 women report stress urinary incontinence [44]. Objective cure rates at 9 weeks were 98.5% in the TVT group and 95.4% in the TVT-O group ($P = 0.1362$). While complication rates were low and similar in both arms of the study, there was a higher incidence of groin pain in the TVT-O group (21 vs 2; $P = 0.0001$).

This data is supported by a recent meta-analysis of the five randomized trials comparing TVT-O with TVT and six randomized trials comparing TVT-O with TVT [45]. Overall, subjective cure rates were identical with the retropubic and transobturator routes. However, adverse events such as bladder injuries (odds ratio [OR] 0.12; 95% CI: 0.05–0.33) and voiding difficulties (OR 0.55; 95% CI: 0.31–0.98) were less common, whereas groin pain (OR 8.28; 95% CI: 2.7–25.4) and vaginal erosions (OR 1.96; 95% CI: 0.87–4.39) were more common after the transobturator approach. Long-term data would also seem to support the durability and efficacy of the transobturator approach. A 3-year followup study of a prospective observational study evaluating the use of TVT-O has recently been reported [46]. Of the 102 patients recruited, 91 (89.2%) were available for followup at a minimum of 3 years. The objective cure rate was 88.4% with an improvement in 9.3% of cases and there was no statistical difference in outcome as compared to the results reported at 1 year. In addition, there also was a significant improvement in subjective outcome, including incontinence severity and quality of life. While four patients required tape division, there were no cases of erosion or persistent pain.

Technique: Transobturator "Inside-out"

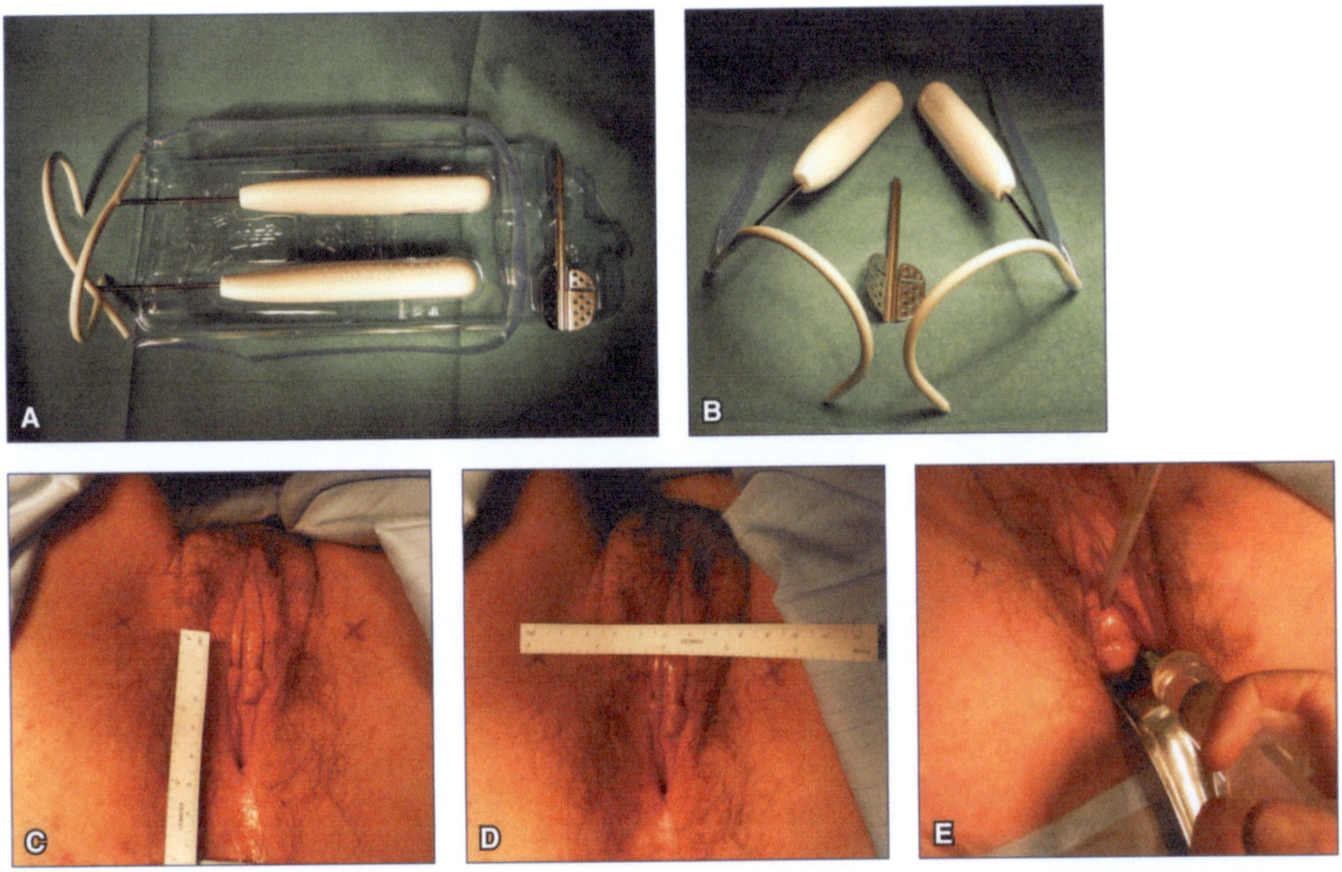

FIGURE 10-14. The tension-free vaginal tape obturator device consists of an 11-mm wide by 40-cm long tape of polypropylene mesh, both ends of which are attached to a plastic sheath that threads over the helical needle introducer (**A**). A winged needle guide is also provided to facilitate passage of the needle through the obturator membrane (**B**).

The procedure may be performed under local or general anesthesia. The patient is placed in the dorsal lithotomy position in 120° hyperflexion. The vagina and thighs are then prepared and an indwelling 12-Fr Foley catheter is inserted into the bladder. Next, two 0.5-cm incisions are made 2 cm superior to a horizontal line level with the urethra and 2 cm lateral to the thigh folds. This marks the exit point for the helical needle introducer (**C** and **D**).

The use of local anesthesia (20 mL Bupivacaine 0.5% with 1 in 200,000 adrenaline, diluted in 100 mL normal saline) allows effective hydrodissection and vasoconstriction while providing effective intra- and postoperative analgesia. Dilute local anesthetic (20 mL) is injected paraurethrally on each side in the direction of the inferior pubic ramus (**E**).

Continued on the next page

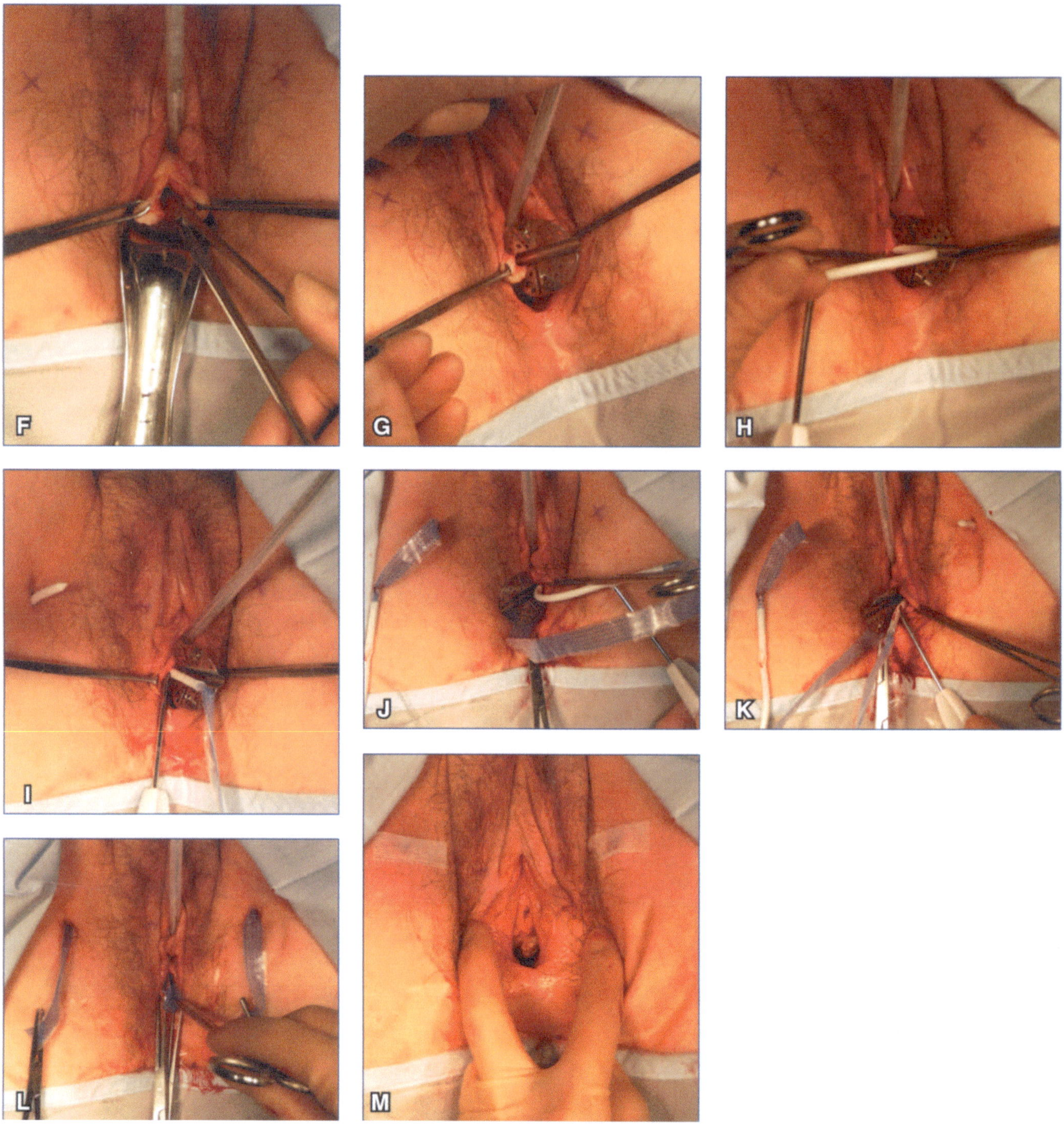

Figure 10-14. *(Continued)* A midline suburethral incision is then made at the midurethra level prior to the paraurethral sharp dissection between the vaginal epithelium and periurethral fascia using McIndoe scissors (**F**). Dissection is continued laterally to the inferior border of the pubic ramus at the midurethra level and the medial aspect of the obturator membrane is perforated.

The winged needle guide is then passed at 45° relative to the sagittal plane of the urethra until reaching the posterior aspect of the inferior pubic ramus and perforating the obturator membrane (**G**). Having mounted the tape onto the helical introducer, the tip is then placed along the guide channel in the winged guide (**H**) to pass through the obturator membrane and is then rotated so that the exit trough is the inner thigh incision (**I**). The tip of the tubing is then clamped and the helical introducer is withdrawn. The procedure is then repeated on the contralateral side (**J**). Once both needles have been passed (**K**) and the tape inserted, a cystoscopy may be performed to exclude bladder or urethral injury.

The tape is then held loosely in position beneath the urethra using a pair of McIndoe scissors while the protective plastic sheaths are removed, ensuring that there is no tension on the urethra and the tape is lying flat (**L**). The vaginal incision is then closed using an absorbable suture and Steri-Strips (3M; St. Paul, MN) are used to close the two small incisions on the thighs (**M**). While an indwelling catheter is not required in all cases, a urethral catheter should be left on free drainage for 48 hours following a bladder injury.

Technique: Transobturator "Outside-in"

This procedure may be performed under local or general anesthesia. The patient is placed in the dorsal lithotomy position in 120° hyperflexion. The vagina and thighs are then prepared and an indwelling 12-Fr Foley catheter is inserted into the bladder. The use of local anesthesia (20 mL Bupivacaine 0.5% with 1 in 200,000 adrenaline, diluted in 100 mL normal saline) allows effective hydrodissection and vasoconstriction while providing effective intra- and postoperative analgesia. Dilute local anesthetic (20 mL) is injected paraurethrally, on each side in the direction of the inferior pubic ramus.

A midline suburethral incision is then made at the midurethra level prior to paraurethral sharp dissection between the vaginal epithelium and periurethral fascia using McIndoe scissors. Dissection is continued laterally to the inferior border of the pubic ramus at the midurethra level and the medial aspect of the obturator membrane is perforated. Next, a small incision is made 1.5 cm lateral to the ischiopubic ramus on each side at the level of the clitoris. The helical needle introducer is then passed "outside-in" through the incision to perforate the medial aspect of the obturator membrane. With an index finger in the vaginal incision palpating the ischiopubic ramus and obturator internus muscle, the tip of the helical needle may then be guided through to the vaginal incision. Care should be taken to avoid perforating the lateral vaginal fornix and the urethra is guarded by the operator's finger. Once the tip of the needle has been passed through the vaginal incision, the tape may then be attached to the needle and pulled through to exit through the thigh incision. The procedure is then repeated on the contralateral side.

The tape is then held loosely in position beneath the urethra using a pair of McIndoe scissors while the protective plastic sheaths are removed, ensuring that there is no tension on the urethra and the tape is lying flat. The vaginal incision is then closed using an absorbable suture and Steri-Strips (3M; St. Paul, MN) are used to close the two small incisions on the thighs. Although an indwelling catheter is not required in all cases, a urethral catheter should be left on free drainage for 48 hours following a bladder injury.

Minimally Invasive Tape Procedures

While the development of the midurethral retropubic and transobturator tapes has transformed the surgical approach to stress urinary incontinence by offering a minimally invasive day case procedure, there has recently been interest in developing a new type of "mini sling" that may offer a truly office-based approach. The tension-free vaginal tape Secur (Gynecare; Ethicon Women's Health & Urology; Somerville, NJ) is the first of these mini slings to be introduced, although there are several other devices currently under investigation and development.

Gynecare TVT Secur

The TVT Secur (Gynecare; Ethicon Women's Health & Urology; Somerville, NJ) was launched in 2006 and currently there is little long-term data to support its use, although several short-term studies have been reported. The first published case series reported on a small sample of 15 women with an overall subjective cure rate of 93% at 1- to 3-month followup [47]. More recently, a multicenter prospective trial has been reported from Italy, in which 95 women with primary stress incontinence had a TVT Secur. Followup at 1 year reported subjective and objective cure rates of 78% and 81%, respectively, while 8% of women complained of voiding difficulties. In addition, there were two cases of mesh erosion [48]. This data is supported by a multicenter prospective observational study in France of 150 patients with 1 year followup. Cure and improvement rates were 76.9% in women with pure stress incontinence, although this fell to 60% in a smaller group with intrinsic sphincter deficiency [49].

The current evidence would appear to suggest that TVT Secur efficacy rates may be slightly inferior to those of the retropubic midurethral tapes [50] and current experience would suggest that the procedure is technically different from a retropubic or obturator approach. Initial success rates have been disappointing in some series and the "learning curve" effect has been clearly documented with objective success rates increasing from 76.2% to 94.7%, depending on the experience of the operating surgeon [51].

From the available clinical evidence available to date, it would appear that TVT-Secur offers an alternative, minimally invasive approach for the treatment of stress urinary incontinence although more data are required to document the long-term efficacy and safety.

Figure 10-15. The TVT Secur device (Gynecare; Ethicon Women's Health & Urology; Somerville, NJ) consists of an 11-mm wide by 8-cm long tape of polypropylene mesh, both ends of which are sandwiched between a fleece pad composed of a woven polyglactin and poly-dioxane fibers. The pads are locked in position on the end of two stainless steel inserters, allowing accurate retropubic placement. After releasing the locking mechanism, the pads may then be released at the time of insertion.

The procedure may be performed under local or general anesthesia. The patient is placed in the dorsal lithotomy position and, having prepared the vagina and suprapubic area, an indwelling 18-Fr Foley catheter is inserted into the bladder. Once the bladder has been emptied, a rigid catheter guide is then inserted down the catheter in order to deflect the bladder away from the passage of the needle introducers. The use of local anesthesia (20 mL Bupivacaine 0.5% with 1 in 200,000 adrenaline, diluted in 100 mL normal saline) allows effective hydrodissection and vasoconstriction while providing effective intra- and postoperative analgesia. Dilute local anesthetic is injected paraurethrally (20 mL) on each side up to the level of the urogenital diaphragm and 5 mL suburethrally.

A 1.5-cm midline suburethral vaginal incision is made and paraurethral dissection is performed using sharp dissection with McIndoe scissors between the vaginal mucosa and pubocervical fascia to a depth of 1 cm. If the placement is retropubic ("U" position), the angle of dissection is 45° although if an obturator ("hammock") placement is planned, dissection is at 90° or horizontal.

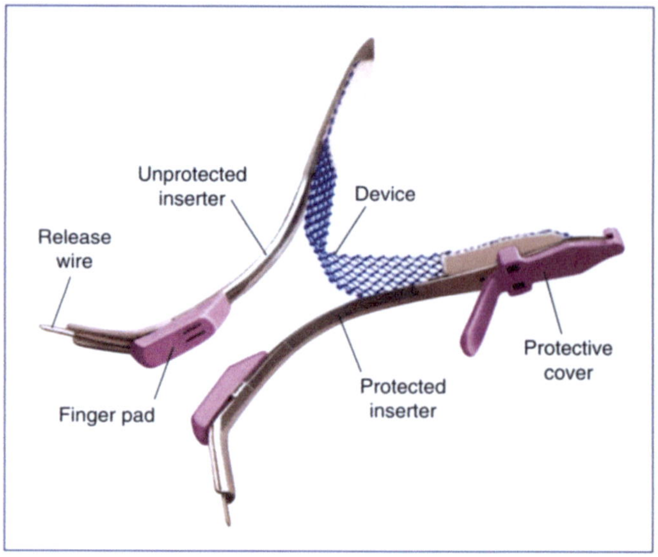

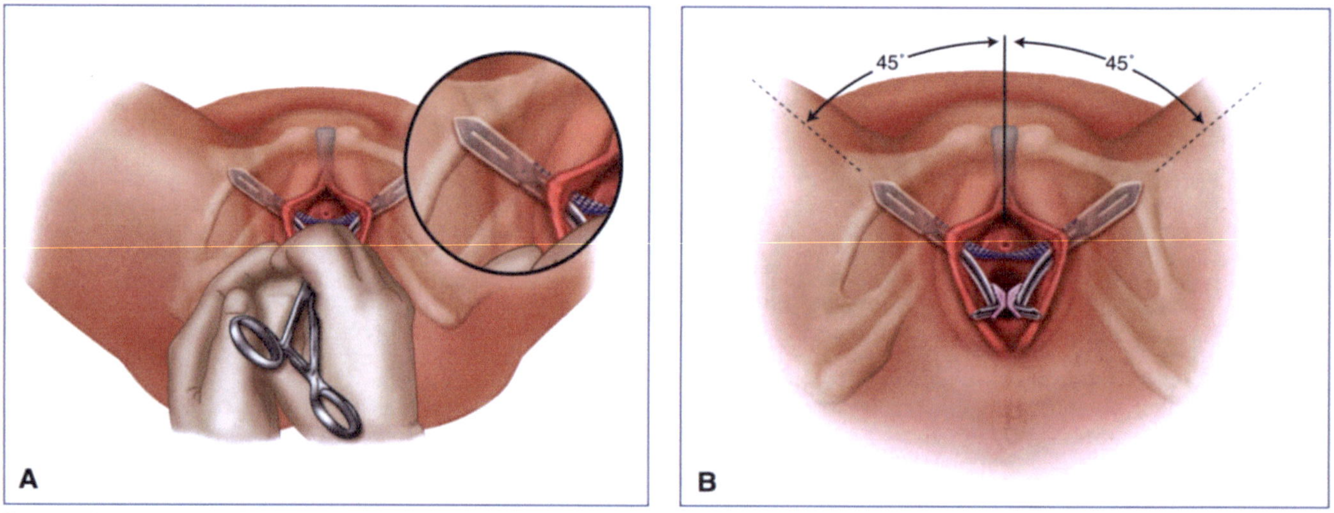

Figure 10-16. U position. Once the protective cover has been removed from the tip, the introducer is then held using a needle holder, making sure the inserter is in line with the handle of the instrument. The tip of the introducer is then carefully placed within the paraurethrally dissected tunnel using the finger pad on the index finger. The inserter should then be pushed 45° toward the ipsilateral shoulder using gentle pressure (**A**). When contact is made with the posterior surface of the pubic bone, the pad is held carefully in place against the bone while the needle holder is released, leaving the inserter in position. The procedure is then repeated on the contralateral side (**B**). (**A** *adapted from* Gynecare TVT SECURE System Professional Education CD-ROM [52].)

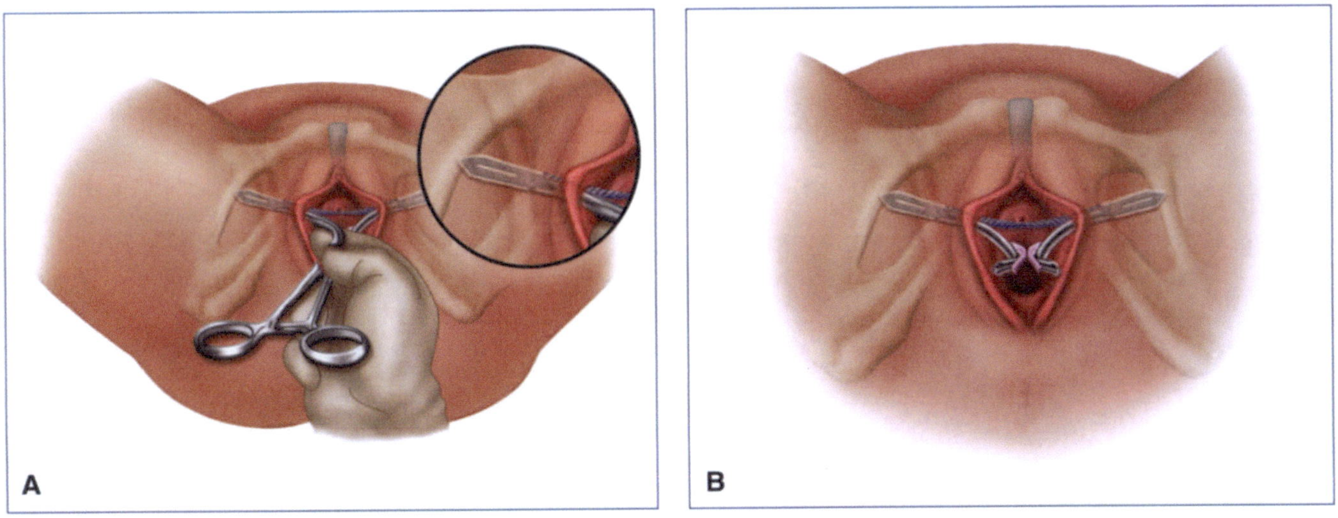

Figure 10-17. Hammock position. Once the protective cover has been removed from the tip, the introducer is then held using a needle holder, making sure the inserter is in line with the handle of the instrument. The tip of the introducer is then carefully placed within the paraurethrally dissected tunnel using the finger pad on the index finger. The inserter tip should then be orientated at 45° from the midline toward the ischiopubic ramus while holding the needle holder parallel to the floor (**A**). Once contact is made with the posterior surface of the pubic bone, the pad is held carefully in place against the bone while the needle holder is released, leaving the inserter in position. The procedure is then repeated on the contralateral side (**B**). (**A** *adapted from* Gynecare TVT SECURE System Professional Education CD-ROM [52].)

After both inserters have been passed, final tape positioning may be performed by adjusting the depth of insertion on each side. Care should be taken to ensure that the inserter tip remains in contact with the posterior surface of the pubic bone on each side and that the tape is flat and lies immediately beneath the urethra. Prior to removal of the inserters, cystourethroscopy should be performed to exclude injury to the bladder or urethra. Should a bladder perforation be noted, the inserter should be removed and replaced.

Once the tape is properly positioned, the first inserter is released by gently pulling on the release wire and then sliding the inserter out from the incision. Care should be taken not to dislodge the anchoring pad from the posterior surface of the pubic bone. The procedure should then be completed on the opposite side.

The vaginal incision is then closed using an absorbable suture. While an indwelling catheter is not required in all cases, a urethral catheter should be left on free drainage for 48 hours following a bladder injury.

Conclusion

Urinary stress incontinence is the most commonly reported type of urinary incontinence in women and is known to have a significant impact on quality of life [53]. While the majority of women will benefit from a conservative approach, surgery initially remains integral in the management of women with moderate to severe symptoms.

The last decade has seen a dramatic change in our approach to continence surgery and, following the description of the integral theory, the focus has shifted from the bladder neck to the midurethral level. With the development of both the retropubic and transobturator tapes, continence surgery has moved from being an inpatient procedure to the day-surgery setting and may now be performed under local or regional anesthesia. Consequently, the number of continence procedures has increased dramatically and the move toward the development of the "mini tapes" may mean that surgical options for stress urinary incontinence become an office-based procedure. An increased choice of surgical procedures and techniques should ultimately benefit both patients and clinicians.

However, despite the rapid pace of innovations in the field of continence surgery, it remains paramount that new procedures should be evidence based and only be introduced following adequate clinical studies demonstrating both efficacy and safety.

References

1. Abrams P, Cardozo L, Fall M, *et al.*: The standardisation of terminology of lower urinary tract function. Report from the standardisation committee of the International Continence Society. *Neurourol Urodyn* 2002, 21:167–178.
2. Hannestad YS, Rortveit G, Sandvik H, Hunskar S: A community-based epidemiological survey of female urinary incontinence: The Norwegian EPINCONT study. *J Clin Epidem* 2000, 53:1150–1157.
3. Rortveit G, Hannnestad YS, Daltveit AK, Hunskaar S: Age and type dependent effects of parity on urinary incontinence: the Norwegian EPINCONT study. *Obstet Gynecol* 2001, 98:1004–1010.
4. Petros P, Ulmsten U: An integral theory of female urinary incontinence. Experimental and clinical considerations. *Acta Obstet Gynecol Scand Suppl* 1990, 153:7–31.
5. Ingelman-Sundberg A: Urinary incontinence in women, excluding fistulas. *Acta Obstet Gynecol Scand* 1952, 31:266–291.
6. Westby M, Asmussen M, Ulmsten U: Location of maximal intraurethral pressure related to urogenital diaphragm in the female subject as studied by simultaneous urethra-cystometry and voiding urethrocystography. *Am J Obstet Gynecol* 1982, 144:408–412.
7. Hilton P: Which operation for which patient? In *Micturition*. Edited by: Drife J, Hilton P, Stanton SL. Berlin: Springer-Verlag; 1990.
8. Marshall VF, Marchetti AA, Krantz KE: The correction of stress incontinence by simple vesicourethral suspension. *Surg Gynecol Obstet* 1949, 88:509–518.
9. Cardozo L, Staskin DR, eds: *Textbook of Female Urology and Urogynaecology*. Abingdon, UK: Taylor & Francis; 2001.
10. Pereyra A: A simplified surgical procedure for the correction of stress incontinence in women. *West J Surg Obstet Gynecol* 1959, 67:223–226.
11. Stamey T: Endoscopic suspension of the vesical neck for urinary incontinence. *Surg Gynecol Obstet* 1973, 136:547–554.
12. Raz S: Modified bladder neck suspension for female stress incontinence. *Urology* 1981, 17:82–85.
13. Burch J: Urethrovaginal fixation to Cooper's ligament for correction of stress incontinence, cystocele, and prolapse. *Am J Obstet Gynecol* 1961, 81:281–290.
14. Cardozo LD, Stanton SL, Williams JE: Detrusor instability following surgery for genuine stress incontinence. *Br J Urol* 1979, 51:204–207.
15. Wiskind AK, Creighton SM, Stanton SL: The incidence of genital prolapse following the Burch colposuspension operation. *Neurourol Urodyn* 1991, 10:453–454.
16. Alcalay M, Monga A, Stanton SL: Burch colposuspension: a 10–20 year follow up. *Br J Obstet Gynaecol* 1995, 102:740–745.
17. Liu CY: Laparoscopic retropubic colposuspension (Burch procedure): a review of 58 cases. *J Reprod Med* 1993, 38:526–530.
18. Burton G: A randomised comparison of laparoscopic and open colposuspension. *Neurourol Urodyn* 1994, 13:497–498.
19. Su T, Wang K, Hsu C, *et al.*: Prospective comparison of laparoscopic and traditional colposuspension in the treatment of genuine stress incontinence. *Acta Obstet Gynecol Scand* 1997, 76:576–582.
20. Carey MP, Goh JT, Rosamilia A, *et al.*: Laparoscopic versus open Burch colposuspension: a randomised controlled trial. *BJOG* 2006, 113:999–1006.
21. Kitchener HC, Dunn G, Lawton V, *et al.*: Laparoscopic versus open colposuspension—results of a prospective randomised controlled trial. *BJOG* 2006, 113:1007–1013.
22. Dumville JC, Manca A, Kitchener HC, *et al.*: Cost effectiveness analysis of open colposuspension versus laparoscopic colposuspension in the treatment of urodynamic stress incontinence. *BJOG* 2006, 113:1014–1022.
23. Guerrero K, Watkins A, Emery S, *et al.*: A randomised controlled trial comparing two autologous fascial sling techniques for the treatment of stress urinary incontinence in women: short, medium and long-term follow-up. *Int Urogynecol J Pelvic Floor Dysfunct* 2007, 18:1263–1270.
24. Ulmsten U, Henriksson L, Johnson P, Varhos G: An ambulatory surgical procedure under local anesthesia for treatment of female urinary incontinence. *Int Urogynecol J Pelvic Floor Dysfunct* 1996, 7:81–85.
25. Nilsson CG: Tension free vaginal tape procedure for treatment of female urinary stress incontinence. In *Textbook of Female Urology and Urogynaecology*. Edited by Cardozo L, Staskin DR. Abingdon, UK: Taylor & Francis. 2001:917– 923.
26. Ulmsten U, Falconer C, Johnson P, *et al.*: A multicenter study of tension free vaginal tape (TVT) for surgical treatment of stress urinary incontinence. *Int Urogynecol J Pelvic Floor Dysfunct* 1998, 9:210–213.
27. Ulmsten U, Johnson P, Rezapour M: A three-year follow up of tension free vaginal tape for surgical treatment of female stress urinary incontinence. *Br J Obstet Gynaecol* 1999, 106:345–350.
28. Nilsson CG, Kuuva N, Falconer C, *et al.*: Long term results of the tension-free vaginal tape (TVT) procedure for surgical treatment of female stress urinary incontinence. *Int Urogynecol J Pelvic Floor Dysfunct* 2001, 12(Suppl 2):S5–S8.
29. Nilsson CG, Falconer C, Rezapour M: Seven-year follow-up of the tension-free vaginal tape procedure for the treatment of urinary incontinence. *Obstet Gynecol* 2004, 104:1259–1262.
30. Nilsson CG, Palva K, Rezapour M, Falconer C: Eleven years prospective follow-up of the tension-free vaginal tape procedure for treatment of stress urinary incontinence. *Int Urogynecol J Pelvic Floor Dysfunct* 2008, 19:1043–1047.
31. Ward K, Hilton P, United Kingdom and Ireland Tension-free Vaginal Tape Trial Group: Prospective multicentre randomised trial of tension-free vaginal tape and colposuspension as primary treatment for stress incontinence. *BMJ* 2002, 325:67.
32. Ward KL, Hilton P, UK and Ireland TVT Trial Group: A prospective multicenter randomized trial of tension-free vaginal tape and colposuspension for primary urodynamic stress incontinence: two-year follow-up. *Am J Obstet Gynecol* 2004; 190:324–331.
33. Ward KL, Hilton P, UK and Ireland TVT Trial Group: Tension-free vaginal tape versus colposuspension for primary urodynamic stress incontinence: 5-year follow up. *BJOG* 2008, 115:226–233.
34. Manca A, Sculpher MJ, Ward K, Hilton P: A cost-utility analysis of tension-free vaginal tape versus colposuspension for primary urodynamic stress incontinence. *BJOG* 2003, 110:255–262.
35. Paraiso MF, Walters MD, Karram MM, Barber MD: Laparoscopic Burch colposuspension versus tension-free vaginal tape: a randomized trial. *Obstet Gynecol* 2004, 104:1249–1258.
36. Staskin DR, Tyagi R: The SPARC sling system. *Atlas Urol Clinic* 2004, 12:185–195.
37. Deval B, Levardon M, Samain E, *et al.*: A French multicenter clinical trial of SPARC for stress urinary incontinence. *Eur Urol* 2003, 44:254–258.
38. Lord HE, Taylor JD, Finn JC, *et al.*: A randomized controlled equivalence trial of short-term complications and efficacy of tension-free vaginal tape and suprapubic urethral support sling for treating stress incontinence. *BJU Int* 2006, 98:367–376.
39. Delorme E: Transobturator urethral suspension: mini-invasive procedure in the treatment of stress urinary incontinence in women. *Prog Urol* 2001, 11:1306–1313.
40. Whiteside JL, Walters MD: Anatomy of the obturator region: relations to a transobturator sling. *Int Urogynecol J Pelvic Floor Dysfunct* 2004, 15:223–226.
41. Costa P, Grise P, Droupy S, *et al.*: Surgical treatment of female stress urinary incontinence with a trans-obturator-tape (T.O.T.) Uratape: short term results of a prospective multicentric study. *Eur Urol* 2004, 46:102–106.
42. Delorme E, Droupy S, De Tayrac R, Delmas V: Transobturator tape (Uratape): a new minimally invasive procedure to treat female urinary incontinence. *Eur Urol* 2004, 45:203–207.
43. Meschia M, Pifarotti P, Bernasconi F, *et al.*: Multicentre randomised trial of tension free vaginal tape (TVT) and transobturator tape in out technique (TVT-O) for the treatment of stress urinary incontinence. *Int Urogynecol J Pelvic Floor Dysfunct* 2006, 17:S92–S93.
44. Laurikainen EH, Valpas A, Kiiholma P, *et al.*: A prospective randomized trial comparing TVT and TVT-O procedures for treatment of SUI: immediate outcome and complications. *Int Urogynecol J Pelvic Floor Dysfunct* 2006, 17:S104–S105.

45. Latthe PM, Foon R, Toozs-Hobson P: Transobturator and retropubic tape procedures in stress urinary incontinence: a systematic review and meta-analysis of effectiveness and complications. *BJOG* 2007, 114:522–531.

46. Waltregny D, Gaspar Y, Reul O, *et al.*: TVT-O for the treatment of female stress urinary incontinence: results of a prospective study after a 3 year minimum follow up. *Eur Urol* 2008, 53:401–408.

47. Martan A, Masata J, Svabik K: TVT-Secur system—tension free support of the urethra in women suffering from stress urinary incontinence—technique and initial experience. *Ceska Gynecol* 2007, 72:42–49.

48. Meschia M, Barbacini P, Ambroqi V, *et al.*: TVT-Secur: a minimally invasive procedure for the treatment of primary stress urinary incontinence. One year data from a multicentre prospective trial. *Int Urogynecol J Pelvic Floor Dysfunct* 2009, 20:313–317.

49. Debodinance P, Lagrange E, Amblard J, *et al.*: TVT-Secur: Prospective study and follow up to 1 year about 150 patients. *Urogynecol J Pelvic Floor Dysfunct* 2008, 19:S11–S12.

50. Molden SM, Lucente VR: New minimally invasive slings: TVT-Secur. *Curr Urol Rep* 2008, 9:358–361.

51. Vervest H, van Dessel N, Lammerink E, *et al.*: TVT-Secur: the learning curve. *Urogynecol J Pelvic Floor Dysfunct* 2008, 19:S3–S4.

52. *Gynecare TVT SECURE System Professional Education* [CD-ROM]. Somerville, NJ: Ethicon Women's Health & Urology; 2006.

53. Kelleher CJ, Cardozo LD, Khullar V, Salvatore S: A new questionnaire to assess the quality of life of urinary incontinent women. *Br J Obstet Gynaecol* 1997, 104:1374–1379.

11 Simple and Complex Urethral Diverticula

Eric S. Rovner and Brett D. Lebed

Urethral diverticula (UD) may represent some of the more challenging diagnostic and reconstructive cases in urology. Women who have lower urinary tract symptoms, pelvic pain, or vaginal masses are often referred to a urologist or gynecologist as diagnostic dilemmas. A portion of these patients are subsequently found to have UD. UD have been reported in as many as 5% of the female population [1]. However, UD represent only one of several types of pathological periurethral masses presenting in the female. Given the rather wide spectrum of lesions and conditions that present in this manner, proper characterization is necessary prior to formulating a therapeutic plan. Proper imaging, including MRI, is important in proper staging and operative planning [2]. Often, but not invariably, UD require surgical intervention. These cases are approached individually and a successful repair may often employ a variety of reconstructive maneuvers including flaps and grafts. Therefore, the operating surgeon should be prepared to be flexible and alter the operative plan according to the findings at operation.

This chapter will review the presentation of patients with UD, describe the anatomic relationship relative to urethra and anterior vaginal walls, explain the pathophysiology of diverticula formation, and show examples of simple and complex diverticula on diagnostic imaging. We also illustrate the principles and technique for the resection of simple and complex urethral diverticula.

Signs and Symptoms of UD

Symptoms	Signs
Vaginal or pelvic mass	Recurrent urinary tract infection
Pelvic pain	Hematuria
Urethral pain	Vaginal or perineal tenderness
Dysuria	Urinary retention
Urinary frequency	Vaginal mass
Postvoid dribbling	Urethral discharge with stripping of the anterior vaginal wall
Dyspareunia	
Urinary urgency	
Incontinence	
Urinary hesitancy	
Vaginal or urethral discharge	
Double voiding	
Sense of incomplete emptying	

Figure 11-1. Signs and symptoms of urethral diverticulum (UD). In patients with suspected UD, the clinician must hold a high index of suspicion for the disease and direct the examination accordingly. At the time of the physical examination, urine analysis and cytology are collected. Cystoscopy can identify alternative sources for lower urinary tract symptoms and could potentially visualize the ostia of UD. If UD is suspected, then the diagnosis should be confirmed with radiologic imaging [3].

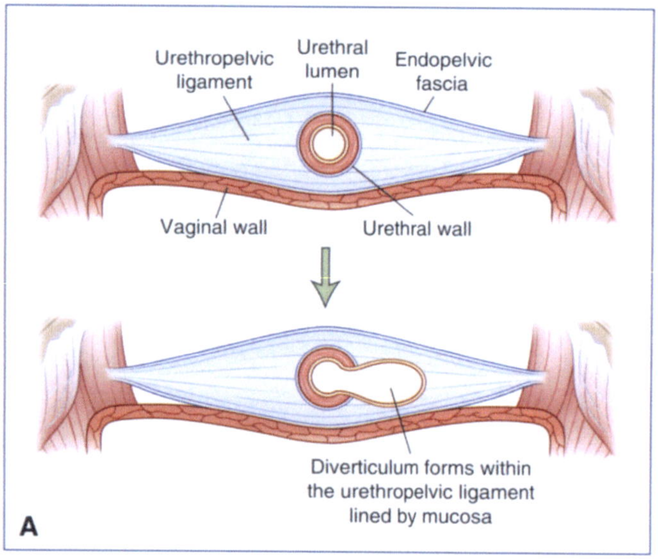

Figure 11-2. Imaging of simple urethral diverticulum (UD). **A,** UD is an epithelialized cavity dissecting within the periurethral fascia and urethropelvic ligament. **B,** The ostia or connection to the urethra is most commonly located in a posterolateral position along the proximal and middle third of the urethra. The adjacent MRI of the pelvis in **B** demonstrates simple UD.

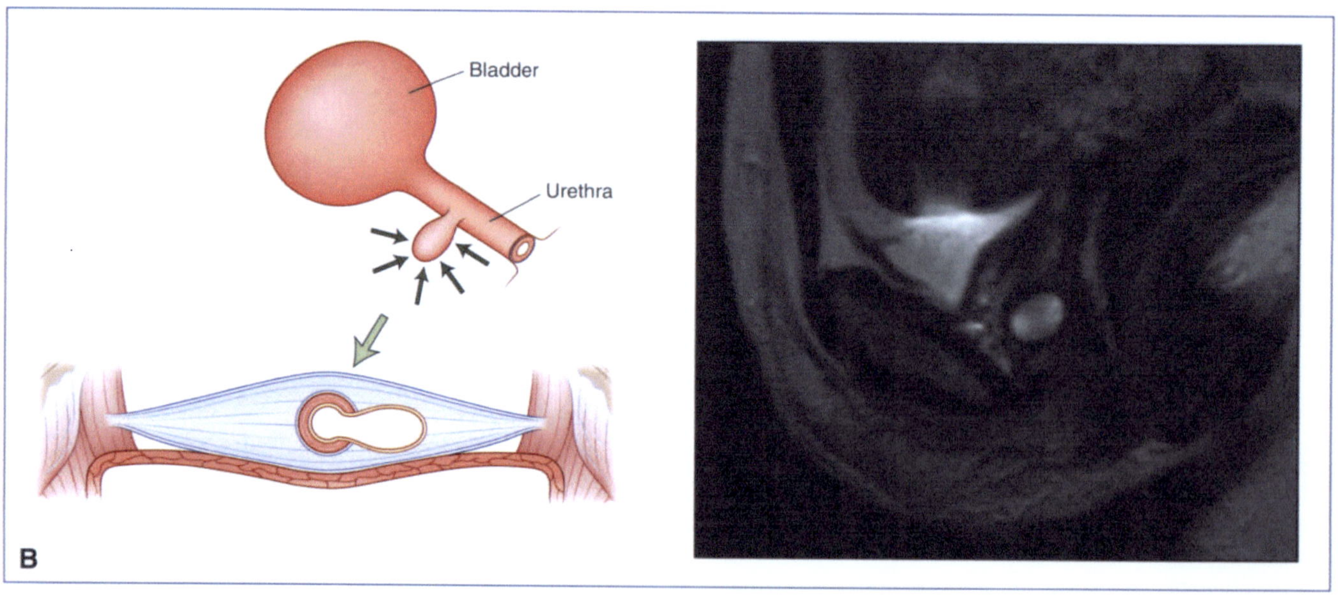

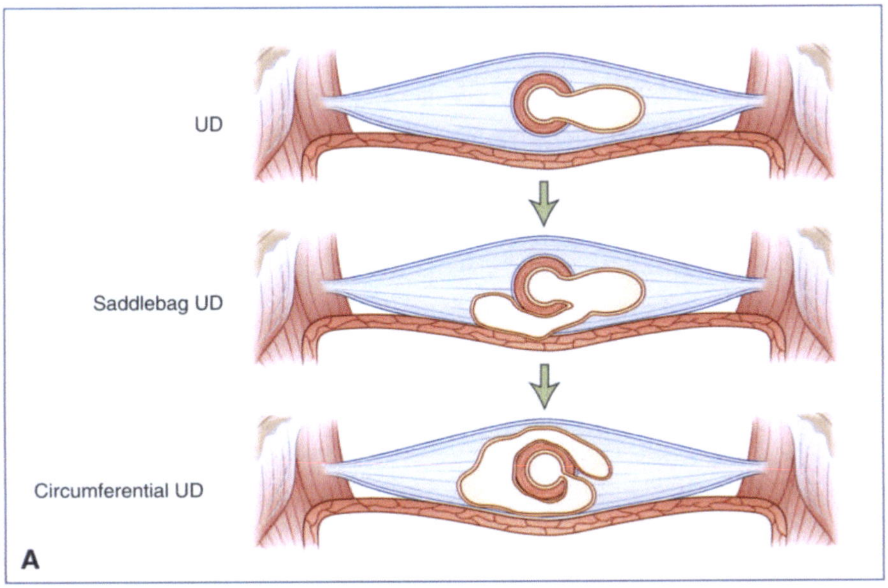

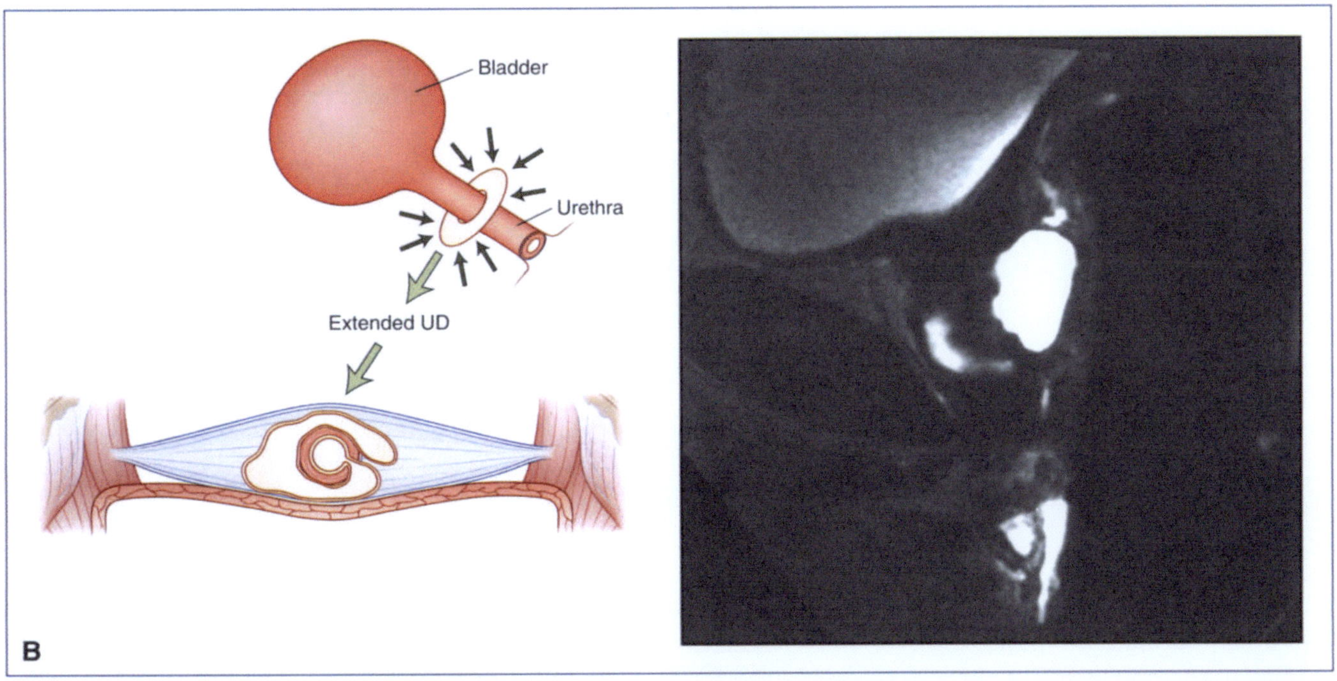

Figure 11-3. The diverticulum most commonly seen will be a single simple cavity. However, there is significant variability in overall size, the number of cavities, relationship to the urethra, and the presence of loculations. These characteristics are important to identify on imaging, as they will influence surgical approaches. **A,** Various types of urethral diverticulum (UD) morphology are shown. **B,** Extended saddlebag diverticula have a complex anatomic structure and relationship to the urethra. The adjacent MRI of the pelvis shows a diverticulum with components anterior and posterior to the urethra within the urethropelvic ligament.

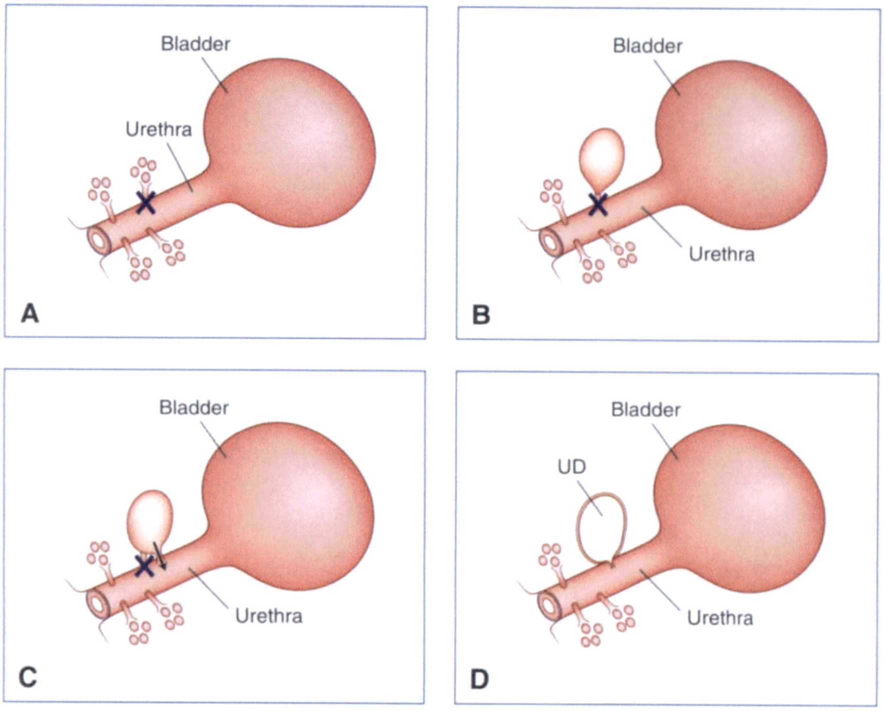

Figure 11-4. Pathophysiology of urethral diverticulum (UD) formation. There are multiple theories of UD formation; however, the most probable origin of acquired UD is from the obstruction of a para-urethral gland [4]. The para-urethral glands are located in the urethral submucosa and drain via ducts to the postero-lateral aspect of the urethral lumen. **A** and **B,** Obstruction of the para-urethral glands is shown. The *blue Xs* mark the site of a para-urethral gland obstruction. **C,** The formation of a para-urethral abscess and its rupture into the urethral lumen is shown. **D,** A residual epithelialized cavity with a narrowed neck is illustrated. Repeated infection, urine stasis, and intermittent obstruction can cause eventual diverticular enlargement and expansion [5].

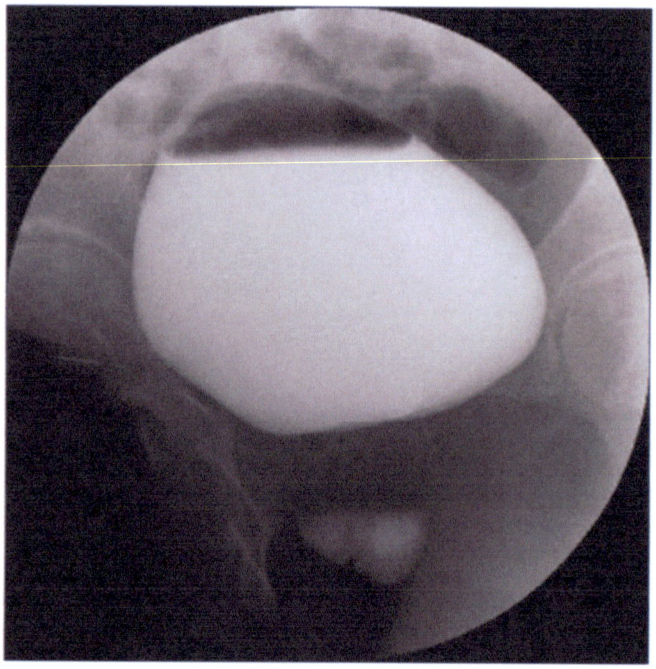

Figure 11-5. Voiding cystourethrogram (VCUG). VCUG is a commonly used radiographic study to diagnose urethral diverticulum (UD) and is dependent on the ability of the patient to void. If voiding does not occur, the urethra and UD will not be visualized. This postvoid film from a VCUG demonstrates a fluid-filled cavity inferior to the bladder, consistent with UD.

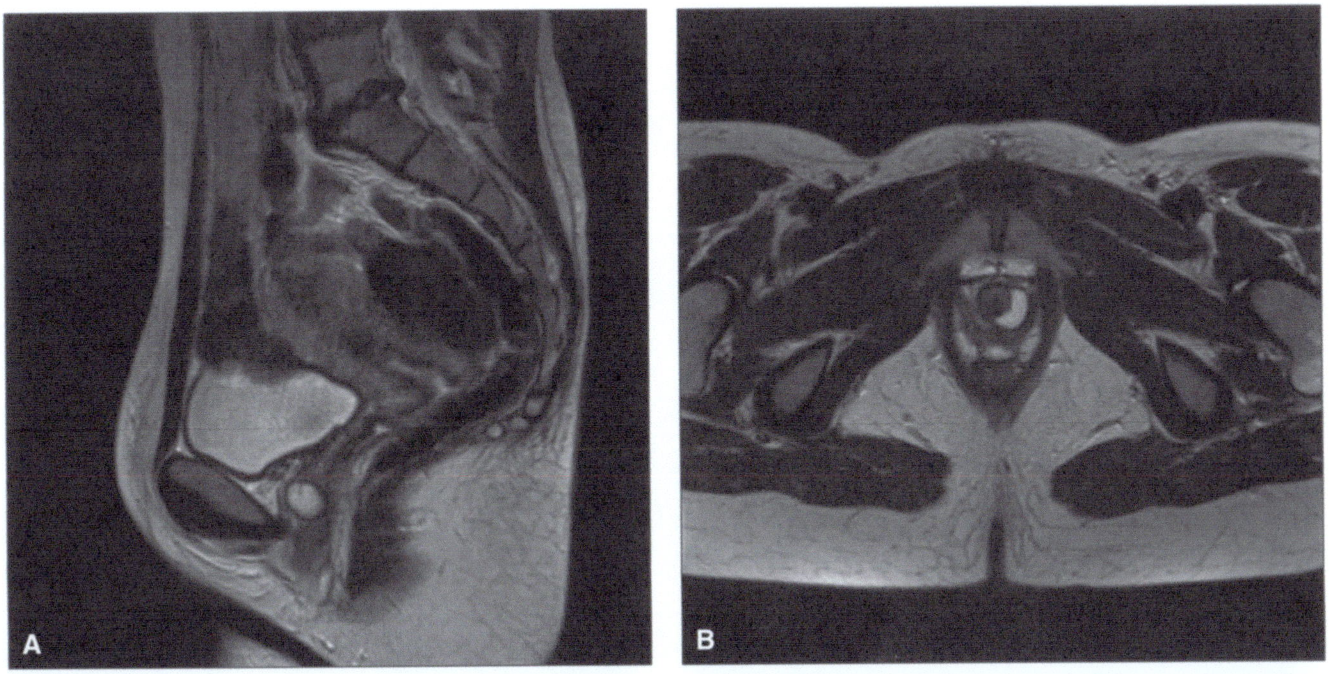

Figure 11-6. MRI of simple urethral diverticulum (UD). MRI is an excellent technique for visualizing UD and evaluating the relevant anatomy. It is independent of voiding [6]. **A,** This T2 weighted sagittal image demonstrates a fluid-filled structure inferior to the bladder, suggestive of simple UD. The differential diagnosis of a fluid-filled mass at this location includes a vaginal wall cyst, Gartner's duct abnormality, Skene's gland cyst or abscess, periurethral injectable agent, or Bartholin's gland obstruction. **B,** This T2 weighted axial image shows simple UD. The diverticulum is in a posterolateral position to the left of the urethra.

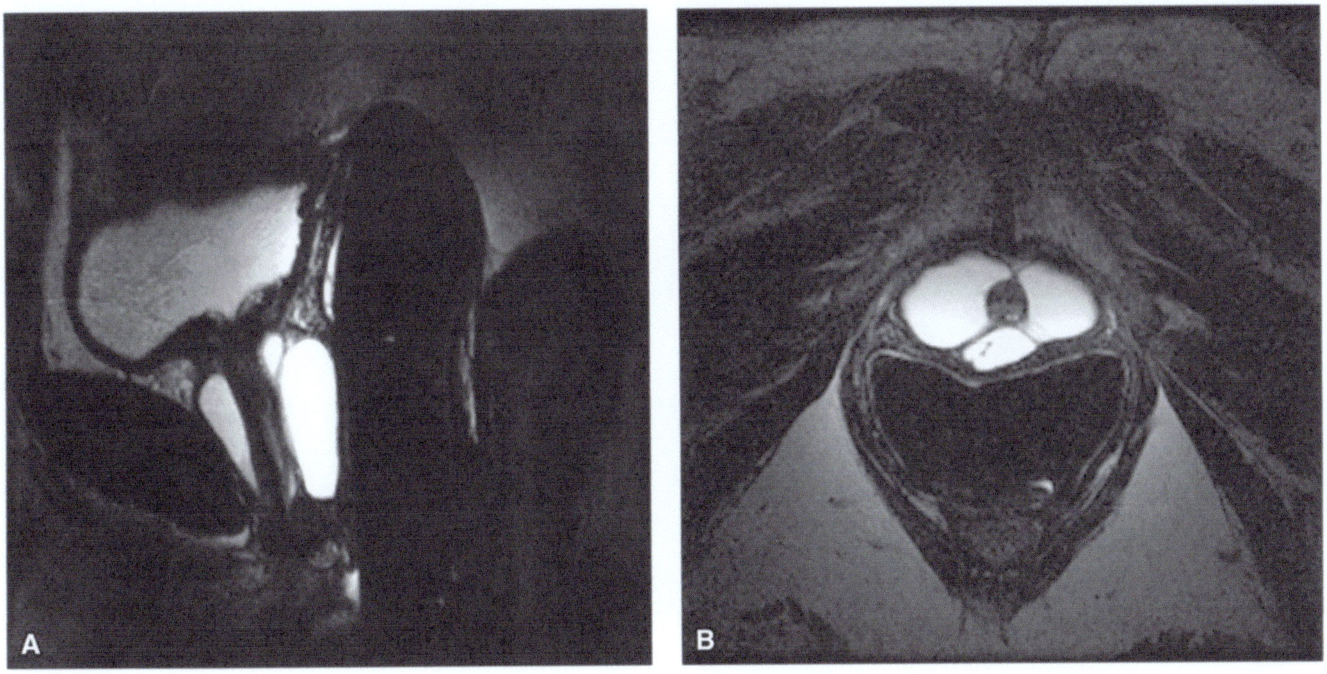

Figure 11-7. MRI of complex circumferential urethral diverticulum (UD). **A,** A T2 weighted sagittal image of complex UD with cavities anterior and posterior to the urethra is shown. **B,** A T2 weighted axial image in the same patient demonstrates the circumferential position of UD around the urethra. The urethral is seen "floating" within the UD.

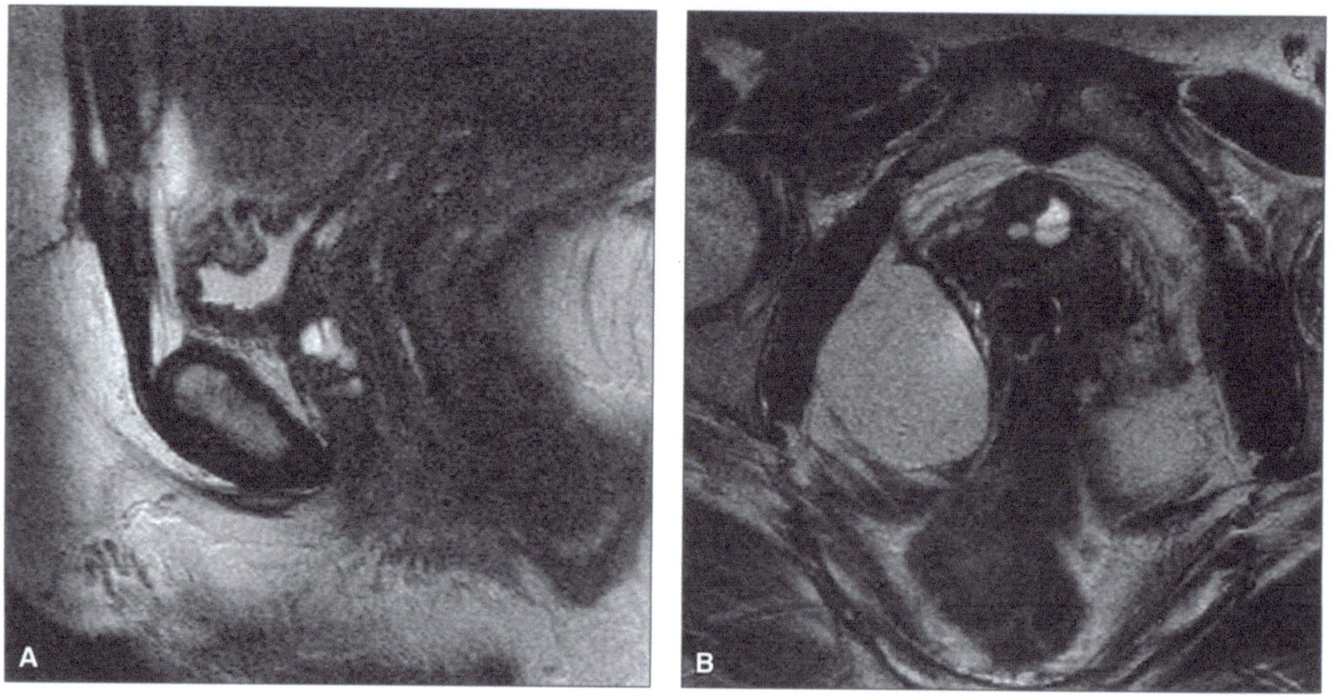

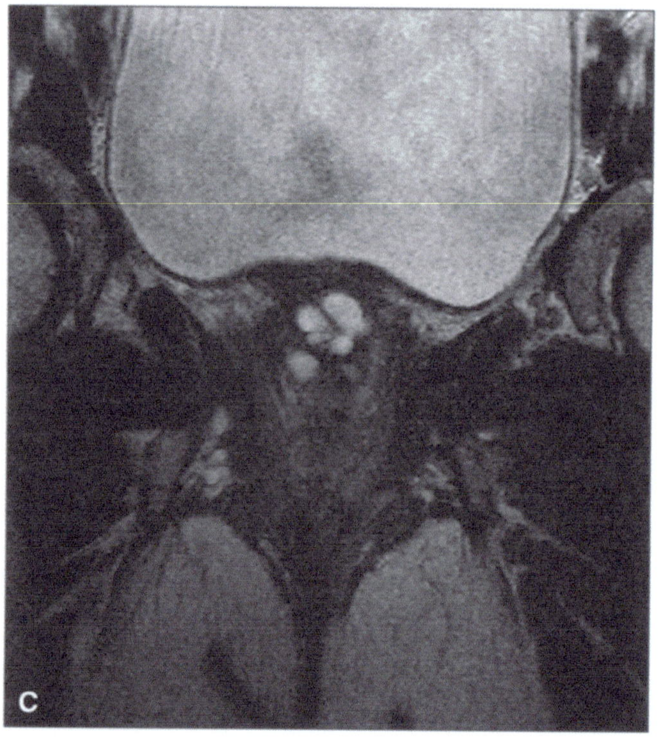

Figure 11-8. MRI of complex loculated urethral diverticulum (UD). **A,** A T2 weighted sagittal image of multiloculated UD is shown. **B,** A T2 weighted axial image of multiloculated UD is shown. **C,** A T2 weighted coronal image of multiloculated UD is shown.

Principles of Urethral Diverticulectomy

- Preservation of the periurethral fascia
  - Closure of dead space
  - Multilayered closure
- Identify and excise the neck or ostia
- Remove entire sac (mucosa)
- Preserve or create continence

Figure 11-9. Basic principles of urethral diverticulectomy. Prior to operative intervention, patients who also have urinary incontinence should undergo urodynamic evaluation. Concomitant anti-incontinence surgery should be considered if there is associated stress urinary incontinence.

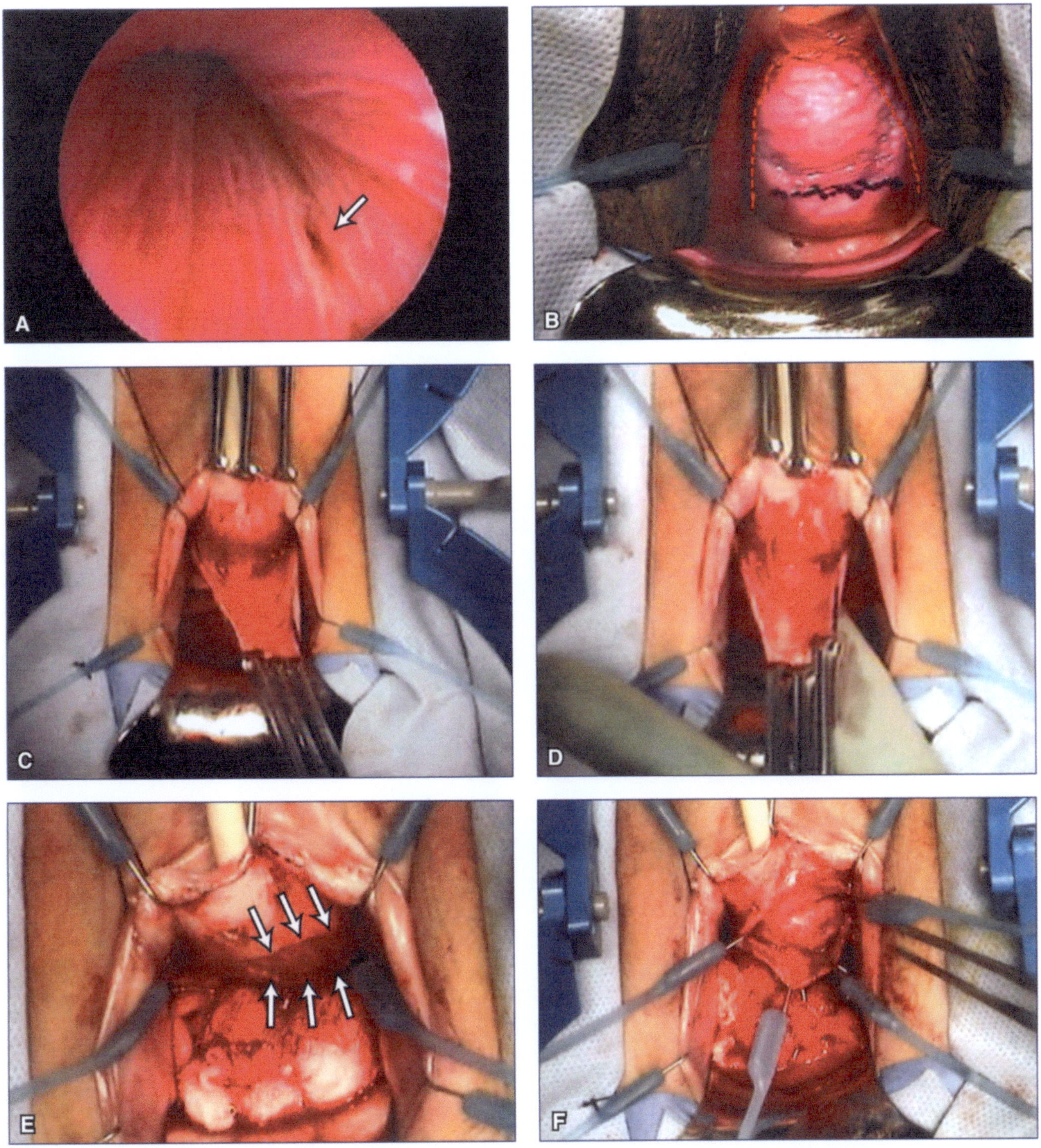

FIGURE 11-10. Surgical technique for urethral diverticulectomy [5,7]. **A,** Urethroscopy. Prior to intervention for urethral diverticulum (UD), a cystoscopy and urethroscopy are performed to identify the ostia of the diverticulum and to evaluate for additional urologic pathology. The *white arrow* shows the location of the UD ostia in this patient.

B, Inverted U-shaped incision. An inverted U-shaped incision (*red dotted line*) is made on the anterior vaginal wall. The bladder neck is delineated by the *blue dotted line*. A ring retractor with hooks and Allis clamps assists with retraction. Prior to the incision, the anterior vaginal wall incision line is injected with sterile saline for hydrodissection.

C, Development of the anterior vaginal wall flap. An anterior vaginal wall flap is created using careful dissection. **D,** Completion of the anterior vaginal wall flap dissection. The vaginal wall flap should be mobilized to the level of the bladder neck. It is important to maintain a broad-based flap to preserve adequate blood supply to the distal portion of the flap. The UD is seen as a subtle bulge within the periurethral fascia.

E, Incision of the periurethral fascia. The periurethral fascia is incised in a transverse fashion over the UD. The edges of the incised periurethral fascia are marked by the *white arrows*. A damp sponge keeps the anterior wall flap moist within the vagina.

F, Dissection of the UD from periurethral fascia. The UD is dissected carefully with the anterior and posterior leaves of periurethral fascia. In this image, hooks are on the edges of the dissected periurethral fascia. The UD is seen as a bulge within the periurethral fascia leaves.

Continued on the next page

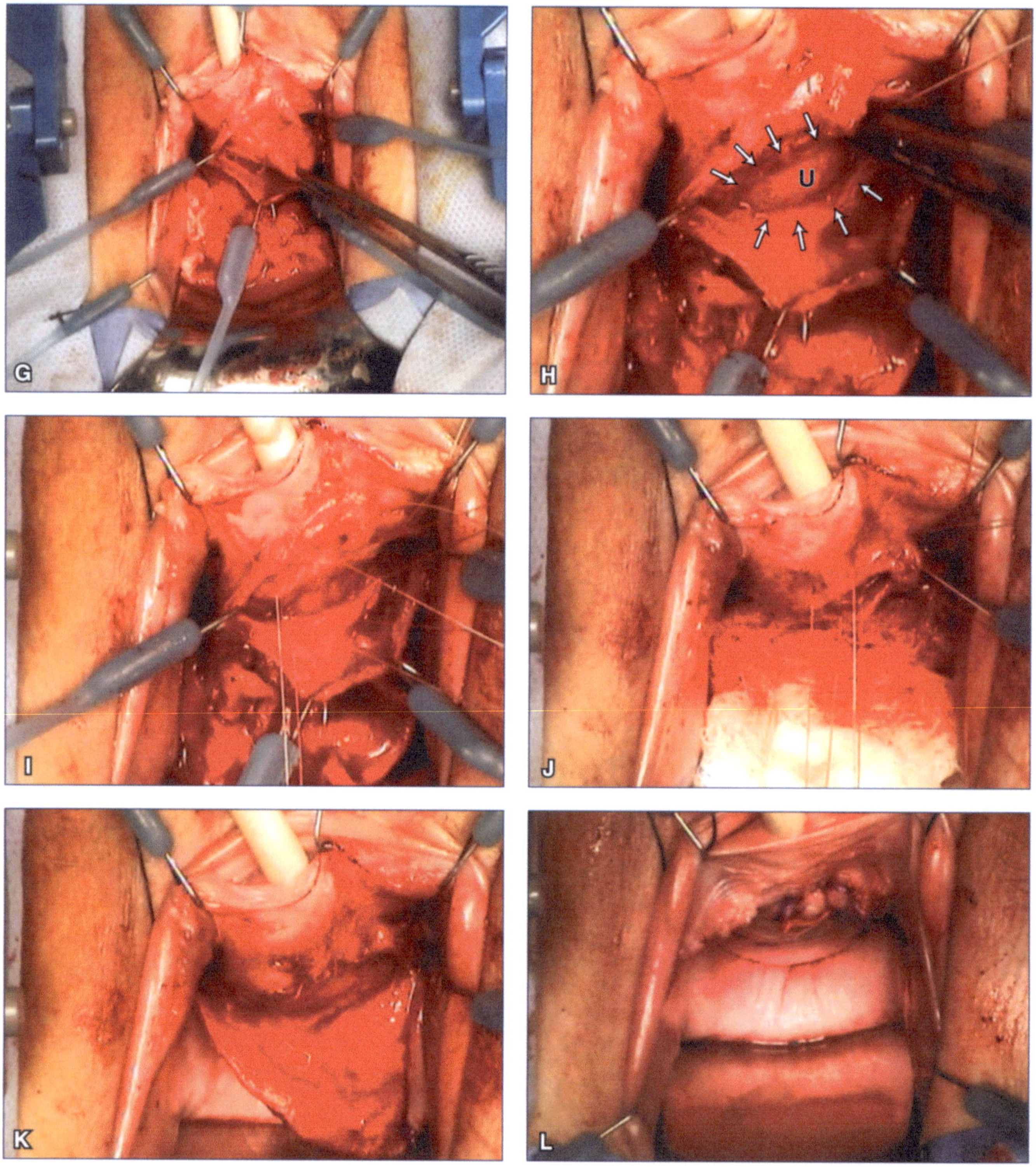

FIGURE 11-10. *(Continued)* **G,** Dissection of the UD from the urethra. The UD is dissected from within the leaves of the periurethral fascia until the urethra is identified. In this image, the UD is grasped with a forceps and is retracted laterally, revealing the ventral urethra.

H, Removal of the UD and closure of the ostia. Following complete mobilization, the UD is sharply excised. Once the diverticulum is excised, the urethral wall is seen (*U*). *White arrows* indicate the edges of the periurethral fascia. The ostia is identified and closed using fine absorbable sutures. The needle driver points in the direction of the ostia (the actual ostia is not seen in this image).

I, Suture placement in the periurethral fascia. The leaves of periurethral fascia are closed transversely with synthetic absorbable sutures. It is important to close all dead space to prevent recurrence of the UD. **J,** Closure of the periurethral fascia. The periurethral fascia is reapproximated as the previously placed sutures are tied down.

K, Advancement of the anterior vaginal wall flap. Once the periurethral fascia is closed, the anterior vaginal wall flap is advanced over the suture line. **L,** Closure. The anterior vaginal wall flap is secured with running, interlocking absorbable sutures.

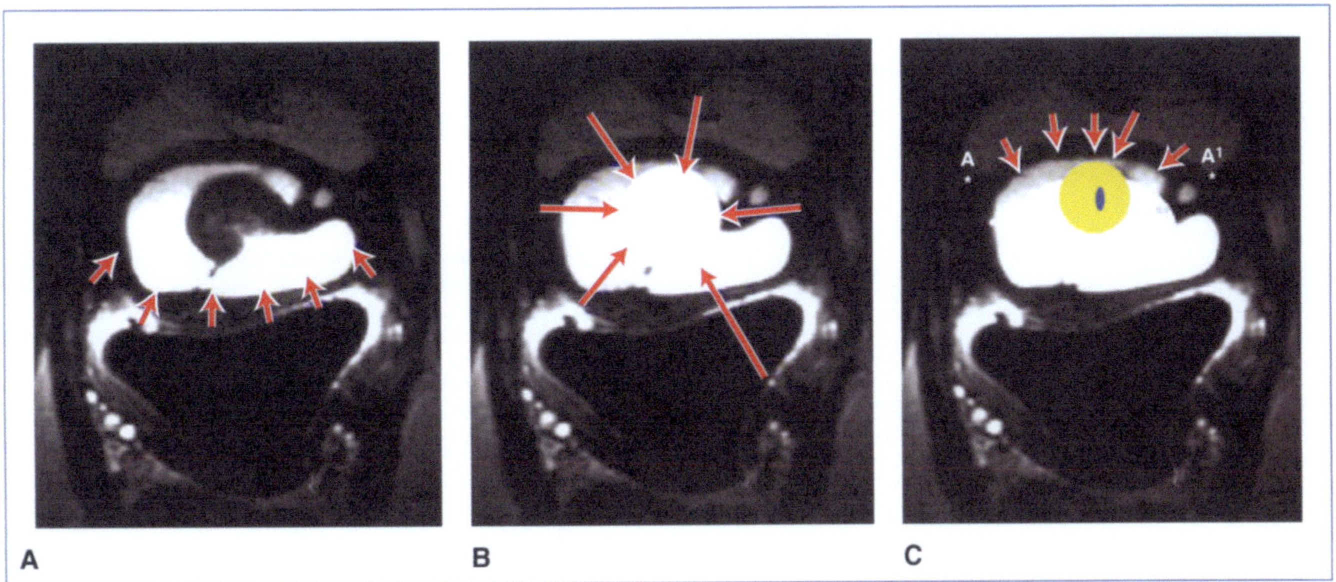

FIGURE 11-11. Circumferential urethral diverticulectomy using MRI imaging. Repairing circumferential urethral diverticulum (UD) is complex. Techniques include a diverticular sac urethroplasty (shown here) or excision and end-to-end urethroplasty. **A,** Once the anterior vaginal wall flap is mobilized and the periurethral fascia is incised and dissected, a posterior aspect of the diverticulum is identified. Once the visualized diverticular wall is separated from the periurethral fascial attachments, the lower (ventral) half of the diverticular wall is excised (*red arrows*). **B,** The urethra traversing through the middle of the UD is then excised for the length of the diverticulum. *Arrows* show the area where the urethra was excised. **C,** A neo-urethra is created using the dorsal wall of the diverticulum (*red arrows*). The remaining diverticular wall (marked at lateral margins A and A1 by the *stars*) is rolled ventrally over a Foley catheter. A Martius flap is used as an additional tissue layer over the closed suture lines. Because the continence mechanism of the female urethra may be compromised during dissection, an autologous pubovaginal fascial sling can be placed in addition to the Martius flap [8].

Excision of the Extended Saddle Bag UD
Potential problems
Exposure of the dorsal portion
Large amount of dead space
Adherence of the sac to the urethral wall
Sphincteric compromise

A

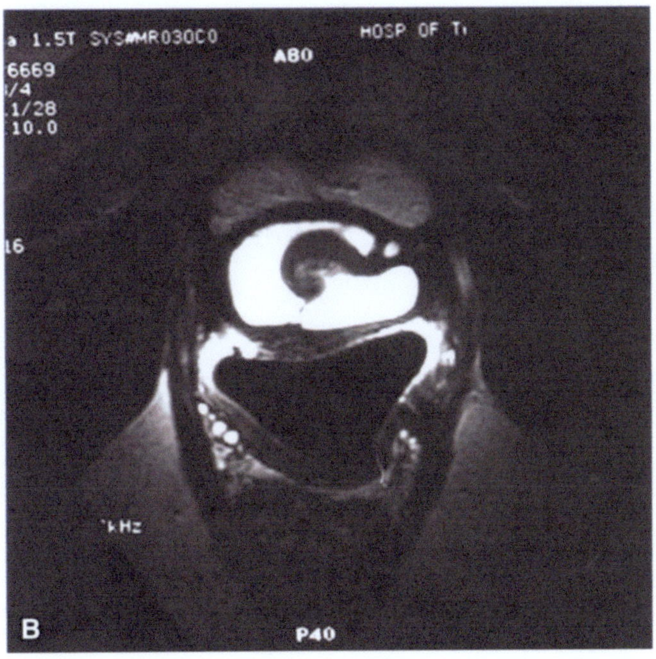

FIGURE 11-12. Challenges associated with surgery for circumferential ("saddle bag") or complex urethral diverticula (UD) that should be addressed at the time of surgery. Complications are listed in **A** and an MRI is shown in **B**.

Complications of Transvaginal Urethral Diverticulectomy
Urinary incontinence
Urethrovaginal fistula
Urethral stricture
Recurrent UD
Recurrent urinary tract infection
Other
Hypospadias/distal urethral necrosis
Bladder or ureteral injury
Vaginal scarring or narrowing: dysparuenia, etc.

FIGURE 11-13. Complications of transvaginal urethral diverticulectomy. Adherence to meticulous surgical technique, including multilayered closure, good hemostasis, nonoverlapping suture lines, and the elimination of dead space, should significantly reduce potential complications. The pre- and intra-operative identification of patients with stress incontinence, significant inflammation, or poor-quality tissues should lead the surgeon to offer simultaneous autologous pubovaginal fascial sling or Martius flap procedures. UD—urethral diverticula.

References

1. Young G, Wahle GR, Raz S: Female urethral diverticulum. In *Female Urology*. Edited by Raz S. Philadelphia: WB Saunders; 1996:477–489.
2. Lorenzo AJ, Zimmern P, Lemack GE, Nurenberg P: Endorectal coil magnetic resonance imaging for diagnosis of urethral and periurethral pathologic findings in women. *Urology* 2003, 61:1129–1133, discussion 1133–1134.
3. Romanzi LJ, Groutz A, Blaivas JG: Urethral diverticulum in women: diverse presentations resulting in diagnostic delay and mismanagement. *J Urol* 2000, 164:428–433.
4. Routh A: Urethral diverticula. *Br Med J* 1890, 1:361–362.
5. Rovner ES: Bladder and urethral diverticula. In *Campbell-Walsh Urology*, edn 9. Edited by Wein AJ, Kavoussi LR, Novick AC, *et al*. Philadephia: Saunders; 2007:2361–2390.
6. Blander DS, Rovner ES, Schnall MD, *et al.*: Endoluminal magnetic resonance imaging in the evaluation of urethral diverticula in women. *Urology* 2001, 57:660–665.
7. Benjamin J, Elliott L, Cooper JF, Bjornson L: Urethral diverticulum in adult female. Clinical aspects, operative procedure, and pathology. *Urology* 1974, 3:1–7.
8. Rovner ES, Wein AJ: Diagnosis and reconstruction of the dorsal or circumferential urethral diverticulum. *J Urol* 2003, 170:82–86, discussion 86.

12 The Male Sling and Artificial Urinary Sphincter I

Simon Y. Kimm and Craig V. Comiter

This chapter describes the surgical approach to treating stress urinary incontinence (SUI) in male patients due to intrinsic sphincter deficiency (ISD). The most common etiology of sphincteric incompetence in men is iatrogenic injury during prostate cancer treatment. While surgical extirpation is associated with the highest risk of SUI, sphincteric damage may occur with brachytherapy, external beam radiotherapy, or cryosurgery. Other less common causes include simple open prostatectomy, transurethral resection of the prostate, traumatic and acquired myelopathy, pelvic trauma, urethral reconstructive surgery, and neurogenic sphincteric incompetence.

Surgical management is indicated for the treatment of SUI in men for ISD that is persistently bothersome despite 6 to 12 months of active conservative management. The artificial urinary sphincter (AUS) and the male sling function by addressing the underactive outlet by increasing urethral resistance during the storage phase. Pressure is applied over a length of the urethra utilizing the sling mesh or the AUS cuff. The surgeon must realize, however, that these forces are also applied to the blood supply of the incorporated and compressed urethral segment and may result in urethral ischemia. Therefore, device construction, component selection, and implantation technique should optimize urethral compression and coaptation while minimizing the risk to urethral viability. Bladder emptying is optimized when the patient has adequate detrusor contractility and when these implants do not significantly impede urinary flow during volitional voiding.

AUS surgery should be avoided in patients who cannot operate the device due to either poor manual dexterity or lack of understanding. Neither AUS nor sling surgery is recommended for patients who have disorders that may jeopardize the upper urinary tract, such as diminished vesical compliance, low-pressure vesicoureteral reflux, and frequent high-pressure detrusor overactivity. Additionally, patients who have urinary tract disorders that may require future transurethral management should weigh their options carefully. If the AUS or male sling would impair transurethral access, or if repeated instrumentation would put the device at risk for erosion or infection (such as stone disease, recurrent transitional cell carcinoma, or unstable urethral stricture disease), then surgery may be contra-indicated. Finally, stress incontinence surgery should be avoided in patients who have untreated low-volume detrusor overactivity that may interfere with symptomatic improvement. Chronic infection of the skin or urine, anatomic abnormalities, immunosuppression, and poor urethral tissue quality are also relative contra-indications.

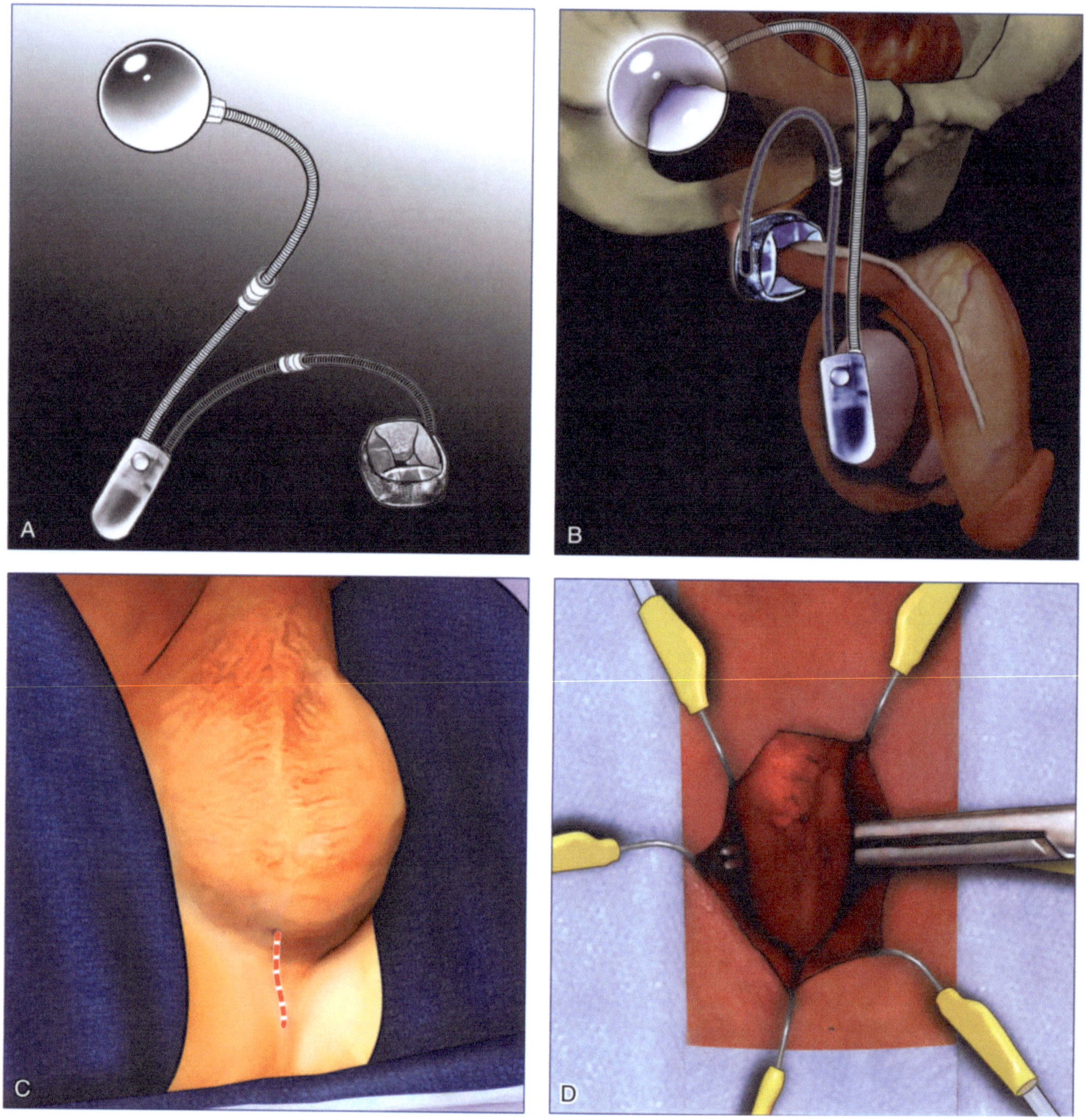

Figure 12-1. A, Surgical placement of the artificial urinary sphincter (American Medical Systems; Minnetonka, MN). **B,** The device consists of three components: a urethral cuff, a scrotal pump, and an abdominal pressure-regulating balloon. **C,** The patient is placed in the lithotomy position and is prepared and draped sterilely. After exposing the urethra, the bulbospongiosus muscle is opened and the corpus spongiosum is exposed. **D,** Circumferential dissection of the urethra is then performed, ultimately permitting a right angle clamp to be passed posterior to the urethra. Care must be taken to avoid injuring the urethra, especially on its dorsal aspect. If inadvertent urethral injury occurs, the procedure should be aborted and a urethral catheter should be left in place until adequate healing occurs. (*Courtesy of* S. Y. Kimm, MD.)

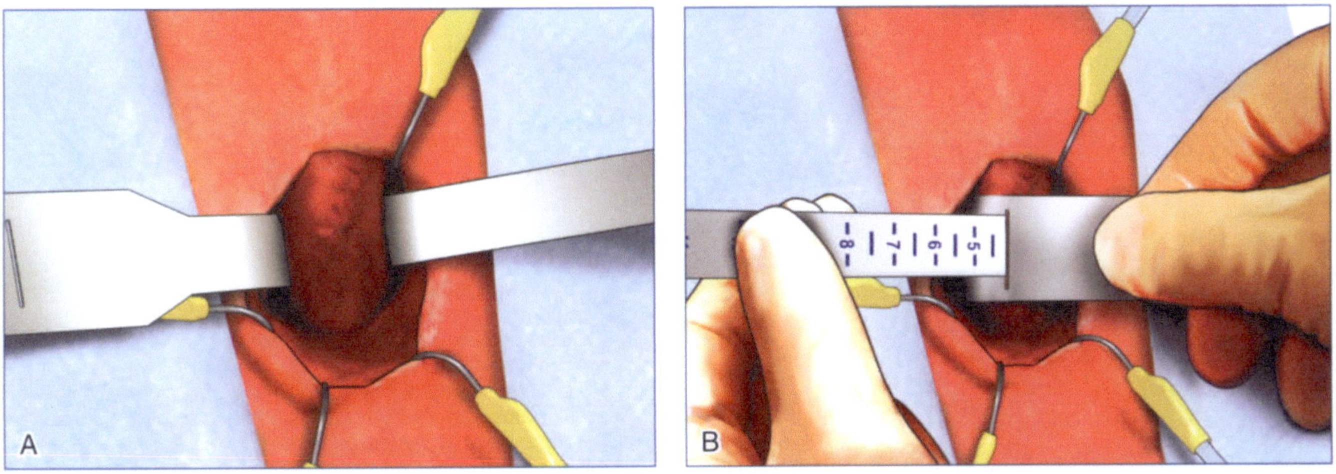

Figure 12-2. **A,** The circumference of the urethra is assessed by passing a flexible measuring device posterior to the urethra. The width of the dorsal dissection should be at least 2 cm, to accommodate the artificial urinary sphincter cuff. **B,** The Foley catheter is removed and the circumference is measured by encircling the urethra with the ruler. In most cases, the urethral circumference measures 4.0 to 4.5 cm. *(Courtesy of S. Y. Kimm, MD.)*

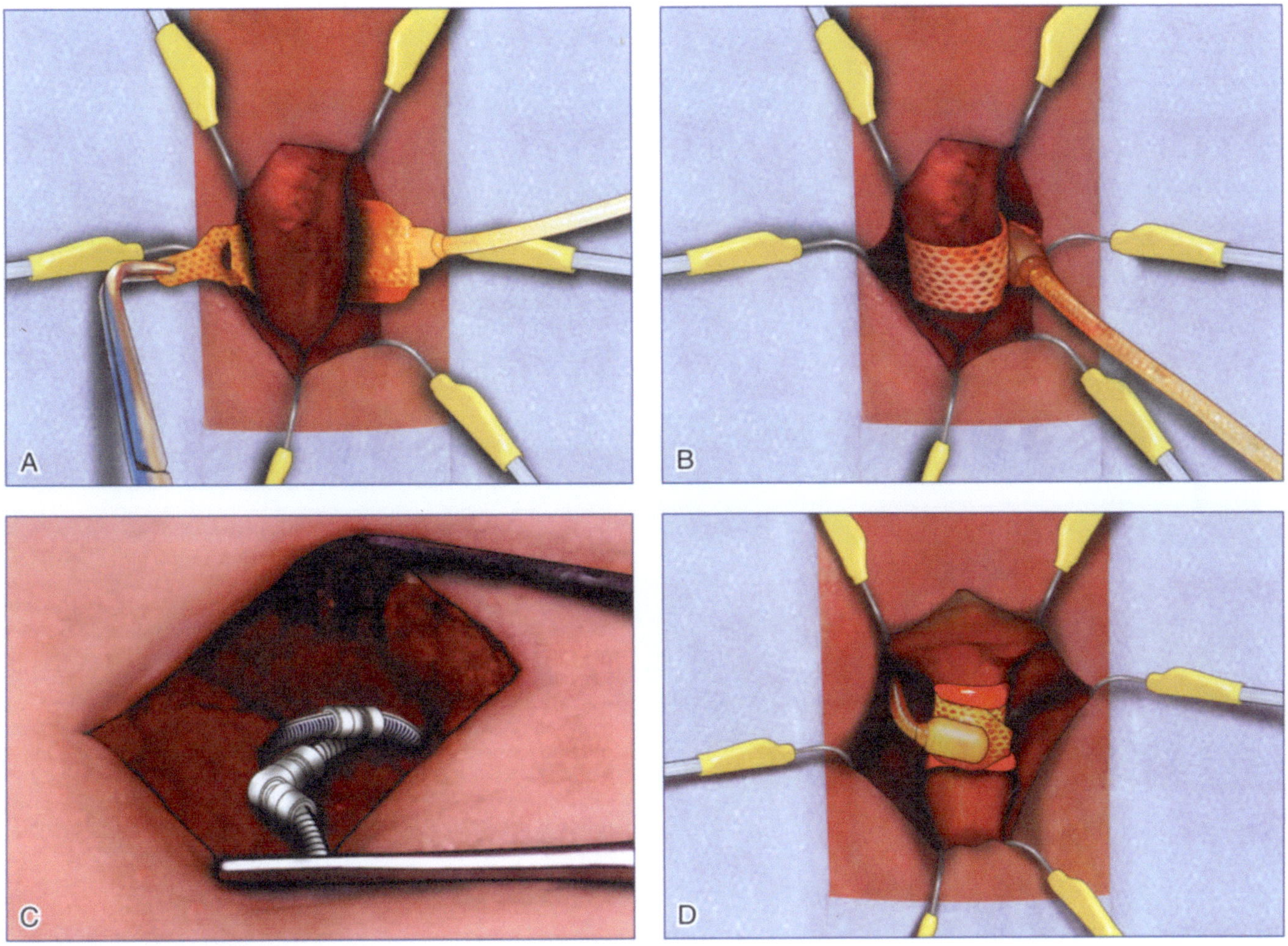

Figure 12-3. **A,** The inflatable cuff is then passed posterior to the urethra. The cuff should be placed without folds on either its superior or inferior edges as any folds may lead to insufficient continence or even urethral obstruction. **B,** The cuff is then wrapped around the urethra and secured in place. **C,** The cuff tubing is then passed prepubically, and the cuff tubing and pressure-regulating balloon tubing are connected to the scrotal pump tubing. **D,** When the cuff is pressurized, the urethra is compressed.

Continued on the next page

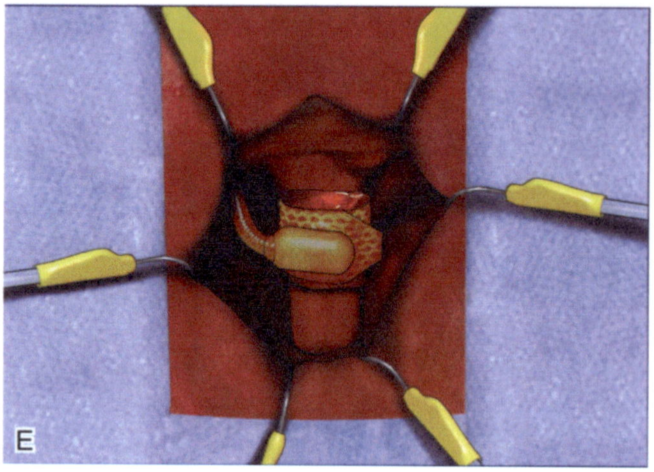

FIGURE 12-3. *(Continued)* **E,** The compressive effect of the artificial urinary sphincter is temporarily relieved when the patient squeezes the scrotal pump, transferring fluid from the urethral cuff to the pressure-regulating balloon, relieving the temporary urethral occlusion. The patient may then void by either detrusor contraction or abdominal straining. In fact, patients who void with Valsalva's maneuver because of an idiopathic underactive or neurologically acontractile bladder do not seem to be at an increased risk of complications [1]. *(Courtesy of* S. Y. Kimm, MD.)

Results of AUS Surgery in Males

Author	Points, *n*	Followup, y	0–1 pads/d
Montague [2]	66	3.2	75%
Perez and Webster [3]	49	3.7	85%
Martins and Boyd [4]	28	2	85%
Fleshner and Herschorn [5]	30	3	87%
Mottet *et al.* [6]	96	1	86%
Madjar *et al.* [7]	71	7.7	59%
Klijn *et al.* [8]	27	3	81%
Haab *et al.* [9]	36	7.2	80%
Trigo *et al.* [10]	40	4.5	90%
Kim *et al.* [11]	124	6.8	82%
Lai *et al.* [12]	218	3.1	69%
Goldwasser *et al.* [13]	42	1.2	82%

FIGURE 12-4. Results of artificial urinary sphincter (AUS) surgery in males with stress urinary incontinence (SUI) following radical prostatectomy with at least 12 months followup are given. In this table, "cure" is defined as no leakage or SUI mild enough to require 0–1 pad/d for protection. Unlike the sling, which is typically recommended for mild to moderate degrees of incontinence, the artificial sphincter is typically efficacious for all degrees of SUI, including total (gravitational) urinary incontinence. While the fixed resistance of a sling may inhibit bladder emptying in men with significant detrusor underactivity, the urethral cuff of the AUS is deflated during voiding, which may allow more efficient bladder emptying in such patients.

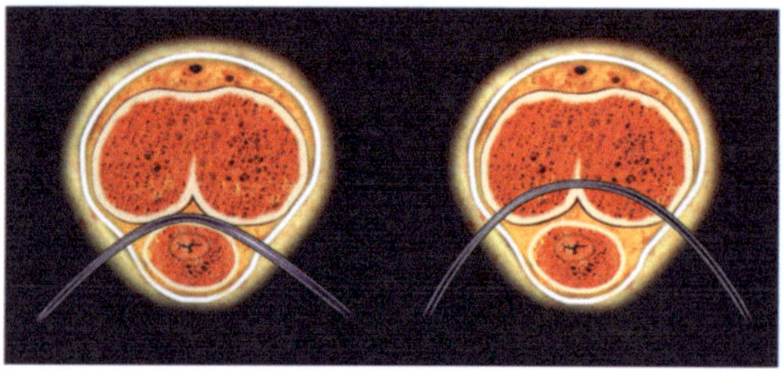

FIGURE 12-5. Urethral atrophy invariably occurs secondarily to corpus spongiosal atrophy [14]. This may lead to recurrent stress urinary incontinence, requiring surgical revision in approximately 17% of patients at 5 years [15]. Several therapeutic options exist to increase the cuff pressure around the atrophied urethral wall: changing the balloon reservoir for one generating at a higher pressure, downsizing the cuff diameter, or increasing the amount of fluid in the system. Another approach consists of placing the cuff inside the corporal tunica albuginea on the dorsal aspect of the urethra (transcorporeal placement) [16]. This allows a safer mobilization of the urethra and adds some supplementary bulk of tissue to the circumference of the urethra, possibly decreasing the risk of urethral erosion. It should be mentioned that there is a risk of reduced erectile function with this technique. The vast majority of such patients, however, already suffer from erectile dysfunction secondary to the prostate cancer surgery. *(Courtesy of* S. Y. Kimm, MD.)

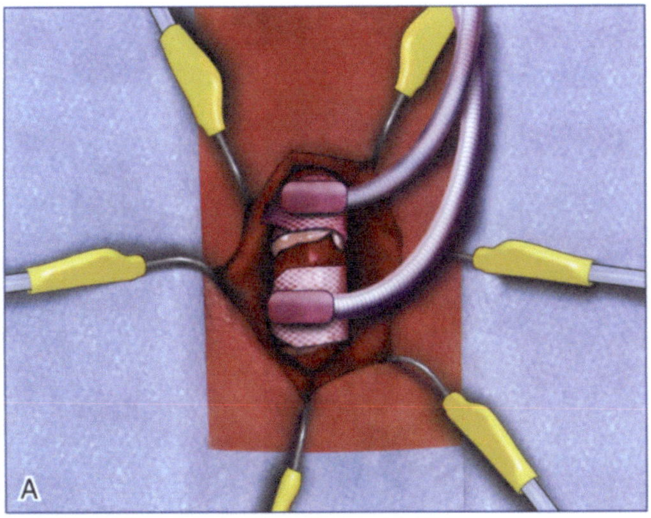

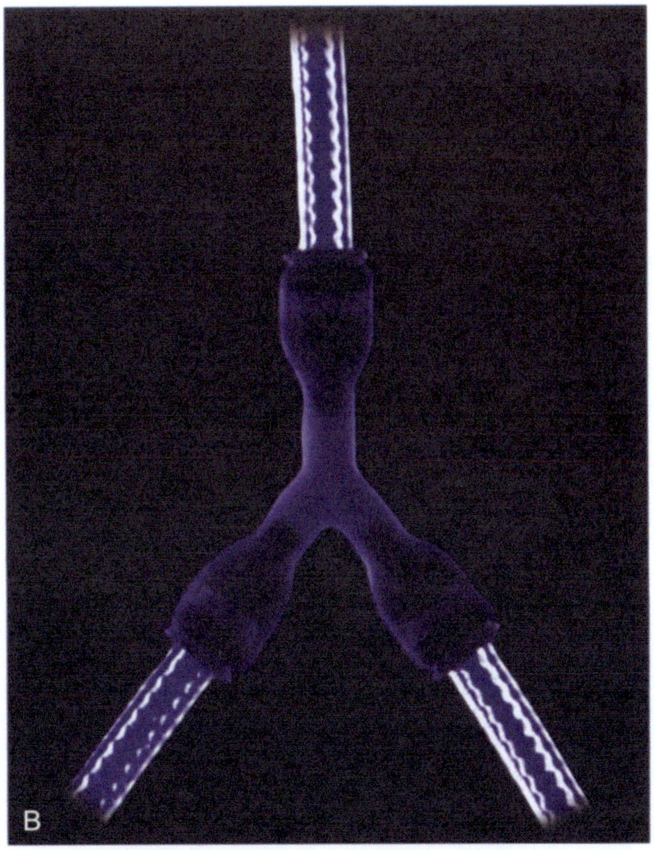

Figure 12-6. The implantation of a double-cuff AMS 800 sphincter (American Medical Systems; Minnetonka, MN) is also a useful salvage procedure, whereby a second cuff is added following a failed previous single cuff, placed 1 to 2 cm distal to the primary cuff (**A**) [17–19], joined to the previous system via a "Y-connector" (**B**). Some investigators have examined the utility of primary double-cuff placement. However, prospective evaluation of this technique revealed an association with a higher complication rate (55% vs 28%) and no significant difference in overall continence and quality of life measures [20]. Therefore, double-cuff placement is recommended as a salvage procedure only. (*Courtesy of* S. Y. Kimm, MD.)

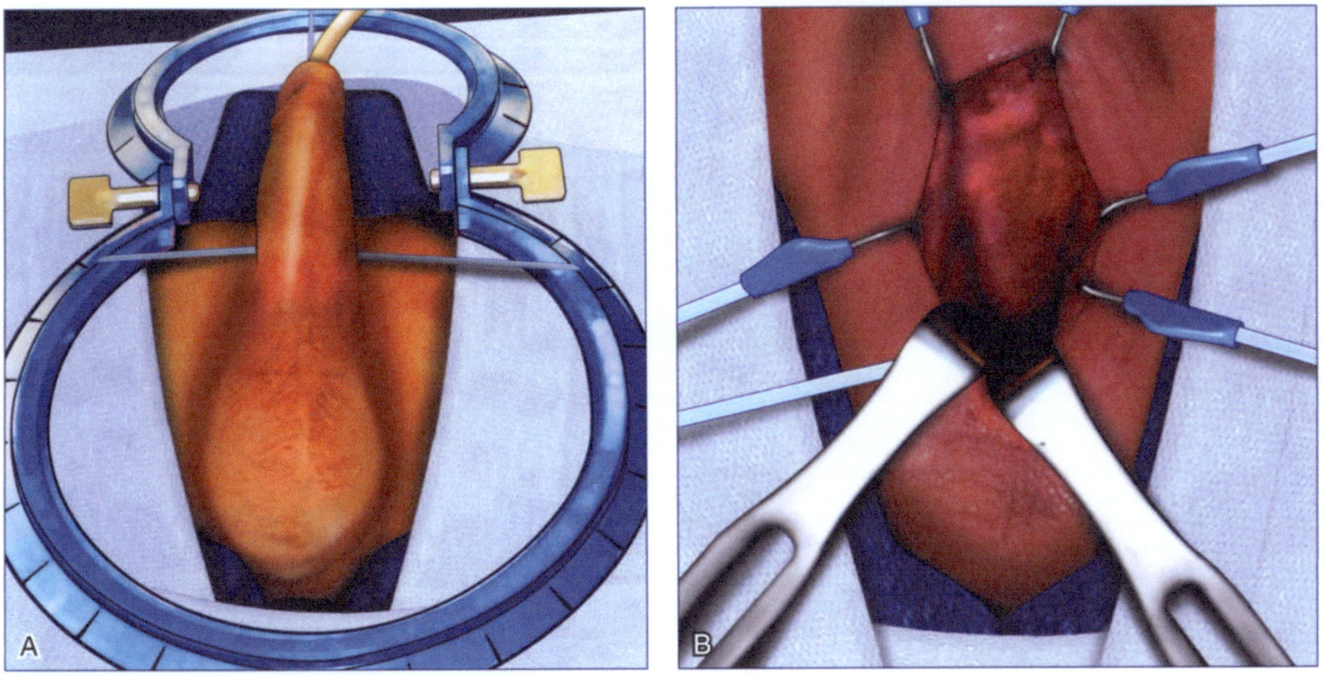

Figure 12-7. As an alternative to the perineal approach, a trans-scrotal procedure may be utilized [21]. **A,** The patient is placed in the supine position, sterilely prepared, and draped. **B,** The urethral is exposed and detaching the bulbous urethral from the perineal body allows proximal urethral exposure.

Continued on the next page

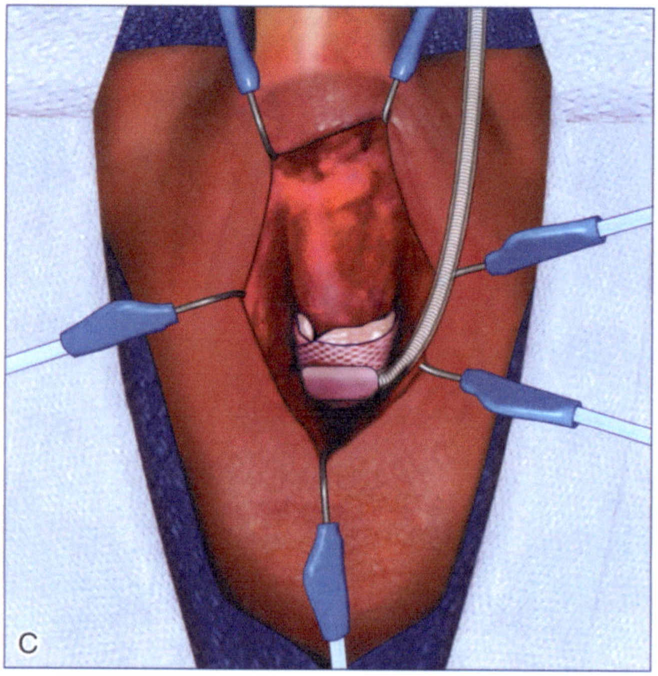

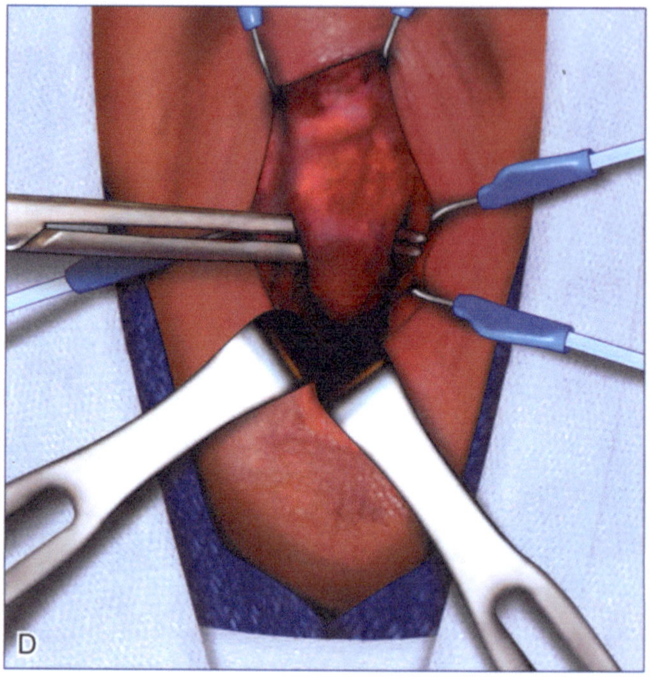

Figure 12-7. *(Continued)* **C,** Similar to the perineal approach, the urethra is dissected circumferentially and a right angle clamp is passed dorsally. **D,** With the trans-scrotal approach, the urethral cuff is placed slightly more proximal than can be achieved with the perineal approach. The advantage of the scrotal approach is that the entire procedure may be performed through a single incision—the scrotal pump is placed in a dartos pouch and the pressure-regulating balloon may be passed through the inguinal canal behind the fascia transversalis. The trans-scrotal approach is particularly useful for the placement of an artificial urinary sphincter (AUS) following previous perineal sling surgery. In the case of suboptimal continence following sling surgery, placing the AUS cuff distal to the sling through a scrotal incision allows the surgeon to avoid the previous operative field, minimizing dissection through potentially scarred tissue. It also leaves the proximally placed sling as a partially effective compressive device in series with the AUS cuff [22]. (*Courtesy of* S. Y. Kimm, MD.)

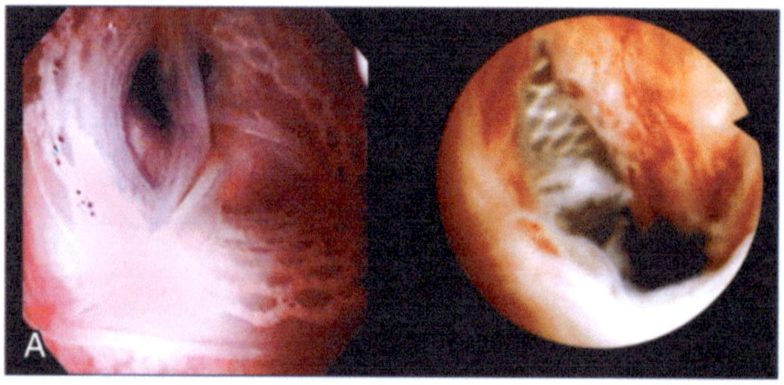

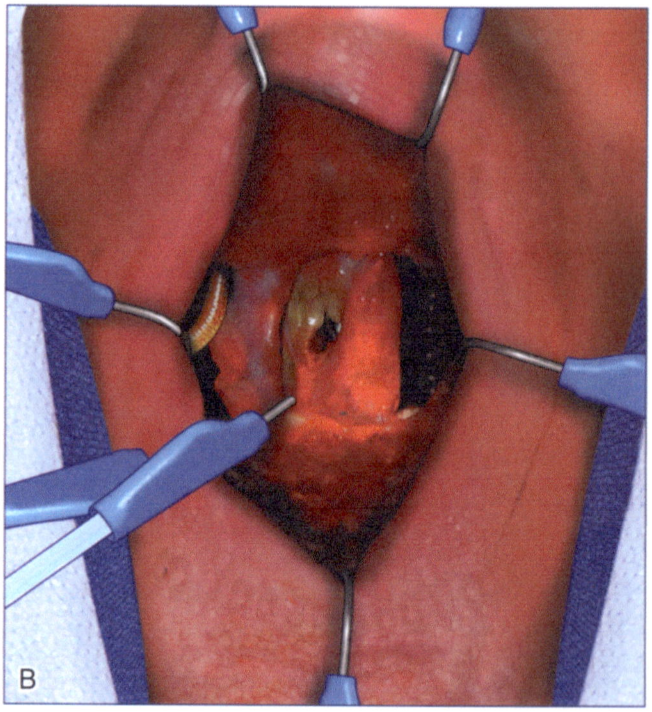

Figure 12-8. Erosion and infection are two major complications that typically necessitate removal of the prosthesis. The incidence of these complications varies from 0% to 24.6% [23–33]. Recent large series report an incidence of infection and erosion generally less than 8% [10–12,34–37]. The most likely etiology of early erosion is intra-operative laceration of the urethra when dissecting it from the corpora cavernosa, where a difficult anatomical plane exists. Whereas it has traditionally been assumed that the majority of postoperative erosions will occur during the first year, Lai *et al.* [12] from the Baylor College of Medicine recently reported that erosion occurred at an average of 19.8 months postoperatively. Other risk factors include urethral catheterization and urethral endoscopic manipulations with an activated sphincter in place [2,33]. **A,** An erosion may be identified endoscopically, which invariably requires surgical explantation. **B,** At the time of surgery, the urethral defect should be repaired and a urethral catheter should be left indwelling until healing is adequate. (**B** *courtesy of* S. Y. Kimm, MD.)

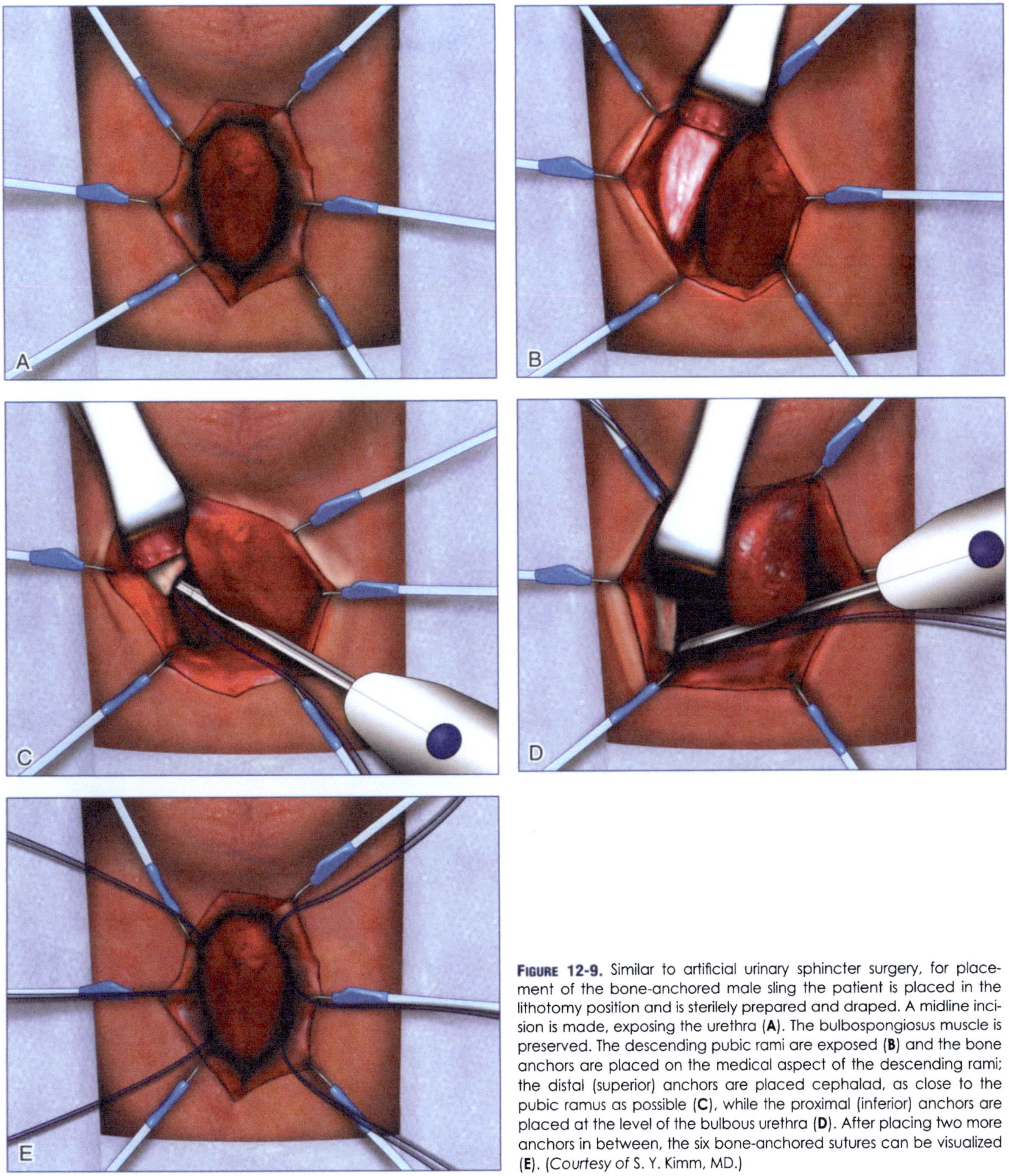

FIGURE 12-9. Similar to artificial urinary sphincter surgery, for placement of the bone-anchored male sling the patient is placed in the lithotomy position and is sterilely prepared and draped. A midline incision is made, exposing the urethra (**A**). The bulbospongiosus muscle is preserved. The descending pubic rami are exposed (**B**) and the bone anchors are placed on the medical aspect of the descending rami; the distal (superior) anchors are placed cephalad, as close to the pubic ramus as possible (**C**), while the proximal (inferior) anchors are placed at the level of the bulbous urethra (**D**). After placing two more anchors in between, the six bone-anchored sutures can be visualized (**E**). (*Courtesy of* S. Y. Kimm, MD.)

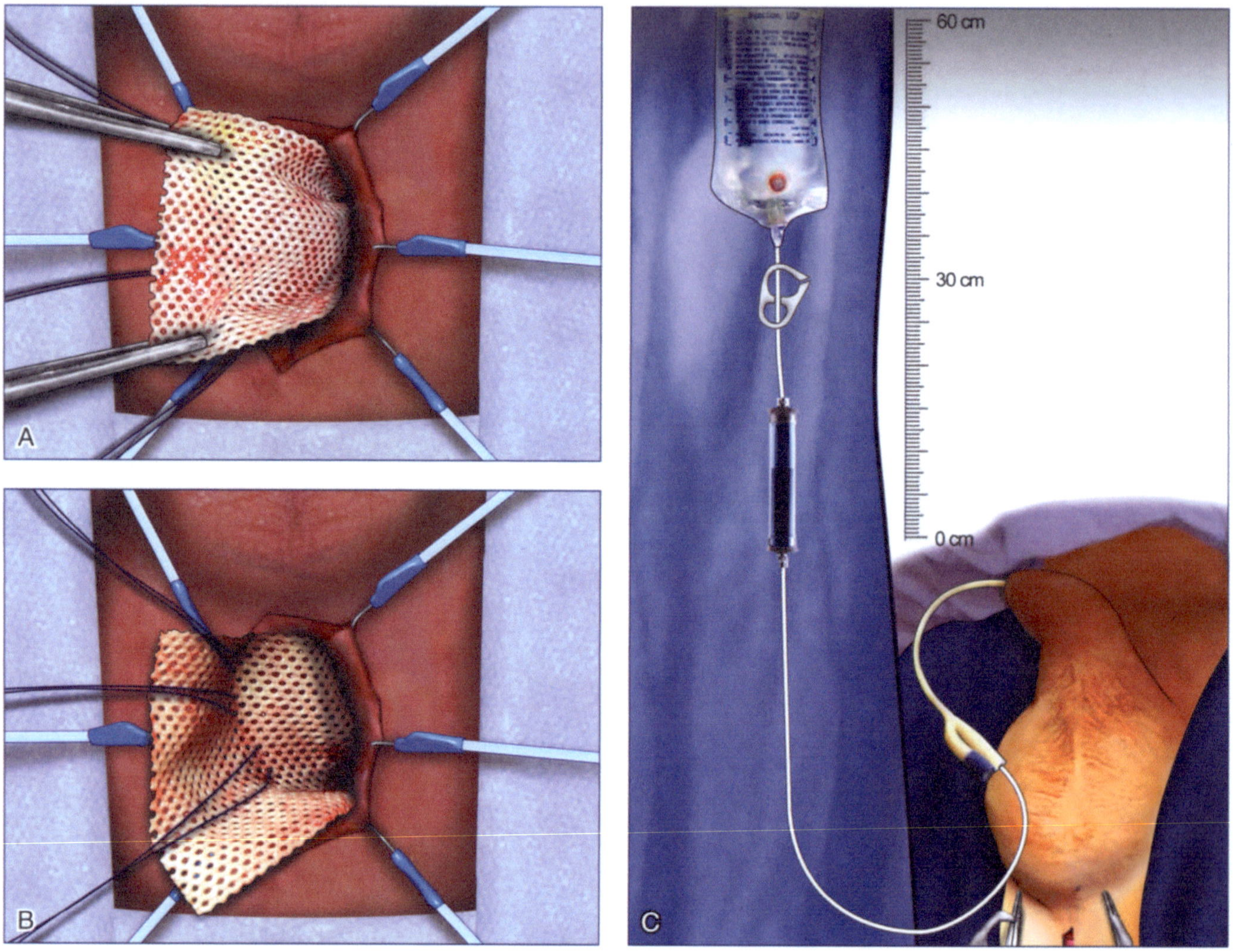

FIGURE 12-10. A 4 × 7-cm synthetic sling is used and the bone-anchored sutures are passed through the sling 0.5 cm from the left edge, equally spaced along the width of the sling, and tied down to the bone (**A**). The contralateral sutures are passed through the right side of the sling (**B**). Sling tension is adjusted by moving the right sutures more medially (tighter) or laterally (looser). A 14-Fr catheter is placed in the distal penile urethra, with the balloon inflated with 1 cc of water. Perfusion sphincterometry is performed by connecting a bag of saline to the catheter via sterile tubing. The bag is elevated until fluid flows from the bag, through the drip chamber, and into the urethra [38]. The retrograde leak point pressure (RLPP) is recorded as the height of the fluid column above the symphysis at which fluid flow begins (**C**). Patients who achieve an RLPP of 60 cm have a better outcome than those who demonstrate a lower compression pressure [39]. Additionally, there have been no instances of prolonged postoperative urinary retention reported when using the 60-cm RLPP as an intraoperative guide to sling tensioning. (*Courtesy of* S. Y. Kimm, MD.)

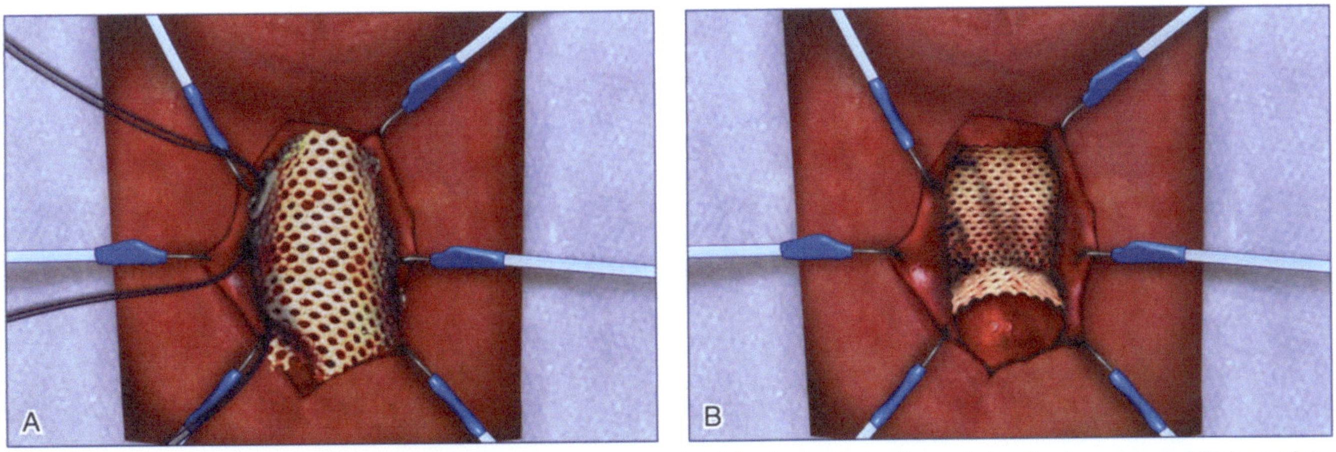

FIGURE 12-11. The contralateral sutures are then tied to maintain appropriate tension. Compared to the urethral position prior to sling placement (**A**), following tensioning the ventral urethra is compressed (**B**), increasing urethral coaptation and resistance. (*Courtesy of* S. Y. Kimm, MD.)

Results of Sling Surgery in Males with SUI

Study	Patients, *n*	Mean followup, *mo*	Sling material	Tensioning method	Cure, %	Cure/ improve, %	Fail, %
Schaeffer *et al.* (1998) [42]	64	18	Synthetic	ALPP/MUCP	56	64	36
Cespedes and Jacoby (2001) [43]	9	13	Organic	Visual	67	78	22
Madjar *et al.* (2001) [44]	16	12	Synthetic or organic	RLPP	86	100	0
Dikranian *et al.* (2004) [45]	36	12	Organic	RLPP	56	87	13
Dikranian *et al.* (2004) [45]	20	12	Synthetic	RLPP	87	100	0
Ullrich and Comiter (2004) [46]	36	25	Synthetic	RLPP	67	92	8
Onur *et al.* (2004) [40]	46	18	Synthetic or organic	Cough	41	76	24
John (2004) [47]	16	14	Synthetic	Cough	69	75	25
Stern *et al.* (2005) [48]	75	48	Synthetic	ALPP	36	68	32
Rajpurkar *et al.* (2005) [49]	46	24	Synthetic or organic	Cough	37	74	26
Comiter (2005) [50]	48	48	Synthetic	RLPP	65	85	15
Castle *et al.* (2005) [51]	42	18	Synthetic	RLPP	16	40	60
Migliari *et al.* (2006) [52]	49	32	Synthetic	RLPP	30	63	37
Fischer *et al.* (2007) [53]	62	56	Synthetic	RLPP	37	58	42
Gallagher *et al.* (2007) [54]	24	15	Synthetic	Visual	38	75	25
Sousa-Escandón *et al.* (2007) [55]	51	32	Synthetic	Visual	65	85	15
Xu *et al.* (2007) [56]	26	28	Synthetic	UPP	85	92	8
Giberti *et al.* (2008) [41]	36	41	Synthetic or organic	RLPP	62	70	30

FIGURE 12-12. Results of sling surgery in males with stress urinary incontinence with at least 12 months followup. Rates of cure depend on the definition of incontinence and the method of evaluation. For these cohorts, "cure" is defined as complete continence or using 0–1 pad/d. "Improved" denotes at least a 50% decrease in pad use. If patients do not achieve at least a 50% reduction in pad use and have continued bothersome leakage, they are considered "treatment failures." The type of sling material utilized affects surgical success rates. Synthetic slings (polypropylene or polyester) have a higher success rate than do organic sling (fascia, dermis, allograft, or xenograft) [40,41]. Unlike sling surgery in women with stress incontinence, the male sling is placed under tension. Thus, re-absorption of organic slings will lead to recurrent incontinence. ALPP—abdominal leak point pressure; MUCP—maximal urethral closure pressure; RLPP—retrograde leak point pressure; UPP—urethral pressure profilometry.

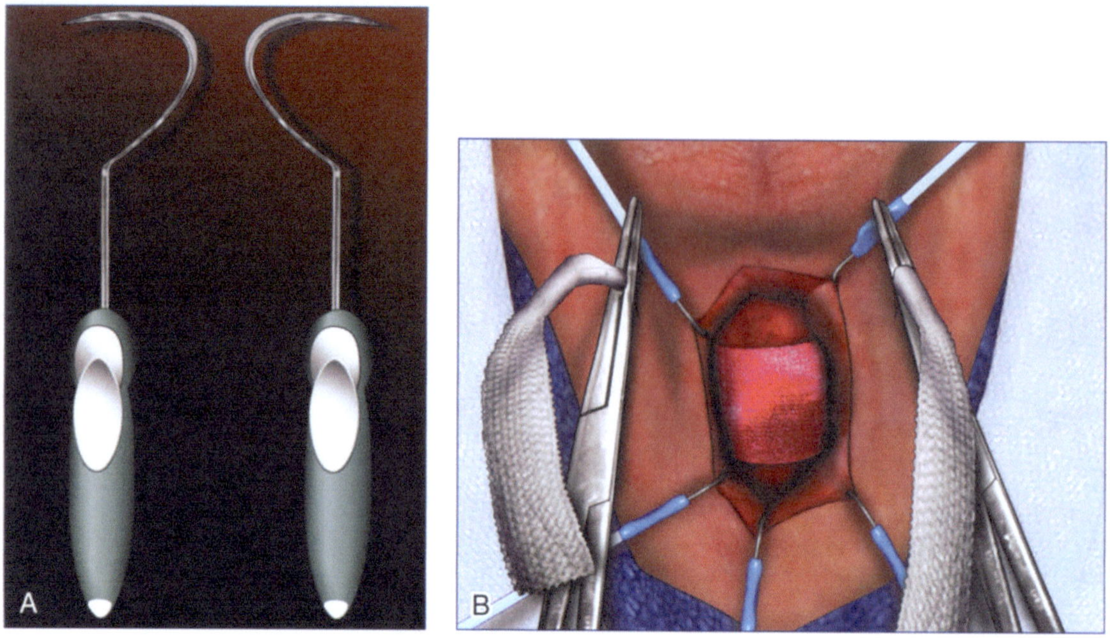

Figure 12-13. A sling that avoids the use of bone screws has recently been introduced, relying more on urethral elevation with only a minor component of bulbous urethral compression [56]. The sling is placed via a transobturator approach. Helical or hooked needle passers (**A**) are passed laterally to medially, through the obturator foramen. Care must be taken during this blind passage to avoid inadvertent injury to the pelvic structures, including nerves, blood vessels, corpora cavernosa, or the urethra. The sling lies under the bulbous urethra (**B**), which has been detached from the perineal body. Tension is applied to the transobturator sling, elevating the urethra, moving the bulbous urethra proximally. Because the sling is much narrower than the bone-anchored sling and provides urethral compression over a substantially smaller area of the bulbous urethra, this transobturator sling is recommended only for cases of mild urinary incontinence. For patients with greater degrees of urinary incontinence, a bone-anchored male sling is recommended. (*Courtesy of* S. Y. Kimm, MD.)

References

1. Gomha MA, Boone TB: Voiding patterns in patients with post-prostatectomy incontinence: urodynamic and demographic analysis. *J Urol* 2003, 169:1766–1769.
2. Montague DK: The artificial urinary sphincter (AS 800): experience in 166 consecutive patients. *J Urol* 1992, 147:380–382.
3. Perez LM, Webster GD: Successful outcome of artificial urinary sphincters in men with post-prostatectomy urinary incontinence despite adverse implantation features. *J Urol* 1992, 148:1166–1170.
4. Martins FE, Boyd SD: Artificial urinary sphincter in patients following major pelvic surgery and/or radiotherapy: are they less favorable candidates? *J Urol* 1995, 153:1188–1193.
5. Fleshner N, Herschorn S: The artificial urinary sphincter for post-radical prostatectomy incontinence: impact on urinary symptoms and quality of life. *J Urol* 1996, 155:1260–1264.
6. Mottet N, Boyer C, Chartier-Kastler E, *et al.*: Artificial urinary sphincter AMS 800 for urinary incontinence after radical prostatectomy: the French experience. *Urol Int* 1998, 60(Suppl 2):25–29.
7. Madjar S, Gousse AE, Lambert MM, Fishman IJ: Artificial urinary sphincter implantation for radical prostatectomy urinary incontinence: which factors influence patient satisfaction? *BJU Int* 2000, 86(Suppl 3):121.
8. Klijn AJ, Hop WC, Mickisch G, *et al.*: The artificial urinary sphincter in men incontinent after radical prostatectomy: 5 year actuarial adequate function rates. *Br J Urol* 1998, 82:530–533.
9. Haab F, Trockman BA, Zimmern PE, Leach GE: Quality of life and continence assessment of the artificial urinary sphincter in men with minimum 3.5 years of followup. *J Urol* 1997, 158:435–439.
10. Trigo Rocha F, Gomes CM, Mitre AI, *et al.*: Prospective study evaluating the efficacy of the artificial sphincter AMS 800 for the treatment of post-radical prostatectomy urinary incontinence and the correlation between preoperative urodynamic and surgical outcomes. *Urology* 2008, 71:85–89.
11. Kim SP, Sarmast Z, Daignault S, *et al.*: Long-term durability and functional outcomes among patients with artificial urinary sphincters: a 10-year retrospective review from the university of Michigan. *J Urol* 2008, 179:1912–1916.
12. Lai HH, Hsu EI, The BS, *et al.*: 13 years of experience with artificial urinary sphincter implantation at Baylor College of Medicine. *J Urol* 2007, 177:1021–1025.
13. Goldwasser B, Furlow WL, Barrett DM: The model AS 800 artificial urinary sphincter: Mayo Clinic experience. *J Urol* 1987, 137:668–671.
14. Bosch JL: The contemporary role of the artificial urinary sphincter. *Curr Opin Urol* 2000, 10:219–223.
15. Elliott DS, Barrett DM: Mayo Clinic long-term analysis of the functional durability of the AMS 800 artificial urinary sphincter: a review of 323 cases. *J Urol* 1998, 159:1206–1208.
16. Guralnick ML, Miller EA, Toh KL, Webster GD: Transcorporal artificial urinary sphincter cuff placement in cases requiring revision for erosion and urethral atrophy. *J Urol* 2002, 167:2075–2078.
17. Kabalin JN: Addition of a second urethral cuff to enhance performance of the artificial urinary sphincter. *J Urol* 1996, 156:1302–1304.
18. Brito CG, Mulcahy JJ, Mitchell ME, Adams MC: Use of a double cuff AMS800 urinary sphincter for severe stress incontinence. *J Urol* 1993, 149:283–285.
19. DiMarco DS, Elliott DS: Tandem cuff artificial urinary sphincter as a salvage procedure following failed primary sphincter placement for the treatment of post-prostatectomy incontinence. *J Urol* 2003, 170:1252–1254.
20. O'Connor RC, Lyon MB, Guralnick ML, Bales GT: Long-term follow-up of single versus double cuff artificial urinary sphincter insertion for the treatment of severe postprostatectomy stress urinary incontinence. *Urology* 2008, 71:90–93.
21. Wilson SK, Delk JR, Henry GD, Siegel AL: New surgical technique for sphincter urinary control system using upper transverse scrotal incision. *J Urol* 2003, 169:261–264.
22. Comiter CV: Surgery insight: surgical management of postprostatectomy incontinence—the artificial urinary sphincter and male sling. *Nat Clin Pract Urol* 2007, 4:615–624.
23. Venn SN, Greenwell TJ, Mundy AR: The long-term outcome of artificial urinary sphincters. *J Urol* 2000, 164:702–706.
24. Roth DR, Vyas PR, Kroovand RL, Perlmutter AD: Urinary tract deterioration associated with the artificial urinary sphincter. *J Urol* 1986, 135:528–530.
25. Aprikian A, Berardinucci G, Pike J, Kiruluta G: Experience with the AS-800 artificial urinary sphincter in myelodysplastic children. *Can J Surg* 1992, 35:396–400.
26. Simeoni J, Guys JM, Mollard P, *et al.*: Artificial urinary sphincter implantation for neurogenic bladder: a multi-institutional study in 107 children. *Br J Urol* 1996, 78:287–293.
27. Light JK, Reynolds JC: Impact of the new cuff design on reliability of the AS800 artificial urinary sphincter. *J Urol* 1992, 147:609–611.
28. Leibovich BC, Barrett DM: Use of the artificial urinary sphincter in men and women. *World J Urol* 1997, 15:316–319.
29. Fishman IJ, Shabsigh R, Scott FB: Experience with the artificial urinary sphincter model AS800 in 148 patients. *J Urol* 1989, 141:307–310.
30. Marks JL, Light JK: Management of urinary incontinence after prostatectomy with the artificial urinary sphincter. *J Urol* 1989, 142:302–304.
31. Nurse DE, Mundy AR: One hundred artificial sphincters. *Br J Urol* 1988, 61:318–325.
32. Webster GD, Sihelnik SA: Troubleshooting the malfunctioning Scott artificial urinary sphincter. *J Urol* 1984, 131:269–272.
33. Martins FE, Boyd SD: Post-operative risk factors associated with artificial urinary sphincter infection-erosion. *Br J Urol* 1995, 75:354–358.
34. Flynn BJ, Webster GD: New advances in the treatment of post-prostatectomy incontinence. *Grand Rounds Urol* 2003, 3:9–15.
35. Montague DK, Angermeier KW: Postprostatectomy urinary incontinence: the case for artificial urinary sphincter implantation. *Urology* 2000, 55:2–4.
36. Petrou SP, Elliott DS, Barrett DM: Artificial urethral sphincter for incontinence. *Urology* 2000, 56:353–359.
37. Hussain M, Greenwell TJ, Venn SN, Mundy AR: The current role of the artificial urinary sphincter for the treatment of urinary incontinence. *J Urol* 2005, 174:418–424.
38. Comiter CV, Sullivan, MP, Yalla SV: Retrograde leak point pressure for evaluating post-radical prostatectomy incontinence. *Urology* 1997, 49:231–236.
39. Ullrich N, Comiter CV: The male sling for stress urinary incontinence: urodynamic and subjective assessment. *J Urol* 2004, 172:204–206.
40. Onur R, Rajpurkar A, Singla A: New perineal bone-anchored male sling: lessons learned. *Urology* 2004, 64:58–61.
41. Giberti C, Gallo F, Schenone M, Cortese P: The bone-anchor sub-urethral sling for the treatment of iatrogenic male incontinence: subjective and objective assessment after 41 months of mean follow-up. *World J Urol* 2008, 26:173–178
42. Schaeffer AJ, Clemens JQ, Ferrari M, Stamey TA: The male bulbourethral sling procedure for post-radical prostatectomy incontinence. *J Urol* 1998, 159:1510–1515.
43. Cespedes RD, Jacoby K: Male slings for postprostatectomy incontinence. *Tech Urol* 2001, 7:176–183.
44. Madjar S, Jacoby K, Giberti C, *et al.*: Bone anchored sling for the treatment of post-prostatectomy incontinence. *J Urol* 2001, 165:72–76.
45. Dikranian AH, Chang JH, Rhee EY, Aboseif SR: The male perineal sling: comparison of sling materials. *J Urol* 2004, 172:608–610.
46. Ullrich NF, Comiter CV: The male sling for stress urinary incontinence: 24-month followup with questionnaire based assessment. *J Urol* 2004, 172:207–209.
47. John H: Bulbourethral composite suspension: a new operative technique for post-prostatectomy incontinence. *J Urol* 2004, 171:1866–1870.
48. Stern JA, Clemens JQ, Tiplitsky SI, *et al.*: Long-term results of the bulbourethral sling procedure. *J Urol* 2005, 173:1654–1656.
49. Rajpurkar AD, Onur R, Singla A: Patient satisfaction and clinical efficacy of the new perineal bone-anchored male sling. *Eur Urol* 2005, 47:237–242.

50. Comiter CV: The male perineal sling: intermediate term results. *Neurourol Urodyn* 2005, 24:648–653.

51. Castle EP, Andrews PE, Itano N, *et al.*: The male sling for postprostatectomy incontinence: mean followup of 18 months. *J Urol* 2005, 173:1657–1660.

52. Migliari R, Pistolesi D, Leone P, *et al.*: Male bulbourethral sling after radical prsotatectomy: intermediate outcomes at 2 to 4-year followup. *J Urol* 2006, 17:2114–2118.

53. Fischer MC, Huckabay C, Nitti VW: The male perineal sling: assessment and prediction of outcome. *J Urol* 2007, 177:1414–1418.

54. Gallagher BL, Dwyer NT, Gaynor-Krupnick DM, *et al.*: Objective and quality-of-life outcomes with bone-anchored male bulbourethral sling. *Urology* 2007, 69:1090–1094.

55. Sousa-Escandón A, Cabrera J, Mantovani F, *et al.*: Adjustable suburethral sling (Male Remeex System) in the treatment of male stress urinary incontinence: a multicentric European study. *Eur Urol* 2007, 52:1473–1479.

56. Xu YM, Zhang XR, Sa YL, *et al.*: Bulbourethral composite suspension for treatment of male-acquired urinary incontinence. *Eur Urol* 2007, 51:1709–1716.

13 Artificial Urinary Sphincter II

George D. Webster and Jack R. Walter

The artificial urinary sphincter (aus), initially described by Scott *et al.* in 1974 [1], is the gold standard for postprostatectomy incontinence. It has undergone several modifications since it was introduced as the AMS 721 (American Medical Systems; Minnetonka, MN) but remains greatly unchanged since 1983, when the AMS 800 was released. Its simplicity in design, patient satisfaction, and durability have made the device popular with surgeons as well as patients.

The aus can be used in virtually all patients and to treat all degrees of stress urinary incontinence. The most frequent use is in treating postprostatectomy incontinence with the cuff placed around the bulbar urethra. Additionally, the cuff can be implanted at the bladder neck, primarily in neurogenic patients, and in the female urethra. The artificial sphincter can be used for fecal incontinence with the cuff implanted around the rectum [2].

Patient selection is critical for successful implantation of the aus. The ideal patient is a male with stress urinary incontinence following radical prostatectomy without prior pelvic radiation therapy or urethral surgery. Caution should be exercised in men with mixed urinary incontinence, as their urgency will not be treated by implantation of the device. Prior pelvic radiation and urethral surgery, including prior aus, increase the risk of complications but still provide acceptable outcomes [3]. Care should be exercised in patients with poorly compliant, low-capacity bladders as they typically have significant frequency of urination, which makes patient satisfaction low and may predispose them to upper tract deterioration. Patients must not have any infection at the time of surgery. Bladder neck anastomotic stricture, a common complication of radical prostatectomy, should be addressed prior to implanting an aus. Refractory anastomotic strictures can be managed with the staged implant of a UroLume wall stent (American Medical Systems; Minnetonka, MN) and subsequent aus [4].

A preoperative evaluation should include the history and physical examination that confirms stress incontinence. A voiding diary assesses bladder capacity and helps define triggers for incontinence. Cystoscopy is necessary to determine if the patient has any obstructive process such as bladder neck contracture or urethral stricture. It also allows one to assess potential sites for cuff implantation. Urodynamics provide additional information that is especially useful in complex patients with mixed incontinence or prior radiation therapy.

There currently are two approaches for implantation of the aus at the bulbar urethra, perineal and transscrotal [5]. We feel that the perineal approach allows improved access to the proximal bulbar urethra, at a location proximal to the symphysis pubis. This location protects the cuff from external perineal pressure and associated deactivation, as well as providing a larger diameter of the urethra to assist in cuff sizing. A description of the perineal approach follows.

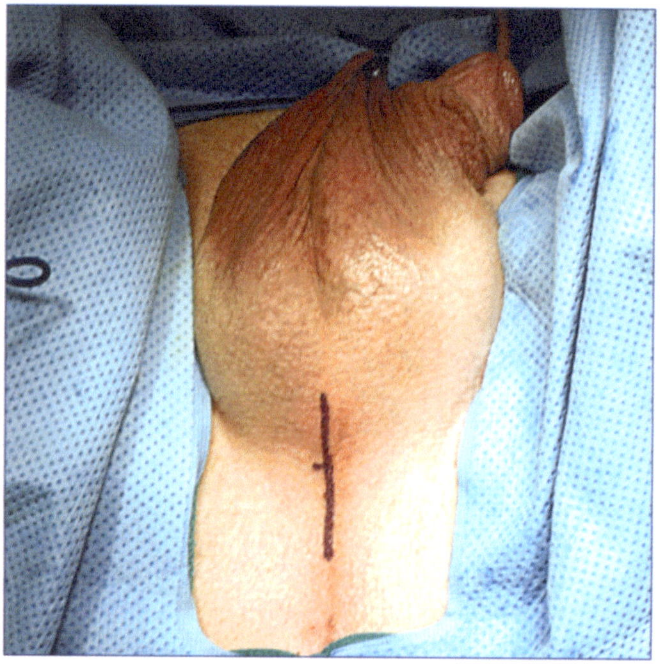

Figure 13-1. The patient is positioned in a modified lithotomy with padded Allen stirrups. The lower abdomen, genitalia, and perineum are shaved of all hair. A 10-minute Betadine preparation is completed. The perineum with the proposed incision is centered over genu of the bulbar urethra, as shown. Rigid endoscopy is repeated to confirm preoperative findings. The bladder is drained with a 16-Fr Foley catheter, which aides in dissection.

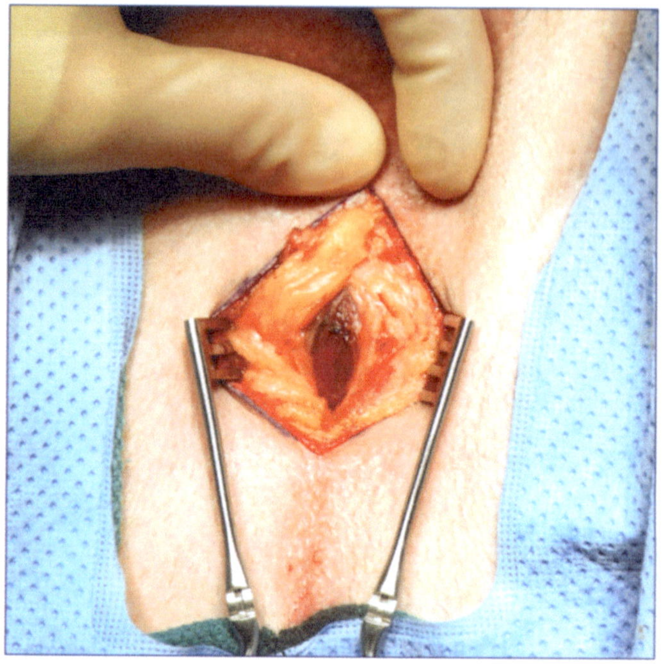

Figure 13-2. A midline perineal incision is made. The subcutaneous tissue, Colles fascia, and bulbospongiosus muscle are split in the midline using electrocautery with a pure cutting current. The Weitlaner Beckman retractor provides excellent exposure.

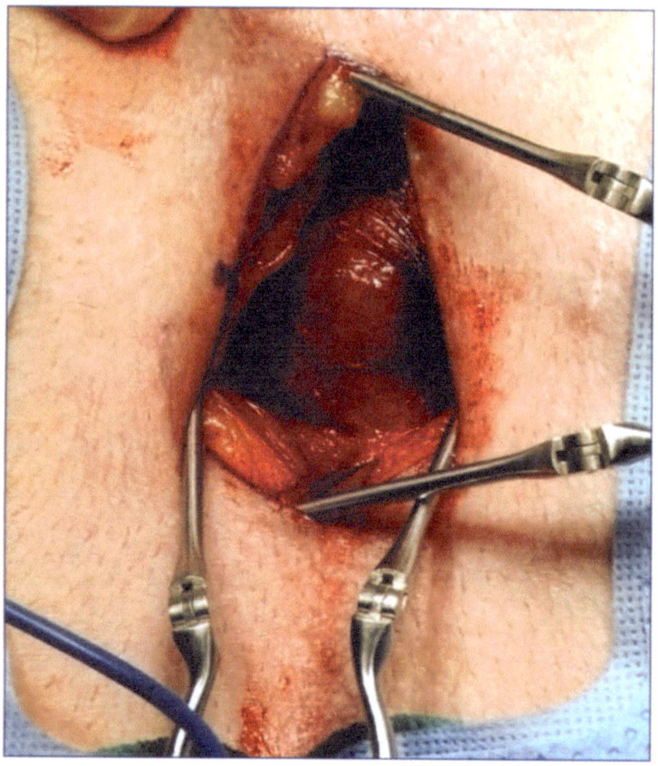

Figure 13-3. The bulbar urethra is exposed using a combination of sharp and blunt dissection. The bulbospongiosus muscle is mobilized laterally at the level of the crus of the corpora cavernosa, exposing Buck's fascia.

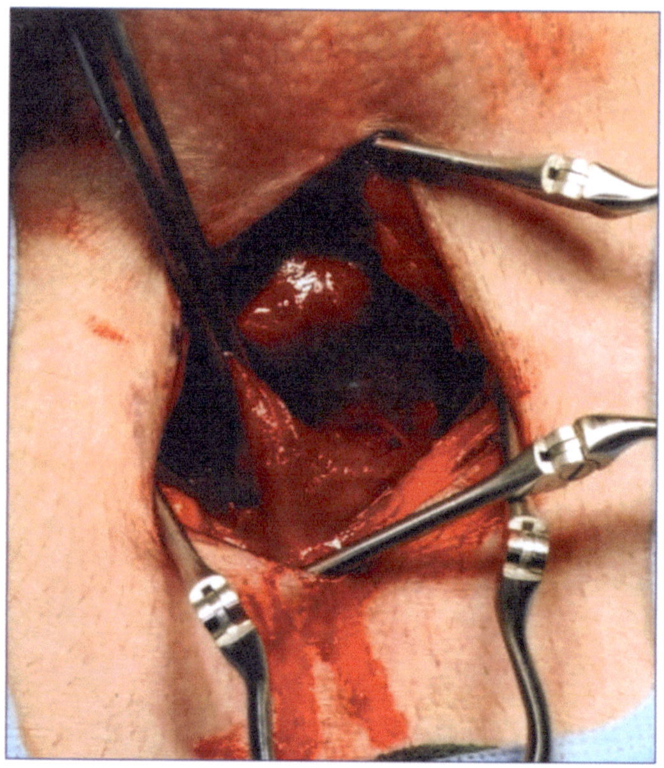

Figure 13-4. By providing gentle traction laterally on the bulbar urethra, Buck's fascia can be easily visualized overlying the corpora cavernosum.

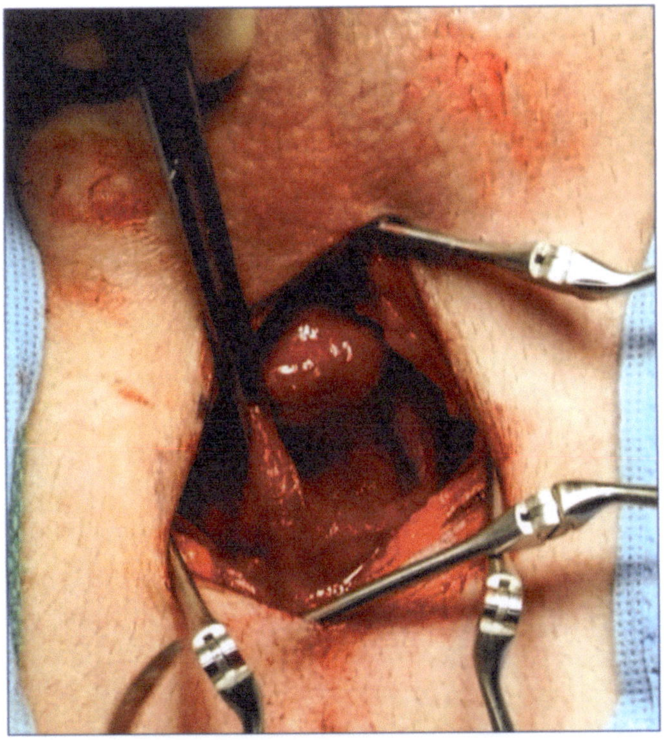

FIGURE 13-5. Buck's fascia has been incised on the left aspect of the urethra. By incising Buck's fascia, a distinct plane can be created dorsal to the urethra. This helps to prevent inadvertent urethrotomies during this portion of the operation.

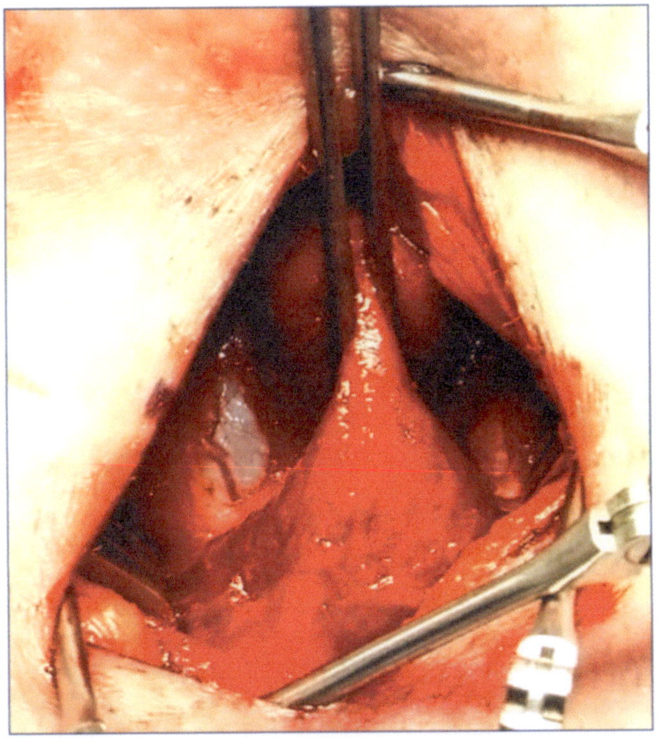

FIGURE 13-6. Buck's fascia, incised bilaterally providing a "safe" dissection plane, is shown. This dissection should be completed sharply as blunt dissection or spreading posterior to the urethra may tear into the urethra. A window approximately 2 cm wide is needed to place the cuff.

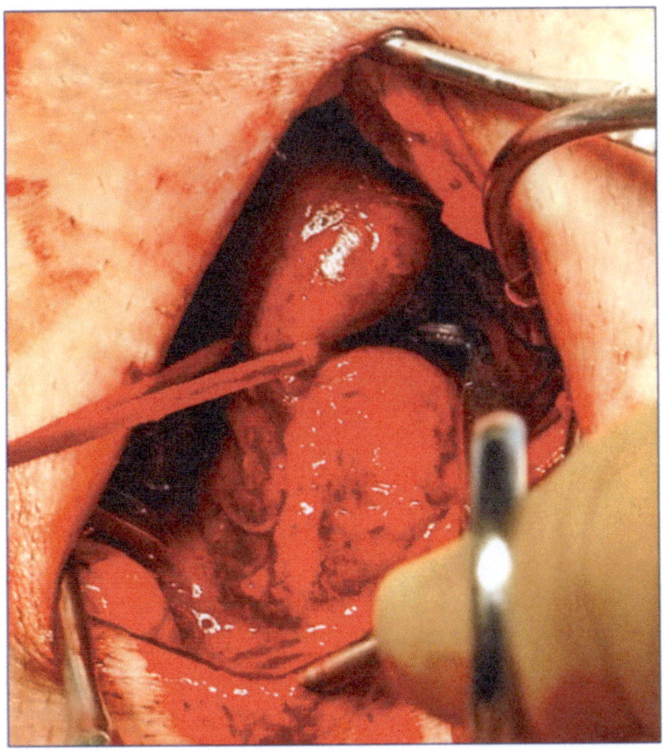

FIGURE 13-7. An umbilical tape is placed around the bulbar urethra, aiding in dissection. The umbilical tape is then cut to the circumference of the urethra and used to select the appropriately sized cuff. One must consider the consistency of the corpora spongiosum when selecting the artificial urinary sphincter cuff. If the spongiosum is indurated, as one sees in prior radiation, consider a size close to the measured length. If the spongiosum is compressible, consider a small cuff size.

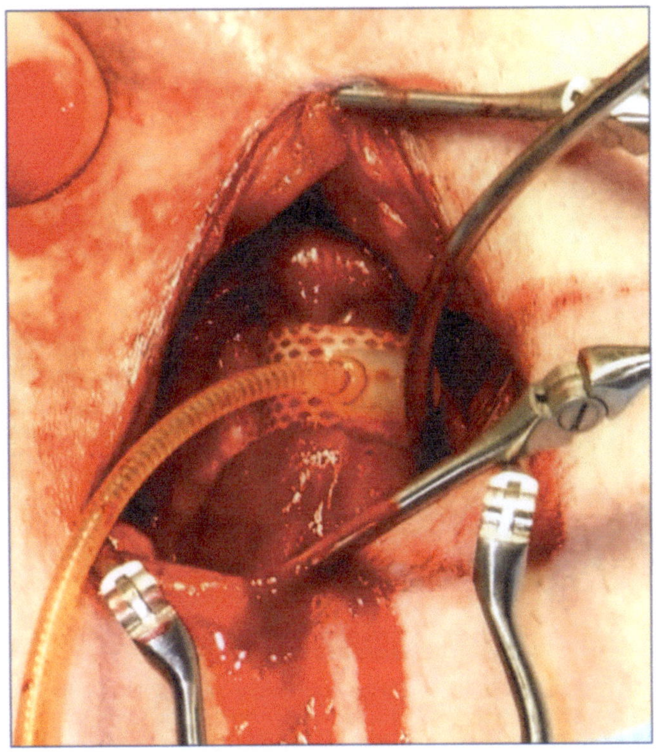

FIGURE 13-8. The artificial urinary sphincter cuff, implanted at the bulbar urethra, provides a snug fit.

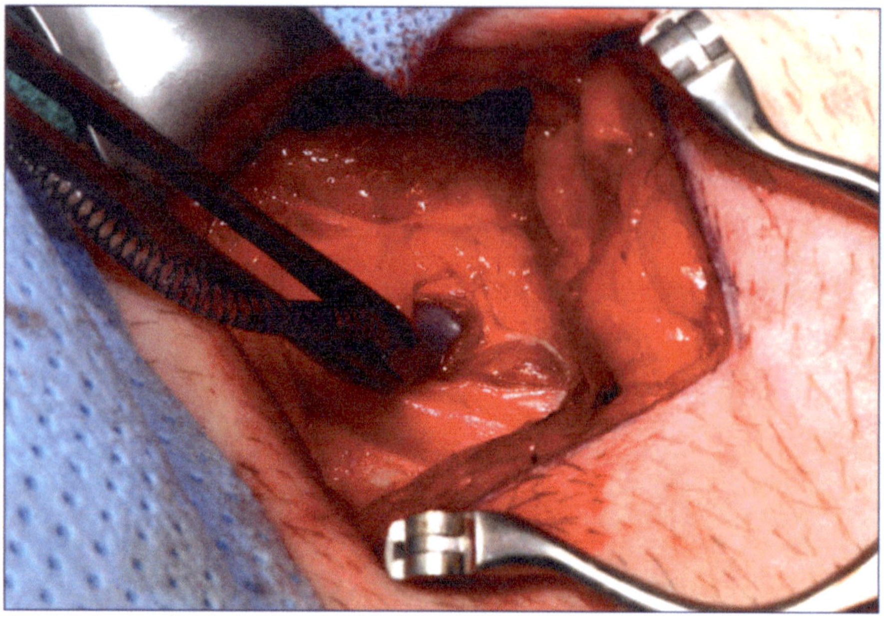

Figure 13-9. A right lower quadrant abdominal incision is made above the inguinal canal. Electrocautery is used to expose the external oblique aponeurosis. The fascia is opened along its fibers and a preperitoneal space is bluntly dissected. A 61–70-cm H_2O pressure regulating balloon is selected, prepared, and implanted at this site. The fascia is closed over the balloon. The balloon is filled with 23 cc of the appropriate contrast material.

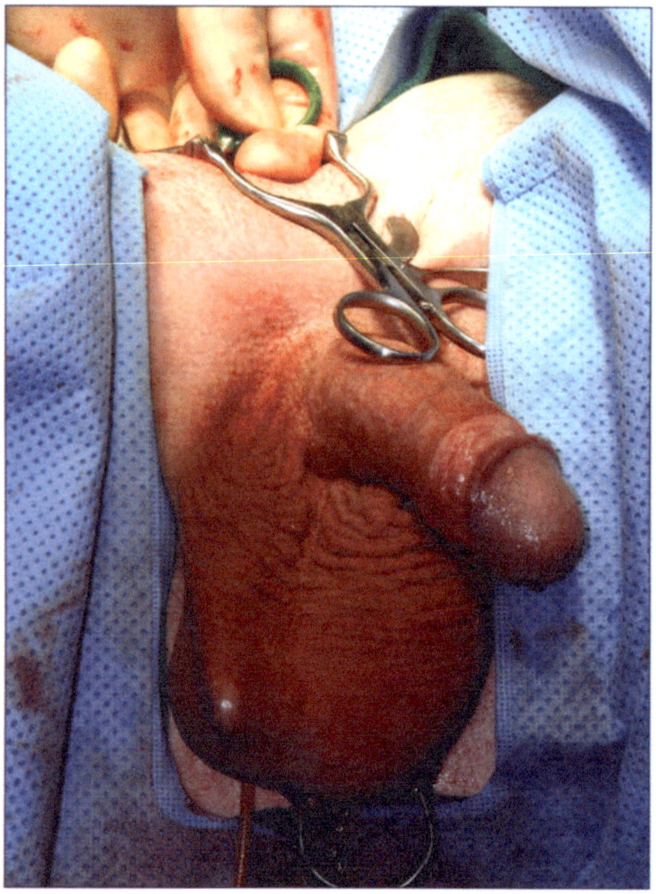

Figure 13-10. From the abdominal incision, a right anterior dependent hemiscrotal pouch is bluntly dissected using a ringed sponge forcep. A pump is prepared and implanted in this location.

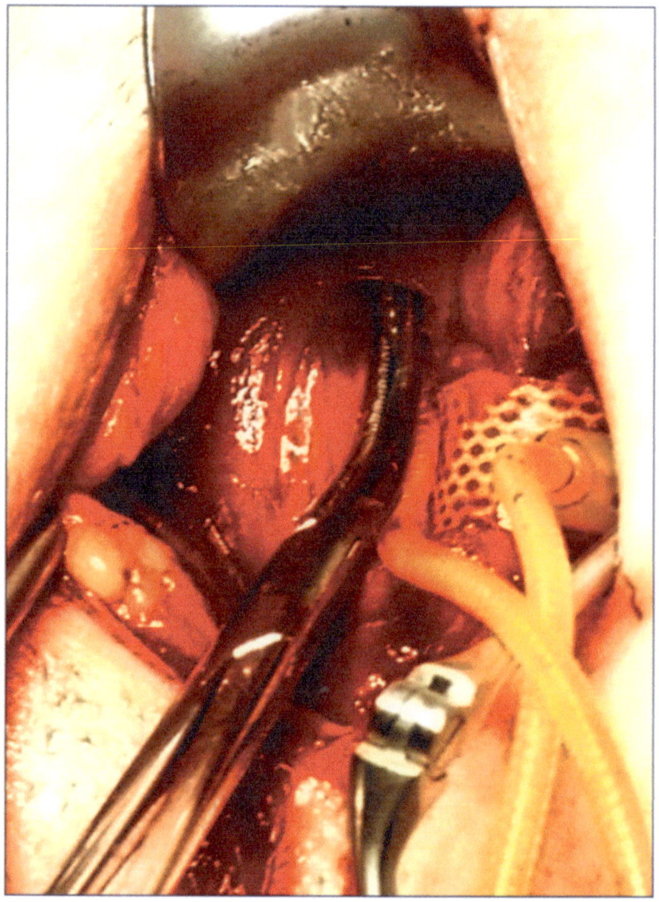

Figure 13-11. The urethral cuff tubing is routed to the abdominal incision over the symphysis pubis, taking care to avoid the spermatic cord structures.

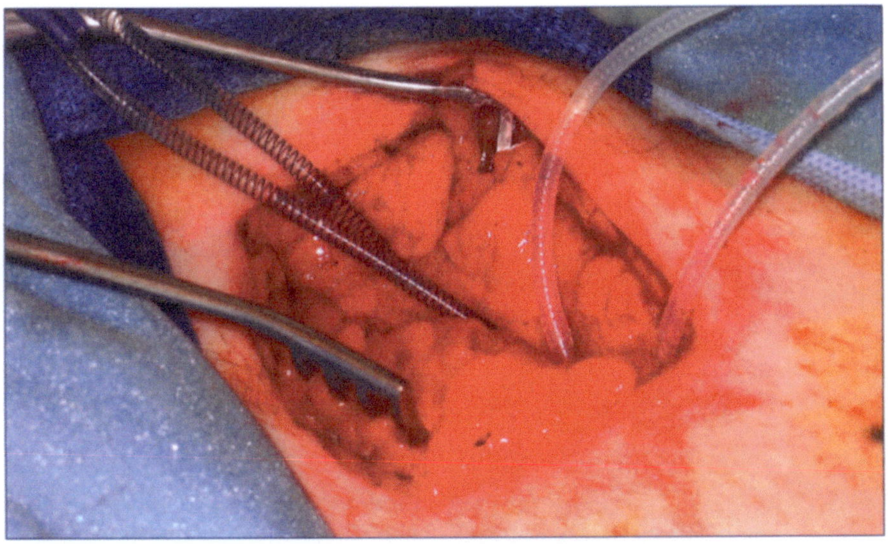

Figure 13-12. All tubing is routed to the lower quadrant abdominal incision, trimmed to length, and prepared for connection. All connections are completed here, allowing easy identification if revision surgery is needed.

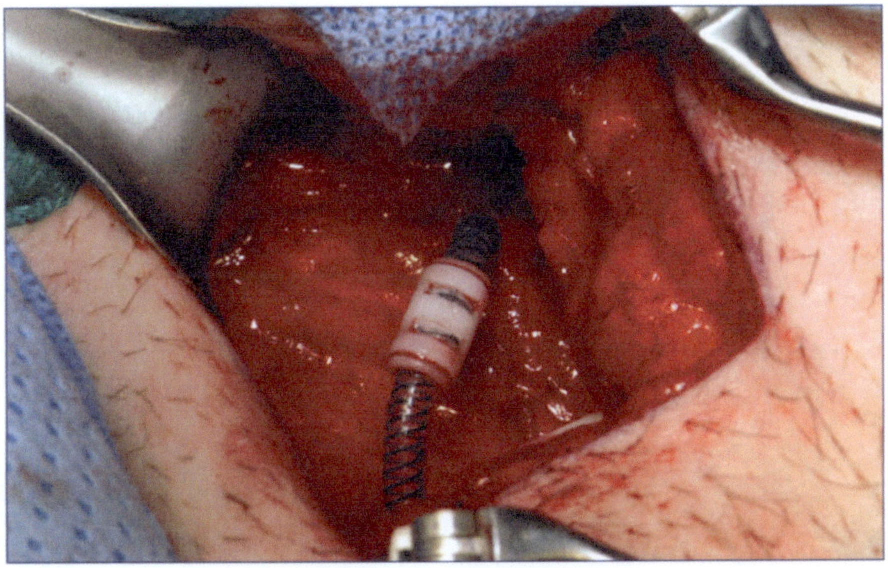

Figure 13-13. The pump tubing is connected to the pressure-regulating balloon and the urethral cuff using the sutureless connector kit. Care is taken in closing Scarpa's fascia, providing a barrier between superficial skin infections and the tubing. Cystoscopy is repeated to confirm that there is no injury to the urethra, appropriate coaptation of the urethra at the cuff location, and adequate lumen to void. The cuff is left in a deactivated, deflated state. If necessary, a small, soft catheter may be left overnight to prevent retention. Sterile dressings are applied. Postoperatively, the patient returns to the clinic for activation in approximately 6 weeks. At this time, the patient is instructed on how to use his device.

Transcorporal Placement of the Artificial Urinary Sphincter

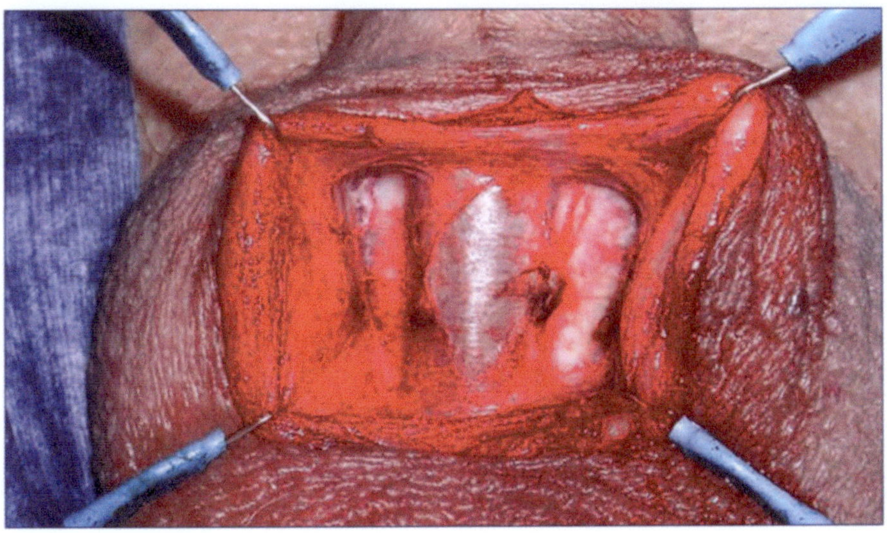

Figure 13-14. If the proximal or midbulbar urethra are not available for artificial urinary sphincterimplantation, alternative approaches are employed. As the urethra proceeds distally, its diameter becomes smaller. To provide an adequately snug cuff, additional tissue is needed. The transcorporeal cuff placement can be used [6]. A penoscrotal incision is made and the distal bulbar urethra and corporal bodies are exposed.

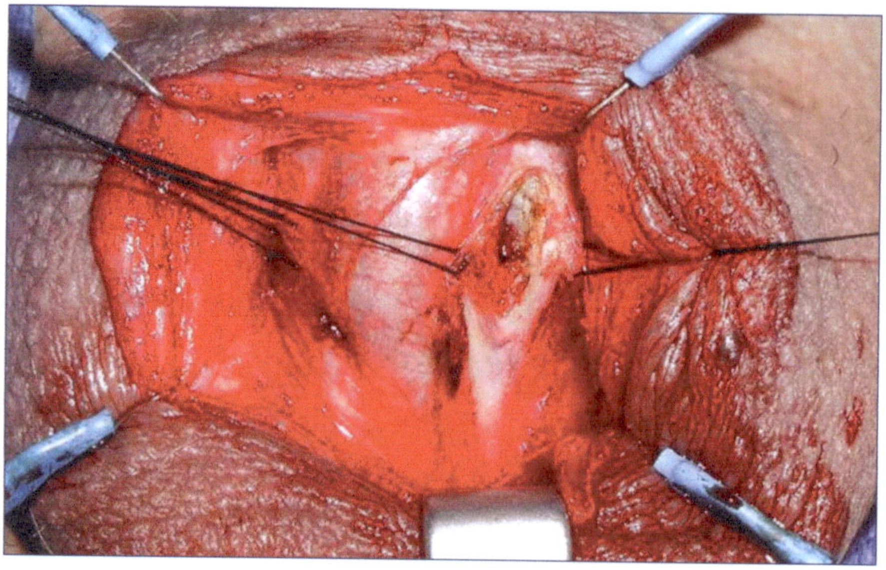

Figure 13-15. Stay sutures are placed in the corpora cavernosa, aiding dissection, and a 2-cm corporotomy is made.

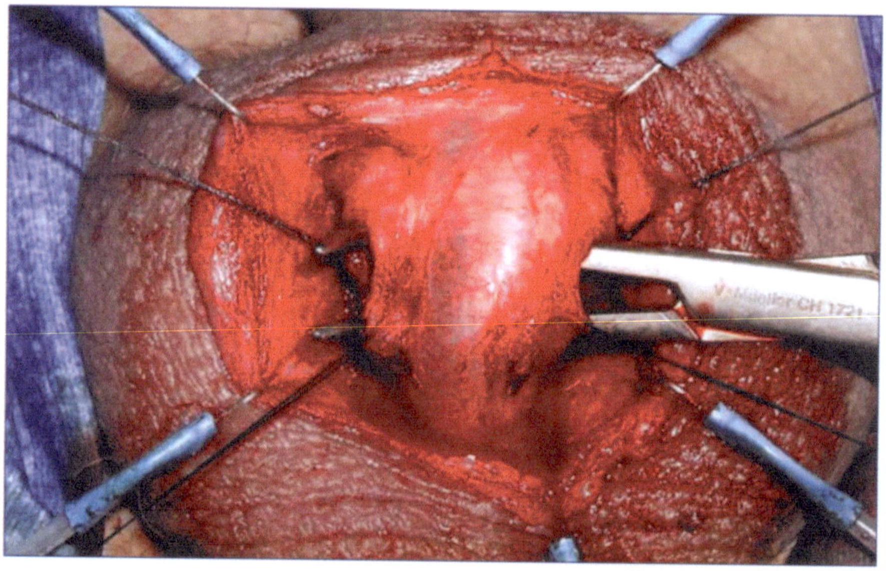

Figure 13-16. A right-angle clamp is placed dorsally to the urethra in a transcorporeal fashion. This allows the added bulk of corporal bodies to aid in the cuff fit.

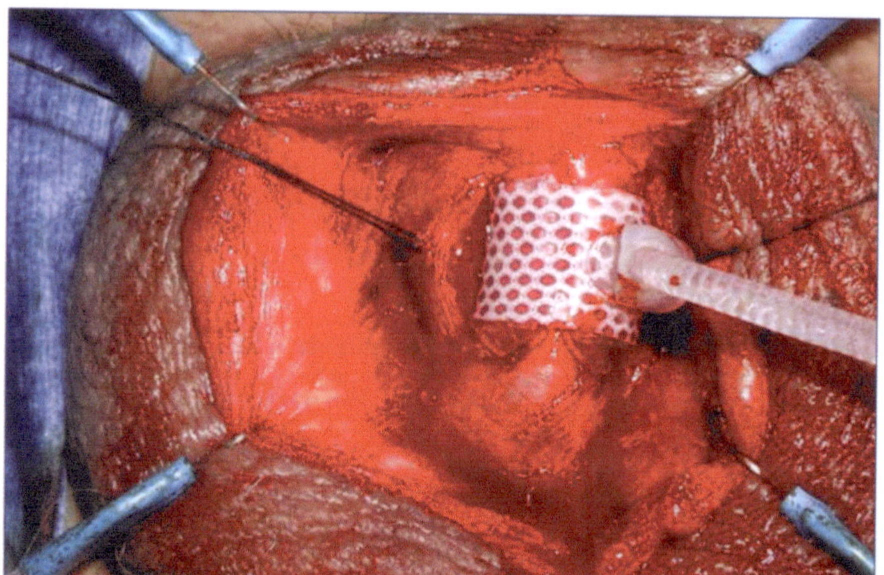

Figure 13-17. The urethral cuff is implanted, providing a snug fit. The remaining portions of the operation are unchanged.

References

1. Scott FB, Bradley WE, Timm GW: Treatment of urinary incontinence by an implantable prosthetic urinary sphincter. *J Urol* 1974, 112:75–80.
2. Wong WD, Jensen LL, Bartolo DC, Rothenberger DA: Artificial anal sphincter. *Dis Colon Rectum* 1996, 39:1345–1351.
3. Raj GV, Peterson AC, Webster GD: Outcomes following erosions of the artificial urinary sphincter. *J Urol* 2006, 175:2186–2190, discussion 2190.
4. Elliott DS, Boone TB: Combined stent and artificial urinary sphincter for management of severe recurrent bladder neck contracture and stress incontinence after prostatectomy: a long-term evaluation. *J Urol* 2001, 165:413–415.
5. Wilson SK, Delk JR II, Henry GD, Siegel AL: New surgical technique for sphincter urinary control system using upper transverse scrotal incision. *J Urol* 2003, 169:261–264.
6. Guralnick ML, Miller E, Toh KL, Webster GD: Transcorporeal artificial urinary sphincter cuff placement in cases requiring revision for erosion and urethral atrophy. *J Urol* 2002, 167:2075–2078, discussion 2079.

14 Bladder Tissue Engineering

L. Spencer Krane and Anthony Atala

Congenital disorders, cancer, trauma, infection, inflammation, iatrogenic injuries, or other conditions of the bladder can lead to organ damage or complete loss of bladder function. These clinical situations eventually require reconstructive procedures, which can be performed with native nonurologic tissues (skin, gastrointestinal segments, or mucosa), homologous tissues from a donor (cadaver or living donor tissue), heterologous tissues or substances (bovine collagen), or artificial materials, which are associated with a number of complications. Implanted tissue is sometimes rejected, and often, the inherently different functional aspects of the different tissues or materials used in reconstructive procedures causes a "mismatch" in the system.

The replacement of lost or deficient urologic structures with biocompatible, functionally equivalent tissues would vastly improve the outcome of reconstructive surgery for the bladder. This may soon be possible with novel tissue engineering techniques. In order to find solutions to the problems with current procedures for reconstructing the urinary tract, physicians and scientists have begun to look to the fields of regenerative medicine and tissue engineering to provide new options for these patients. These fields strive to develop biologic substitutes that can significantly improve the quality of life of the urologic patient by eliminating the need for intensive grafting procedures or transplant surgery.

Tissue engineering, one of the major components of regenerative medicine, follows the principles of cell transplantation, materials science, and engineering to develop biologic substitutes that can restore and maintain normal organ function. This chapter reviews the major components of most tissue engineering techniques, and describes how these techniques are being applied to the reconstruction and regeneration of the urinary bladder.

Use of Autologous Nonurologic Tissue in Bladder Reconstructive Surgery	
Advantages	**Disadvantages**
Material readily available	Metabolic disturbances (GI)
No immunologic response	Mucous production (GI)
	Stone formation (GI)
	Infection
	Not functionally equivalent
	Secondary malignancy

FIGURE 14-1. Advantages and disadvantages to using nonurologic tissues in the urinary tract. Current methods of replacing bladder tissue with gastrointestinal (GI) segments can be problematic because bladder epithelium and intestinal epithelial tissue are designed to handle solutes in opposite ways. Urologic tissue normally excretes material, and, especially in the case of the bladder, prevents the reabsorption of these materials. In contrast, GI tissue readily absorbs these same molecules, and this natural function continues even when a GI segment is introduced into the urinary tract. This mismatch is often a serious problem and leads to metabolic complications as well as infection, stone formation, excess mucous production, and in some cases, malignancy.

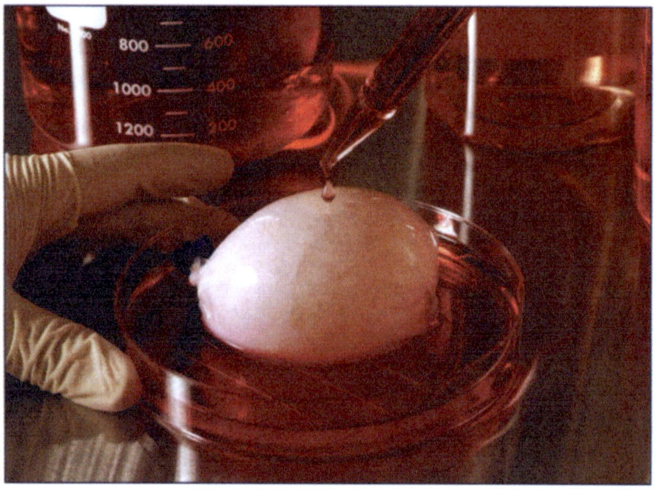

FIGURE 14-2. Tissue engineering strategies. Tissue engineering strategies generally fall into two categories: the use of acellular matrices designed to encourage the body's own infiltrating cells to regenerate damaged tissue, and the use of matrices seeded with cells in the laboratory. These seeded scaffolds are then cultured in specific ways to produce novel tissues and organs that can eventually be implanted into the patient. Acellular tissue matrices are usually prepared by manufacturing artificial scaffolds, or by removing cellular components from donor tissues via mechanical and chemical manipulation to produce collagen-rich matrices [1–4]. When implanted in vivo, either type of matrix can serve to attract host cells and unlock their regenerative potential. hese matrices are designed to slowly degrade after implantation as the extracellular matrix (ECM) proteins secreted by the ingrowing cells begin to support the new tissue. The scaffold pictured here demonstrates a bladder matrix being developed for eventual implantation. In addition, techniques using cells themselves for therapy have been developed. These cells are most often delivered via direct injection to the damaged tissue, although studies investigating the ability of cells to home to damaged areas after a systemic injection are underway.

Cell-based Therapies

Advantages and Disadvantages of Autologous Cell Sources	
Autologous cells for urologic tissue engineering	
Advantages	**Disadvantages**
Identical structure and function	Potential paucity of functional cells for expansion
No immune response	
In vitro capabilities to grow bladder, ureter, and renal pelvis	

FIGURE 14-3. Autologous cell sources. The source of the donor tissue used to produce cells for tissue engineering and regenerative medicine applications can be heterologous, allogeneic, or autologous. Ideally, autologous cells are used, because in this case both structural and functional tissue replacement will usually occur with minimal complications [2,5–12]. The use of autologous cells may cause a transient inflammatory response, but it avoids rejection, and thus the deleterious side effects of lifelong immunosuppression can be avoided. However, for many patients with extensive end-stage organ failure, a tissue biopsy may not yield enough normal cells for expansion and transplantation. In other instances, primary autologous cells cannot be expanded from a particular organ, such as the pancreas.

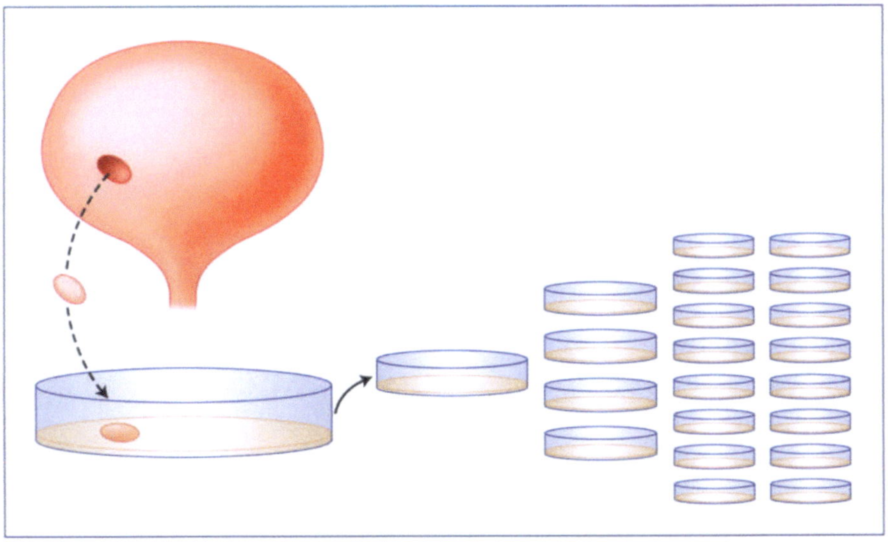

Figure 14-4. In vitro expansion of native cells. By studying the privileged sites for committed precursor cells in these organs, as well as by exploring the conditions that promote differentiation and/or self-renewal of these cells, it has been possible to overcome some of the obstacles that limit cell expansion in vitro. One example is the urothelial cell. Urothelial cells could be grown in the laboratory setting in the past, but only with limited success. Several protocols were developed over the past two decades that identify the undifferentiated cells in a mixed culture of cells isolated from the urinary tract, and keep them undifferentiated during their growth phase [11,13–16]. Using these methods of cell culture, it is now possible to expand a urothelial culture that initially covered a surface area of 1 cm^2 to one covering a surface area of 4202 m^2 (the equivalent of one football field) within 8 weeks [11] as is demonstrated here. These studies indicated that it should be possible to collect autologous bladder cells from human patients, expand them in culture, and return them to the donor in sufficient quantities for reconstructive purposes [11,14–19].

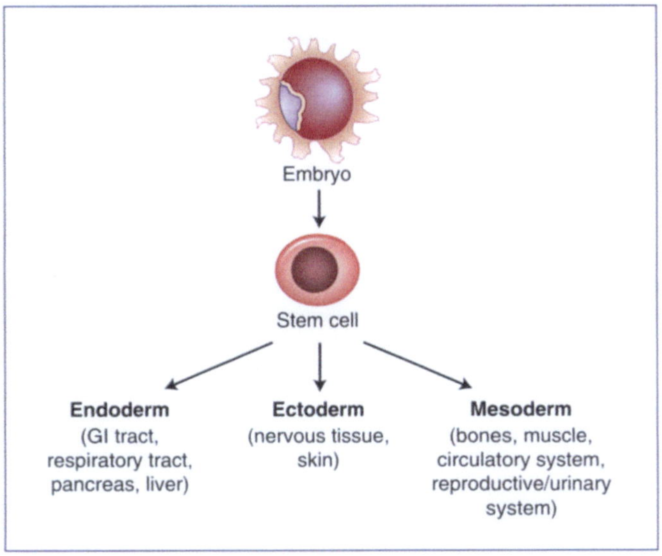

Figure 14-5. Human embryonic stem cells. In 1981, pluripotent cells were found in the inner cell mass of the human embryo, and the term *human embryonic stem cell* was coined [20]. These cells are able to differentiate into all cells of the human body, excluding placental cells (only cells from the morula are totipotent, *ie*, able to develop into all cells of the human body including the placenta). Embryonic stem cells could be an ideal resource for tissue engineering because of their fundamental properties: the ability to self renew indefinitely and the ability to differentiate into cells from all three embryonic germ layers. Skin and neurons have been formed, indicating ectodermal differentiation [21–24]. Blood, cardiac cells, cartilage, endothelial cells, and muscle have been formed, indicating mesodermal differentiation [25–27]. Finally, pancreatic cells have been formed, indicating endodermal differentiation [28]. In addition, as further evidence of their pluripotency, embryonic stem cells can form embryoid bodies, which are cell aggregations that exist in culture and contain all three embryonic germ layers, and they can also form teratomas in vivo [29]. These cells have demonstrated longevity in culture and can maintain their undifferentiated state for at least 80 passages when grown using current published protocols [30,31]. These cells have great therapeutic potential, but their use is limited by both biologic and ethical factors. GI—gastrointestinal.

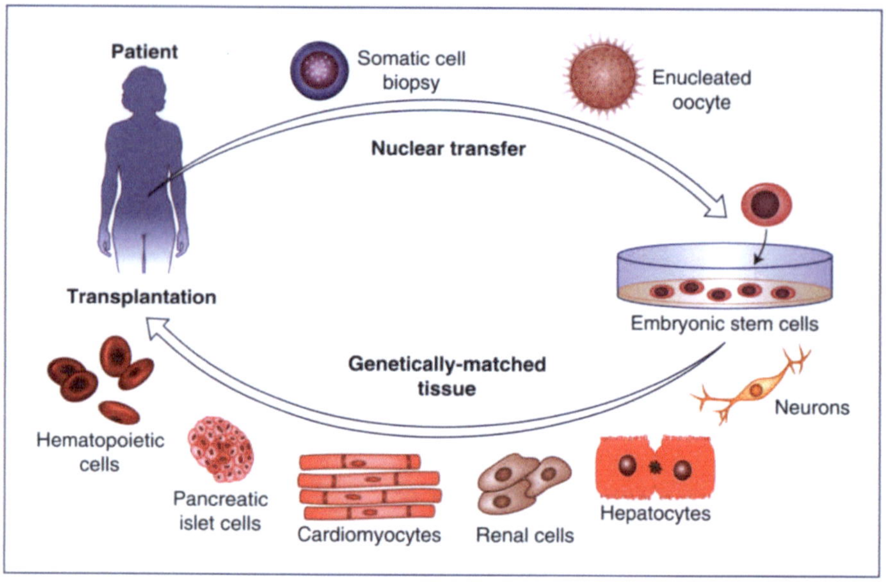

Figure 14-6. The use of cloning technology to produce stem cells for regenerative medicine techniques. Somatic cell nuclear transfer (SCNT), or therapeutic cloning, entails the removal of an oocyte nucleus in culture, followed by its replacement with a nucleus derived from a somatic cell obtained from a patient. Activation with chemicals or electricity stimulates cell division up to the blastocyst stage, and embryonic stem cells that are genetically identical to the patient can be obtained from the newly generated inner cell mass. To use SCNT to produce cells for regenerative medicine strategies, a biopsy is taken from the patient, and cells are derived from this tissue. A nucleus from one of these somatic cells is then inserted into an enucleated oocyte and, after physical and chemical manipulation, this hybrid cell can develop into a blastocyst. Embryonic stem cells are then derived from the inner cell mass of the resulting blastocyst and cultured. Like embryonic stem cells derived from a blastocyst that result from fertilization, these "cloned" embryonic stem cells can be differentiated into the specific type of cell needed for treatment (neurons for neurologic disease, renal cells for kidney disease, and the like). Because these cells are genetically identical to the patient, they can then be transplanted back into the patient without fear of rejection and without the need for immunosuppressant medication. It has been shown that embryonic stem cells derived from the nuclei of fibroblasts, lymphocytes, and olfactory neurons are pluripotent and can generate live pups after injection into blastocysts. This shows that cells generated by SCNT have the same developmental potential as blastocysts that are fertilized and produced naturally [32–35]. Lanza *et al.* [36] demonstrated that the mitochondrial DNA present in the SCNT does not induce a T-cell response in cloned renal cells.

Therapeutic Versus Reproductive Cloning

	Initial step	Next step	Goal of technique	Potential cell lineages	Ethical concerns
Reproductive cloning	Insertion of donor DNA into an enucleated oocyte	Implantation of embryo into uterus of pseudopregnant female	Develop offspring identical to parent	Pluripotent	Many; illegal in most countries
Therapeutic cloning	Insertion of donor DNA into an enucleated oocyte	Oocyte used to generate blastocytes that are explanded in culture ex vivo	Develop autologous cell lines for potential therapies	Pluripotent	Few; cell division arrested at 100-cell stage; routinely used for developing embryonic stem cell

Figure 14-7. Therapeutic versus reproductive cloning. It is extremely important to differentiate between the two types of cloning that exist—reproductive cloning and therapeutic cloning. Both involve the insertion of donor DNA into an enucleated oocyte to generate an embryo that has identical genetic material to its DNA source. However, the similarities end there. In reproductive cloning, the embryo is then implanted into the uterus of a pseudopregnant female to produce an infant that is a clone of the donor. A world-famous example of this type of cloning resulted in the birth of a sheep named Dolly in 1997 [37].

Limitations to Somatic Cell Nuclear Transfer

Limitations of human SCNT
Ethical concerns
Has not been successful in humans
Low success rate of SCNT
Availability of human oocytes
Concerns for translocation in reproducing SCNT cells

Figure 14-8. Limitations to somatic cell nuclear transfer (SCNT). Although promising, SCNT has certain limitations that must be overcome before it can be applied clinically. In addition, ethical considerations regarding the potential of SCNT-derived embryos to develop into offspring if implanted into a uterus must be addressed. First and foremost, this technique has not yet been shown to work in humans. The initial failures and fraudulent reports of nuclear transfer in humans reduced excitement in the scientific community and suggested SCNT may not be ideal for human applications [38–40], although it was recently reported that nonhuman primate embryonic stem cell lines were generated by SCNT of nuclei from adult skin fibroblasts [41,42]. In addition, before SCNT-derived embryonic stem cells can be used for any type of clinical therapy, careful assessment of the quality of the generated cell lines must be determined. The low "success rate" of SCNT (only 0.7% of the nuclear transfers result in a viable blastocyst) and the inadequate supply of human oocytes further hinder the therapeutic potential of this technique. Still, these studies have renewed the hope that ethically neutral embryonic stem cell lines could one day be generated from human cells to produce patient-specific stem cells for use in tissue engineering and regenerative medicine applications.

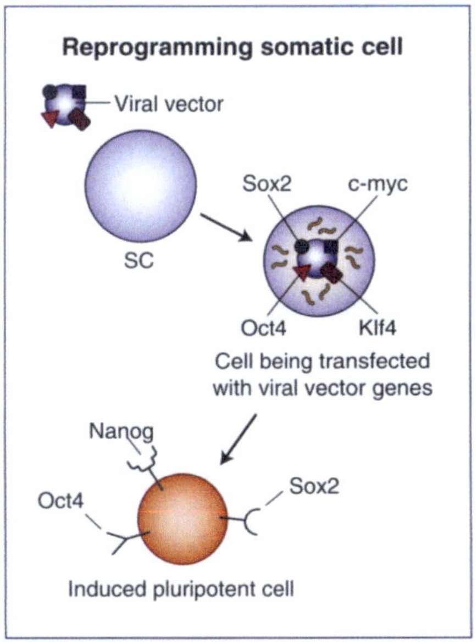

FIGURE 14-9. Reprogramming of adult somatic cells (SCs). Reprogramming is a technique that involves de-differentiation of adult SCs to produce patient-specific pluripotent stem cells, thus eliminating the need to create embryos to obtain stem cells. Takahashi and Yamanaka [43] were the first to discover that mouse embryonic fibroblasts and adult mouse fibroblasts could be reprogrammed into an "induced pluripotent state" (iPS). These iPS cells possessed the immortal growth characteristics of self-renewing embryonic stem cells, expressed genes specific for embryonic stem cells, and generated embryoid bodies in vitro and teratomas in vivo. However, although iPS cells selected in this way were pluripotent, they were not identical to embryonic stem cells. Gene expression profiles of the iPS cells showed that they possessed a distinct gene expression signature that was different from that of embryonic stem cells. These results were improved significantly by Wernig *et al.* [44] in July 2007. In their reprogrammed cells, the DNA methylation pattern, gene expression profiles, and chromatin state were similar to those of embryonic stem cells. Teratomas induced by these cells contained differentiated cell types representing all three embryonic germ layers. Most importantly, the reprogrammed cells from this experiment were able to form viable chimeras and contribute to the germ line like true embryonic stem cells, suggesting that these iPS cells were completely reprogrammed.

Advantages and Disadvantages of Reprogramming Adult Somatic Cells

Advantages	Disadvantages
Identical immune markers	Has not reliably been demonstrated in human cell lines
Does not require oocytes	Concerns for viral introduction of genetic material
Fewer ethical concerns	

FIGURE 14-10. Advantages and disadvantages of reprogramming adult somatic cells. Stem cells generated by reprogramming would be genetically identical to the somatic cells used to create them—and thus the patient who donated those cells—and would not be rejected. It has recently been shown that reprogramming of human cells is possible [45,46]. Yamanaka [43] generated human induced pluripotent state (iPS) cells that are similar to human embryonic stem (hES) cells in terms of morphology, proliferation, gene expression, surface markers, and teratoma formation. Thompson's [46] group showed that retroviral transduction of the stem cell markers OCT4, SOX2, NANOG, and LIN28 could generate pluripotent stem cells. However, in both studies, the human iPS cells were similar but not identical to hES cells, and there is always cause for concern when viruses are introduced into cell lines, since the long-term effects of the presence of a retroviral genome in engineered cells and tissues is unclear at present. Although reprogramming is an exciting phenomenon, our limited understanding of the mechanism underlying it currently limits the clinical applicability of the technique, but the future potential of reprogramming is quite intriguing.

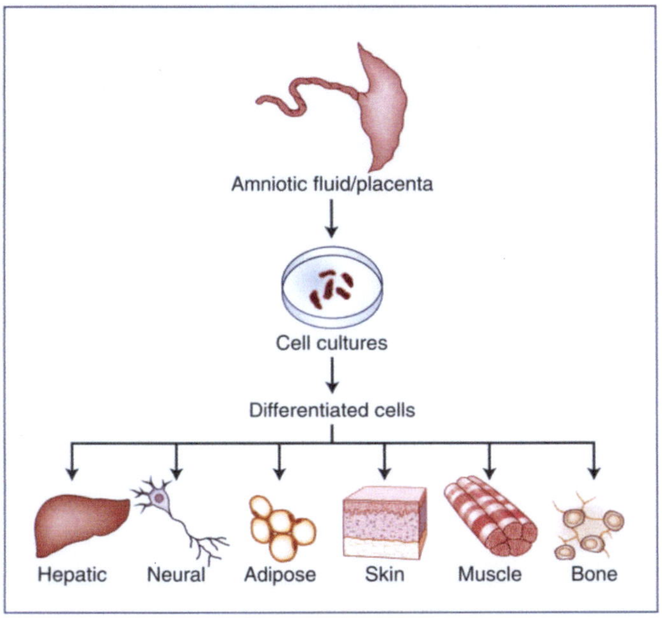

FIGURE 14-11. Amniotic fluid and placental stem cells (AFPSC). Pluripotent cells may be derived from the amniotic fluid and placenta. AFPSC express embryonic and adult stem cell markers [47]. The cells can be obtained either from amniocentesis or chorionic villus sampling in the developing fetus, or from the placenta at the time of birth. The undifferentiated stem cells expand extensively without a feeder cell layer and double every 36 hours. Unlike human embryonic stem cells, the AFPSC do not form tumors in vivo. Lines maintained for over 250 population doublings retained long telomeres and a normal complement of chromosomes. Amniotic fluid stem cells are broadly multipotent, and human lines can be induced to differentiate into cell types representing each embryonic germ layer, including cells of adipogenic, osteogenic, myogenic, endothelial, neuronal, hepatic, and renal lineages. Examples of differentiated cells derived from amniotic fluid stem cells and displaying specialized functions include neuronal cells that secrete the neurotransmitter L-glutamate or express G-protein–gated inwardly rectifying potassium channels, hepatic lineage cells that produce urea, and osteogenic cells that can form tissue engineered bone. In this respect, AFPSC meet a commonly accepted criterion for pluripotent stem cells, without implying that they can generate every adult tissue.

FIGURE 14-12. The ideal biomaterial. The ideal biomaterial should be biodegradable, bioresorbable, and support the replacement of normal tissue without inducing inflammation. Incompatible materials are destined for an inflammatory or foreign-body response that eventually leads to rejection and/or necrosis. Degradation products, if produced, should be removed from the body via normal metabolic pathways at an adequate rate so that the concentration of these degradation products in the tissue remains at a tolerable level [48]. The biomaterial should also provide an environment in which appropriate regulation of cell behavior (adhesion, proliferation, migration, and differentiation) can occur. Cell behavior in the newly formed tissue has been shown to be regulated by multiple interactions of the cells with their microenvironment, including interactions with cell-adhesion ligands [49] and with soluble growth factors. Since biomaterials provide temporary mechanical support while the cells undergo spatial reorganization into tissue, the properly chosen biomaterial should allow the engineered tissue to

Properties of The Ideal Biomaterial
Biodegradable
Bioresorbable
Noninflammatory
Degradation products removed via natural pathway
Provide environment for endogenous cellular activity
Allow delivery of bioactive materials
Maintenance of cell phenotypes
Mechanical integrity

FIGURE 14-13. Types of biomaterials. Generally, three classes of biomaterials have been used for engineering tissues: naturally derived materials (*eg*, collagen and alginate), acellular tissue matrices (*eg*, bladder submucosa and small intestinal submucosa), and synthetic polymers such as polyglycolic acid (PGA), polylactic acid (PLA), and poly(lactic-co-glycolic acid) (PLGA). These classes of biomaterials have been tested in respect to their biocompatibility [51,52]. Naturally derived materials and acellular tissue matrices have the potential advantage of biologic recognition. However, synthetic polymers can be produced reproducibly on a large scale with controlled properties such as strength, degradation rate, and microstructure, which would aid in the preparation of easily used, "off-the-shelf" scaffold material.

Types of Biomaterials

Naturally derived materials	Acellular tissue matrices	Synthetic polymers
Collagen	Bladder submucosa	PGA
Alginate	Small intestine submucosa	PLA
		PLGA

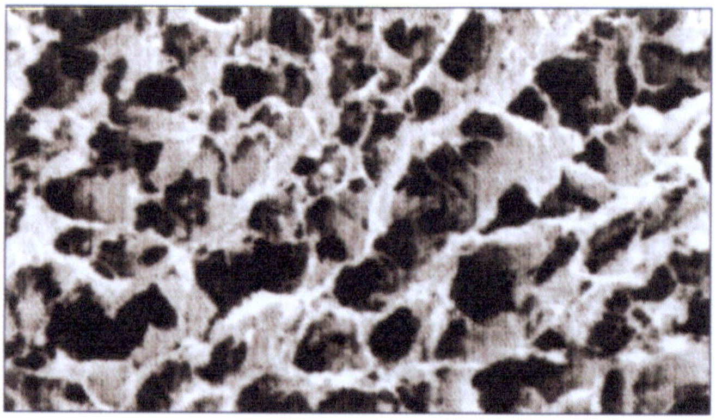

FIGURE 14-14. Collagen and alginate. Collagen is the most abundant and ubiquitous structural protein in the body, and may be readily purified from both animal and human tissues with an enzyme treatment and salt/acid extraction [53]. Collagen implants, under normal conditions, degrade through a process involving phagocytosis of collagen fibrils by fibroblasts [54]. This is followed by sequential attack by lysosomal enzymes including cathepsins B1 and D. Under inflammatory conditions, the implants can be rapidly degraded largely by matrix metalloproteins and collagenases [54]. However, controlling the density of the implant and the extent of intermolecular crosslinking can regulate the in vivo resorption rate of a collagen implant. Collagen contains cell adhesion domain sequences (*eg*, RGD) that may assist to retain the phenotype and activity of many types of cells, including fibroblasts [55] and chondrocytes [56]. Alginate, a polysaccharide isolated from seaweed, has been used as an injectable cell delivery vehicle [57] and a cell immobilization matrix [58] owing to its gentle gelling properties in the presence of divalent ions such as calcium. Alginate is relatively biocompatible and is approved by the US Food and Drug Administration for human use as wound dressing material. Alginate is a family of copolymers of D-mannuronate and L-guluronate. The physical and mechanical properties of alginate gel are strongly correlated with the proportion and length of polygluronic block in the alginate chains [57]. Pictured here is an electron microscope image of a collagen sponge.

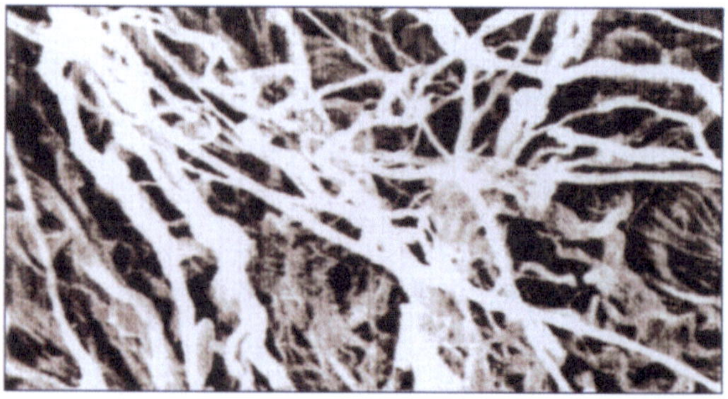

FIGURE 14-15. Acellular tissue matrix. Acellular tissue matrices are collagen-rich matrices prepared by removing cellular components from tissues. The matrices are often prepared by mechanical and chemical manipulation of a segment of tissue [1–4]. These matrices slowly degrade upon implantation, and are replaced and remodeled by extracellular matrix proteins synthesized and secreted by transplanted or growing cells.

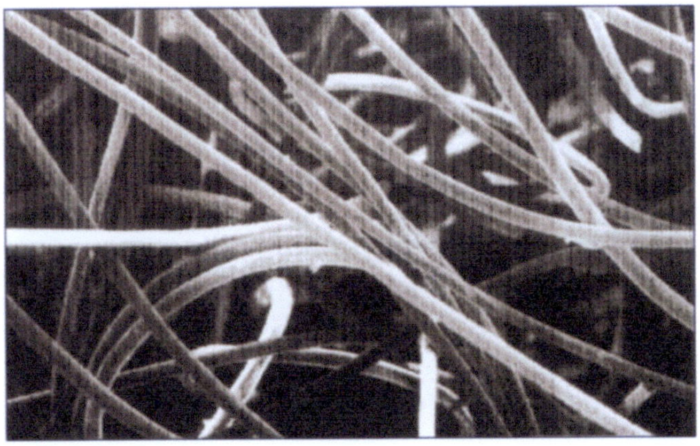

FIGURE 14-16. Synthetic polymers. Polyesters of naturally occurring α-hydroxy acids, including polyglycolic acid (PGA), polylactic acid (PLA), and poly(lactic-co-glycolic acid (PLGA), are widely used in tissue engineering. These polymers are US Food and Drug Administration–approved for a variety of applications, including sutures [59]. The ester bonds in these polymers are hydrolytically labile, and they degrade by nonenzymatic hydrolysis. The degradation products of PGA, PLA, and PLGA are nontoxic natural metabolites and are eventually eliminated from the body in the form of carbon dioxide and water [59]. The degradation rate of these polymers can be tailored to the application by altering crystallinity, initial molecular weight, and the copolymer ratio of lactic to glycolic acid. Generally, the optimal degradation time ranges from several weeks to several years. Since these polymers are thermoplastics, they can be easily formed into a three-dimensional scaffold with a desired microstructure, gross shape, and dimension by various techniques, including molding, extrusion, solvent casting [60], phase separation techniques, and gas foaming techniques [61]. Many applications in tissue engineering often require a scaffold with high porosity and ratio of surface area to volume. Other biodegradable synthetic polymers, including poly(anhydrides) and poly(ortho-esters), can also be used to fabricate scaffolds for tissue engineering with controlled properties [62].

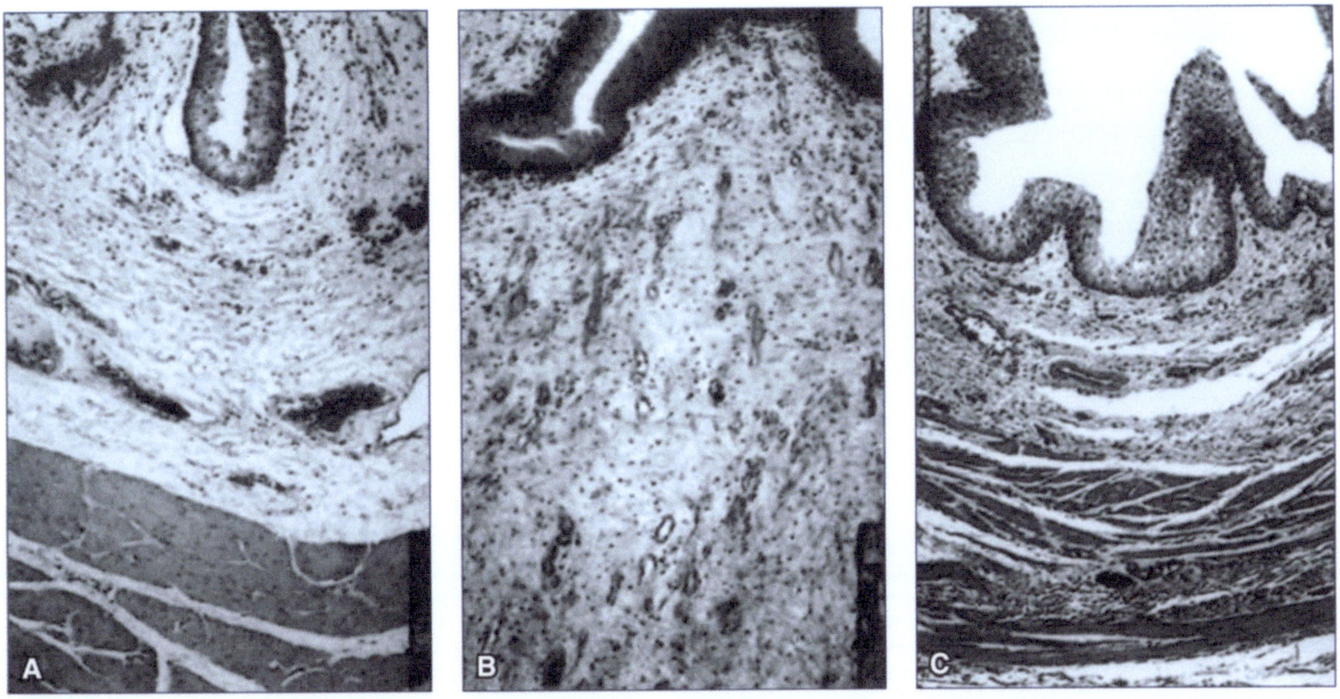

FIGURE 14-17. Seeded scaffolding. In the most common tissue engineering procedures, isolated cells are seeded onto a scaffold composed of an appropriate biomaterial. These biomaterials replicate the biologic and mechanical function of the native extracellular matrix (ECM) found in tissues in the body by serving as an artificial ECM. Biomaterials provide a three-dimensional space for the cells to develop into new tissues with appropriate structure and function. They can also allow delivery of appropriate bioactive factors (*eg*, cell adhesion peptides, growth factors) to the developing tissue [50] to help regulate cellular function. As the majority of mammalian cell types are anchorage-dependent and will die if no cell adhesion substrate is available, biomaterials provide this substrate that can deliver cells to specific sites in the body with high loading efficiency. Biomaterials can also provide mechanical support against in vivo forces so that the predefined three-dimensional structure of the engineered implant is maintained during tissue development. Shown here is hematoxylin and eosin staining 6 months after surgery in canines subjected to subtotal cystectomy (**A**), subtotal cystectomy with replacement by acellular scaffold (**B**), and subtotal cystectomy with replacement by scaffolding seeded with autologous urothelial and smooth muscle cells (**C**). **A**, Normal canine bladder. **B**, The bladder dome of the bladder reconstructed with cell-free polymer consists of normal urothelium over a thickened layer of collagen and fibrotic tissue; only scarce muscle fibers are apparent. **C**, The tissue-engineered neo-organ has a histomorphologically normal appearance. A trilayered architecture consisting of urothelium, submucosa, and smooth muscle is evident.

Problems Associated with Using Gastrointestinal Segments in Bladder Reconstruction

Segment	Metabolic disturbance
Stomach	Metabolic alkalosis
Jejunum	Hyperkalemia, hypochloremia, metabolic acidosis
Ileum/colon	Hyperchloremia, metabolic acidosis
All	Infections
	Renal/diversion calculi
	Renal damage
	Altered sensorium
	Abnormal drug metabolism
	Malabsorption and associated syndromes
	Secondary malignancy

FIGURE 14-18. Problems associated with using gastrointestinal segments in bladder reconstruction. Currently, gastrointestinal segments are commonly used for bladder replacement or repair. However, gastrointestinal tissues are designed to absorb solutes that urinary tissue excretes, and due to this difference in function, multiple complications may ensue, such as infection, metabolic disturbances, urolithiasis, perforation, increased mucus production, and malignancy [63–65]. Because of the problems encountered with the use of gastrointestinal segments, numerous investigators have attempted alternative reconstructive procedures for bladder replacement or repair. The use of tissue expansion, seromuscular grafts, matrices for tissue regeneration, and tissue engineering with cell transplantation have been investigated.

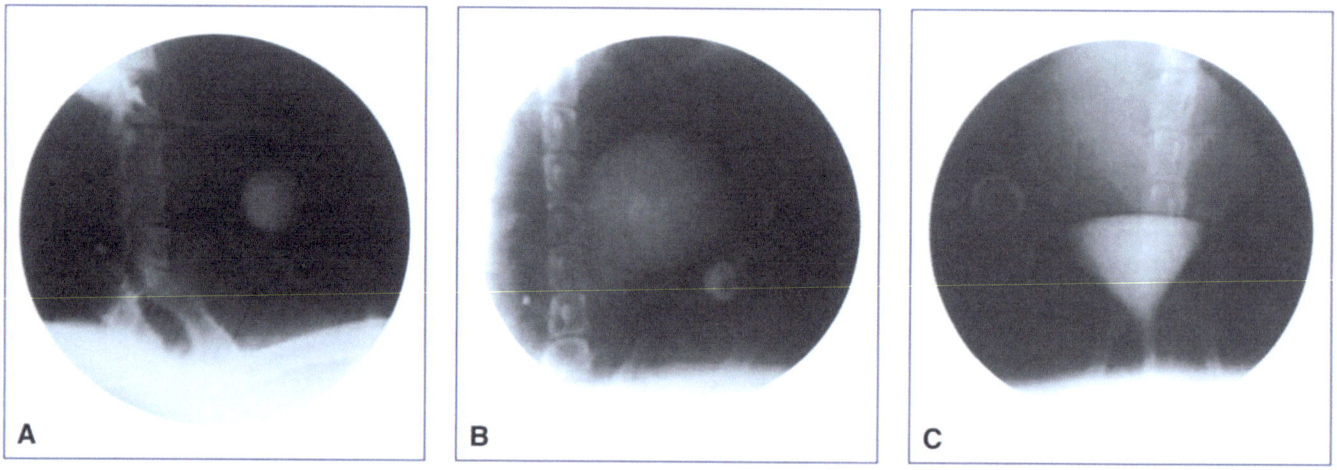

FIGURE 14-19. Tissue expansion for bladder augmentation. A system of progressive dilation for ureters and bladders has been proposed as a method of bladder augmentation but has not yet been attempted clinically. Augmentation cystoplasty performed with dilated ureteral segments in animals has resulted in an increased bladder capacity ranging from 190% to 380% [66,67]. A system for the progressive expansion of native bladder tissue has also been used for augmenting bladder volumes in animals. Within 30 days after progressive dilation, the neoreservoir volume was expanded at least 10-fold. Urodynamic studies showed normal compliance in all animals and microscopic examination of the expanded neoreservoir tissue showed a normal histology. A series of immunocytochemical studies demonstrated that the dilated bladder tissue maintained normal phenotypic characteristics [67]. Progressive bladder dilation can be performed with adequate increases in capacity. Cystography of bladder neoreservoir before progressive dilation (**A**) is compared with cystography results after progressive dilation (**B**) and with cystogram showing dilated neoreservoir and intact bladder segment (**C**).

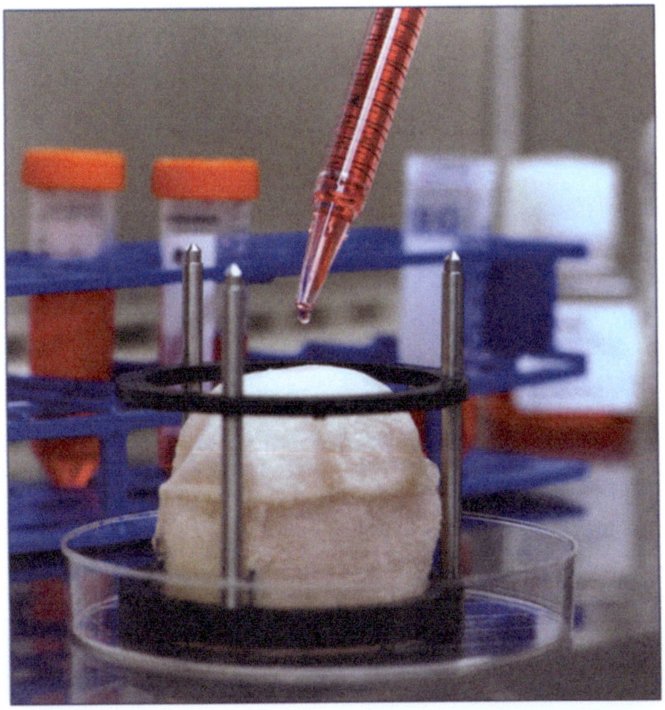

FIGURE 14-20. Matrices for bladder regeneration. Nonseeded allogeneic acellular matrices have served as scaffolds for the ingrowth of host bladder wall components. The matrices are prepared by mechanically and chemically removing all cellular components from bladder tissue [2,3,74,75]. The matrices serve as vehicles for partial bladder regeneration, and relevant antigenicity is not evident. One example is small intestine submucosa (SIS), a biodegradable, acellular, xenogeneic collagen-based tissue matrix [70]. Animal studies have shown that the nonseeded SIS matrix used for bladder augmentation is able to regenerate in vivo [71,72]. In multiple studies using various materials as nonseeded grafts for cystoplasty, the urothelial layer was able to regenerate normally, but the muscle layer, although present, was not fully developed [2,68,69,72]. Often the grafts contracted to 60% to 70% of their original size with little increase in bladder capacity or compliance [73,74]. Studies involving acellular matrices that may provide the necessary environment to promote cell migration, growth, and differentiation are being conducted. Recently, bladder regeneration has been shown to be more reliable when the SIS was derived from the distal ileum [71]. With continued research in this area, these matrices may have a clinical role in bladder replacement in the future.

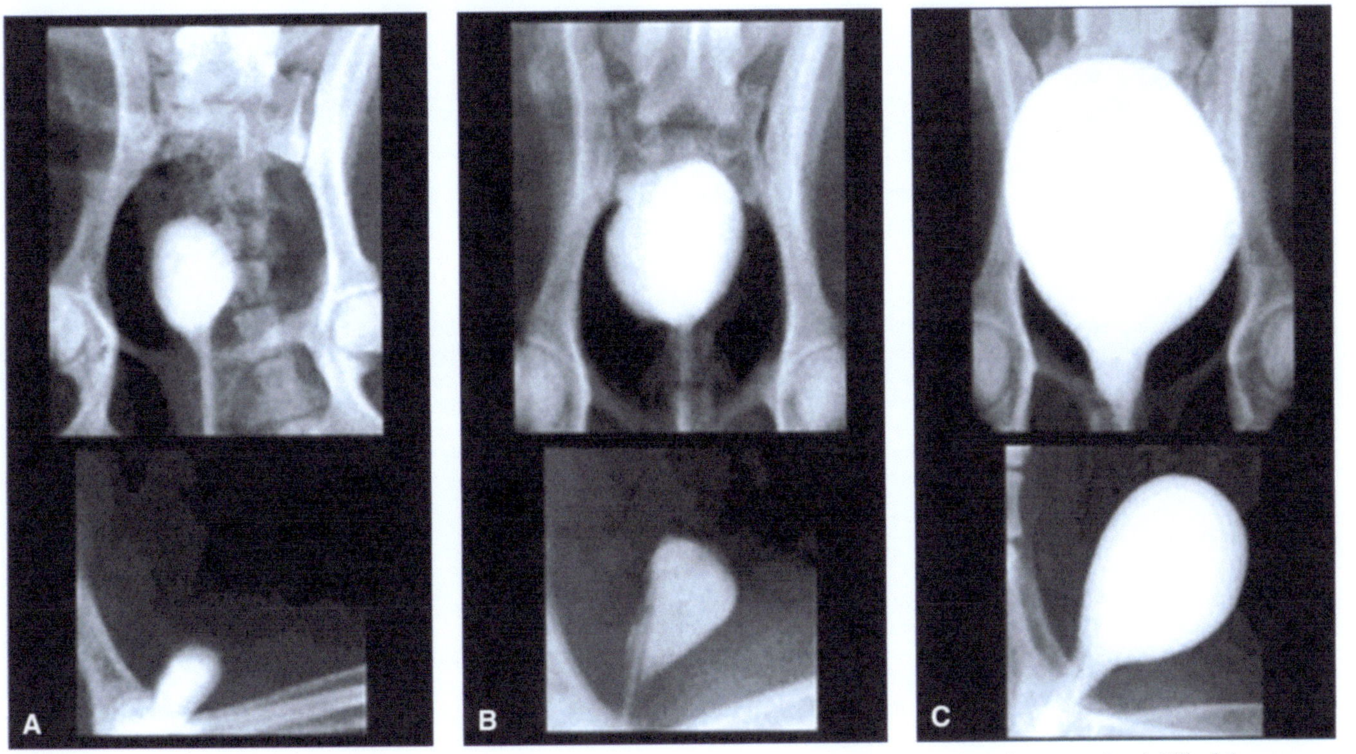

FIGURE 14-21. Cystographic images from canines 11 months following cystectomy. Cell-seeded allogeneic acellular bladder matrices have been used for bladder augmentation in dogs. A group of experimental dogs underwent a trigone-sparing cystectomy and were randomly assigned to one of three groups. One group underwent closure of the trigone without a reconstructive procedure, another underwent reconstruction with a nonseeded bladder-shaped biodegradable scaffold, and the last underwent reconstruction using a bladder-shaped biodegradable scaffold that was seeded with autologous urothelial and smooth muscle cells [12]. The cystectomy-only bladder (**A**) had a capacity of 22% of the preoperative value and a decrease in bladder compliance to 10% of the preoperative value. The nonseeded, scaffold-only controls (**B**) demonstrated a capacity of 46% of the preoperative value and a decrease in bladder compliance to 42% of the preoperative value; however, significant scarring and fibrosis is evident in the gross specimen. In sharp contrast to these results, an average bladder capacity of 95% of the original precystectomy volume was achieved when cell-seeded tissue engineered bladder replacements were used (**C**). The compliance was almost no different from the preoperative values that had been obtained when the native bladder was present (106%). In addition, bladder tissue resembling a normal organ had formed by 11 months postsurgery. This tissue was made up of a urothelial cell layer, a transitional cell layer, and a well-organized layer of smooth muscle cells resembling normal detrusor tissue.

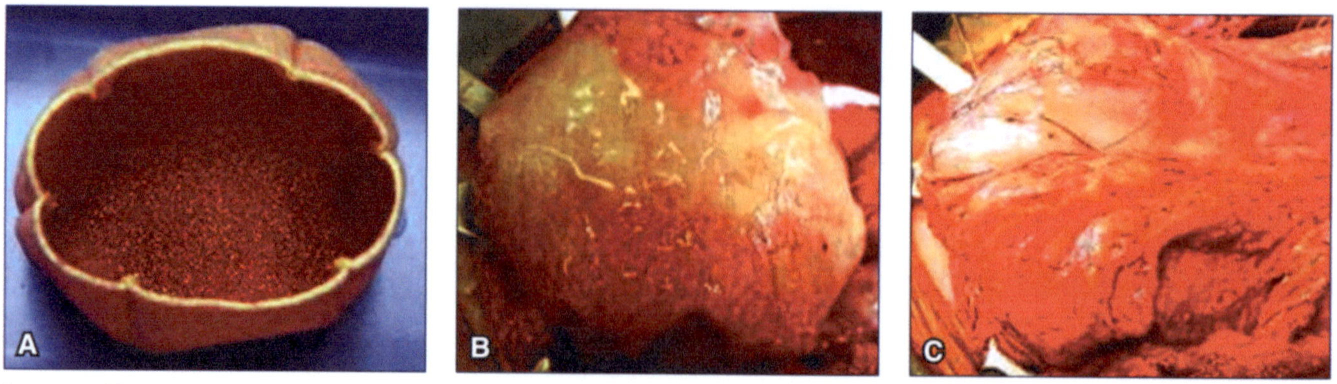

FIGURE 14-22. Seeded scaffolding and surgical demonstration of placement of bladder augmentation. A clinical experience involving engineered bladder tissue for cystoplasty reconstruction was conducted starting in 1999. A small pilot study of seven patients was reported, using a collagen scaffold seeded with cells either with or without omentum coverage, or a combined polyglycolic acid–collagen scaffold seeded with cells and omental coverage. **A,** A bladder-shaped scaffold was created and seeded with cells derived from a biopsy of the patient's own bladder tissue. This seeded scaffold was cultured in the laboratory until adequate cell coverage was achieved, and then it was implanted into the patient. **B,** The engineered bladder was anastomosed to the native bladder tissue with running 4-0 polyglycolic sutures. **C,** The implant was covered with fibrin glue and omentum and fixed in place.

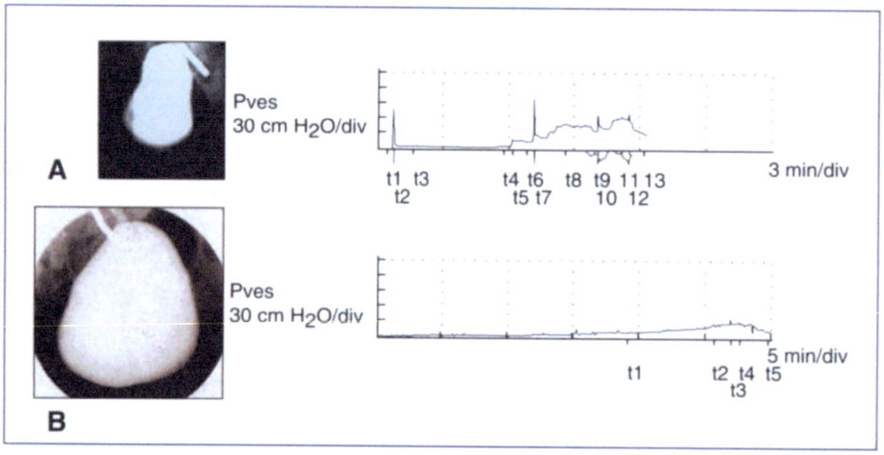

FIGURE 14-23. Cystograms and urodynamic studies of a patient before and after implantation of the tissue engineered bladder. The patients reconstructed with the engineered bladder tissue created with the polyglycolic acid–collagen cell-seeded scaffolds showed increased compliance, decreased end-filling pressures, increased capacities, and longer dry period [75]. Although the experience is promising in terms of showing that engineered tissues can be implanted safely, it is just a start in terms of accomplishing the goal of engineering fully functional bladders. Further experimental and clinical work is being conducted. **A,** Preoperatively, a cystogram indicates an irregular, misshapen bladder. Additionally, abnormal bladder pressures during bladder filling were measured via urodynamic study. **B,** Postoperatively, these findings were significantly improved. A larger bladder appears on the cystogram, and bladder filling pressures are within normal ranges.

References

1. Dahms SE, Piechota HJ, Dahiya R, *et al.*: Composition and biomechanical properties of the bladder acellular matrix graft: comparative analysis in rat, pig and human. *Br J Urol* 1998, 82:411.
2. Yoo JJ, Meng J, Oberpenning F, *et al.*: Bladder augmentation using allogenic bladder submucosa seeded with cells. *Urology* 1998, 51:221.
3. Piechota HJ, Dahms SE, Nunes LS, *et al.*: In vitro functional properties of the rat bladder regenerated by the bladder acellular matrix graft. *J Urol* 1998, 159:1717.
4. Chen F, Yoo JJ, Atala A: Acellular collagen matrix as a possible "off the shelf" biomaterial for urethral repair. *Urology* 1999, 54:407.
5. Amiel, G. E., Atala, A.: Current and future modalities for functional renal replacement. *Urol Clin North Am* 1999, 26:235.
6. Amiel GE, Komura M, Shapira O, *et al.*: Engineering of blood vessels from acellular collagen matrices coated with human endothelial cells. *Tissue Eng* 2006, 12:2355.
7. Yoo JJ, Park HJ, Lee I, *et al.*: Autologous engineered cartilage rods for penile reconstruction. *J Urol* 1999, 162:1119.
8. Atala A: Autologous cell transplantation for urologic reconstruction. *J Urol* 1998, 159:2.
9. Atala A: Bladder regeneration by tissue engineering [see comment]. *BJU Int* 2001, 88:765.
10. Atala A: Creation of bladder tissue in vitro and in vivo. A system for organ replacement. *Adv Exp Med Biol* 1999, 462:31.
11. Cilento BG, Freeman MR, Schneck FX, *et al.*: Phenotypic and cytogenetic characterization of human bladder urothelia expanded in vitro. *J Urol* 1994, 152:665.
12. Oberpenning F, Meng J, Yoo JJ, *et al.*: De novo reconstitution of a functional mammalian urinary bladder by tissue engineering [see comment]. *Nat Biotechnol* 1999, 17:149.
13. Scriven SD, Booth C, Thomas DF, *et al.*: Reconstitution of human urothelium from monolayer cultures. *J Urol* 1997, 158:1147.
14. Liebert M, Hubbel A, Chung M, *et al.*: Expression of mal is associated with urothelial differentiation in vitro: identification by differential display reverse-transcriptase polymerase chain reaction. *Differentiation* 1997, 61:177.

15. Liebert M, Wedemeyer G, Abruzzo LV, *et al.*: Stimulated urothelial cells produce cytokines and express an activated cell surface antigenic phenotype. *Semin Urol* 1991, 9:124.

16. Puthenveettil JA, Burger MS, Reznikoff CA: Replicative senescence in human uroepithelial cells. *Adv Exp Med Biol* 1999, 462:83.

17. Freeman MR, Yoo JJ, Raab G, *et al.*: Heparin-binding EGF-like growth factor is an autocrine growth factor for human urothelial cells and is synthesized by epithelial and smooth muscle cells in the human bladder. *J Clin Invest* 1997, 99:1028.

18. Nguyen HT, Park JM, Peters CA, *et al.*: Cell-specific activation of the HB-EGF and ErbB1 genes by stretch in primary human bladder cells. *In Vitro Cell Dev Biol Anim* 1999, 35:371.

19. Harriss DR: Smooth muscle cell culture: a new approach to the study of human detrusor physiology and pathophysiology. *Br J Urol* 1995, 75(Suppl 1):18.

20. Martin GR: Isolation of a pluripotent cell line from early mouse embryos cultured in medium conditioned by teratocarcinoma stem cells. *Proc Natl Acad Sci U S A* 1981, 78:7634.

21. Reubinoff BE, Itsykson P, Turetsky T, *et al.*: Neural progenitors from human embryonic stem cells [see comment]. *Nat Biotechnol* 2001, 191134.

22. Schuldiner M, Eiges R, Eden A, *et al.*: Induced neuronal differentiation of human embryonic stem cells. *Brain Res* 2001, 913:201.

23. Schuldiner M, Yanuka O, Itskovitz-Eldor J, *et al.*: Effects of eight growth factors on the differentiation of cells derived from human embryonic stem cells. *Proc Natl Acad Sci U S A* 2000, 97:11307.

24. Zhang SC, Wernig M, Duncan ID, *et al.*: In vitro differentiation of transplantable neural precursors from human embryonic stem cells [see comment]. *Nat Biotechnol* 2001, 19:1129.

25. Kaufman D S, Hanson ET, Lewis RL, *et al.*: Hematopoietic colony-forming cells derived from human embryonic stem cells. *Proc Natl Acad Sci U S A* 2001, 98:10716.

26. Kehat I, Kenyagin-Karsenti D, Snir M, *et al.*: Human embryonic stem cells can differentiate into myocytes with structural and functional properties of cardiomyocytes.[see comment]. *J Clin Invest* 2001, 108:407.

27. Levenberg S, Golub JS, Amit M, *et al.*: Endothelial cells derived from human embryonic stem cells. *Proc Natl Acad Sci U S A* 2002, 99:4391.

28. Assady S, Maor G, Amit M, *et al.*: Insulin production by human embryonic stem cells. *Diabetes* 2001, 50:1691.

29. Itskovitz-Eldor J, Schuldiner M, Karsenti D, *et al.*: Differentiation of human embryonic stem cells into embryoid bodies compromising the three embryonic germ layers. *Mol Med* 2000, 6:88.

30. Reubinoff BE, Pera MF, Fong CY, *et al.*: Embryonic stem cell lines from human blastocysts: somatic differentiation in vitro [see comment] [erratum appears in *Nat Biotechnol* 2000,18(5):559]. *Nat Biotechnol* 2000, 18:399.

31. Thomson JA, Itskovitz-Eldor J, Shapiro SS, *et al.*: Embryonic stem cell lines derived from human blastocysts [see comment] [erratum appears in *Science* 1998, 282(5395):1827]. *Science* 1998, 282:1145.

32. Brambrink T, Hochedlinger K, Bell G, *et al.*: ES cells derived from cloned and fertilized blastocysts are transcriptionally and functionally indistinguishable. *Proc Natl Acad Sci U S A* 2006, 103:933.

33. Rideout WM III, Hochedlinger K, Kyba M, *et al.*: Correction of a genetic defect by nuclear transplantation and combined cell and gene therapy. Cell 2002, 109:17.

34. Hochedlinger K, Jaenisch R: Monoclonal mice generated by nuclear transfer from mature B and T donor cells. *Nature* 2002, 415:1035.

35. Eggan K, Baldwin K, Tackett M, *et al.*: Mice cloned from olfactory sensory neurons 1. *Nature* 2004, 428:44.

36. Lanza RP, Chung HY, Yoo JJ, *et al.*: Generation of histocompatible tissues using nuclear transplantation. *Nat Biotechnol* 2002, 20 689.

37. Wilmut I, Schnieke AE, McWhir J, *et al.*: Viable offspring derived from fetal and adult mammalian cells [see comment] [erratum appears in *Nature* 1997, 386(6621):200]. *Nature* 1997, 385:810.

38. Hwang WS, Roh SI, Lee BC, *et al.*: Patient-specific embryonic stem cells derived from human SCNT blastocysts. *Science* 2005, 3081777.

39. Simerly C, Dominko T, Navara C, *et al.*: Molecular correlates of primate nuclear transfer failures. *Science* 2003, 300:297.

40. Hwang WS, Ryu YJ, Park JH, *et al.*: Evidence of a pluripotent human embryonic stem cell line derived from a cloned blastocyst. *Science* 2004, 303:1669.

41. Byrne J, Pedersen D, Clepper L, *et al.*: Producing primate embryonic stem cells by somatic cell nuclear transfer. *Nature* 2007, 450:497.

42. Mitalipov S: Reprogramming following somatic cell nuclear transfer in primates is dependent upon nuclear remodeling. *Hum Reprod* 2007, 22:2232.

43. Takahashi K, Yamanaka S: Induction of pluripotent stem cells from mouse embryonic and adult fibroblast cultures by defined factors. *Cell* 2006, 126:663.

44. Wernig M, Meissner A, Foreman R, *et al.*: In vitro reprogramming of fibroblasts into a pluripotent ES-cell-like state. *Nature* 2007, 448:318.

45. Takahashi K, Tanabe K, Ohnuki M, *et al.*: Induction of puripotent stem cells from adult human fibroblasts by defined factors. *Cell* 2007, 131:861.

46. Yu J, Vodyanik MA. Smuga-Otto K, *et al.*: Induced pluripotent stem cell lines derived from human somatic cells. *Science* 2007, 1151:526.

47. De Coppi P, Bartsch G, Jr, Siddiqui MM, *et al.*: Isolation of amniotic stem cell lines with potential for therapy [see comment]. *Nat Biotechnol* 2007, 25:100.

48. Bergsma JE, Rozema FR, Bos RR, *et al.*: In vivo degradation and biocompatibility study of in vitro pre-degraded as-polymerized polyactide particles [see comment]. *Biomaterials* 1995, 16:267.

49. Hynes RO: Integrins: versatility, modulation, and signaling in cell adhesion. *Cell* 1992, 69:11.

50. Kim BS, Mooney DJ: Development of biocompatible synthetic extracellular matrices for tissue engineering. *Trends Biotechnol* 1998, 16:224.

51. Pariente JL, Kim BS, Atala A: In vitro biocompatibility assessment of naturally derived and synthetic biomaterials using normal human urothelial cells. *J Biomed Mater Res* 2001, 55:33.

52. Pariente JL, Kim BS, Atala A: In vitro biocompatibility evaluation of naturally derived and synthetic biomaterials using normal human bladder smooth muscle cells. *J Urol* 2002, 167:1867.

53. Li ST: Biologic biomaterials: tissue derived biomaterials (collagen). In *The Biomedical Engineering Handbook*. Edited by Bronzino JD. Boca Raton, FL: CRS Press; 1995:627–647.

54. Arora PD, Manolson MF, Downey GP, *et al.*: A novel model system for characterization of phagosomal maturation, acidification, and intracellular collagen degradation in fibroblasts. *J Biol Chem* 2000, 275:35432.

55. Silver FH, Pins G: Cell growth on collagen: a review of tissue engineering using scaffolds containing extracellular matrix. *J Long Term Eff Med Implants* 1992, 2:67.

56. Sams AE, Nixon AJ: Chondrocyte-laden collagen scaffolds for resurfacing extensive articular cartilage defects. *Osteoarthritis Cartilage* 1995, 3:47.

57. Smidsrod O, Skjak-Braek G: Alginate as immobilization matrix for cells. *Trends Biotechnol* 1990, 8:71.

58. Lim F, Sun AM: Microencapsulated islets as bioartificial endocrine pancreas. *Science* 1980, 210:908.

59. Gilding D: Biodegradable polymers. In *Biocompatibility of Clinical Implant Materials*. Edited by Williams D. Boca Raton, FL: CRC Press; 1981:209–232.

60. Mikos AG, Lyman MD, Freed LE, *et al.*: Wetting of poly(L-lactic acid) and poly(DL-lactic-co-glycolic acid) foams for tissue culture. *Biomaterials* 1994, 15:55.

61. Harris LD, Kim BS, Mooney DJ: Open pore biodegradable matrices formed with gas foaming. *J Biomed Mater Res* 1998, 42:396.

62. Peppas NA, Langer R: New challenges in biomaterials [see comment]. *Science* 1994, 263:1715.

63. McDougal WS: Metabolic complications of urinary intestinal diversion. *J Urol* 1992, 147:1199.

64. Kaefer M, Hendren WH, Bauer SB, *et al.*: Reservoir calculi: a comparison of reservoirs constructed from stomach and other enteric segments [see comment]. *J Urol* 1998, 160:2187.

65. Kaefer M, Tobin MS, Hendren WH, *et al.*: Continent urinary diversion: the Children's Hospital experience. *J Urol* 1997, 157:1394.

66. Lailas NG, Cilento B, Atala A: Progressive ureteral dilation for subsequent ureterocystoplasty. *J Urol* 1996, 156:1151.

67. Satar N, Yoo JJ, Atala A: Progressive dilation for bladder tissue expansion. *J Urol* 1999, 162:829.

68. Probst M, Dahiya R, Carrier S, *et al.*: Reproduction of functional smooth muscle tissue and partial bladder replacement. *Br J Urol* 1997, 79:505.

69. Sutherland RS, Baskin LS, Hayward SW, *et al.*: Regeneration of bladder urothelium, smooth muscle, blood vessels and nerves into an acellular tissue matrix. *J Urol* 1996, 156:571.

70. Badylak SF, Lantz GC, Coffey A, *et al.*: Small intestinal submucosa as a large diameter vascular graft in the dog. *J Surg Res* 1989, 47:74.

71. Kropp BP, Cheng EY, Lin HK, *et al.*: Reliable and reproducible bladder regeneration using unseeded distal small intestinal submucosa. *J Urol* 2004, 172:1710.

72. Kropp BP, Rippy, MK, Badylak SF, *et al.*: Regenerative urinary bladder augmentation using small intestinal submucosa: urodynamic and histopathologic assessment in long-term canine bladder augmentations. *J Urol* 1996, 155:2098.

73. Portis AJ, Elbahnasy AM, Shalhav AL, *et al.*: Laparoscopic augmentation cystoplasty with different biodegradable grafts in an animal model. *J Urol* 2000, 164:1405.

74. Landman J, Olweny E, Sundaram CP, *et al.*: Laparoscopic mid sagittal hemicystectomy and bladder reconstruction with small intestinal submucosa and reimplantation of ureter into small intestinal submucosa: 1-year followup. *J Urol* 2004, 171:2450.

75. Atala A, Bauer SB, Soker S, *et al.*: Tissue-engineered autologous bladders for patients needing cystoplasty. *Lancet* 2006, 367:1241.

15 Bladder Cancer

E. Jason Abel and Ashish M. Kamat

Bladder cancer is a major health problem in the United States, with an estimated 69,810 new cases and 14,100 deaths in 2008. While it usually occurs in older men (median age 73 years), the incidence in younger patients and women has been increasing. At presentation, the majority (about 70%) of bladder tumors are nonmuscle invasive (confined to epithelium or lamina propria) with the remaining patients having either muscle-invasive or more advanced disease.

Bladder cancer has the highest recurrence rate of any solid tumor; the natural history of nonmuscle-invasive disease involves frequent recurrences and the risk of progression, which requires careful and constant surveillance and frequent interventions. Thus, from an analysis of Medicare costs, bladder cancer is the most expensive cancer to treat from diagnosis to death, with an estimated annual cost of 2.9 billion dollars.

There are various major histologic subtypes of bladder cancer: the three most common are urothelial carcinoma (also known as transitional cell carcinoma), squamous cell carcinoma, and adenocarcinoma. In the United States, urothelial carcinoma accounts for the vast majority of cases (a variant of urothelial carcinoma, known as micropapillary bladder cancer, is gaining in recognition). In some countries, squamous cell carcinoma is the dominant subtype because of chronic infection with *S. hematobium*, but accounts for only 3% to 7% of bladder cancer in the United States. Adenocarcinoma is the rarest histologic subtype and is responsible for less than 2% of bladder cancer cases. Other less common types of bladder cancer include small cell carcinoma, carcinosarcoma, neurofibroma, pheochromocytoma, lymphoma, sarcomas, and metastatic lesions.

Bladder cancer is almost never found incidentally at autopsy, as most cases will eventually become symptomatic. Clinically, bladder cancer is usually detected during an evaluation for painless gross hematuria, microscopic hematuria, or irritative voiding symptoms. The workup for suspected bladder cancer involves a cystoscopic examination of the bladder as well as imaging studies to evaluate the kidneys and urothelium.

The first step in diagnosis and treatment is an endoscopic transurethral resection of the tumor; further treatment is dependent on the stage and grade. Options for the treatment of nonmuscle-invasive disease include intravesical instillation of immunotherapy (Bacillus Calmette-Guérin) or chemotherapy, or cystectomy, depending on the stage, grade, and risk factors. (In patients with muscle-invasive disease at diagnosis, surgical therapy with radical cystectomy is the mainstay of treatment, often including neoadjuvant or adjuvant chemotherapy. Patients who present with more advanced disease undergo chemotherapy as the primary treatment modality, with select patients undergoing surgery as part of multimodal therapy.

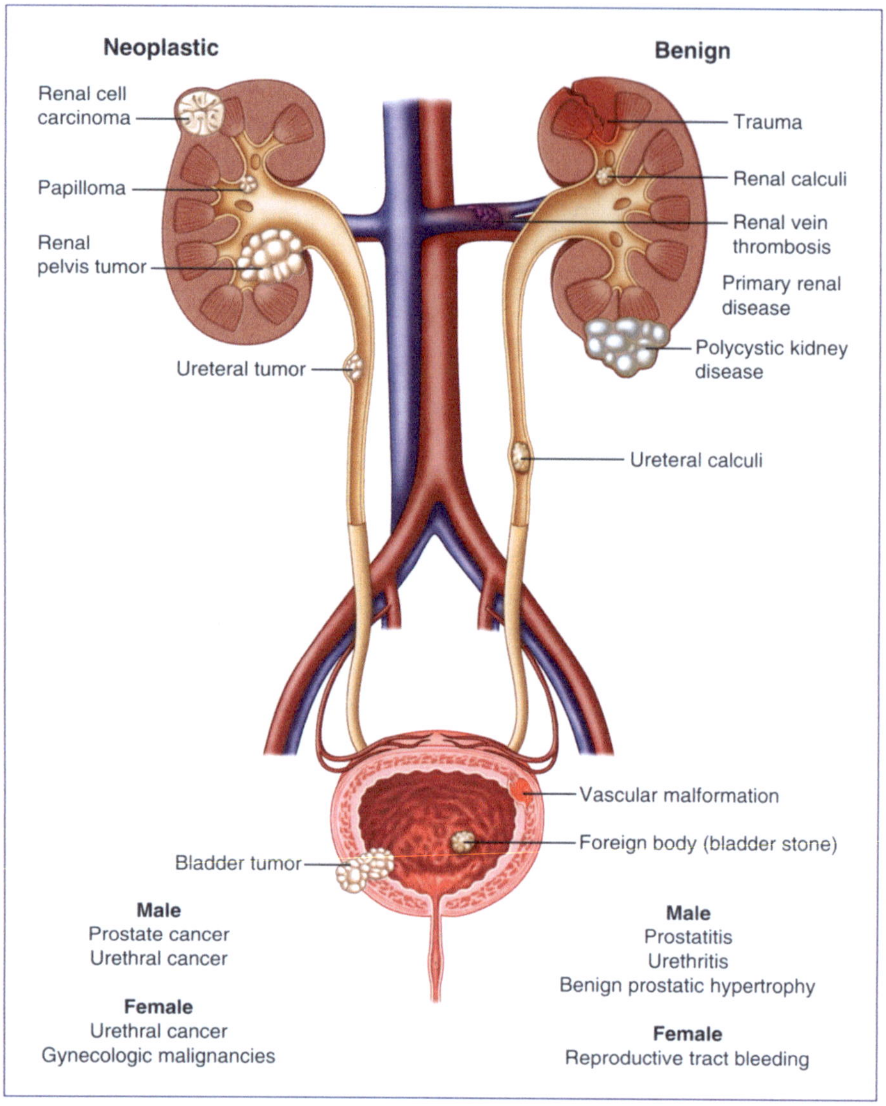

FIGURE 15-1. Causes of hematuria. Blood in the urine (hematuria) may originate from any point in the urinary tract. Characteristically, bleeding due to bladder cancer is painless, frequently intermittent, and may be gross or microscopic. The most common causes of hematuria are benign and include infection, calculi, and kidney disease, but a complete evaluation is required to rule out malignancy. A delay in appropriate evaluation, especially in women, can lead to missed diagnoses.

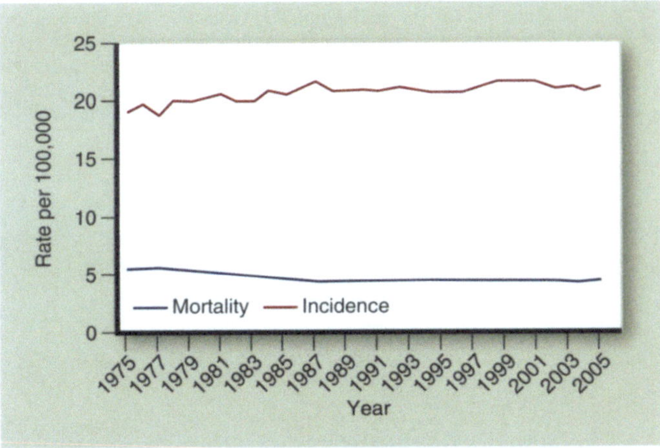

FIGURE 15-2. Age-adjusted incidence and mortality of bladder cancer in the United States. The incidence of bladder cancer in the United States has increased slightly over the last 30 years. While men are three times more likely to develop bladder cancer than women, women have increased mortality rates as compared to men. Similarly, while white men are almost twice as likely to develop bladder cancer as age-matched black men, black patients usually present with more advanced-stage disease and have worse survival rates. Bladder cancer is more common in older individuals with a peak incidence in the eighth decade. Younger patients who develop bladder cancer have a better prognosis because they more often present with superficial low-grade lesions as compared to older patients [1].

Risk Factors for Carcinoma of the Bladder

Risk factor	Association
Behavioral	
Cigarette smoking	XXXX
Cigar, pipe, and secondhand smoking	X
Urban and industrial residence	XX
Demographic	
Male gender	XX
White race	X
Age	XX
Family history	X
Exposure	
Arsenic	XX
Artificial sweeteners (saccharin and cyclamates at high doses)	+/-
Hair dyes	X
Aristolochia Fanchi	X
Cyclophosphamide	X
Phenacetin	+/-
Pelvic radiation	X
Occupational	
Aromatic amines	XX
Chemical dyes	XX
Other	
Shistosoma hematobium infection	XX
Chronic UTI, bladder stones	X

FIGURE 15-3. Risk factors for carcinoma of the bladder. Tobacco is the most commonly recognized risk factor for bladder cancer; exposure to smoking increases the risk of developing bladder cancer two- to fourfold. Risk is related to the dose, duration, and type of tobacco exposure. It is estimated that half of all bladder cancers in men and one-third of all bladder cancers in women are related to smoking. Furthermore, smoking cessation can reduce the risk of developing a bladder tumor.

A high-risk occupation is the second greatest risk factor for developing bladder cancer; workplace exposures are estimated to account for 5% to 25% of all bladder cancer cases. Occupational exposure to aromatic amines has been identified as a major risk factor and patients may experience increased risk if they have worked in the following industries: dyestuff manufacturing, rubber manufacturing, paint manufacturing, textile manufacturing, leather, metal, coal gasification, diesel exhaust, and carbon electrode production.

In several studies, a family history of bladder cancer increased risk, but it is unclear whether this is a genetically conferred risk or exposure to a common environmental risk factor. Several syndromes with mutations in proto-oncogenes (H-Ras) or tumor-suppressor genes (p53, Rb) demonstrate an increased risk of bladder cancer and have helped to elucidate the carcinogenesis of bladder cancer [2–5]. UTI—urinary tract infection.

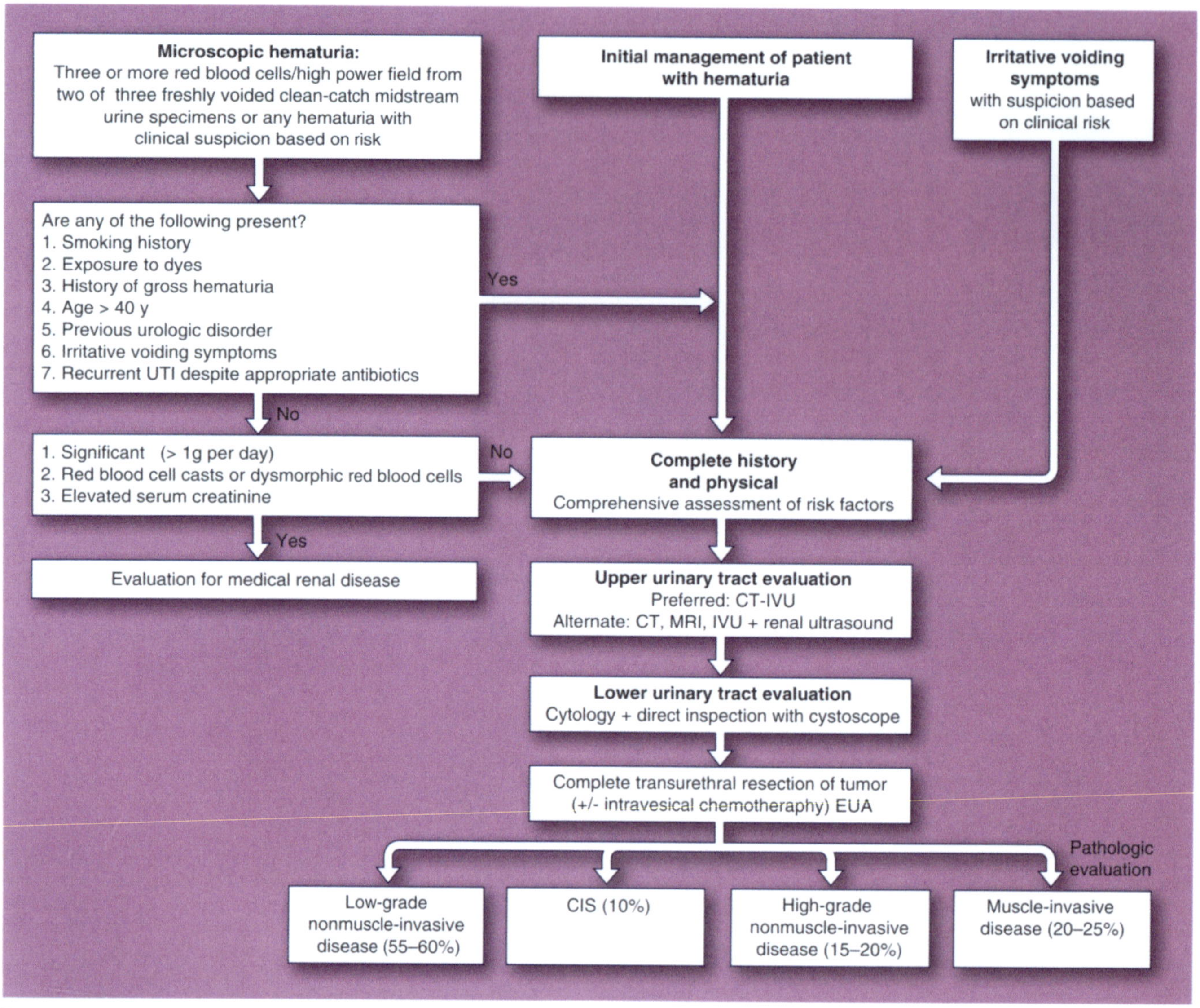

FIGURE 15-4. Initial evaluation of a patient with bladder cancer. A careful history and physical examination with an assessment of risk factors is essential for evaluating patients with hematuria. Hematuria should be confirmed using a microscopic evaluation of urine, since many medical conditions and medications can cause the urine to appear red without true hematuria. In addition, conditions such as myoglobinuria may cause false dipstick readings for hematuria. Factitious hematuria (originating from sites outside the urinary tract) can be excluded when using catheterized urine specimens. Patients with risk factors for bladder cancer, including older patients and those with exposure to risk factors, deserve special attention. In patients with an initial negative evaluation for hematuria, continued periodic evaluation with urinalysis, voided urine cytology, and blood pressure is recommended for 3 years [6–8]. CIS—carcinoma in situ; EUA—examination under anesthesia; CT-IVU—computed tomography intravenous urogram; UTI—urinary tract infection.

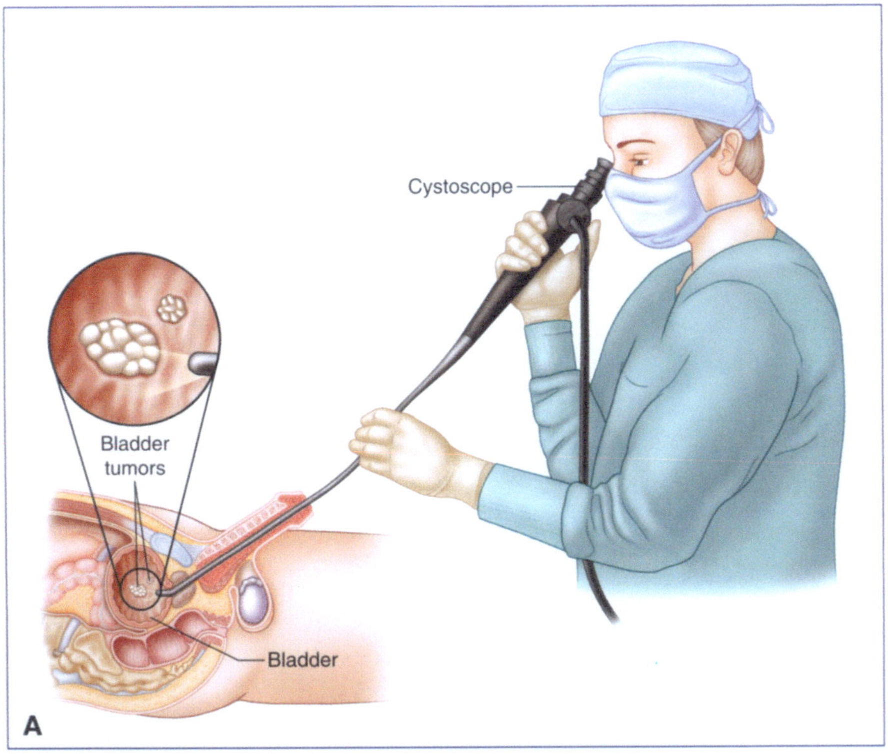

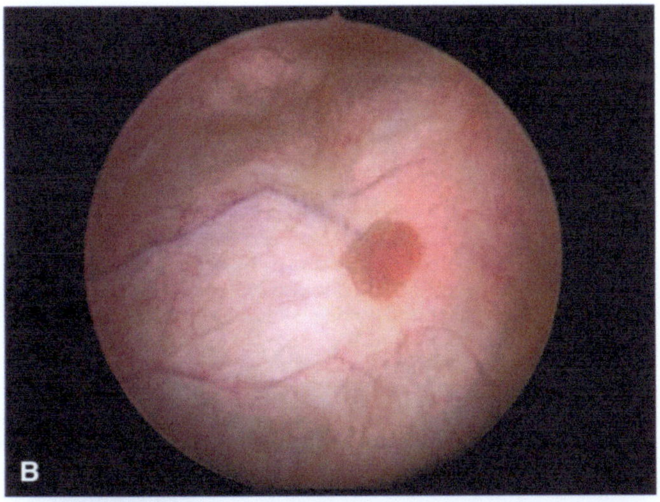

Figure 15-5. **A,** Cystoscopy. Cystoscopy allows direct inspection of the urothelium of the bladder in a patient with hematuria. Small-caliber flexible cystoscopes can be used in an office setting with only a local anesthetic in the majority of patients.

B, Small low-grade papillary tumor as seen through a cystoscope. Several studies have shown improved detection of bladder tumors using fluorescence cystoscopy.

C, This lesion is identified using hexaminolevulinate fluorescence cystoscopy [9]. **D,** Stage Ta urothelial carcinoma using white light illumination. (**C** and **D** *from* Grossman *et al.* [9], *with permission.*)

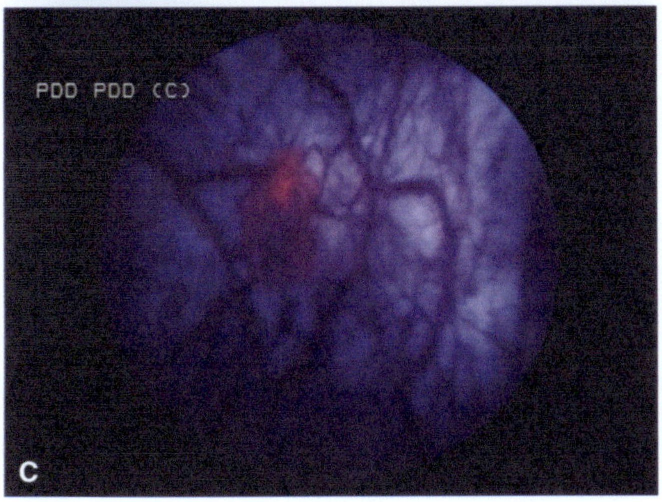

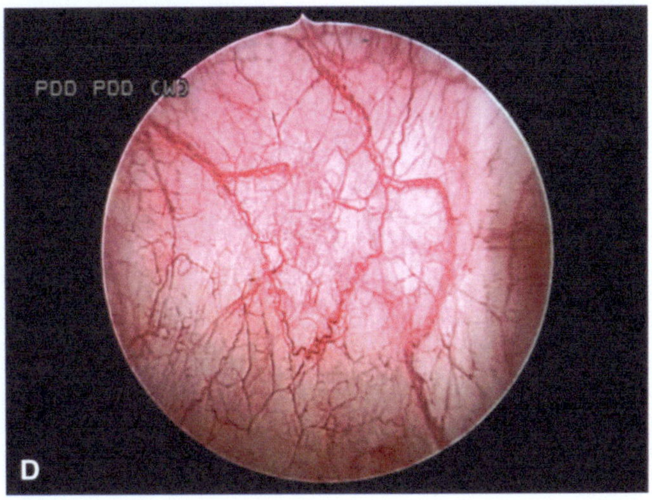

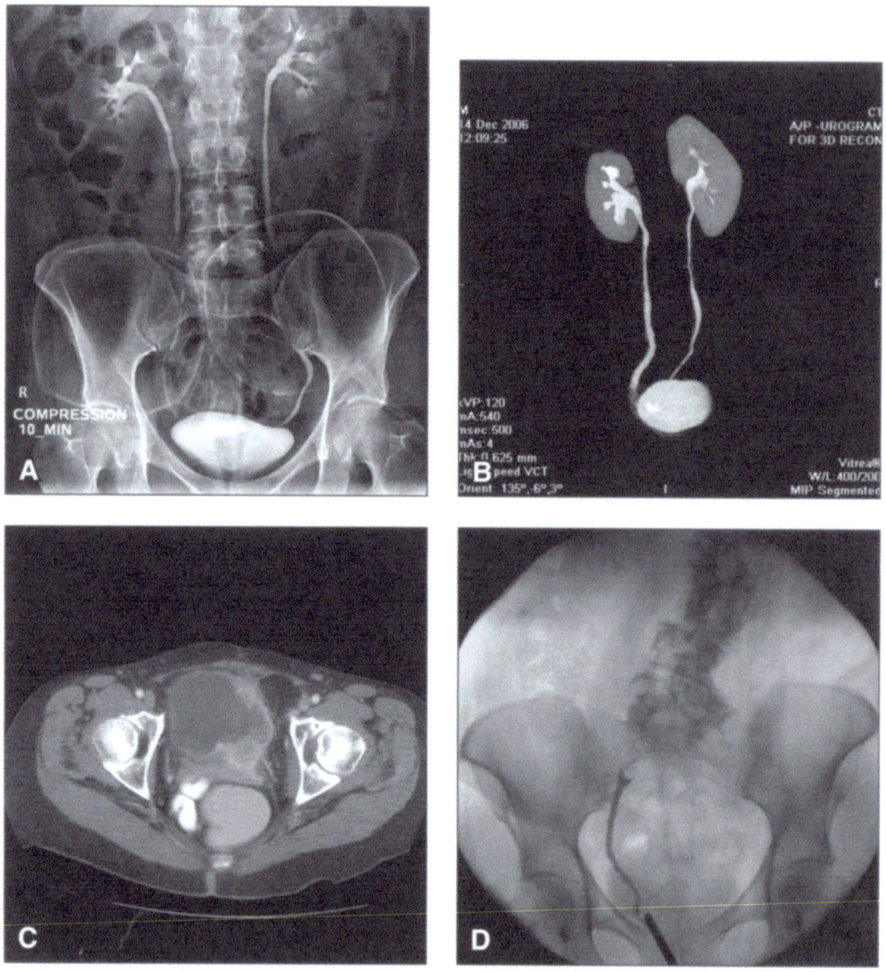

FIGURE 15-6. A, Upper tract evaluation. A workup for hematuria is incomplete until the entire urothelium has been evaluated. Imaging of the upper urinary tracts facilitates diagnosis of kidney calculi as well as of neoplasms. Radiologic imaging is preferred to direct visualization of the urothelium of the upper tracts because ureteroscopy requires general anesthesia and is not an appropriate screening test.

B, Normal intravenous urogram. (*Note*: the entire length of ureters is not seen in this example.) Intravenous urograms are inexpensive and provide radiologic visualization of the upper urinary tracts. Multiple images are produced to examine the kidneys and the passage of contrast along the ureters over time.

Computed tomography urograms (CTUs) are more expensive but provide more information about parenchymal lesions and are more sensitive for sessile urothelial lesions and small calculi. **C,** CTU showing a left distal ureteral tumor. Upper tract urothelial tumors comprise 5% of all urothelial carcinomas and may present with synchronous bladder tumors. Axial imaging from CTU can also provide information about the extent of bladder tumors (**C**), which is important for the clinical staging of large bladder masses.

D, Retrograde pyelogram. In patients with equivocal imaging, renal failure, or contrast allergy, retrograde pyelograms may be performed to evaluate the upper urinary tracts. In this procedure, contrast is injected up into each ureter via a small flexible catheter by the urologist. This retrograde pyelogram shows a classic "goblet sign" of ureteral tumor. Disadvantages of this technique are the lack of visualization of kidney parenchyma and a frequent need for sedation or anesthesia. (*Courtesy of* Carl Sandler, MD.)

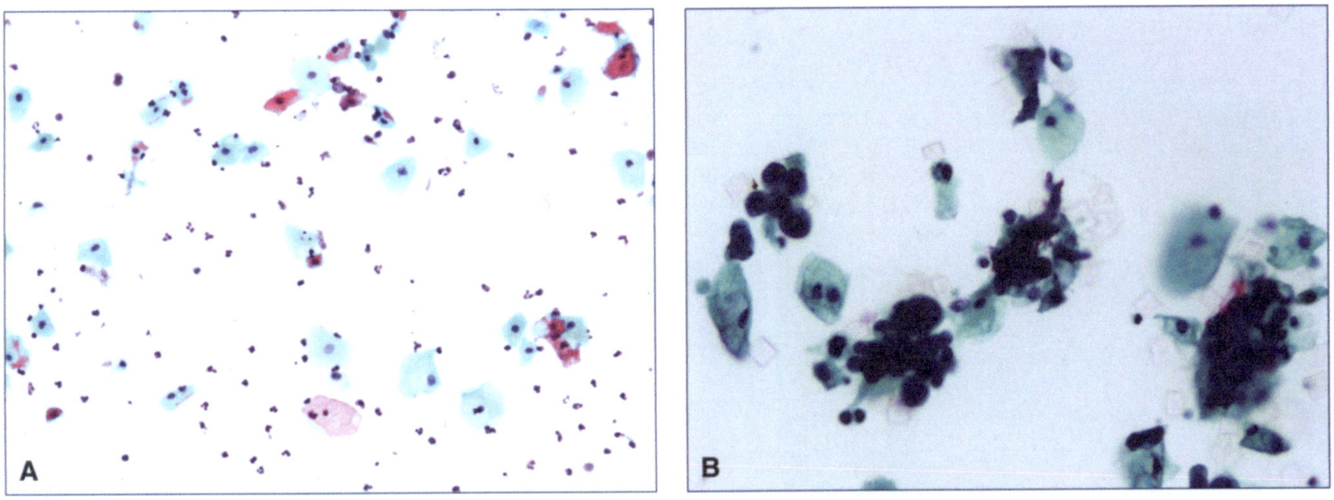

FIGURE 15-7. Cytology. **A,** Normal urine cytology: superficial (umbrella) cells and squamous cells. **B,** High-grade urothelial carcinoma: clusters of high-grade cells with a high nuclear:cytoplasmic ratio, prominent nucleoli hyperchromasia, pleomorphism, and irregular nuclear membranes. (*Courtesy of* Tatjana Antic, MD.)

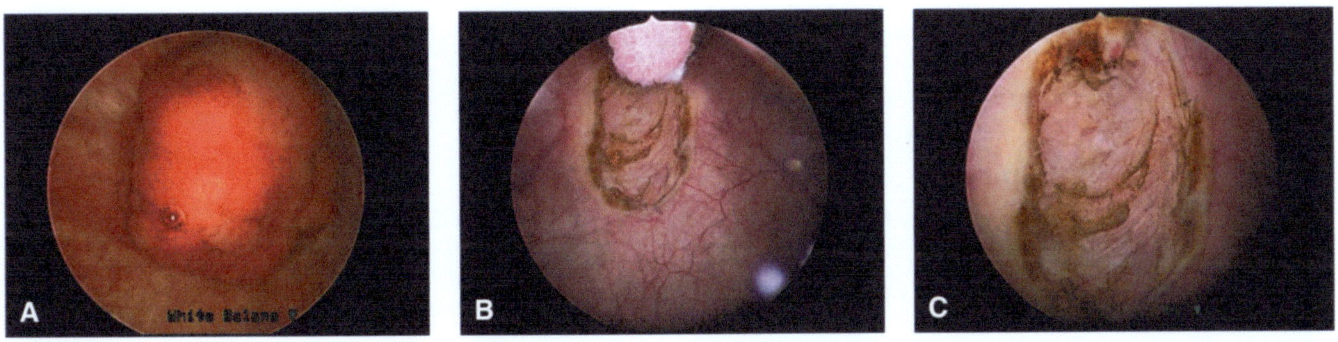

FIGURE 15-8. Transurethral resection. **A,** Papillary bladder mass. A papillary bladder mass as seen through a resectoscope is shown. The initial treatment and staging for bladder tumors is complete transurethral resection of all visible tumor. **B,** Resection. Complete resection should include muscularis propria, which is often evident as whitish fibers among glistening "fat globules" of perivesical adipose tissue. **C,** Tumor after complete resection. The appearance of the tumor base after a complete resection is shown. This specimen showed abundant muscularis propria on pathologic examination.

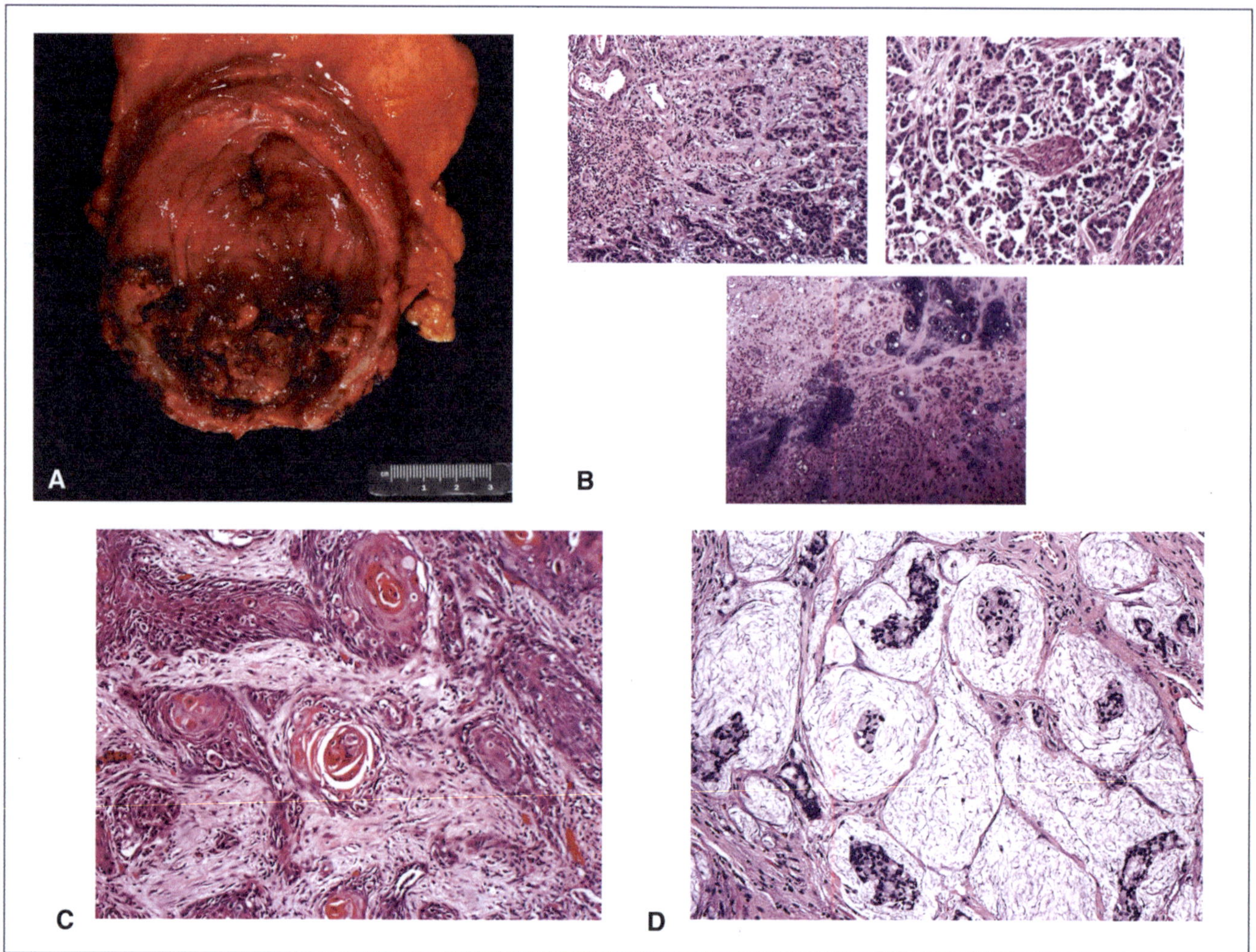

Figure 15-9. Pathology. **A,** Radical cystectomy specimen. Radical cystectomy involves the removal of the intact bladder along with perivesical fat and the prostate in men or the uterus, ovaries, urethra, and anterior vagina in women. A complete pelvic node dissection is integral to surgery. (For details of the radical cystectomy surgery please see Chapter 16.)

B, Urothelial carcinoma is the most common histologic subtype of bladder cancer in the United States.

Left: A high-grade invasive tumor with nests of cells with large hyperchromatic nuclei and high mitotic rate is shown. *Middle*: Micropapillary bladder cancer is a rare aggressive variant of urothelial carcinoma, as demonstrated by Kamat *et al.* [10]. Histologically, there are infiltrating clusters of micropapillary tumor without central vascular cores. Intravesical Bacillus Calmette-Guérin is ineffective in these patients. It has been suggested that patients with micropapillary histology should be offered immediate radical cystectomy because of observed rapid progression even in the absence of muscle invasion on transurethral resection. *Right*: Sarcomatoid bladder cancer is another aggressive variant that contains epithelial and mesenchymal elements. Patients with this variant have a poor prognosis and often present at a more advanced stage.

C, Squamous cell carcinoma of the bladder accounts for the majority of bladder cancer in areas where schistosomiasis is endemic. In Western countries, squamous cell carcinoma represents less than 5% of cases and is associated with spinal cord injury and indwelling urinary catheter. Histologically, keratin production is seen in these tumors and the degree of differentiation is estimated by keratinization.

D, Mucinous adenocarcinoma of the bladder. This uncommon tumor accounts for less than 1% of cases in the United States. It may be associated with the urachus (urachal tumor) or the bladder wall and has secondary involvement of the epithelium. Under microscopy, tumor cells appear with a background of mucin. (*Courtesy of* Charles Guo, MD.)

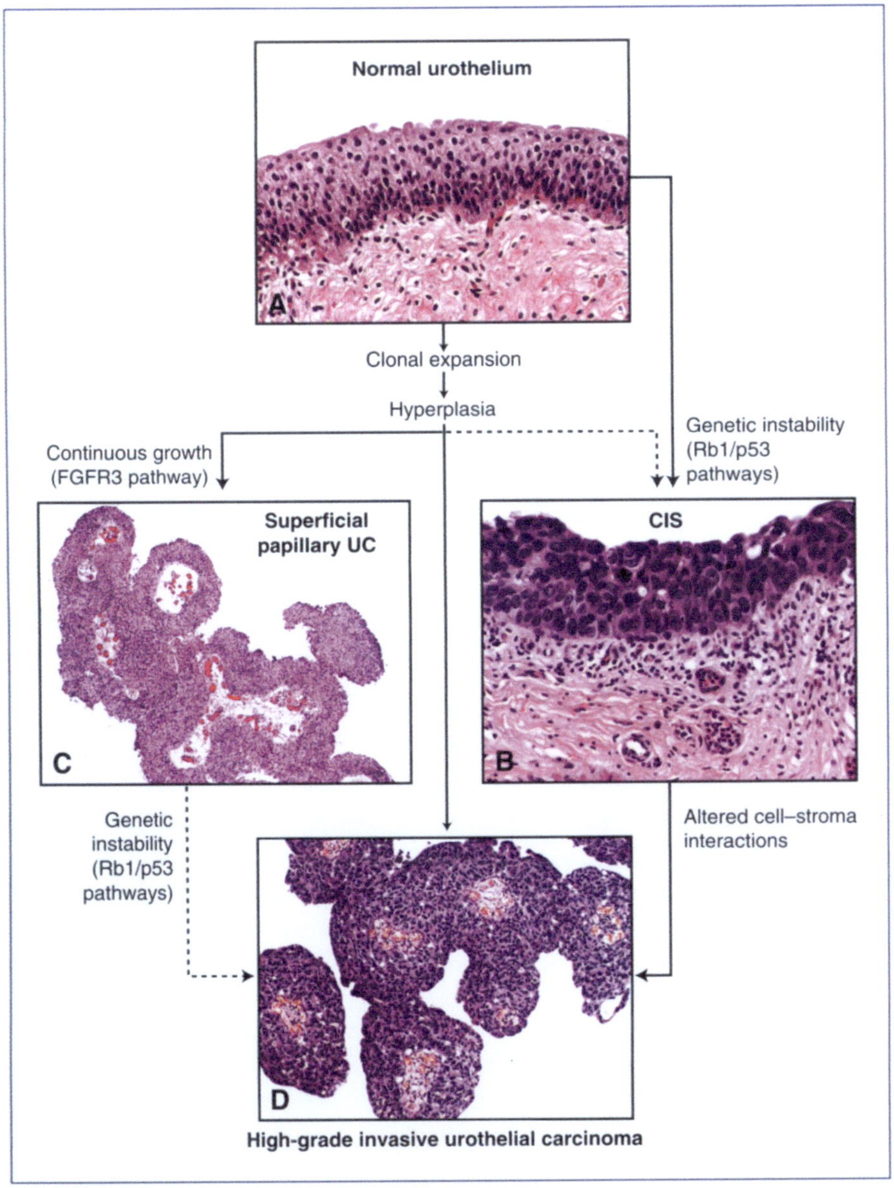

FIGURE 15-10. Pathology normal to high grade. **A**, Normal urothelial lining. **B**, Carcinoma in situ. **C**, Low grade. **D**, High grade.

The normal bladder urothelium is a transitional epithelium with five to seven cell layers composed of umbrella, intermediate, and basal cells. Various hypotheses of bladder cancer pathogenesis have been put forward. In the most commonly accepted, a dual-tract concept of bladder carcinogenesis/urothelial cancers arise from two distinct pathways with some overlap between subtypes. The majority (80%) of cancers are papillary and exophytic; these tumors recur frequently, but rarely become invasive. Microscopically, these lesions appear papillary with fibrovascular stalks and rare cytologic atypia or mitoses. The most common genetic abnormality is a loss of all or part of chromosome 9, but overall low-grade tumors rarely have chromosomal abnormalities. In addition, a variety of mutations in the fibroblast growth factor receptor 3 (FGFR3) have been described, which are primarily associated with low-grade papillary urothelial carcinoma or precursor lesions (urothelial papilloma).

Alternatively, tumors may progress through a nonpapillary pathway to form high-grade lesions. The genetic alterations involved include p53 and Rb. Carcinoma in situ shows severe cytologic atypia, a pleomorphic appearance with numerous mitoses, and noncohesive cells, which allows detection using cytology. High-grade lesions have a high mitotic rate and frequently become invasive. Mutations of FGFR3 and tumor p53 (associated with high-grade lesions) typically have an inverse relationship, which provides further evidence that high-grade tumors evolve along a separate pathway from low-grade tumors [11,12]. (*Courtesy of* Charles Guo, MD.)

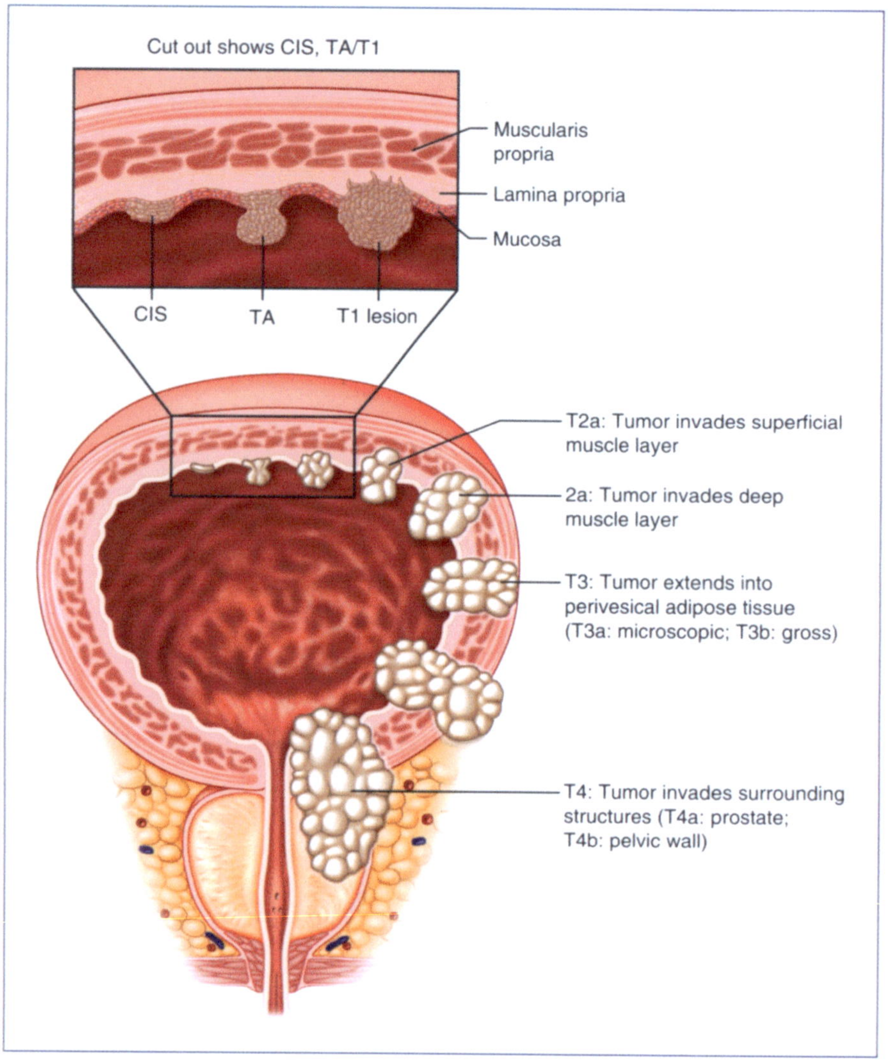

Figure 15-11. Staging system for bladder cancer. Staging information is provided from the physical examination (including bimanual examination under anesthesia), axial imaging, and from a pathologic examination of the resected tumor. Stage is a primary prognostic factor for survival. Patients who have disease confined to the bladder (T2) have a significantly improved survival compared to advanced stages.

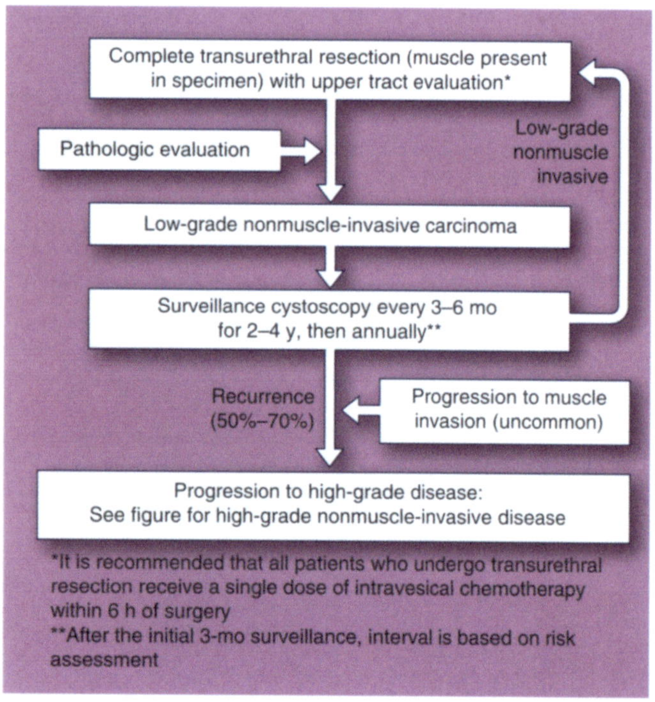

Figure 15-12. Management of low-grade nonmuscle-invasive bladder cancer. Low-grade tumors, while not immediately life threatening, require appropriate treatment. Although tumors frequently recur (50%–70%), they rarely progress to high-grade lesions (less than 7%) or become invasive. Thus, the majority of patients can be treated with repeated transurethral resection with or without intravesical chemotherapy or immunotherapy. Radical cystectomy is appropriate for patients who progress or have extensive functional damage to their bladder from repeated resections.

All patients undergoing a transurethral resection of a bladder tumor should be considered for perioperative chemotherapy instilled into the bladder, ideally within the first 6 hours and certainly within 24 hours of resection. A meta-analysis of 1476 patients showed that a single dose of intravesical mitomycin after transurethral resection decreased the odds of recurrence by 39%. Patients who develop multiple recurrences may be considered for induction and maintenance therapy with intravesical immunotherapy (Bacillus Calmette-Guérin) or chemotherapy.

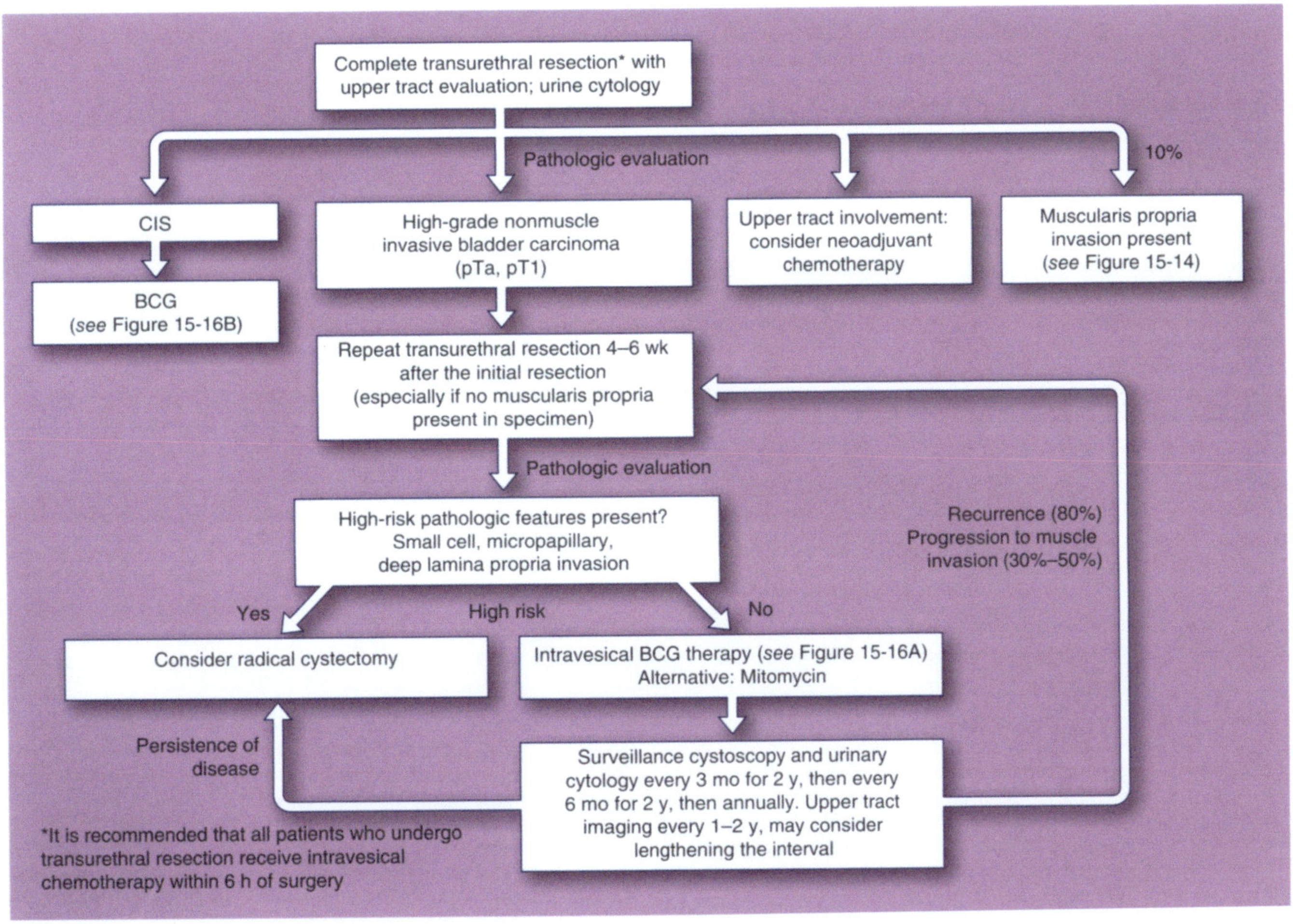

Figure 15-13. Management of high-grade nonmuscle-invasive bladder cancer. High-grade tumors may be confined to epithelium or lamina propria. High-grade tumors have increased potential to become invasive and metastasize. Up to 50% of tumors invading the lamina propria may eventually progress.

After the initial resection, careful evaluation of the specimen is required. All patients with high-grade tumors initially staged as T1 should be re-resected at 4 to 6 weeks postsurgery. Repeat transurethral resection is especially important in T1 tumors without muscle present in the specimen, since as many as half of patients may be understaged.

Induction and maintenance with Bacillus Calmette-Guérin immunotherapy is the treatment of choice (see Figure 15-16) for patients who elect initial conservative management of high-grade nonmuscle-invasive bladder cancer. In a subset of patients who are at high risk for disease progression, a more aggressive treatment with early radical cystectomy is considered to be appropriate. It is known that a significant percentage of patients with low-stage high-grade disease will ultimately require cystectomy and patients who have cystectomy at a lower stage have improved survival when compared to patients with muscle-invasive disease. In addition, cystectomy provides accurate staging and theoretically treats patients at an earlier point in the course of the disease. Early radical cystectomy should be discussed with all patients and pursued in patients with a high risk of disease [13–17].

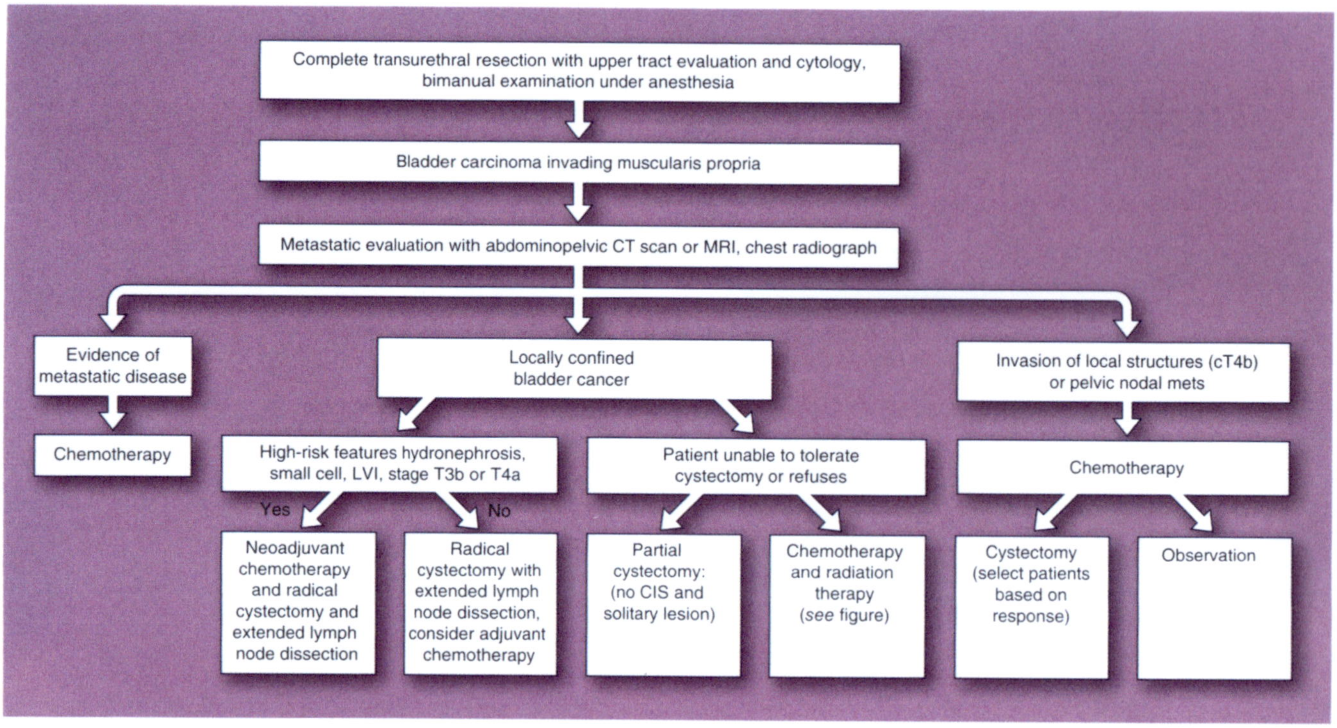

FIGURE 15-14. Management of muscle-invasive bladder cancer. Up to 25% of patients will present with bladder tumors that invade into or beyond the muscularis propria. Bimanual examination under anesthesia and axial imaging (*eg*, with a CT scan) are important to evaluate the extent of disease. Unfortunately, current imaging modalities have poor accuracy to detect extravesical extension and micrometastatic disease when compared to surgical pathology; thus, an assessment of risk factors must be made using clinical data.

Standard therapy for muscle-invasive bladder cancer is radical cystoprostatectomy in males and anterior pelvic exenteration in females, along with extended lymph node dissection. Neoadjuvant chemotherapy has been shown in randomized trials to provide a survival advantage and should be offered to all patients with muscle-invasive disease and especially to patients with high-risk features, including pathologic lymphovascular invasion, hydronephrosis, and stage T3 disease or greater. Patients may be offered adjuvant chemotherapy if advanced stage or lymph node metastases are discovered after surgery.

Patients who present with tumors that invade local structures or who have metastatic disease at presentation have a poor prognosis and should be offered chemotherapy as first-line therapy. Select patients who respond to chemotherapy can be offered radical cystectomy since a proportion of patients will derive benefit from such multimodal therapy [18–23].

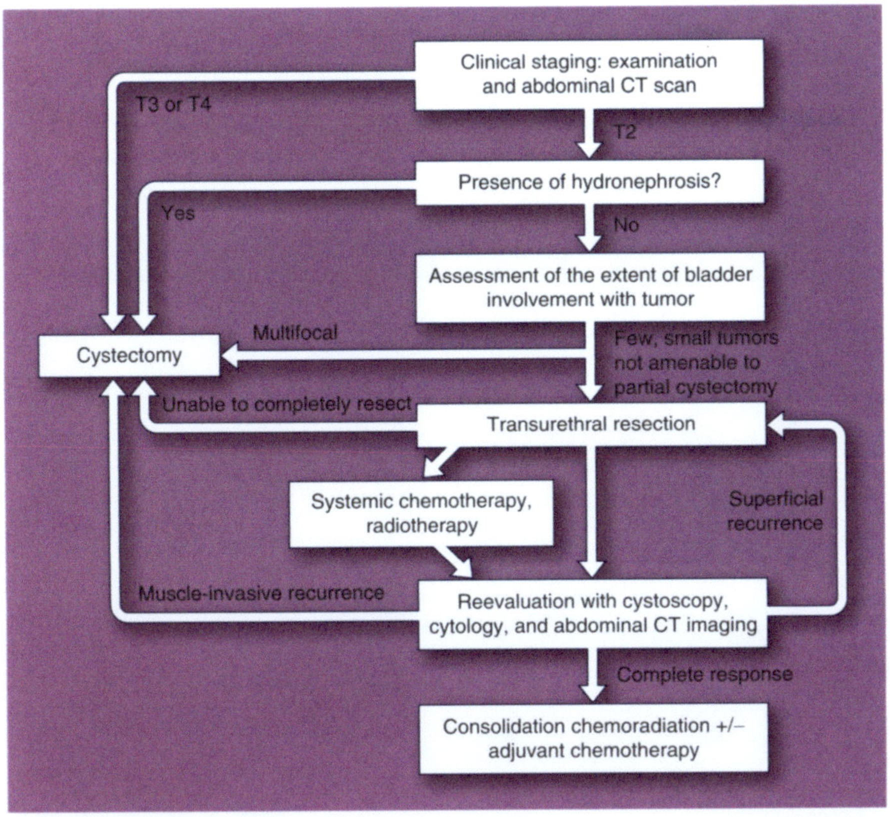

Figure 15-15. Chemoradiation for bladder cancer. Radical cystectomy is the gold standard of care for muscle-invasive bladder cancer in most patients. However, certain patients who are not candidates for radical surgery or refuse surgery may be considered for radiation therapy. In patients who undergo bladder-preservation protocols, induction radiation is initiated after appropriate transurethral resection and risk assessment. The radiation field includes the tumor site, the entire bladder, and regional lymph nodes. In patients with a complete response to induction, consolidation chemoradiation is performed. Select retrospective series [25] have shown similar disease-specific survival to radical cystectomy in pT2-4 patients, but this therapeutic approach has not been widely adopted in the United States [24,25].

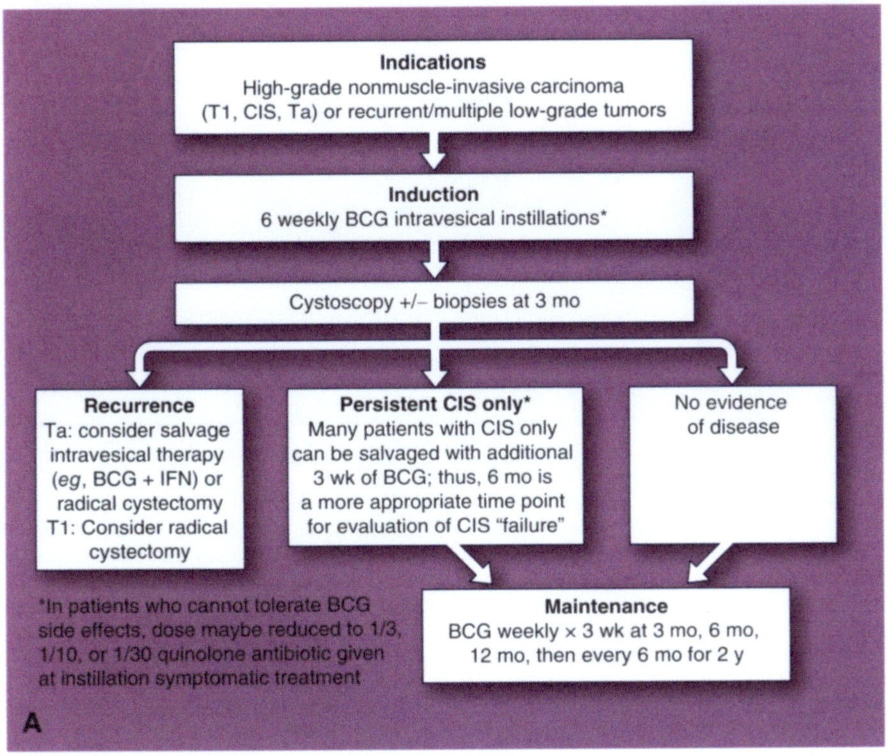

Figure 15-16. **A,** Intravesical immunotherapy for bladder cancer. Bacillus Calmette-Guérin (BCG) is an attenuated form of Mycobacterium tuberculosis, which is effective therapy for appropriately selected patients with non-muscle-invasive bladder cancer.

Continued on the next page

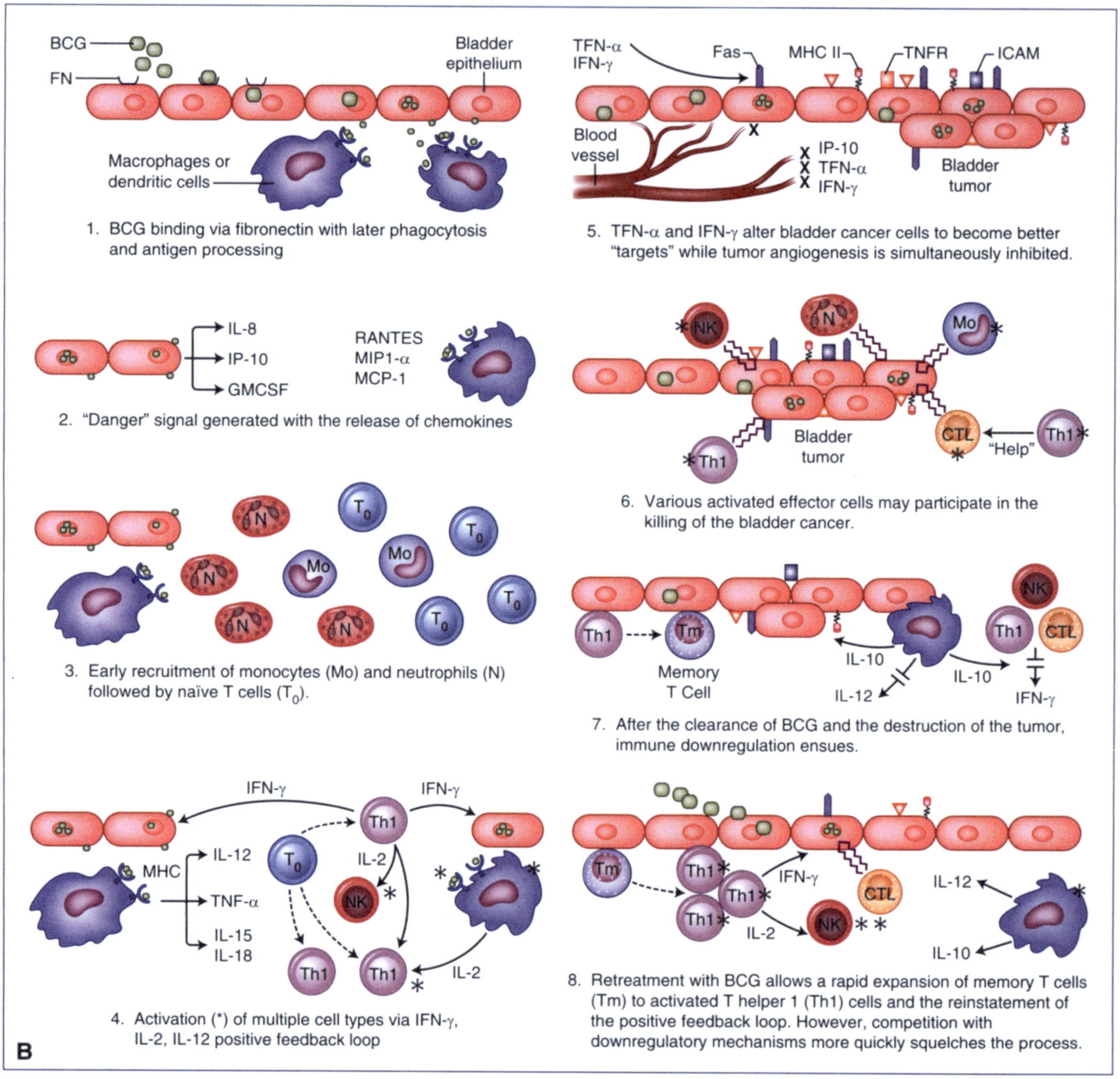

1. BCG binding via fibronectin with later phagocytosis and antigen processing

2. "Danger" signal generated with the release of chemokines

3. Early recruitment of monocytes (Mo) and neutrophils (N) followed by naïve T cells (T_0).

4. Activation (*) of multiple cell types via IFN-γ, IL-2, IL-12 positive feedback loop

5. TFN-α and IFN-γ alter bladder cancer cells to become better "targets" while tumor angiogenesis is simultaneously inhibited.

6. Various activated effector cells may participate in the killing of the bladder cancer.

7. After the clearance of BCG and the destruction of the tumor, immune downregulation ensues.

8. Retreatment with BCG allows a rapid expansion of memory T cells (Tm) to activated T helper 1 (Th1) cells and the reinstatement of the positive feedback loop. However, competition with downregulatory mechanisms more quickly squelches the process.

Figure 15-16. *(Continued)* While BCG has been used for bladder cancer since the 1970s, the exact mechanism of action remains unknown to this date. A proposed mechanism is displayed in **B**. *(Adapted from* O'Donnell and Burns [36].)

BCG immunotherapy is effective only when the therapy is administered appropriately. After a standard 6-week induction course (weekly instillation into the bladder), most patients should receive maintenance therapy. While many regimens have been put forward, the most effective is that reported by the Southwest Oncology Group, which involves 3 weekly instillations at 3 and 6 months, and then every 6 months. Although maintenance therapy has shown benefit in prospective studies, many patients cannot complete the entire regimen because of adverse effects of treatment. A variety of strategies have been devised in order to decrease symptoms and allow the patient to continue therapy by minimizing symptoms. Rarely, severe febrile reactions may require emergent systemic treatment.

Patients who fail initial BCG therapy are at a high risk for disease progression. While several "salvage" regimens have been tried, at this time there is no effective therapy for patients failing two courses of BCG; these patients should be considered for radical cystectomy [13,15]. CTL—cytotoxic T lymphocyte; GMCSF—granulocyte macrophage colony-stimulating factor; ICAM—intercellular adhesion molecule; IFN-γ—interferon-γ; IL-2—interleukin-2; IL-8—interleukin-8; IL-12—interleukin-12; IL-15—interleukin-15; IL-18—interleukin-18; IP-10—interferon-inducible protein-10; MCP-1—monocyte chemotactic protein-1; MHC—major histocompatability complex; MIP1-α—macrophage inflammatory protein; NK—natural killer; RANTES—regulated on activation, normal T expressed and secreted; TFN-α—tumor necrosis factor-α; Th1—T helper cell subset 1; TNFR—tumor necrosis factor receptor.

Five-Year Survival Rates (%) after Radical Cystectomy, by Stage				
Study	**Patients, no**	**pT2**	**pT3**	**pT4**
Richie, 1975	134	40	20	—
Mathur, 1981	58	77	33	29
Skinner, 1984	197	64	44	36
Montie *et al.*, 1984 [26]	99	69	57	—
Giuliani, 1985	202	56	19	0
Roehrborn, 1991	280	63	36	24
Pagano *et al.*, 1991 [21]	261	57	15	21
Wishnow, 1992	188	79	46	33
Waehre *et al.*, 1993 [27]	227	61	36	29
Vieweg *et al.*, 1999 [28]	686	58	22	15
Stein *et al.*, 2001 [23]	633	72	48	33
Dalbagni *et al.*, 2001 [19]	284	59	29	25
Madersbacher, 2003	507	74	52	36
Grossman *et al.*, 2003 [20]	154	75	—	28

FIGURE 15-17. Five-year survival rates after radical cystectomy, by stage. Survival after radical cystectomy in a contemporary series is increased when compared to historical series. This increased survival is attributed to improved surgical techniques, and to perioperative and postoperative care. This table is a summary of survival data from various trials. (*Adapted from* Herr *et al.* [18].)

Approved Urinary Markers for Bladder Cancer					
Marker	**Description**	**Sensitivity**	**Specificity**	**Advantages**	**Disadvantages**
Hematuria	Dipstick or microscropic evaluation	47%–74% initial, 90%–95% serial testing		Inexpensive, widely available	Poor sensitivity and specificity
Cytology	Microscropic analysis of cells in urine	80%–90% high grade, 35%–65% in low grade	90%–100%	Very specific, good for high grade and CIS	Not sensitive for low-grade disease, requires trained pathologist
BTA-Stat, BTA-TRAK	Assay for human complement factor-H–related protein	43%–89%	19%–70%	Inexpensive, BTA-Stat available point of care	False positive with hematuria or inflammation
NMP-22	ELISA for nuclear matrix protein	47%–100%	60%–80%	Inexpensive, able to identify lesions not seen on cystoscopy	False positive with hematuria or inflammation
BladderChek	ELISA for nuclear matrix protein	50%–85%	40%–90%	Point of care, inexpensive	Expensive, false-positives high in "real world" situations
FISH	Probes for polysomy of Chr 3,7,17 or loss of 9p21	73%–87%	90%–96%	Sensitive in occult disease	Expensive, false positives high in "real world" situations
Immunocyt, uCyt	Monoclonal antibodies applied to cytology	40%–95%	60%–70%	Sensitive for low-grade cancer	Expensive

FIGURE 15-18. Summary of available urinary tests for bladder cancer. While cystoscopy is described as the gold standard for the diagnosis of bladder cancer, it is poor for detecting carcinoma in situ and may miss small papillary lesions. Several biomarkers have been approved to help increase bladder cancer detection. Cytology has been used for many years and is highly specific, but lacks sensitivity. Newer biomarkers have improved sensitivity but are associated with more false negatives and false positives. The clinical utility and proper role in detecting initial and recurrent disease is being investigated; however, current data (and author experience) suggest that, in experienced hands, cystoscopy remains the gold standard and adjunct tests should be reserved for situations where an early detection of recurrence (*eg*, high-grade T1 lesions) would change patient management. CIS—carcinoma in situ. (*Adapted from* Shirodkar and Lokeshwar [29].)

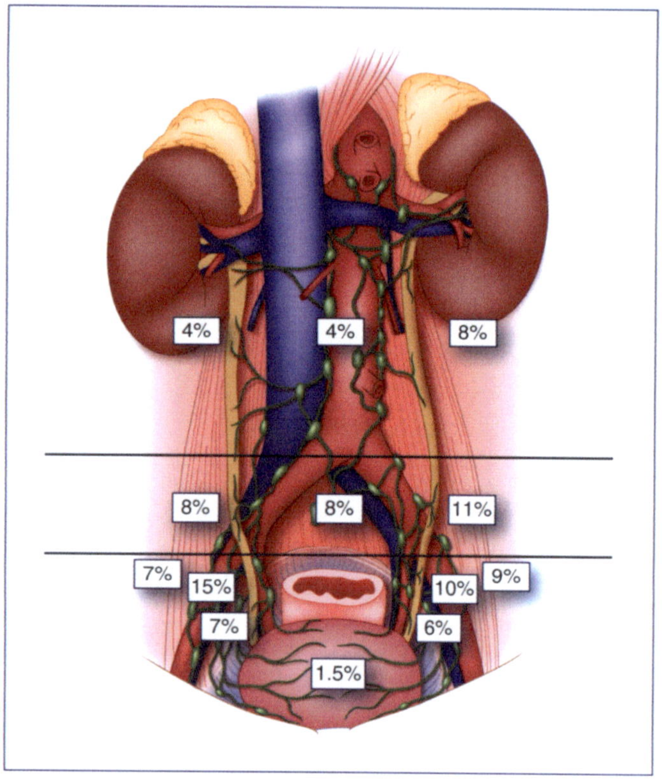

FIGURE 15-19. Sites of nodal metastases observed after lymph node dissection. The percentage yield of lymph nodes in an extended lymphadenectomy (based on 599 nodal metastases in 290 patients [4]) is shown. The risk of lymph node metastases increases as stage increases. Obturator and external iliac lymph nodes are the most commonly involved with metastatic disease, while metastases to the common iliac and presacral lymph nodes are seen less frequently.

Extended pelvic lymphadenectomy is an important diagnostic and therapeutic component to surgical treatment for bladder cancer and may extend long-term survival. The extent of lymphadenectomy has been suggested to influence survival as the increased total number of lymph nodes removed correlates with increased survival. Such a lymphadenectomy should involve the distal preaortic and precaval lymph nodes, as well as the presacral nodes. Meticulous dissection is needed in all patients regardless of clinical stage, because isolated metastatic disease in less common sites has been reported in patients without lyphadenopathy in common sites. In addition, lymph node density (the total number of positive nodes divided by the total number of lymph nodes removed) is a sensitive predictor of disease specific survival in node positive patients [28,31,32]. (*Percentages from* Leissner *et al.* [30].)

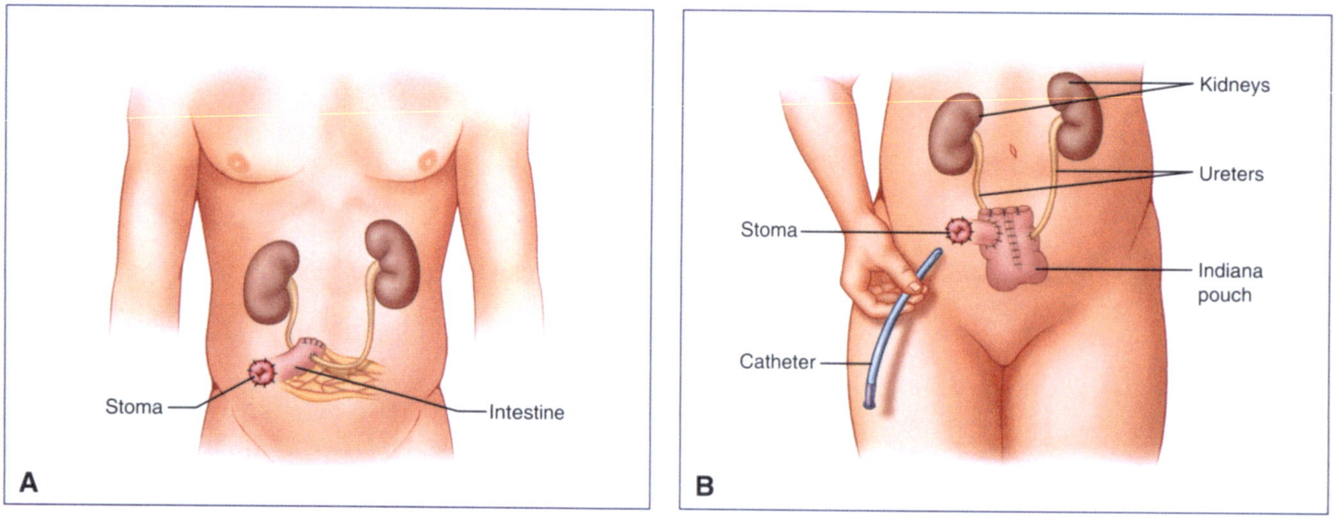

FIGURE 15-20. Cystectomy and urinary diversion. Radical cystoprostatectomy in males and anterior pelvic exenteration in females is the gold standard for patients with muscle-invasive bladder tumors, as well as for some nonmuscle-invasive high-grade tumors. Recent modifications to the neurovascular bundle in appropriately selected males may allow for recovery of postoperative sexual function. In addition, some female patients with no involvement of the bladder neck may be candidates for urethral sparing.

There are many options available for urinary diversions after cystectomy. An ileal conduit (**A**) is a common diversion in which a small segment of small bowel (usually terminal ileum) is resected and connected to the ureters on the proximal end. The distal end is brought out though the abdominal wall and an ostomy is created. Although it requires an external appliance to collect urine, patients report excellent quality of life with this type of diversion, with minimal maintenance. Another option is the creation of a cutaneous catheterizable pouch. There are many options using different bowel segments and multiple approaches have been devised to recreate a continence mechanism that will function with repeated catheterization. One example is the "Indiana pouch" (**B**), which is created using the cecum, ascending colon, and a buttressed ileocecal valve as a continence mechanism.

Continued on the next page

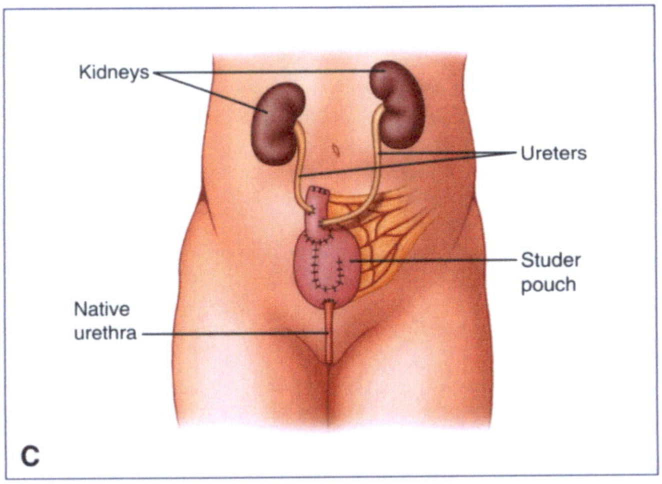

FIGURE 15-20. *(Continued)* With the advent of the "orthotopic neobladder," many patients are able to void via the urethra. A common method used for the orthotopic continent diversion is the neobladder, shown in **C**. Herein, a section of ileum is resected and detubularized to serve as a reservoir for urine collection. The ureters are connected to the bowel in the afferent limb and the neobladder is connected to the urethra distally through an opening created in the bowel wall. Patients with a functioning external sphincter apparatus after surgery have high rates of daytime continence.

Summary/Comparison of the Two Commonly Used Chemotherapeutic Regimens in Urothelial Cancer

	MVAC	GC
Regimen (28-d cycles)	Methotrexate 30 mg/m^2 days 1, 15, 22 Vinblastine 3 mg/m^2 days 2, 15, 22 Adriamycin 30 mg/m^2 day 2 Cisplatin 70 mg/m^2 day 2	Gemcitabine 1000 mg/m^2 days 1, 15, 22 Cisplatin 70 mg/m^2 day 2
N	202	203
Median overall survival (months)	15.2	14
5-y overall survival	15.30%	13%
Side effects	Neutropenia; mucositis; nausea and vomiting; anemia; thrombocytopenia; renal, cardiac, and neurologic toxicity; alopecia	Thrombocytopenia, renal toxicity, anemia, neutropenia, nausea and vomiting, alopecia
Drug-related mortality	3%	1%
Response rate	46%	49%

FIGURE 15-21. Chemotherapy for bladder cancer. Chemotherapy for bladder cancer may be given in the neoadjuvant, adjuvant, or palliative setting. The two most common regimens are MVAC (methotrexate, vinblastine, doxorubicin) or GC (gemcitabine plus cisplatin), as shown in this table. In a multicenter randomized trial of patients with stage IV bladder cancer, there was no statistically significant difference in the response rate or survival between the two groups. In the GC group, there were more patients with grade 3 or 4 thrombocytopenia compared with the MVAC group, who had more neutropenia, neutropenic fever, sepsis, and mucositis. The quality of life was similar between the groups.

The results of randomized clinical trials with neoadjuvant MVAC have demonstrated an overall survival advantage, which led to recommendations that neoadjuvant chemotherapy be given to patients with muscle-invasive bladder cancer. Another advantage to neoadjuvant therapy is that it may be easier for patients to tolerate chemotherapy prior to surgery and it allows timely therapy. [20,33,34]. (*Adapted from* von der Maase *et al.* [35].)

References

1. Jemal A, Siegel R, Ward E, *et al.*: Cancer statistics, 2008. *CA Cancer J Clin* 2008, 58:71–96.
2. Jankovic S, Radosavljevic V: Risk factors for bladder cancer. *Tumori* 2007, 93:4–12.
3. Mueller CM, Caporaso N, Greene MH: Familial and genetic risk of transitional cell carcinoma of the urinary tract. *Urol Oncol* 2008, 26:451–464.
4. Olfert SM, Felknor SA, Delclos GL: An updated review of the literature: risk factors for bladder cancer with focus on occupational exposures. *South Med J* 2006, 99:1256–1263.
5. Scelo G, Brennan P: The epidemiology of bladder and kidney cancer. *Nat Clin Pract Urol* 2007, 4:205–217.
6. Agarwal PK, Black PC, Kamat AM: Considerations on the use of diagnostic markers in management of patients with bladder cancer. *World J Urol* 2008, 26:39–44.
7. Grossfeld GD, Litwin MS, Wolf JS, *et al.*: Evaluation of asymptomatic microscopic hematuria in adults: the American Urological Association best practice policy—part I: definition, detection, prevalence, and etiology. *Urology* 57: 2001, 599–603.
8. Messing EM, Vaillancourt A: Hematuria screening for bladder cancer. *J Occup Med* 1990, 32:838–845.
9. Grossman HB, Gomella L, Fradet Y, *et al.*: A phase III, multicenter comparison of hexaminolevulinate fluorescence cystoscopy and white light cystoscopy for the detection of superficial papillary lesions in patients with bladder cancer. *J Urol* 2007, 178:62–67.
10. Kamat AM, Dinney CP, Gee JR, *et al.*: Micropapillary bladder cancer: a review of the University of Texas M. D. Anderson Cancer Center experience with 100 consecutive patients. *Cancer* 2007, 110:62–67.

11. Dinney CP, McConkey DJ, Millikan RE, *et al.*: Focus on bladder cancer. *Cancer Cell* 2004, 6:111–116.

12. Knowles MA: Role of FGFR3 in urothelial cell carcinoma: biomarker and potential therapeutic target. *World J Urol* 2007, 25:581–593.

13. Brassell SA, Kamat AM: Contemporary intravesical treatment options for urothelial carcinoma of the bladder. *J Natl Compr Canc Netw* 2006, 4:1027–1036.

14. Hall MC, Chang SS, Dalbagni G, *et al.*: Guideline for the management of nonmuscle invasive bladder cancer (stages Ta, T1, and Tis): 2007 update. *J Urol* 2007, 178:2314–2330.

15. Kamat AM: Intravesical BCG for bladder cancer: how much is enough? *Cancer* 2008,113:674–676.

16. Metwalli AR, Kamat AM: Controversial issues and optimal management of stage T1G3 bladder cancer. *Expert Rev Anticancer Ther* 2006, 6:1283–1294.

17. Sylvester RJ, Oosterlinck W, van der Meijden AP: A single immediate post-operative instillation of chemotherapy decreases the risk of recurrence in patients with stage Ta T1 bladder cancer: a meta-analysis of published results of randomized clinical trials. *J Urol* 2004,171:2186–190, quiz 2435.

18. Herr HW, Dotan Z, Donat SM, Bajorin DF: Defining optimal therapy for muscle invasive bladder cancer. *J Urol* 2007, 177:437–443.

19. Dalbagni G, Genega E, Hashibe M, *et al.*: Cystectomy for bladder cancer: a contemporary series. *J Urol* 2001, 165:1111–1116.

20. Grossman HB, Natale RB, Tangen CM, *et al.*: Neoadjuvant chemotherapy plus cystectomy compared with cystectomy alone for locally advanced bladder cancer. *N Engl J Med* 2003, 349:859–866.

21. Pagano F, Bassi P, Galetti TP, *et al.*: Results of contemporary radical cystectomy for invasive bladder cancer: a clinicopathological study with an emphasis on the inadequacy of the tumor, nodes and metastases classification. *J Urol* 1991, 145:45–50.

22. Shariat SF, Karakiewicz PI, Palapattu GS, *et al.*: Outcomes of radical cystectomy for transitional cell carcinoma of the bladder: a contemporary series from the Bladder Cancer Research Consortium. *J Urol* 2006, 176:2414–2222; discussion 2422.

23. Stein JP, Lieskovsky G, Cote R, *et al.*: Radical cystectomy in the treatment of invasive bladder cancer: long-term results in 1,054 patients. *J Clin Oncol* 2001,19:666–675.

24. Coen JJ, Zietman AL, Kaufman DS, Shipley WU: Benchmarks achieved in the delivery of radiation therapy for muscle-invasive bladder cancer. *Urol Oncol* 2007, 25:76–84.

25. Shipley WU, Kaufman DS, Zehr E, *et al.*: Selective bladder preservation by combined modality protocol treatment: long-term outcomes of 190 patients with invasive bladder cancer. *Urology* 2002, 60:62–67; discussion 67–68.

26. Montie JE, Straffon RA, Stewart BH: Radical cystectomy without radiation therapy for carcinoma of the bladder. *J Urol* 1984, 131:477–482.

27. Waehre H, Ous S, Klevmark B, *et al.*: A bladder cancer multi-institutional experience with total cystectomy for muscle-invasive bladder cancer. *Cancer* 1993, 72:3044–3051.

28. Vieweg J, Gschwend JE, Herr HW, Fair WR: The impact of primary stage on survival in patients with lymph node positive bladder cancer. *J Urol* 1999,161:72–76.

29. Shirodkar SP, Lokeshwar VB: Bladder tumor markers: from hematuria to molecular diagnostics—where do we stand? *Expert Rev Anticancer Ther* 2008, 8:1111–1123.

30. Leissner J, Ghoneim MA, Abol-Enein H, *et al.*: Extended radical lymphadenectomy in patients with urothelial bladder cancer: results of a prospective multicenter study. *J Urol* 2004, 171:139–144.

31. Kassouf W, Agarwal PK, Herr HW, *et al.*: Lymph node density is superior to TNM nodal status in predicting disease-specific survival after radical cystectomy for bladder cancer: analysis of pooled data from MDACC and MSKCC. *J Clin Oncol* 2008, 26:121–126.

32. Leissner J, Ghoneim MA, Abol-Enein H, *et al.*: Extended radical lymphadenectomy in patients with urothelial bladder cancer: results of a prospective multicenter study. *J Urol* 2004, 171:139–144.

33. Sternberg CN, Donat SM, Bellmunt J, *et al.*: Chemotherapy for bladder cancer: treatment guidelines for neoadjuvant chemotherapy, bladder preservation, adjuvant chemotherapy, and metastatic cancer. *Urology* 2007, 69:62–79.

34. von der Maase H, Hansen SW, Roberts JT, *et al.*: Gemcitabine and cisplatin versus methotrexate, vinblastine, doxorubicin, and cisplatin in advanced or metastatic bladder cancer: results of a large, randomized, multinational, multicenter, phase III study. *J Clin Oncol* 2000,18:3068–3077.

35. von der Maase H, Sengelov L, Roberts JT, *et al.*: Long-term survival results of a randomized trial comparing gemcitabine plus cisplatin, with methotrexate, vinblastine, doxorubicin, plus cisplatin in patients with bladder cancer. *J Clin Oncol* 2005, 23:4602–4608.

36. O'Donnell MA, Burns J: Intravesical BCG in treatment and prophylaxis of urothelial bladder cancer. In *Urothelial Tumors: American Cancer Society Atlas of Clinical Oncology*. Edited by Droller MJ. Hamilton, ON, Canada: BC Decker; 2004;219–247.

16 Robotic-Assisted Laparoscopic Radical Cystectomy

Declan G. Murphy and Prokar Dasgupta

Open radical cystectomy with pelvic lymph node dissection remains the gold standard for muscle-invasive or high-risk nonmuscle-invasive bladder cancer in patients who are fit for surgery [1,2]. However, significant morbidity is associated with this procedure in 20% to 50% of patients [3,4] and hospital stays in the United Kingdom average 18.7 days [5].

Therefore, urologists are exploring minimally invasive options to reduce this morbidity. Laparoscopic radical cystectomy (LRC) has been reported in over 500 patients and evidence suggests that the laparoscopic approach may allow for less blood loss, decreased postoperative pain, and quicker recovery compared with open surgery [6,7]. However, LRC has not yet enjoyed widespread popularity, largely due to the technical difficulty involved and the lack of long-term oncological outcomes.

The introduction of robotic assistance using the da Vinci surgical system (Intuitive Surgical Inc.; Mountain View, CA) offers technical advantages that may be of use during LRC [8]. Three-dimensional vision with 10× magnification, wristed instruments that offer an improved range of motion, motion scaling, and superior ergonomics all are of benefit when performing complex pelvic laparoscopic surgery. Robotic-assisted radical cystectomy (RARC) was first reported by Menon *et al.* [9] in 2003. The operative times ranged from 260 to 308 minutes, depending on whether or not an ileal conduit or orthotopic neobladder was formed. Blood loss was less than 150 mLs and surgical margins were clear in all cases.

Since then, a number of other small series have been reported. Guru *et al.* [10] reported on their experience with RARC and extracorporeal urinary diversion in 20 patients. The mean total operative time for the series was 442 minutes, including 133 minutes for the urinary diversion. Pruthi and Wallen [11] also reported on a series of 20 patients who underwent RARC with extracorporeal urinary diversion. The mean total operative time for this series was 366 minutes and the complication rate was 30%, which included one rectal injury (repaired intra-operatively), one postoperative hemorrhage requiring laparotomy, and one parastomal hernia requiring repair.

Rhee *et al.* [12] compared seven RARCs to 23 open radical cystectomies (ORCs). They utilized a midline incision to extract the specimen and fashion the ileal conduit, and also performed pelvic lymphadenectomy through this incision. The mean operative durations were 638 and 507 minutes for the RARC and open radical cystectomy, respectively, and the hospital stays averaged 11 and 13 days, respectively.

Wang *et al.* [13] compared their series of 33 RARCs with 21 ORCs. Operative times were longer (390 vs 300 minutes) but blood loss (400 vs 750 mL) and hospital stays (5 vs 8 days) were shorter in the RARC group. Complication rates were similar.

In our initial experience, we reported on 23 patients who underwent RARC and extracorporeal urinary diversion [14]. The mean total operative time was 397 minutes with a mean hospital stay of 11.6 days. Only one patient required a blood transfusion.

Although RARC with completely intracorporeal urinary diversion has been reported [15,16], long operating times have prevented the widespread adoption of this approach and most units prefer an extracorporeal approach for urinary diversion [6,17].

These early experiences of RARC are encouraging and, as larger series are reported, it is possible that the robotic-assisted laparoscopic approach will develop a defined role for radical cystectomy. At this time, however, RARC must still be considered an investigational intervention as the procedure continues to evolve and longer-term outcomes are awaited.

In the procedure illustrated in this chapter, RARC is performed on a male patient using a three-arm da Vinci surgical system (Intuitive Surgical Inc.; Sunnyvale, CA). Procedural modifications for a four-arm robot and for a female patient are included where appropriate.

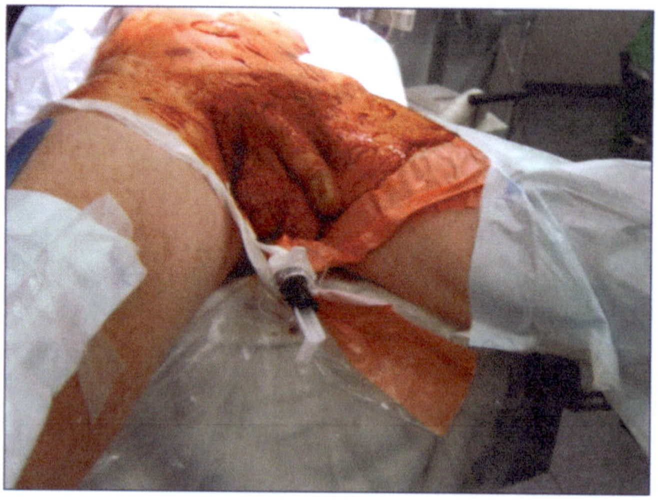

FIGURE 16-1. Patient position for robotic-assisted laparoscopic radical cystectomy. A pneumatic leg-compression system is used for prophylaxis of deep vein thrombosis. The bladder is catheterized and the patient's legs are secured in a modified lithotomy position using Yellofin stirrups (Allen Medical; Acton, MA) with Gelfoam padding (Pfizer; New York, NY). All pressure points are carefully padded with the arms by the patient's side and the patient is secured to the table using heavy elastic tape. A Bair Hugger warming system (Arizant Ltd; Yorkshire, UK) is used to control the patient's upper body temperature. The table is placed in the 45-degree Trendelenburg position and the patient is checked to ensure that he or she remains secure in the desired position. The hips are extended enough to allow subsequent docking of the robot. The table can be returned to the neutral position until the port is inserted.

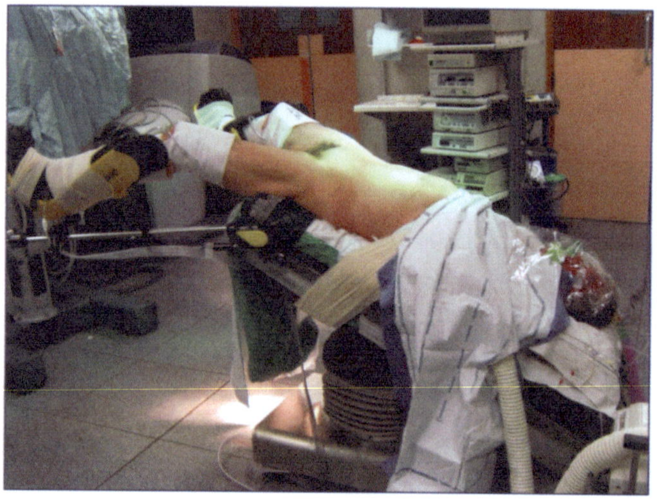

FIGURE 16-2. Disposable sigmoidoscope in the rectum. In male patients, a disposable sigmoidoscope is inserted into the rectum to aid in its subsequent identification. This is placed during patient positioning and is secured in place using adhesive tapes. The sigmoidoscope is covered with sterile drapes during patient preparation but is still readily maneuverable by the assistant during the procedure, thereby allowing the rectum to be identified and retracted posteriorly during dissection between the bladder and rectum.

In women, a methylene blue-soaked swab stick is placed in the vagina during patient positioning, which can be similarly maneuvered to aid in dissection between the bladder and vagina.

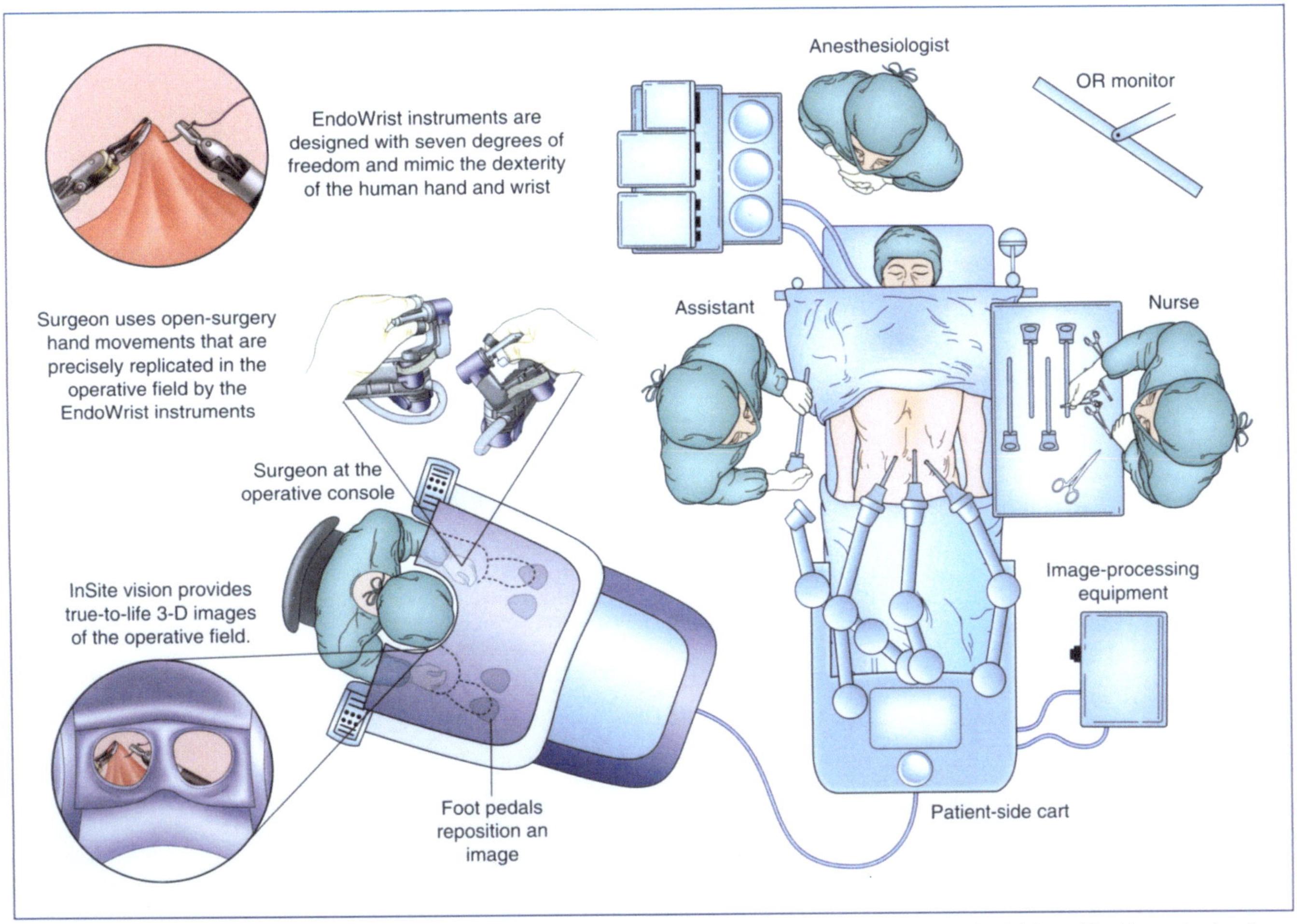

FIGURE 16-3. Theater setup for robotic-assisted laparoscopic radical cystectomy (RARC). A typical setup for RARC using a four-arm da Vinci surgical system (Intuitive Surgical Inc.; Sunnyvale, CA) is illustrated here. For a three-arm system, a second patient-side assistant is required on the right side. EndoWrist—Intuitive Surgical Inc.; Mountain View, CA; InSite Vision—Intuitive Surgical Inc.; Mountain View, CA; OR—operating room.

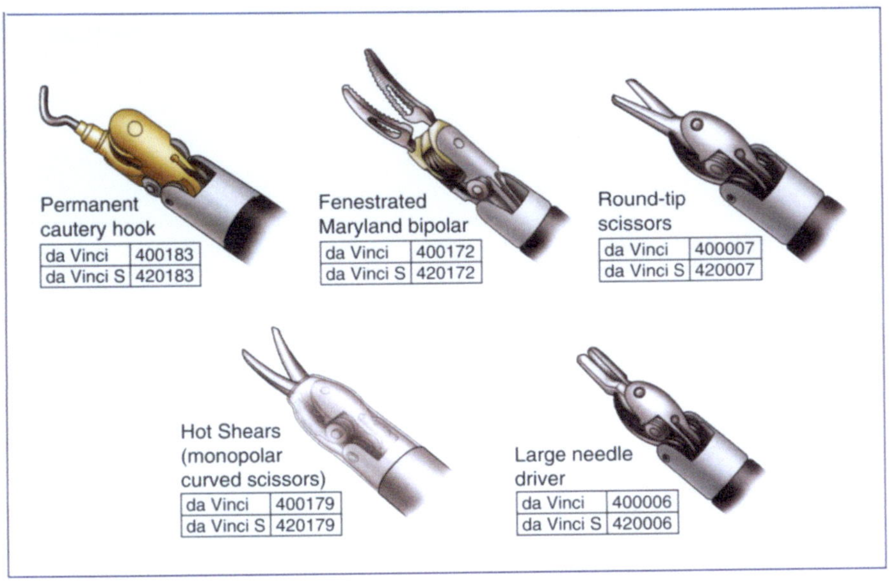

FIGURE 16-4. EndoWrist (Intuitive Surgical Inc.; Mountain View, CA) instruments used during robotic-assisted laparoscopic radical cystectomy (RARC). The precise selection of EndoWrist instruments for use during RARC is at the discretion of the surgeon. Typically, we prefer the Maryland bipolar instrument on the left arm and the monopolar cautery hook on the right. However, the monopolar shears may be preferred to the hook. The large needle holders are required for suturing. da Vinci system—Intuitive Surgical Inc.; Mountain View, CA.

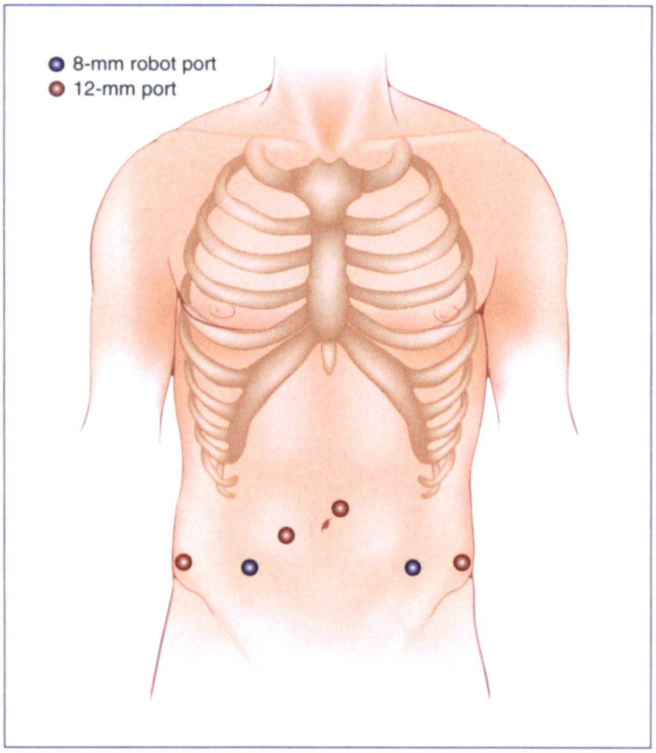

FIGURE 16-5. Port positions. A six-port transperitoneal approach is used. The first 12-mm port is placed in the midline 2 cm above the umbilicus using the Hasson technique. The pneumoperitoneum is established at a pressure of 14 mm Hg and insufflation is maintained at high flow throughout the procedure. Subsequent ports are placed under vision with the patient in a slight Trendelenburg position. The 8-mm robotic ports are placed 10 cm from the midline camera port. For a three-arm robot, two 12-mm assistant ports are placed on the right side of the abdomen with a further 5-mm assistant port on the left side. For a four-arm robot, the most lateral port on the right is an 8-mm robot port for the fourth arm. Depending on the patient's habitus, most of these ports are located on a transverse line 1 to 2 cm below the umbilicus. The exception is the medial assistant port on the right side, which is placed higher to prevent clashing with the robotic arms. An extra-long 45-cm laparoscopic suction device allows this port to be placed above the umbilicus if necessary, to prevent clashing between the assistant and robotic ports on the right.

The key difference to bear in mind between port positions for robotic prostatectomy and radical cystectomy is that the ports must be placed higher for cystectomy to allow adequate exposure for pelvic lymphadenectomy. However, when using the original da Vinci system (Intuitive Surgical Inc.; Mountain View, CA), the left and right robotic ports must be no more than 16 cm from the symphysis pubis to prevent problems in reaching the urethra later in the procedure. The newer da Vinci S robot features multiquadrant access, which makes it easier to access the bifurcation of the iliac vessels and to dissect more cranially from there. The instruments are also 5 cm longer, which allows more flexibility when choosing port positions.

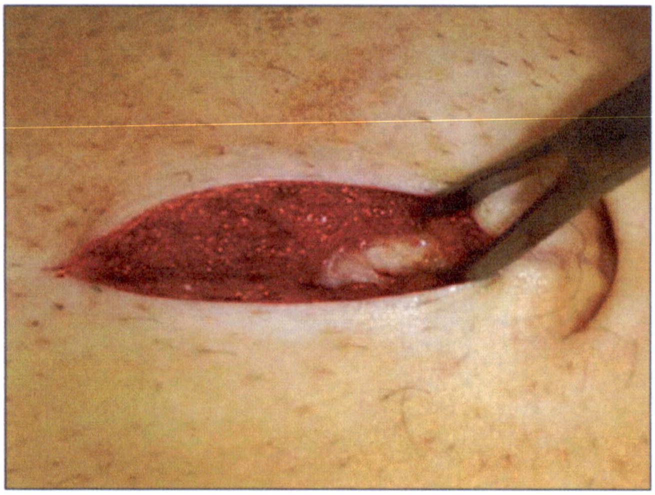

FIGURE 16-6. Hasson access above the umbilicus. An open Hasson technique is preferred for accessing the abdomen for insertion of the first port and for insufflation. This incision is placed 2 cm above the umbilicus in the midline. The rectus sheath is exposed, grasped, and incised. The peritoneum is exposed; it is opened between clips and a finger is introduced to ensure there are no nearby adhesions. A 12-mm disposable port is placed and the skin is approximated using a 1/0 suture to prevent any gas leaks. Insufflation is then started and the 0-degree telescope is introduced for laparoscopic inspection of the abdomen.

The 0-degree telescope may be used for the duration of the procedure, although depending on the patient's habitus it may be advantageous to change to the 30-degree up- or down-angle telescope at certain stages of the dissection.

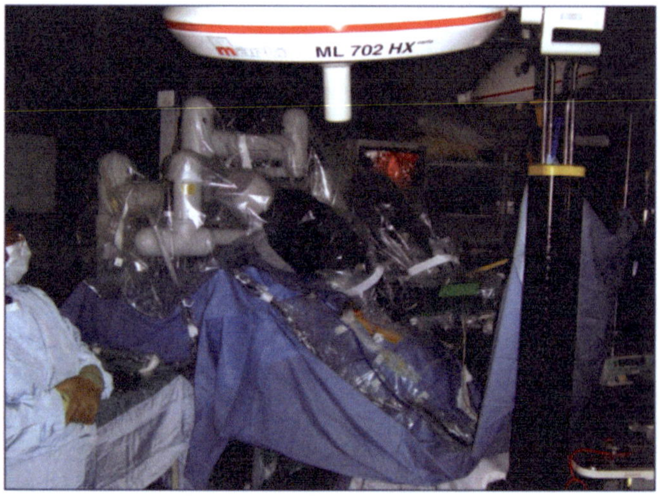

FIGURE 16-7. Docking of the robotic cart. Once all the ports have been inserted, the patient is moved to the steep Trendelenburg position and the hips are extended. The robotic cart is then docked to the ports as shown. Care is taken to ensure all pressure points remain safely protected and that the robotic arms are not in contact with the patient's knees. A sterile drape is used to shield the anaesthetic team at the head of the table (*right* of picture). The instruments are introduced under vision before the console surgeon takes control of the robotic arms.

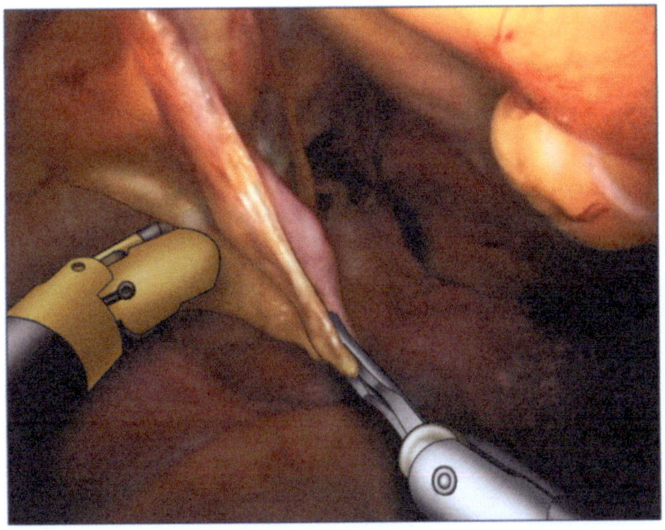

FIGURE 16-8. Mobilization of the right ureter. The ureters can often be seen through the peritoneum as they course over the iliac bifurcation. In more obese patients, the pulsation of the common iliac artery is the guide to where the peritoneal incision should be made.

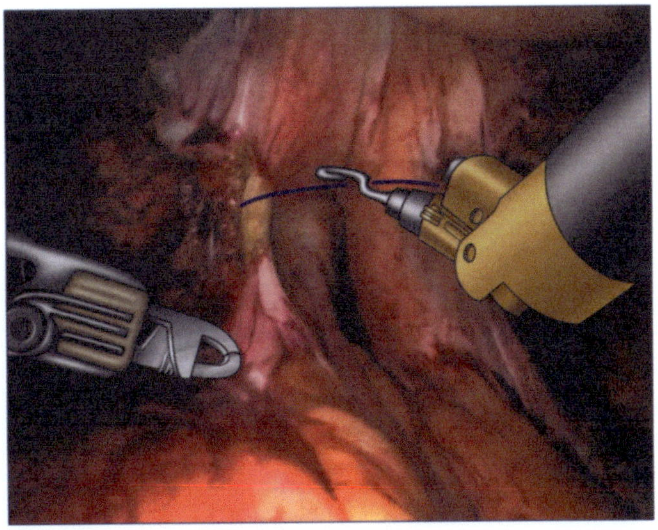

FIGURE 16-9. Ligation and division of the right ureter. Once the base of the bladder has been reached, the ureter is clipped using a large Hem-o-lok locking clip (Weck Closure Systems; Research Triangle Park, NC). The ureter is divided proximally to the clip.

The right ureter is mobilized by incising the overlying peritoneum and identifying the vermiculating ureter. Care is taken when dissecting the ureter to leave adequate peri-ureteric adventitia reached and cranially to the iliac bifurcation.

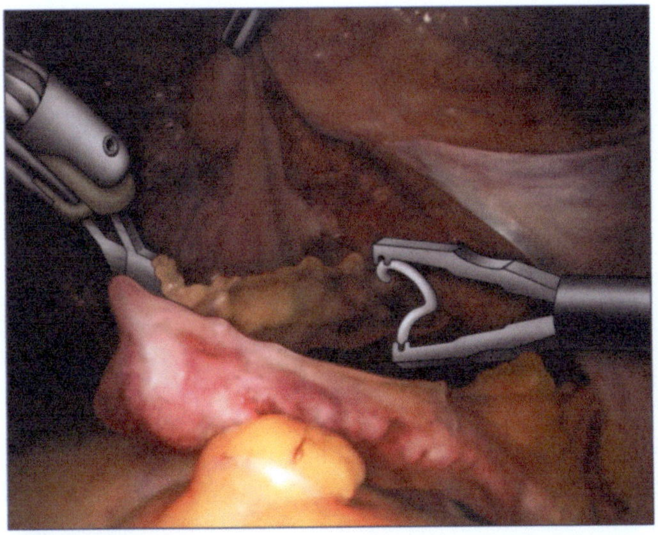

FIGURE 16-10. Frozen section analysis. Once the ureter has been divided, the distal ureteric margin is excised and sent for frozen section analysis to ensure that the distal margin is clear of malignancy. The free end of the ureter is not clipped. The left ureter is then mobilized, ligated, and divided in an identical fashion and the distal margin is sent for frozen section analysis.

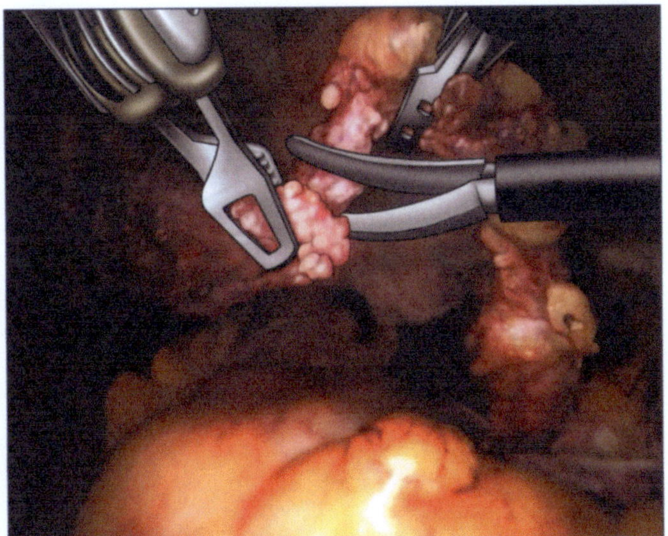

Posterior dissection 1. Attention is now directed to dissecting the posterior plane between the bladder and rectum.

Upward retraction of the bladder is maintained by the left-side assistant (or fourth arm). A transverse peritoneotomy is made in the pouch of Douglas by using monopolar cautery and is extended laterally until the peritoneal incision overlying the ureters is reached. Denonvilliers fascia is incised in the midline. The left-side assistant also manipulates the disposable sigmoidoscope to retract the rectum posteriorly.

In women, the posterior vaginal fornix is opened using monopolar cautery, revealing the methylene blue-soaked swab stick. The lateral vaginal walls are transected using a combination of monopolar cautery and ultrasonic energy with the Harmonic ACE scalpel (Ethicon Endosurgery; Livingston, UK). The vagina is then closed longitudinally by continuous intracorporeal suturing with 2-0 polyglactin on a CT-1 needle.

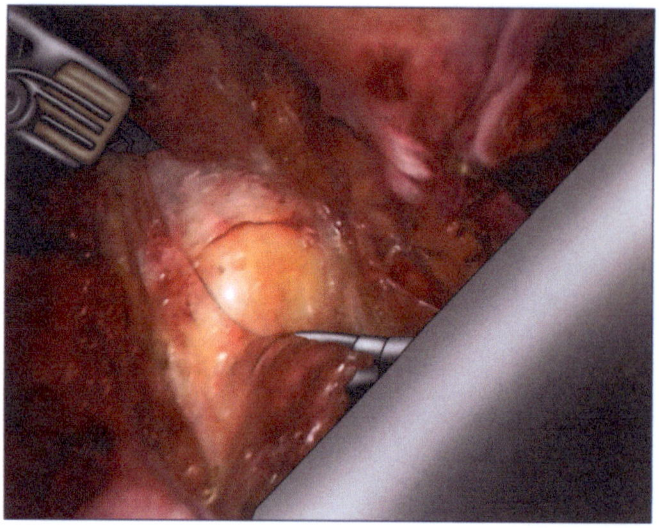

FIGURE 16-12. Posterior dissection 2. Once the Denonvilliers fascia has been incised, the perirectal fat is identified by its characteristic yellow appearance. The plane between the prostate (or vagina) and the rectum is developed using a combination of blunt and sharp dissection. The seminal vesicles are identified on the undersurface of the bladder. While the right-side assistant retracts the rectum posteriorly using the suction device, the console surgeon develops the plane and advances under the bladder toward the prostate. If this plane proves difficult to develop, the rectum may be identified by asking the left-side assistant to maneuver the sigmoidoscope. Small vessels are controlled with bipolar or monopolar cautery. The assistant advances the suction device as the plane is developed, which creates tissue tension for dissection and keeps the rectum out of the dissection plane. The left-side assistant maintains anterior retraction of the bladder. The lateral border of the posterior dissection is determined by the bladder pedicles, which are not ligated at this stage. Posterior dissection continues until no further progress is possible and attention then moves to the lateral dissection.

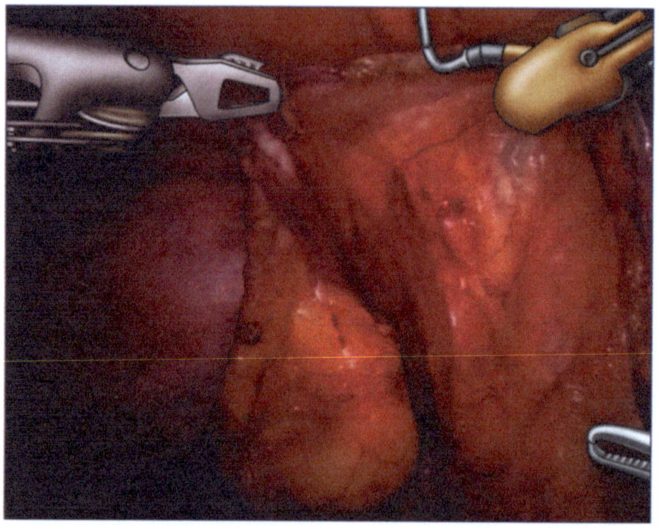

FIGURE 16-13. Right lateral dissection 1. The bladder is mobilized laterally by entering the space of Retzius on both sides. The peritoneum lateral to the medial umbilical ligament is incised from its most superior aspect and continued posteriorly until the vas is encountered. This is divided using cautery. The extraperitoneal space is then entered and developed using blunt dissection.

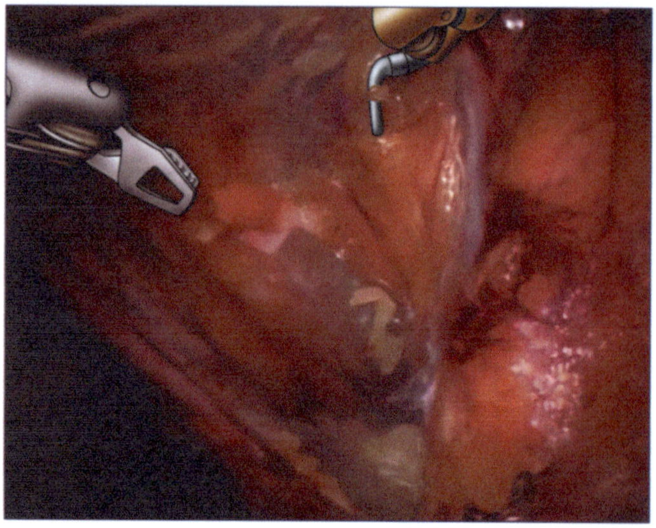

FIGURE 16-14. Right lateral dissection 2. Dissection is continued medial to the external iliac vein to preserve the obturator nerves and to expose the lateral pelvic wall. The endopelvic fascia is seen posteriorly and the lateral aspect of the prostate may be appreciated. The posterior and lateral dissection allows the lateral pedicles to the bladder (and uterus in women) to be delineated. The same procedure is subsequently performed on the left side to allow the left bladder pedicle to be demonstrated.

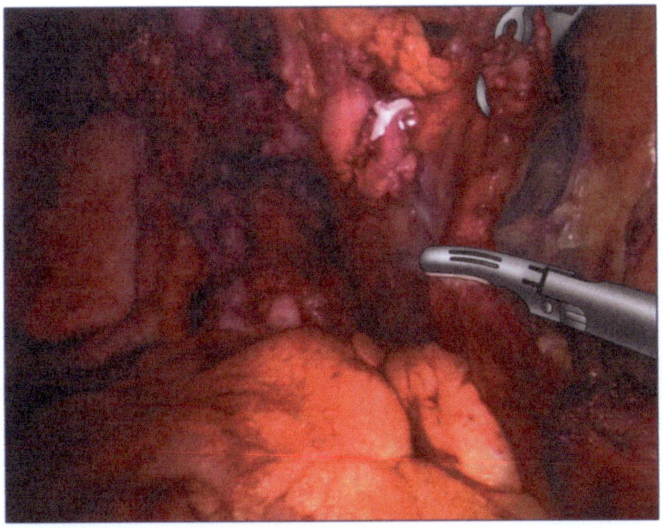

Figure 16-15. Ligation of right bladder pedicle 1. There are a number of options for ligation of the vascular pedicle. We have previously used a vascular linear stapler and the LigaSure bipolar device (Valleylab; Boulder, CO). An extra-large–sized Hem-o-lok locking clip (Weck Closure Systems; Research Triangle Park, NC) may also be used. However, we prefer the Harmonic ACE scalpel (Ethicon Endosurgery; Livingston, UK), which is used by the right-side assistant to ligate the vascular pedicles (demonstrated on the right bladder pedicle in this figure).

Whichever modality is chosen, it is important to have a laparoscopically experienced right-side assistant as he/she will be performing this step of the procedure. The vascular pedicles of the bladder are put on tension by the left-side assistant retracting the bladder anteriorly and contralaterally, while the console surgeon maintains countertraction and sweeps the rectum away. The right-side assistant then proceeds to ligate the pedicle on each side, thereby fully mobilizing the lateral aspect of the bladder.

The Harmonic scalpel is not used in patients undergoing a nerve-sparing procedure who instead undergo athermal ligation of the pedicles using Hem-o-lok clips or a linear stapler.

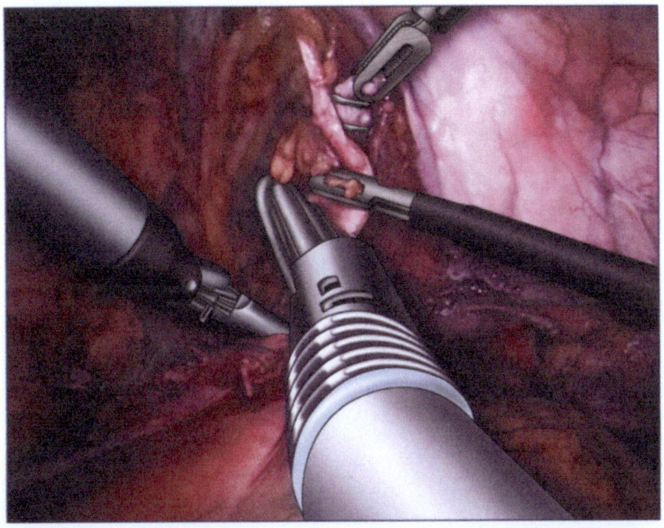

Figure 16-16. Ligation of left bladder pedicle 2. This figure demonstrates ligation of the left bladder pedicle using a vascular linear stapler. Three or four reloads of the stapler are typically required for each side.

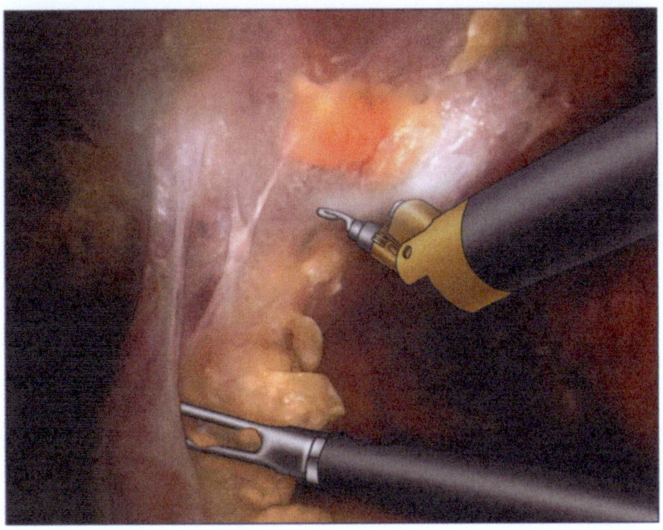

Figure 16-17. Anterior dissection 1. Attention is now directed toward anterior mobilization of the bladder. The bladder is filled with 200 mL of formol–saline solution to aid in the identification of the correct plane. Using an inverted U-shaped incision through the peritoneum overlying the urachus, the bladder is dropped off the anterior abdominal wall. Bipolar and monopolar cautery is used to divide the urachus where it meets the anterior abdominal wall. The left-side assistant then retracts the bladder posteriorly, allowing the console surgeon to continue the anterior mobilization until the previously dissected lateral margins are encountered.

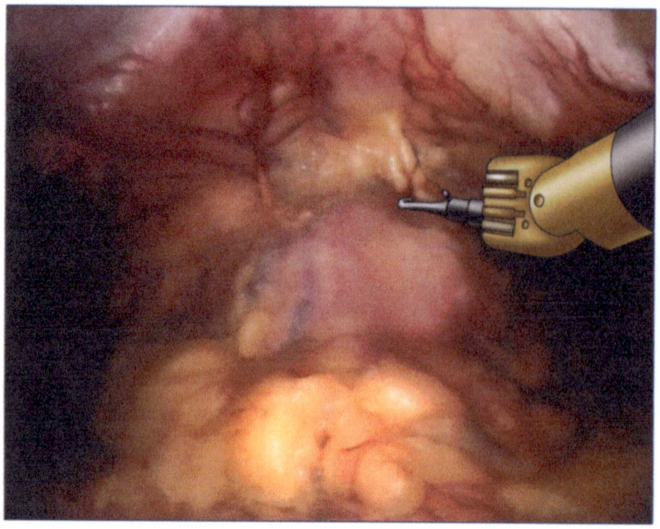

FIGURE 16-18. Anterior dissection 2. Once the anterior mobilization has been completed, the formol–saline solution is drained through the Foley catheter. The symphysis pubis is now clearly seen (*top*) and the prostate has been cleared of fat. The superficial dorsal vein is controlled using bipolar cautery. Any remaining fat is cleared off the endopelvic fascia laterally. Slight cranial traction is placed on the bladder by the left-side assistant (or fourth arm).

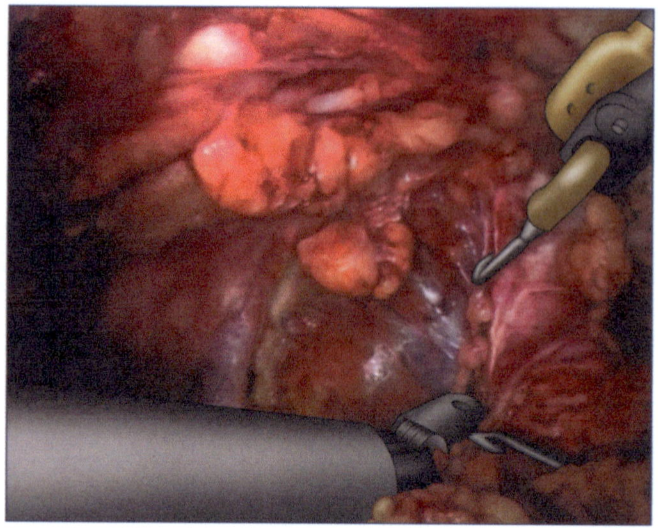

FIGURE 16-19. Incision of left endopelvic fascia. These steps of the procedure are identical to the corresponding steps during robotic-assisted laparoscopic radical prostatectomy. Opening of the left endopelvic fascia is demonstrated in this illustration. The right-side assistant puts countertraction on the base of the prostate as the console surgeon opens the endopelvic fascia using the scissors or monopolar hook. The endopelvic fascia is opened at the base where the prostate is most widely separated from the levator ani. Dissection proceeds toward the apex of the prostate by continuing the incision in the endopelvic fascia and sweeping the levator ani fibres laterally until the apex of the prostate is reached and the dorsal vein becomes apparent. The puboprostatic ligament is incised using monopolar cautery to allow the apex of the prostate to drop away.

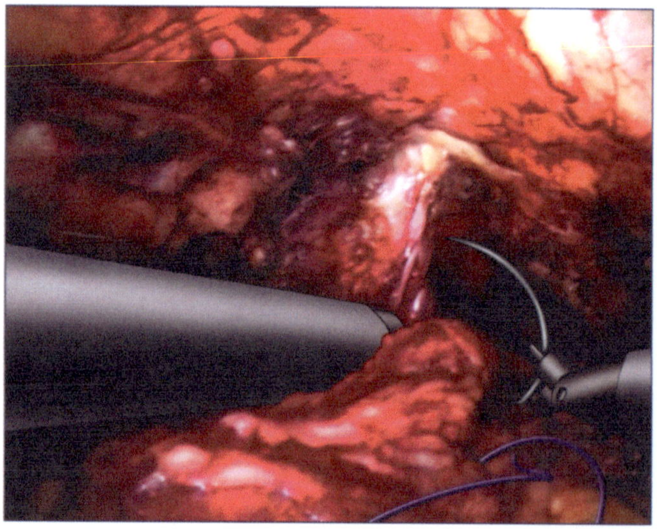

FIGURE 16-20. Ligation of dorsal venous complex. Once the endopelvic fascia has been opened bilaterally and the puboprostatic ligaments have been transected, the notch between the dorsal vein and the urethra should be clearly visible. The large EndoWrist needle holders (Intuitive Surgical Inc.; Mountain View, CA) are loaded onto the robotic arms and a 20-cm length of 1/0 polyglactin suture on a CT-1 needle is passed through the right assistant port. The needle is grasped two-thirds of the way back and positioned at a slight downward angle. The dorsal vein is then ligated using a figure-eight–style suture. The assistants play an important role in exposing the entry and exit points of the needle as it is passed between the dorsal vein and urethra.

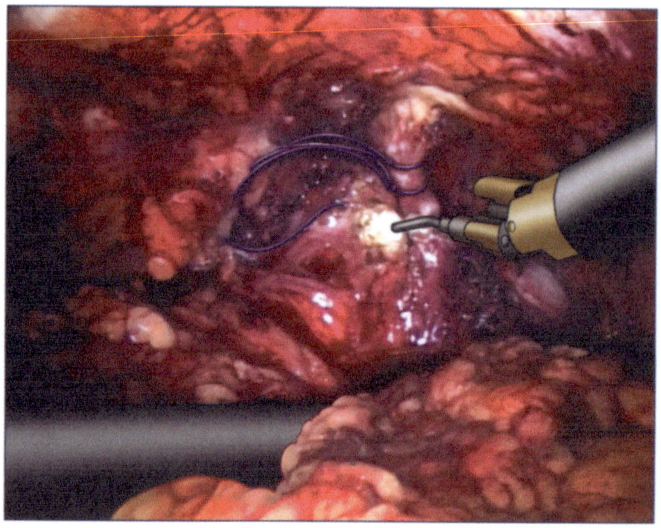

FIGURE 16-21. Division of dorsal venous complex. The dorsal vein complex is divided 4 to 5 mm proximal to the ligature using monopolar cautery.

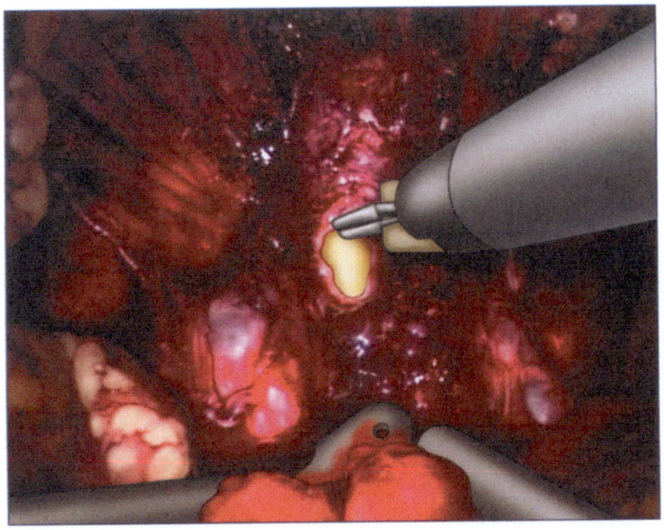

FIGURE 16-22. Division of the urethra. The anterior urethral wall is divided with scissors, exposing the Foley catheter within. The catheter is withdrawn until it just disappears into the distal urethra, thereby exposing the mucosa of the posterior wall of the urethra that is then divided. The distal urethral margin is sent for frozen section analysis and the bladder neck is sealed with a Hem-o-lok locking clip (Weck Closure Systems; Research Triangle Park, NC) to prevent contamination. Any remaining attachments are then divided, leaving the specimen fully mobilized.

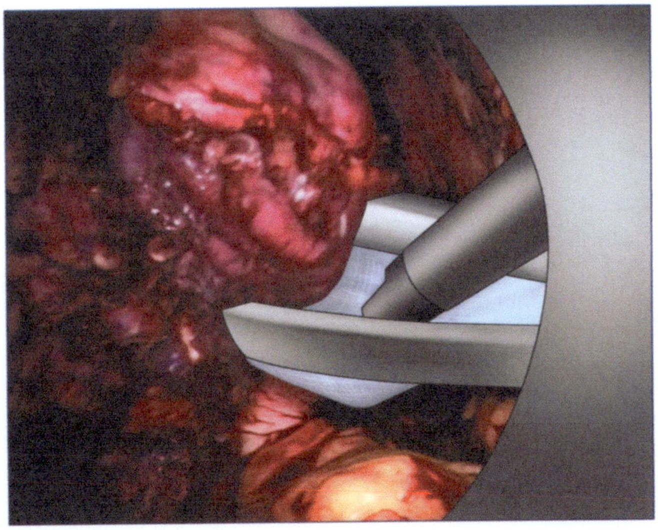

FIGURE 16-23. Entrapment of the specimen. A 15-mm EndoCatch II bag (Tyco Healthcare; Hampshire, UK) is introduced through the right-side assistant's lateral port. The cystoprostatectomy specimen is entrapped within the bag, which is then closed and positioned in the upper abdomen for later retrieval.

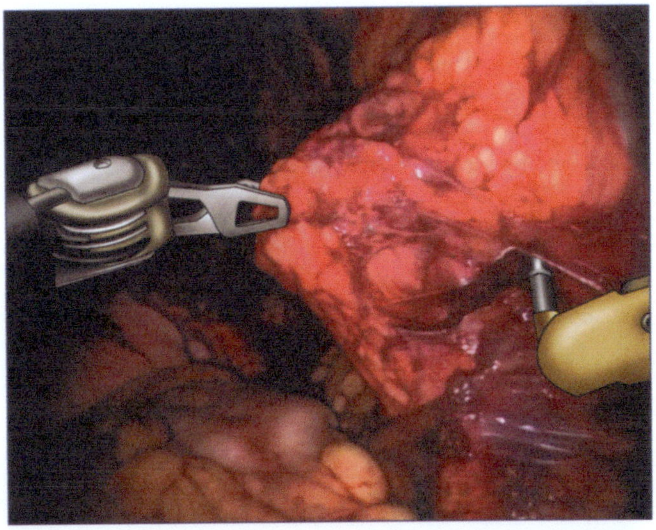

FIGURE 16-24. Pelvic lymphadenectomy. Either a standard or extended lymphadenectomy is performed, depending on the surgeon's preference and local guidelines. Our policy is to perform a standard lymphadenectomy as suggested by the guidelines of the European Urological Association. Our margins for lymphadenectomy are the genitofemoral nerve laterally, the bifurcation of the common iliac artery proximally, the obturator nerve inferiorly, and the node of Cloquet distally.

The lymph node dissection is performed using a combination of blunt and sharp dissection. Dissection of the right obturator and external iliac lymph node packet overlying the right external iliac vein is shown. We prefer the EndoWrist monopolar hook (Intuitive Surgical Inc.; Mountain View, CA) for lymph node dissection, as it is an effective tool for blunt dissection and allows the use of monopolar cautery when necessary. Hem-o-lok locking clips or titanium clips are used to ligate lymph trunks when it is required. However, the EndoWrist monopolar shears may also be used effectively for this purpose. Take care when dissecting around the obturator nerve and iliac vessels to prevent inadvertent injury. The external iliac artery and vein, and the obturator nerve, are skeletonized to the level of the common iliac bifurcation to complete a standard lymphadenectomy.

Extended lymph node dissection (to the bifurcation of the aorta) may also be undertaken, but it requires the multiquadrant of the newer da Vinci S robot (Intuitive Surgical Inc.; Mountain View, CA), rather than the previous machine. It also requires placing the working ports close to the level of the umbilicus.

The lymph node specimens are placed in separately marked 10-mm EndoCatch bags (Tyco Healthcare; Hampshire, UK). An Endoloop (Ethicon Endo-surgery; Livingston, UK) is applied on the distal end of the left ureter, which is then transposed under the sigmoid mesocolon by pulling the Endoloop through a window in the mesentry anterior to the sacrum. A ratcheted laparoscopic grasper is passed through the most lateral right-side assistant port and used to grasp the distal ends of both ureters. This grasper is left in position until the incision has been made for specimen retrieval, as it facilitates the subsequent identification of the ureters in preparation for the urinary diversion.

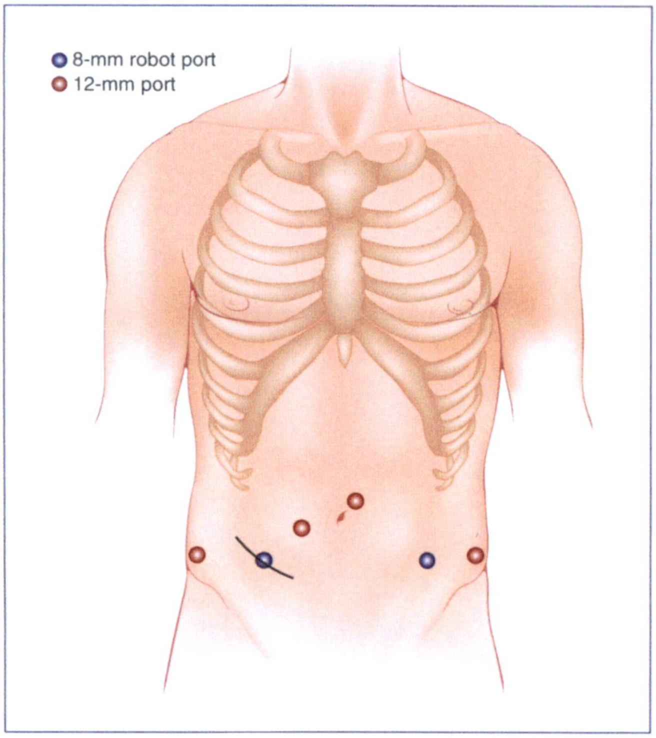

FIGURE 16-25. Incision for specimen extraction and ileal conduit urinary diversion. The incision for specimen removal depends on the type of urinary reconstruction planned. Two types of diversions are commonly used: ileal conduit incontinent diversion and Studer pouch orthotopic neobladder. All diversions are performed extracorporeally using a Deaver retractor (Thomas Medical; Indianapolis, IN) to aid exposure. A detailed description of each of these diversions is beyond the scope of this chapter, but we briefly describe our approach and refer to standard descriptions.

For ileal conduits, a 5- to 7-cm muscle-splitting incision (Lanz) is made in the right iliac fossa, usually incorporating the right robotic port or lateral assistant port site. This allows extraction of the specimens and extracorporeal fashioning of the urinary diversion. In obese patients (body mass index > 30 kg/m^2), a lower midline incision may be used for easier access to the left ureter. Uretero–ileal anastomosis using 4/0 Monocryl is performed over 8-Fr ureteric stents using a Wallace I or Bricker technique. The distal end of the conduit is fashioned as a stoma at a previously marked site on the abdominal wall.

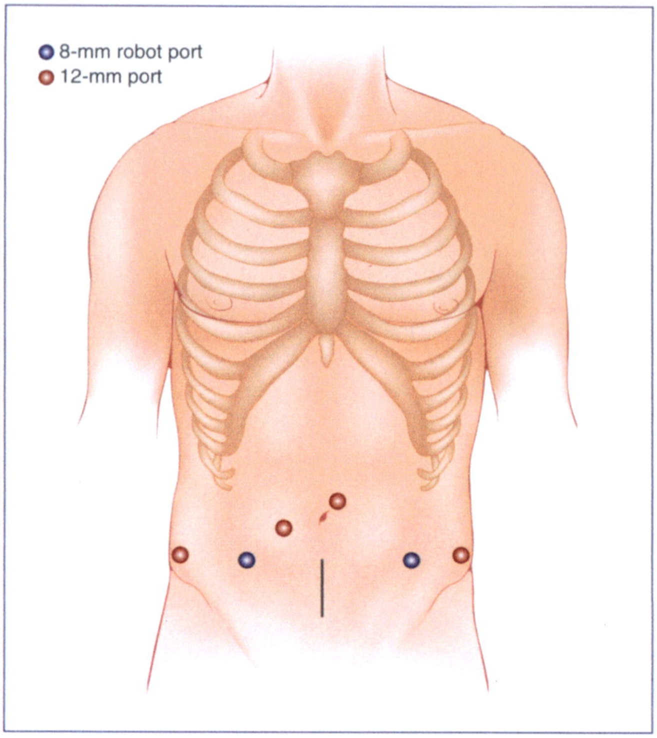

FIGURE 16-26. Incision for specimen extraction and Studer pouch urinary diversion. Orthotopic neobladders are fashioned through a 5- to 7-cm lower midline incision as described by Studer [18]. The more posterior urethral sutures are placed laparoscopically using robotic assistance prior to undocking the da Vinci robot (Intuitive Surgical Inc.; Mountain View, CA). The remaining urethral and neobladder sutures are placed using an open surgery approach through the lower midline incision. The pouch is then "parachuted" down to the urethra over an 18-Fr urethral catheter. Further management of urinary catheters is as described by Studer.

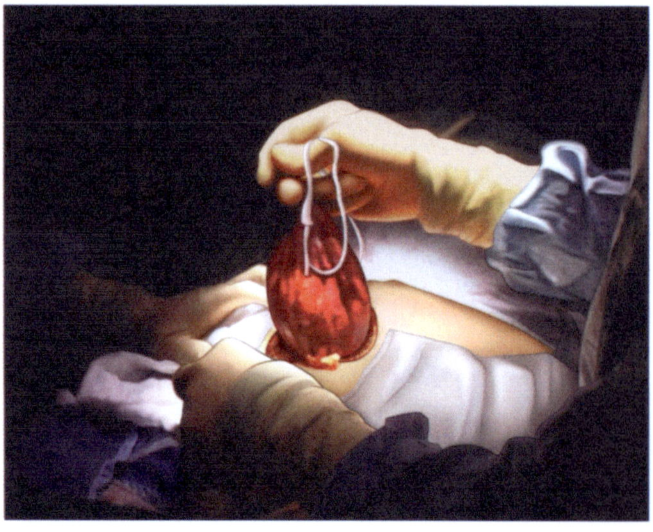

FIGURE 16-27. Specimen extraction. The cystoprostatectomy and right and left lymph node dissection specimens are delivered separately within their EndoCatch bags (Tyco Healthcare; Hampshire, UK). Even quite bulky specimens can be delivered through a 5- to 7-mm incision.

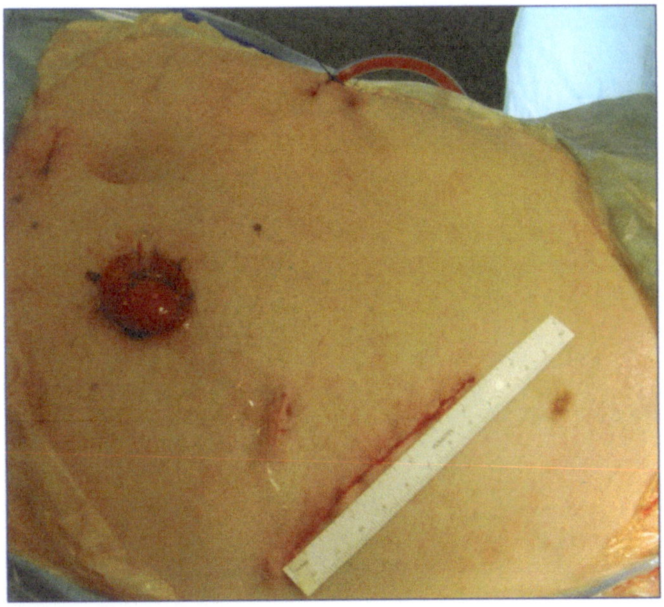

FIGURE 16-28. Closure of wounds. The fascia of the right iliac fossa or midline incision is closed with 1/0 polydioxone and the skin incisions closed with 3/0 Monocryl. A 20-Fr nonsuction drain is placed through the left-side assistant port.

Postoperative care: These patients are managed using the Enhanced Recovery After Surgery program, coordinated by our anesthetic team [19]. Regional anesthesia is used as appropriate, high inspired oxygen concentrations are used intra-operatively, and early postoperative feeding and mobilization are encouraged. Typically, patients start oral fluids on postoperative day one, semi-solids on day two, and solids on day three. Our standard care plan aims to discharge patients on postoperative day five or six.

References

1. Stein JP, Lieskovsky G, Cote R, Groshen S, *et al.*: Radical cystectomy in the treatment of invasive bladder cancer: long-term results in 1,054 patients. *J Clin Oncol* 2001, 19:666–675.
2. Herr HW, Bochner BH, Dalbagni G, *et al.*: Impact of the number of lymph nodes retrieved on outcome in patients with muscle invasive bladder cancer. *J Urol* 2002, 167:1295–1298.
3. Konety BR, Allareddy V, Herr H: Complications after radical cystectomy: analysis of population-based data. *Urology* 2006, 68:58–64.
4. Novotny V, Hakenberg OW, Wiessner D, *et al.*: Perioperative complications of radical cystectomy in a contemporary series. *Eur Urol* 2007, 51:397–402.
5. Nuttall MC, van der Meulen J, McIntosh G, *et al.*: Changes in patient characteristics and outcomes for radical cystectomy in England. *BJU Int* 2005, 95:513–516.
6. Haber GP, Colombo JR Jr, Aron M, *et al.*: Laparoscopic radical cystectomy and urinary diversion: status in 2006. *Eur Urol Suppl* 2006, 5:950–955.
7. Basillote JB, Abdelshehid C, Ahlering TE, Shanberg AM: Laparoscopic assisted radical cystectomy with ileal neobladder: a comparison with the open approach. *J Urol* 2004, 172:489–493.
8. Raychaudhuri B, Khan MS, Challacombe B, *et al.*: Minimally invasive radical cystectomy. *BJU Int* 2006, 98:1064–1067.
9. Menon M, Hemal AK, Tewari A, *et al.*: Nerve-sparing robot-assisted radical cystoprostatectomy and urinary diversion. *BJU Int* 2003, 92:232–236.
10. Guru KA, Kim HL, Piacente PM, Mohler JL: Robot-assisted radical cystectomy and pelvic lymph node dissection: initial experience at Roswell Park Cancer Institute. *Urology* 2007, 69:469–474.
11. Pruthi RS, Wallen EM: Robotic assisted laparoscopic radical cystoprostatectomy: operative and pathological outcomes. *J Urol* 2007, 178:814–818.
12. Rhee JJ, Lebeau S, Smolkin M, Theodorescu D: Radical cystectomy with ileal conduit diversion: early prospective evaluation of the impact of robotic assistance. *BJU Int* 2006, 98:1059–1063.
13. Wang GJ, Barocas DA, Raman JD, Scherr DS: Robotic vs open radical cystectomy: prospective comparison of perioperative outcomes and pathological measures of early oncological efficacy. *BJU Int* 2008, 101:89–93.
14. Murphy DG, Challacombe BJ, Elhage O, *et al.*: Robotic-assisted laparoscopic radical cystectomy with extracorporeal urinary diversion: initial experience. *Eur Urol* 2008, 54:570–580.
15. Beecken WD, Wolfram M, Engl T, *et al.*: Robotic-assisted laparoscopic radical cystectomy and intra-abdominal formation of an orthotopic ileal neobladder. *Eur Urol* 2003, 44:337–339.
16. Sala LG, Matsunaga GS, Corica FA, Ornstein DK: Robot-assisted laparoscopic radical cystoprostatectomy and totally intracorporeal ileal neobladder. *J Endourol* 2006, 20:233–236.
17. Cathelineau X, Jaffe J: Laparoscopic radical cystectomy with urinary diversion: what is the optimal technique? *Curr Opin Urol* 2007, 17:93–97.
18. Studer UE, Varol C, Danuser H: Orthotopic ileal neobladder. *BJU Int* 2004, 93:183–193.
19. Blake L, Sicinski M, Gulati S: Anaesthesia and robotic surgery. In *Urologic Robotic Surgery in Clinical Practice*. Edited by Dasgupta P. Guildford, UK: Springer; 2008:181–194.

17 Robotic Sacrocolpopexy: Suspension of the Bladder and Vagina

Shawn M. McGee, George K. Chow, and Daniel S. Elliott

The anatomy of the female pelvis changes after childbirth and with advancing age, which affects the support of the bladder and vagina. Poor pelvic floor support in the female pelvis may result in symptomatic pelvic organ prolapse (POP) with or without concomitant urinary incontinence. POP is a generalized description of the vaginal canal's anatomic disruption seen upon physical examination due to bowel (enterocele or rectocele) or bladder (cystocele), or both. More specific anatomic terms, such as anterior, posterior, or apical vaginal prolapse are typically used to assist in determining the appropriate management of POP.

Surgical management of urinary incontinence or POP is estimated to occur in 10% of women over their lifetime [1]. Multiple procedures and routes of repair are described for POP. Sacrocolpopexy is a procedure indicated for the repair of symptomatic high-grade, posthysterectomy apical vaginal prolapse. A comprehensive review of transabdominal sacrocolpopexy has shown it to be a durable procedure, with approximately 90% of patients experiencing no recurrence on long-term followup [2]. Over the decades, surgeons have moved toward less invasive surgery and utilized other routes for performing sacrocolpopexy, such as the transvaginal, laparoscopic, and more recently robot-assisted laparoscopic sacrocolpopexy (RALS). The Urology Department at the Mayo Clinic has recently described the long-term results for RALS. This technique has demonstrated greater than 90% durability in repair, as defined by no recurrent POP [3–5]. In addition, it has been shown that RALS has decreased hospital stays, resulted in less postoperative pain, and has similar postoperative morbidity when compared to the transabdominal route [4,6–8]. This chapter focuses on RALS, which has evolved since it was first described at the Mayo Clinic in patients with high-grade, posthysterectomy, apical POP [9]. As the reader will see, the success of RALS is dependent not only on reapproximating the vaginal canal's normal anatomic location, but performing the procedure with respect to the adjacent female pelvic anatomy.

Pelvic Organ Prolapse

Definitions of Pelvic Organ Prolapse

POP Description

Types of prolapse	Common anatomic cause(s)	Typical surgical repair(s)
Anterior	Cystocele	Anterior colporrhaphy
Posterior	Rectocele	Posterior colporrhaphy
Apical	Uterine prolapse	Sacrocolpopexy or sacrouteropexy
	Vault prolapse after hysterectomy	Pelvic ligament suspension or fixation
	Enterocele	

Figure 17-1. Pelvic organ prolapse (POP) described. The term *POP* is a general description of the altered vaginal anatomy that is applied broadly to its multiple causes. In addition, POP also represents a spectrum of changes to the vaginal canal's anatomy that may be an asymptomatic incidental finding or may be seen as complete vaginal eversion on the pelvic exam. The majority of women will undergo no therapy or nonsurgical management of their diagnosis of POP. When surgery is indicated, the appropriate management of POP is highly dependent on the clinician to correctly classify the specific type and cause of POP. This figure briefly describes the common anatomic causes of POP and their typical surgical management.

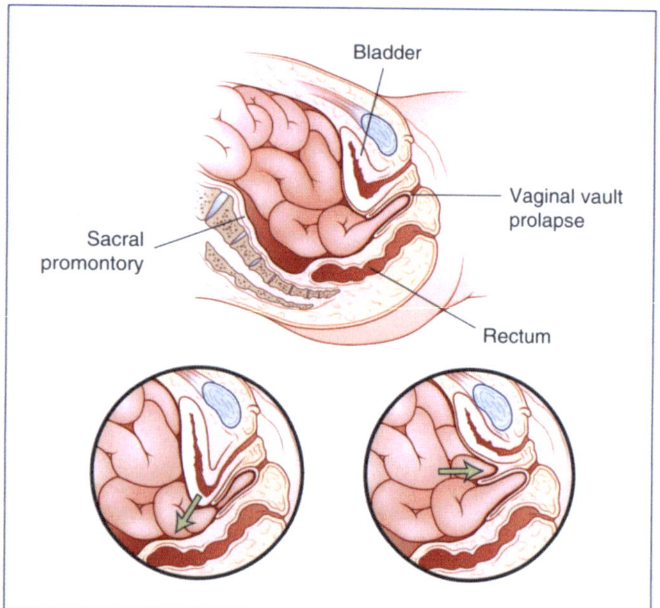

Figure 17-2. Vaginal vault prolapse after hysterectomy. The term *apical vaginal vault prolapse* is used to specifically describe the disruption of the middle and proximal support of the vaginal wall, represented by an enterocele, uterine prolapse, or vault prolapse after hysterectomy. Prolapse of the vaginal canal after hysterectomy has variations and is dependent on the surrounding pelvic organs in the female pelvis. In some women, the urinary bladder can conceal the boundary of the prolapsed anterior wall of the vaginal canal as it drapes over the apex of the vagina (*left lower inset*), whereas in other women the bladder's posterior wall is associated with the mid portion of the anterior vaginal wall (*right lower inset*). These anatomic variations have been witnessed by our surgical group and are important to recognize to dissuade inadvertent perforation to the vaginal canal or bladder during surgical repair. (*Courtesy of* Mayo Clinic, Rochester, MN.)

Grading of POP

Baden-Walker system	POP-Q system
Grade 1: apex of the vaginal canal descends halfway to the hymenal ring	Stage I: most distal portion of the prolapse > 1 cm above the level of the hymenal ring
Grade 2: apex of the vaginal canal is level with the hymenal ring	Stage II: most distal portion of the prolapse < 1 cm above or below the level of the hymenal ring
Grade 3: apex of the vaginal canal extends past the hymenal ring, but the vagina is not completely everted	Stage III: most distal portion of the prolapse > 1 cm below the level of the hymenal ring, but is not completely everted
Grade 4: complete vaginal eversion	Stage IV: complete vaginal eversion

Figure 17-3. Grading of pelvic organ prolapse (POP). Most patients who eventually have their POP managed surgically typically have high-grade or higher stage prolapse associated with symptoms. Multiple authors have proposed staging systems to systematically assess the degree of POP and allow communication between practitioners. Prior to the last decade, various staging systems, including the Baden-Walker system [10], were routinely used to assess POP. Regardless of the staging system used, the degree of prolapse is based on a thorough pelvic examination that utilizes a split bivalved speculum to independently visualize the anterior and posterior vaginal walls. Recently, a validated staging system called the Pelvic Organ Prolapse Quantification (POP-Q) has been proposed and applied successfully to patients with POP [11]. This system does not rely on the anatomic cause of POP, but instead defines the stage of vaginal vault descent based on specific points along the vaginal canal.

Surgical Correction of High-Grade Apical POP: RALS

Operative Preparation

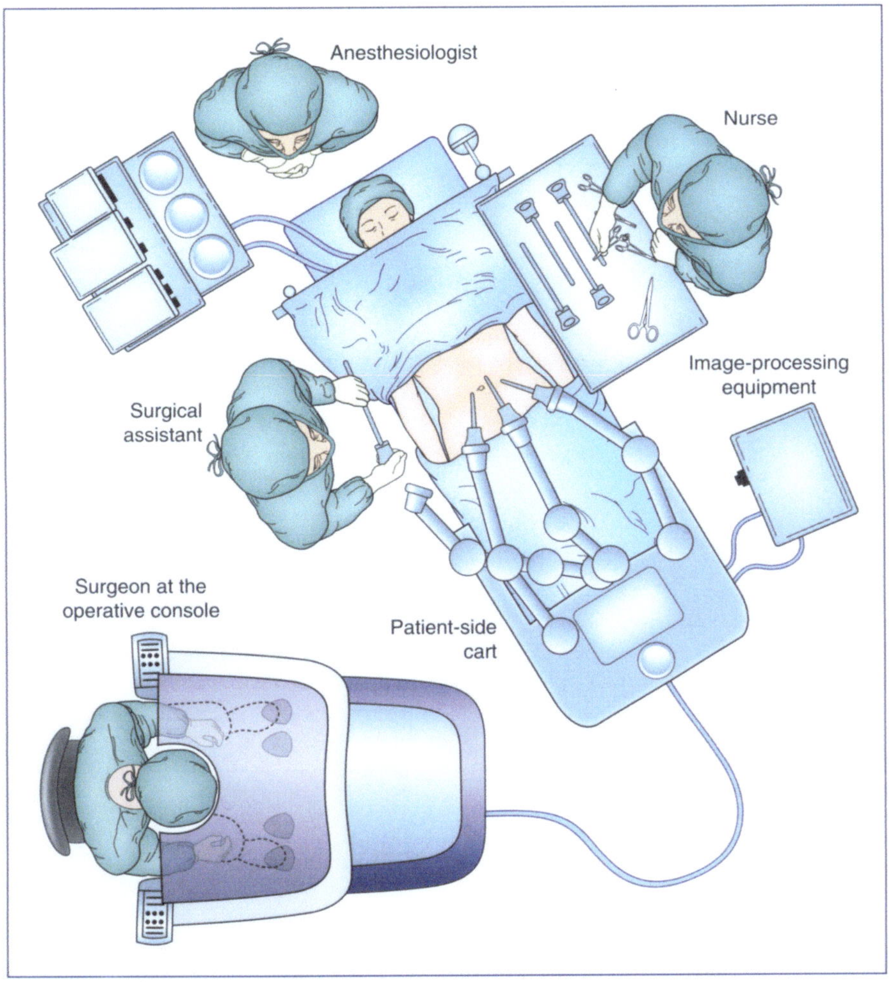

FIGURE 17-4. Operative suite setup. The da Vinci system (Intuitive Surgical; Sunnyvale, CA) is a remote-control, integrated, computer-based system consisting of two or three interactive robotic arms and a camera arm that has three-dimensional vision capability. The da Vinci system uses instruments with six degrees of freedom, which provides intracorporal flexibility in a laparoscopic procedure that is similar to the human wrist. Setting up the operative suite with the da Vinci system is different than the open and other standard laparoscopic procedures and should be thought out prior to the procedure, to expedite operative times. Our surgical group places the surgeon console in the corner of the room toward the foot of the operating table, as shown. The patient cart, when rolled in, should have its center column between the legs of the patient, with the base of the patient cart straddling the base of the operating table. The surgical assistant stands on the right side of the patient, which allows access to the perineum during the procedure.

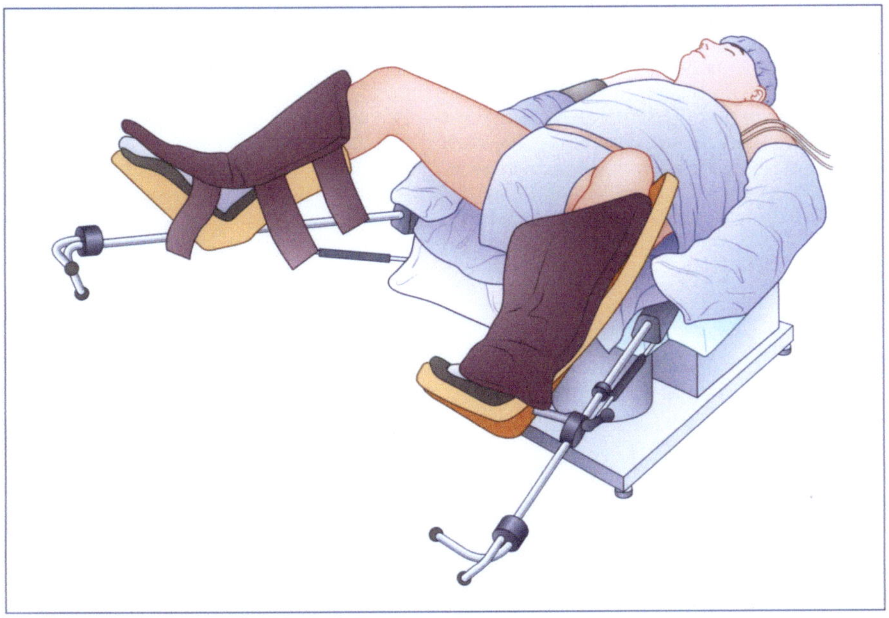

FIGURE 17-5. Patient positioning. Patient positioning for robot-assisted laparoscopic sacrocolpopexy is different from other described laparoscopic procedures. The patient's legs are placed in cushioned, fully supporting stirrups to keep the patient in the dorsal lithotomy position for the entire procedure and to allow access to the vagina before and after the patient cart is rolled in, as shown here. The lower extremities' pressure points are padded, paying specific attention to the region behind the knees. The stirrups should not place the lower extremities in excessive angles, to dissuade plexus injuries. The patient is then placed in the Trendelenburg position (between 15° and 20°) after a strap is securely placed across the chest below the level of the breasts. The patient's arms are tucked beside the torso on arm boards after padding the arms' pressure points. A urethral catheter is placed into the bladder and attached to drainage, which will remain until the first postoperative morning. The abdomen below the level of the breasts, pelvis, vagina, and perineum are prepped for surgery. The vagina is left exposed during draping to allow placement of a vaginal retractor during the case.

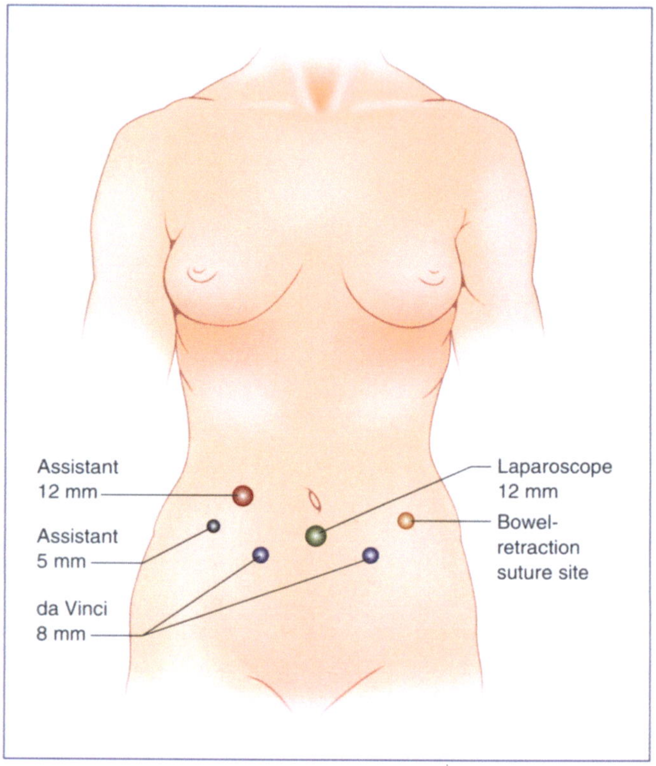

FIGURE 17-6. Trocar placement. Initial placement of the central camera port is based on the patient's pubic symphysis and umbilicus, as shown. Generally, the initial central camera port is placed 12 to 15 cm above the pubic symphysis, but below the umbilicus. All measurements are generalized and can change based on a patient's body habitus. The placement of trocars is initiated by placing the 12-mm disposable camera port (*green circle*). The right and left da Vinci arms (Intuitive Surgical; Sunnyvale, CA) reusable 8-mm ports (*blue circles*) are then placed laterally to the rectus muscles, two fingerbreadths superior to the level of the anterior superior iliac spine and approximately 10 to 12 mm from the central camera port. An assistant 12-mm port (*red circle*) is placed two fingerbreadths below the subcostal margin and one handbreadth (8–10 cm) away from the right robotic 8-mm instrument port. A second assistant 5-mm port (*black circle*) is then placed one handbreadth (8–10 cm) inferior, lateral from the assistant 12-mm port at approximately the level of the umbilicus. The bowel-retraction suture site (*orange circle*) is not an actual laparoscopic port; this suture site extracorporeally holds the sigmoid colon away from the pelvis with a hemostat.

Laparoscopic and Robotic Instruments Used in RALS

Standard laparoscopic instruments	Robotic instruments
Curved monopolar scissors with cautery	Needle driver
Needle driver	Prograsp dissector
Maryland grasper	Monopolar scissors with or without cautery
Suction irrigator	

A

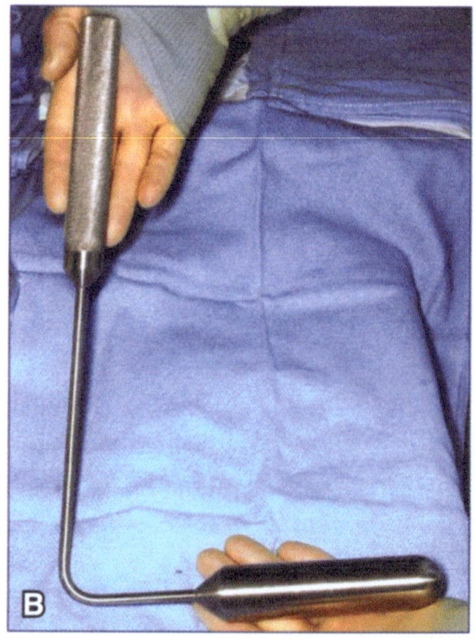

FIGURE 17-7. Surgical instrumentation. Standard laparoscopic instruments, as well as robotic instruments, are utilized in our description of robot-assisted laparoscopic sacrocolpopexy (RALS). The laparoscopic and robotic instruments commonly used during our procedure are listed in **A**. Depending on the patient's body habitus and prior intra-abdominal procedures, the standard laparoscopic or robotic instruments assist in initially taking down adhesions prior to dissecting the vagina from the posterior wall of the bladder. Dissection of the vagina is then done with the robotic arms and instruments. Regardless of what method is used, the sacrocolpopexy depends on the correct identification of the vaginal apex and the ability to retract the vagina inferiorly during dissection of the anterior vaginal plane. At the Mayo Clinic, a specialized instrument was engineered and utilized, which is called the "handheld vaginal retractor" to visualize the plane between the vagina and bladder (**B**).

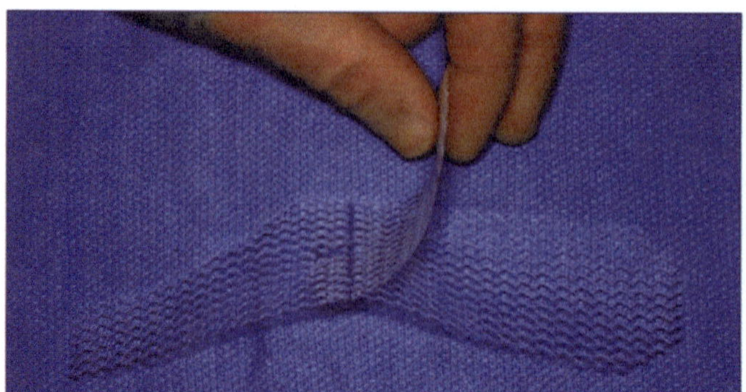

FIGURE 17-8. Mesh. In the literature, synthetic meshes are used in the majority of patients undergoing a sacrocolpopexy as described by Nygaard *et al.* [2]. Current literature has reported that polypropylene mesh is superior to cadaveric fascia lata when comparing prolapse failure based on the postoperative Pelvic Organ Prolapse Quantification stage [12]. At the Mayo Clinic, the preference is to use synthetic mesh (polypropylene) because of its initial pliability and long-term durability. Overall, in a large review of the transabdominal sacrocolpopexy, the mesh erosion rate is 3.4% [2]. Currently, in our series of robot-assisted laparoscopic sacrocolpopexy, we have reported two patients with mesh erosion (3.8%) [8].

Steps of Robot-Assisted Laparoscopic Sacrocolpopexy

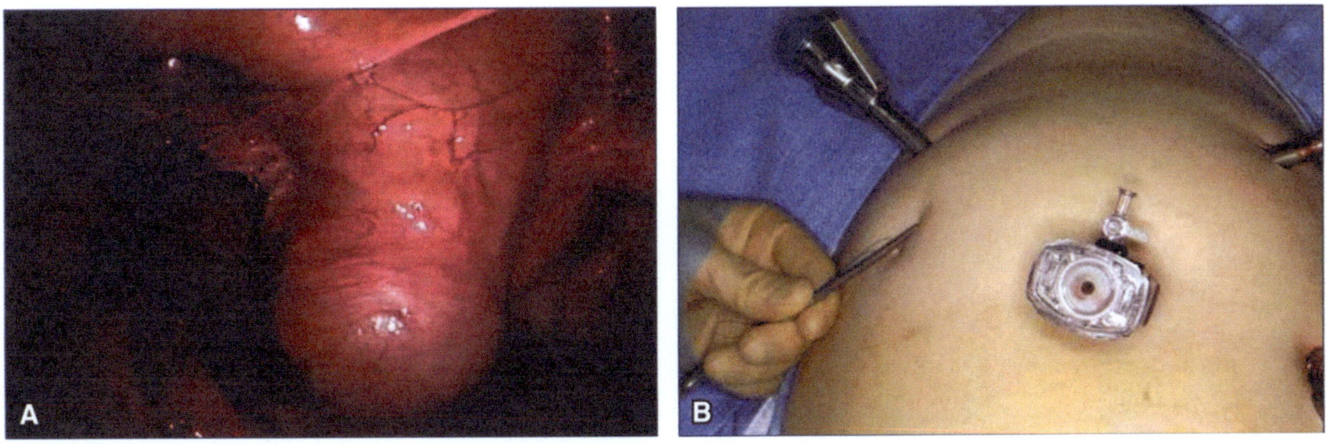

FIGURE 17-9. Vaginal retractor placement and sigmoid bowel retraction. Utilizing the assistant ports, adhesions are taken down in the abdomen and pelvis with a Maryland grasper and curved scissors with cautery. Adhesion takedown should allow exposure of the vagina and sigmoid. To assist in dissection, the handheld vaginal retractor is placed in the previously prepped vaginal canal by the assistant to expose the vaginal apex (**A**). Prior to vaginal dissection, the sigmoid colon is reflected superior-laterally to the patient's left with a retracting suture that is brought out from the anterior abdominal wall at approximately 10 cm lateral to the camera port at the level of the umbilicus (**B**). The sigmoid retraction suture is placed with the da Vinci system (Intuitive Surgical; Sunnyvale, CA) using ProGrasp forceps (Intuitive Surgical; Sunnyvale, CA) and a large needle driver.

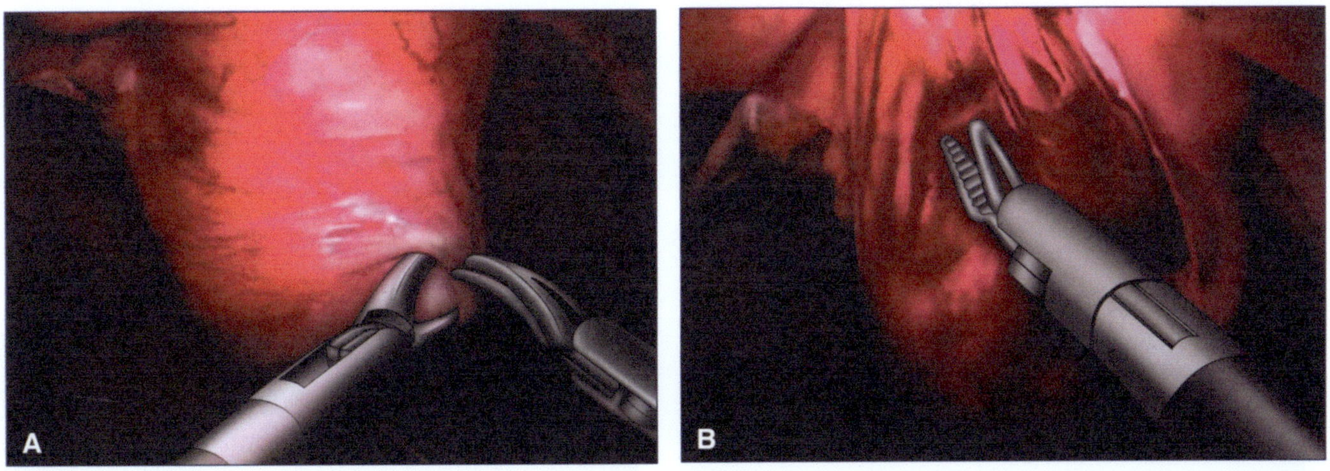

FIGURE 17-10. Vaginal vault and bladder dissection. The plane between the anterior vagina and the posterior bladder wall is dissected beginning with cautery to gently score the surface of the vagina (**A**). This dissection is achieved with ProGrasp forceps (Intuitive Surgical; Sunnyvale, CA) and curved scissors with cautery. Hereafter, no cautery is used to dissuade devascularization of the vaginal wall. During the vaginal vault dissection, the handheld vaginal retractor is used to deflect the vaginal apex inferiorly, to allow better visualization of the plane between the vagina and bladder. Utilizing the robotic instruments noted, the plane between the anterior vagina and bladder is dissected with a spread-and-cut technique. The left-hand instrument should be grasping the tissue anterior to the vagina and retracting superiorly, to allow visualization of the apex of the vagina (**B**). If the surgeon is in the right plane, this dissection is generally bloodless. This plane between the anterior vagina and bladder wall is continued distally, as close as possible to the introitus, to maximize the support given by the Y-mesh graft (AMS; Minnetonka, MN). The plane between the rectum and posterior vagina can be dissected with the same instruments and the technique can be utilized as described above for the anterior dissection.

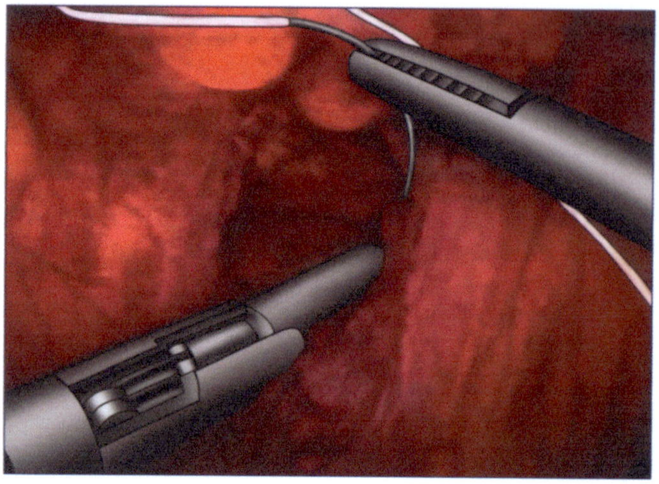

FIGURE 17-11. Exposing the sacral promontory and placing sutures. Utilizing ProGrasp forceps (Intuitive Surgical; Sunnyvale, CA) and curved scissors with cautery, the peritoneal reflection above the proximal sacrum is gently scored with cautery to begin the dissection. The dissection is continued through the tissues underlying the peritoneal reflection to visualize the sacral promontory. It is important to note that severe bleeding is described by authors who have dissected and sutured mesh below the S-2 level in the transabdominal sacrocolpopexy [13]. Because of this, our technique stays proximal on the sacrum during the dissection and suture placement for mesh fixation. During this part of the procedure, the surgical assistant typically uses a suction irrigator in the right hand (5-mm assistant port) and a Maryland grasper in the left hand (12-mm assistant port) to help with exposure. Then, using large needle drivers on both robotic arms, individual 2-0 GORE-TEX sutures (Gore; Newark, DE) on a CV-2 needle approximately 7 cm in length are placed horizontally into the sacrum above the S-2 level. The suture should be placed deep enough into the sacral promontory to sufficiently withstand moderate traction. A total of three or four sutures with the needles left attached remain in the abdomen for mesh fixation.

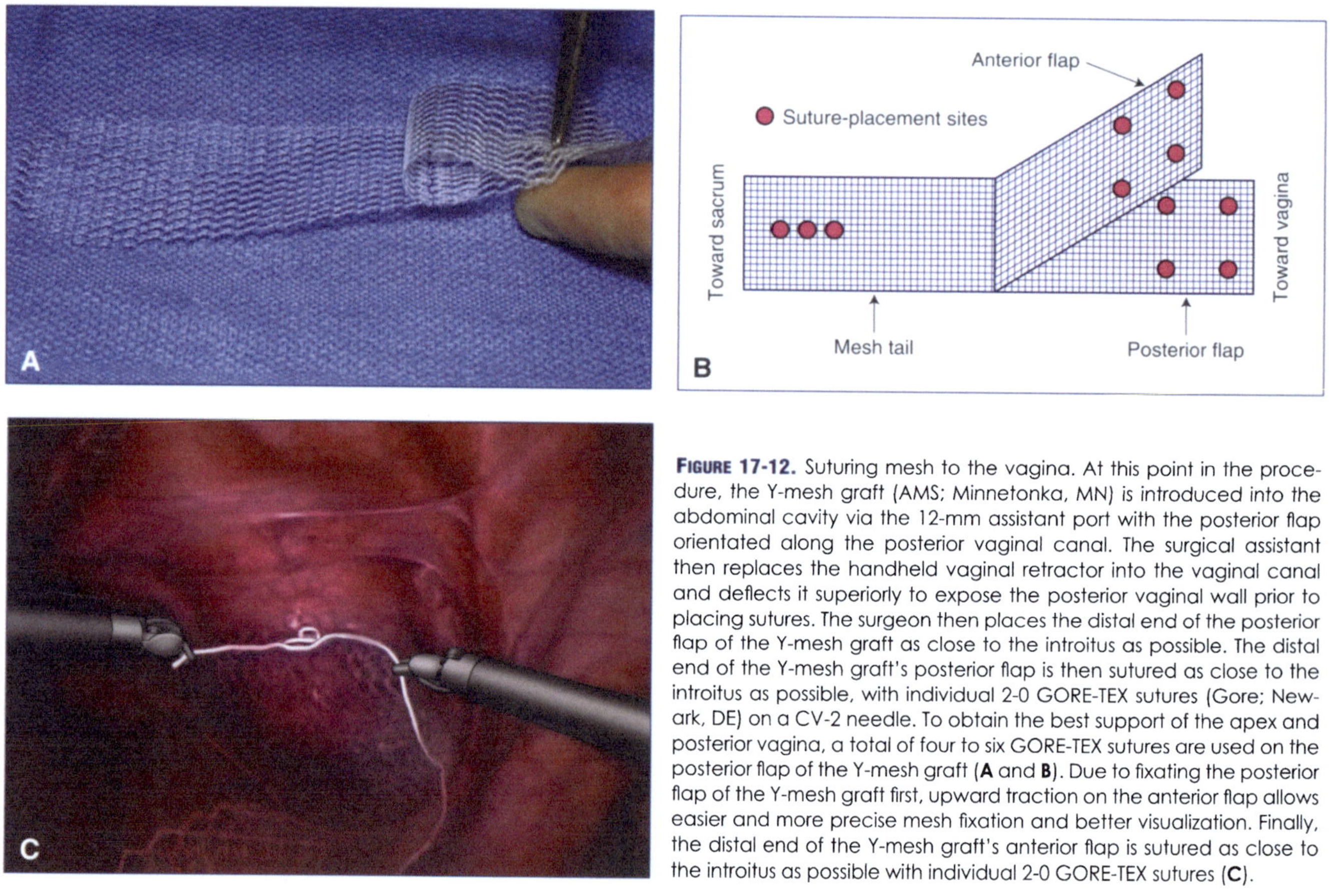

FIGURE 17-12. Suturing mesh to the vagina. At this point in the procedure, the Y-mesh graft (AMS; Minnetonka, MN) is introduced into the abdominal cavity via the 12-mm assistant port with the posterior flap orientated along the posterior vaginal canal. The surgical assistant then replaces the handheld vaginal retractor into the vaginal canal and deflects it superiorly to expose the posterior vaginal wall prior to placing sutures. The surgeon then places the distal end of the posterior flap of the Y-mesh graft as close to the introitus as possible. The distal end of the Y-mesh graft's posterior flap is then sutured as close to the introitus as possible, with individual 2-0 GORE-TEX sutures (Gore; Newark, DE) on a CV-2 needle. To obtain the best support of the apex and posterior vagina, a total of four to six GORE-TEX sutures are used on the posterior flap of the Y-mesh graft (**A** and **B**). Due to fixating the posterior flap of the Y-mesh graft first, upward traction on the anterior flap allows easier and more precise mesh fixation and better visualization. Finally, the distal end of the Y-mesh graft's anterior flap is sutured as close to the introitus as possible with individual 2-0 GORE-TEX sutures (**C**).

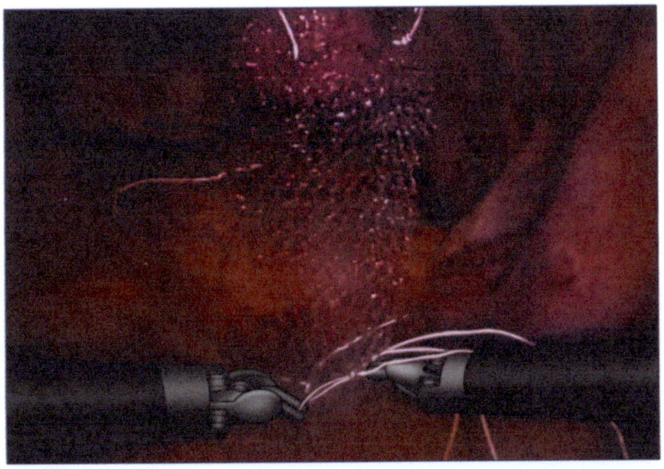

FIGURE 17-13. Suturing mesh to the sacrum. Utilizing needle drivers in the right and left hands of the robot, the previously placed sacral sutures are used to tie the tail of the Y-mesh graft (AMS; Minnetonka, MN) to the sacrum. The mesh should not be under tension, but should approximate the apex of the vagina into a more normal anatomical position. By using the handheld vaginal retractor, the assistant directs the vaginal apex into the normal anatomical configuration, which allows the surgeon to tie the sutures without tension. The excess stem of the Y-mesh graft is excised and removed through the assistant port along with the GORE-TEX needles (Gore; Newark, DE).

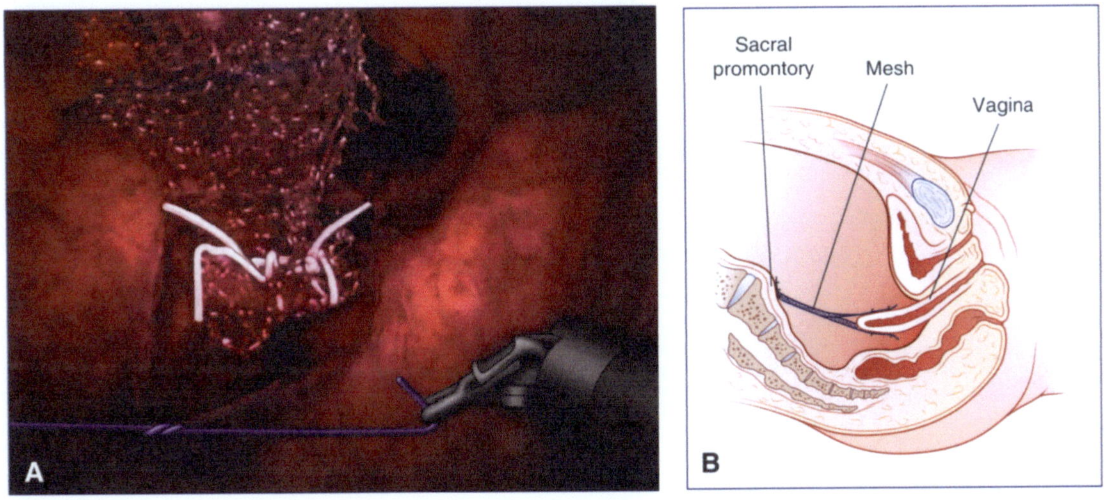

FIGURE 17-14. Retroperitonealize the mesh. With the needle drivers on the robotic arms, a running 2-0 Vicryl suture on a CT-1 needle (7 cm in length) is used to reapproximate the peritoneal reflection over the Y-mesh graft (AMS; Minnetonka, MN), which is now tied to the sacrum (**A**). The Y-mesh graft should approximate the vagina in a more normal anatomical position but also support the anterior and posterior walls of the vaginal canal (**B**). After confirming hemostasis, a port-site closure is done in the usual manner, using a port-site closure device to close all wounds greater than 5 mm in diameter. (**B** *adapted from* Mayo Clinic, Rochester, MN.)

Results from the Robot-assisted Laparoscopic Sacrocolpopexy

RALS Results

Study	Age, *y*	BMI, *kg/m²*	Operative time, *min*	Estimated blood loss, *mL*	Hospital stay, *d*	Complication, *n* (%)	Prolapse recurrence, *n* (%)
Elliott *et al.* [4]	66.3 (43–83)	26.7 (18–40)	179 (105–285)	49.1 (0–200)	1.0 (1–2)	8 (15%)	3 (6%)
Daneshgari *et al.* [7]	64 (50–79)	NR	317 (258–363)	81 (50–150)	2.4 (1–7)	1 (8%)	0
Geller *et al.* [6]	60.2 ± 10.3	27.0 ± 6.5	328 ± 55	103 ± 96	1.3 ± 0.8	13 (18%)	NR
Akl *et al.* [15]	66.5 ± 8.3	NR	197.9 ± 66.8	96.8 (25–300)	2.6	11 (14%)	3 (4%)

FIGURE 17-15. Robot-assisted laparoscopic sacrocolpopexy (RALS) results. Results of RALS are encouraging, as shown here. Investigators have reported decreased blood loss and overall hospitalization duration when compared to the gold standard, transabdominal sacrocolpopexy. In addition, the overall complication rate is low and the durability of repair greater than 90% when considering all prolapse recurrences reported postoperatively. Also, our department has found that an increased body mass index (BMI) does not compromise the durability of repair and complication rate [14].

References

1. Olsen AL, Smith VJ, Bergstrom JO, *et al.*: Epidemiology of surgically managed pelvic organ prolapse and urinary incontinence. *Obstet Gynecol* 1997, 89:501–506.
2. Nygaard IE, McCreery R, Brubaker L, *et al.*: Abdominal sacrocolpopexy: a comprehensive review. *Obstet Gynecol* 2004, 104:805–823.
3. Elliott DS, Siddiqui SA, Chow GK: Assessment of the durability of robot-assisted laparoscopic sacrocolpopexy for treatment of vaginal vault prolapse. *J Robot Surg* 2007, 1:163–168.
4. Elliott DS, Krambeck AE, Chow GK: Long-term results of robotic assisted laparoscopic sacrocolpopexy for the treatment of high grade vaginal vault prolapse. *J Urol* 2006, 176:655–659.
5. McGee SM, Chow GK, Elliott DS: Comparison of prolapse repair durability between robotically-assisted versus transabdominal sacrocolpopexy. World Congress of Endourology. Shanghi, China, 2008.
6. Geller EJ, Siddiqui NY, Wu JM: Short-term outcomes of robotic sacrocolpopexy compared with abdominal sacrocolpopexy. *Obstet Gynecol* 2008, 112:1201–1206.
7. Daneshgari F, Kefer JC, Moore C, *et al.*: Robotic abdominal sacrocolpopexy/sacrouteropexy repair of advanced female pelvic organ prolapse (POP): utilizing POP-quantification-based staging and outcomes. *BJU Int* 2007, 100:875–879.
8. McGee SM, Chow GK, Elliott DS: Surgical complications of the robotically-assisted versus transabdominal sacrocolpopexy: World Congress of Endourology. Shanghi, China, 2008.
9. DiMarco DS, Chow GK, Gettman MT, *et al.*: Robotic-assisted laparoscopic sacrocolpopexy for treatment of vaginal vault prolapse. *Urology* 2004, 63:373–376.
10. Baden WF, Walker TA: Genesis of the vaginal profile: a correlated classification of vaginal relaxation. *Clin Obstet Gynecol* 1972, 15:1048–1054.
11. Bump RC, Mattaisson A, Bo K, *et al.*: The standardization of terminology of female pelvic organ prolapse and pelvic floor dysfunction. *Am J Obstet Gynecol* 1996, 175:10–17.
12. Culligan PJ, Blackwell L, Goldsmith LJ, *et al.*: A randomized controlled trial comparing fascia lata and synthetic mesh for sacral colpopexy. *Obstet Gynecol* 2005, 106:29–37.
13. Sutton GP, Addison WA, Livengood C, *et al.*: Life-threatening hemorrhage complicating sacrocolpopexy. *Am J Obstet Gynecol* 1981, 140:836–837.
14. McGee SM, Priyanka G, Siddiqui SA, *et al.*: Impact of obesity on surgical outcomes after robotic-assisted laparoscopic sacrocolpopexy: World Congress of Endourology. Shanghi, China, 2008.
15. Akl MN, Long JB, Giles DL, *et al.*: Robotic-assisted sacrocolpopexy: technique and learning curve. *Surg Endosc* 2009. (Epub ahead of print).

18 Bladder Neck Reconstruction Following Minimally Invasive Radical Prostatectomy

Jay K. Jhaveri, Gerald Y. Tan, and Ashutosh K. Tewari

Prostate cancer remains the most common cancer in men in the Western hemisphere. In 2009, it is estimated that 192,000 men will be diagnosed and over 27,000 men will die from it in the United States alone [1–3]. Radical prostatectomy has emerged as a popular treatment option for organ-confined cancer, with technical and technological advances in the last decade significantly improving functional and pathologic outcomes for patients undergoing this surgery [4–6]. Nonetheless, urinary incontinence following radical prostatectomy remains a primary concern of patients, causing significant social and psychological distress in the post-operative period.

In recent years, several investigators have made significant progress in overcoming the problem of postprostatectomy urinary incontinence through the study of real-time intra-operative video and cadaveric anatomy, histopathological analysis of final prostatectomy specimens, and data analysis of functional outcomes [7–15]. Our group [16] has identified seven major principles for optimizing early continence recovery following radical prostatectomy, as shown in Figure 18-1: 1) preservation of anterior fibrotendinous support structures, chiefly the arcus tendineus and the puboprostatic ligaments; 2) optimization of functional membranous urethral length; 3) reinforcement of unstable posterior bladder neck in the unsupported retrotrigonal fossa left by excised seminal vesicles; 4) reinforcement of the posteriorly deficient Ω-shaped urethral sphincter complex for suspensory support; 5) fashioning of a tension-free, stable vesico-urethral anastomosis; 6) prevention of urethral stump recession and optimizing mucosal coaptation; and 7) ameliorating pelvic descent and downward pressure of the bladder on the anastomosis during micturition. Our approach to bladder neck reconstruction following minimally invasive radical prostatectomy, incorporating surgical modifications to address each of these concerns, is described.

Principles for Early Continence Recovery

1) Preserve anterior fibrotendinous support structures, ie, arcus tendineus and puboprostatic ligaments
2) Optimize functional membranous urethral length
3) Reinforce the unstable posterior bladder neck in unsupported retrotrigonal fossa left by excised seminal vesicles
4) Reinforce the posteriorly deficient Ω-shaped remnant urethral sphincteric complex for suspensory support
5) Fashion tension-free, stable vesico-urethral anastomosis
6) Prevent urethral stump recession and optimize mucosal coaptation
7) Prevent pelvic descent and downward pressure of the bladder on the anastomosis during micturition

A

Key Steps of the Anatomic Restoration Technique

1) a) Preserve the arcus tendineus during endopelvic fascia dissection (Delaney principle); b) perform a puboprostatic ligament-sparing
2) Precise apical dissection and preparation of thick and long remnant urethral stump (Myers principle)
3) Dissect out the retrotrigonal layer behind the bladder neck and reinforce it with buttressing sutures after seminal vesicle excision (modified Pagano/Libertino principle) [17]
4) Suture the distal flap of Denonvilliers fascia to reinforce the posterior bladder neck close to the urethral stump (modified Rocco/Bartsch principle) [18–20]
5) Tension taken off the vesico-urethral anastomosis by steps 5), 6), and 7) (Mundy urethroplasty principle)
6) Perform a continous running suture for vesicourethral anastomosis (modified van Velthoven/Menon principle) [15]
7) Hitch bladder up to the arcus tendineus and puboprostatic collar (modified Lapides/Walsh principle)

B

Figure 18-1. **A,** Seven major principles for augmenting early recovery of urinary continence and **B,** seven key steps of the anatomic restorative technique following radical prostatectomy are provided.

Minimally Invasive Access to the Prostate

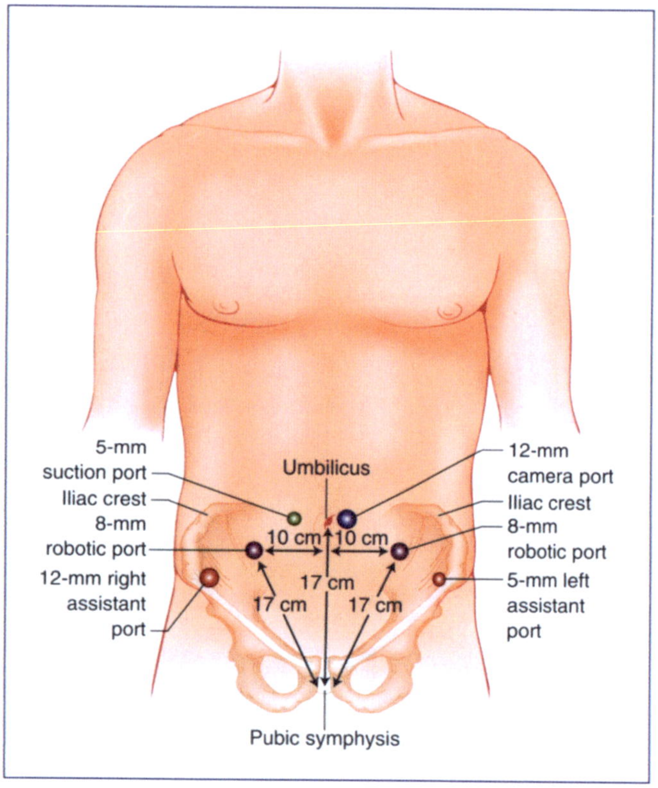

Figure 18-2. We utilize a six-port transperitoneal approach to perform robotic-assisted radical prostatectomy using the da Vinci surgical platform (Surgical Intuitive Inc.; Sunnyvale, CA), as illustrated. The 12-mm camera port is inserted around the level of the umbilicus using the Hassan technique. The two 8-mm robotic ports for robotic arms are placed 10 cm lateral to midline below the level of the umbilicus lateral to rectus muscle on either side after insufflation with carbon dioxide. The 12-mm right assistant port is placed 2 to 3 cm above the right iliac crest under direct laparoscopic guidance. The one 5-mm left assistant port is similarly placed 2 to 3 cm above the left iliac crest under direct visualization. The 5-mm suction port is sited between the camera port and the right robotic port at the level of the umbilicus.

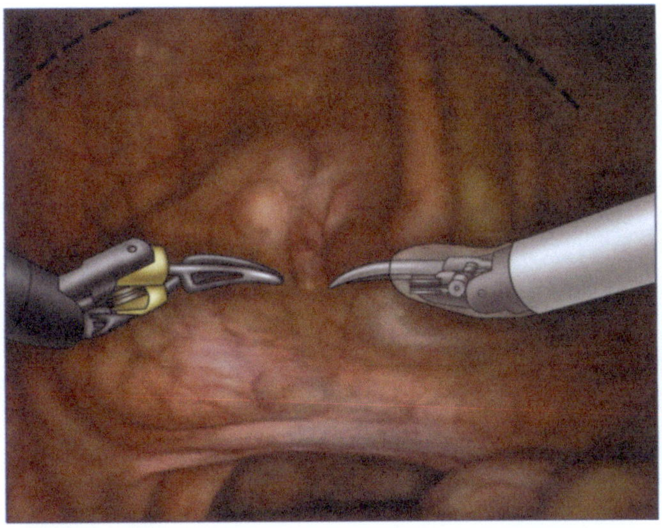

Figure 18-3. Following insertion of the transperitoneal ports and establishment of pneumoperitoneum, the pelvis is surveyed and key landmarks are identified. If adhesiolysis is required, it is carefully performed. We adopt an anterior approach to the prostate, incising the anterior peritoneum over the pubis (*dotted line*). In our experience, approaching the prostate anteriorly provides optimal exposure of key structures such as the puboprostatic ligaments and arcus tendineus fasciae pelvis.

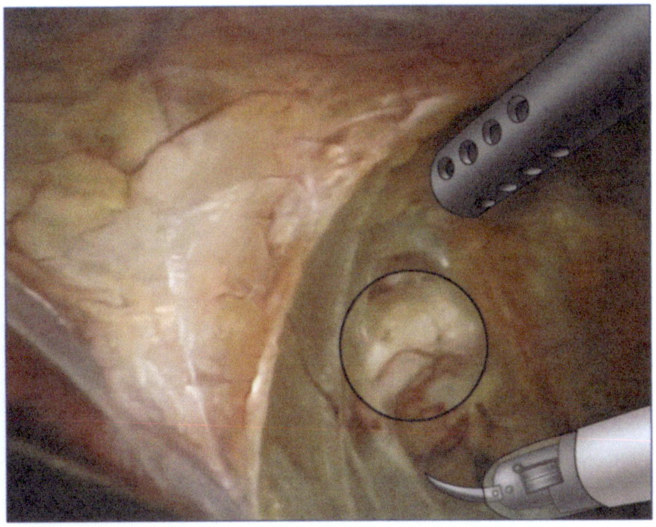

Figure 18-4. Following the incision of the anterior peritoneum, the left side of the pubis is exposed (*circle*). Dissection in the same plane on the contralateral side is similarly performed. Subsequent transection of the median umbilical ligament permits the development of a bloodless surgical plane to the anterior surface of the prostate gland.

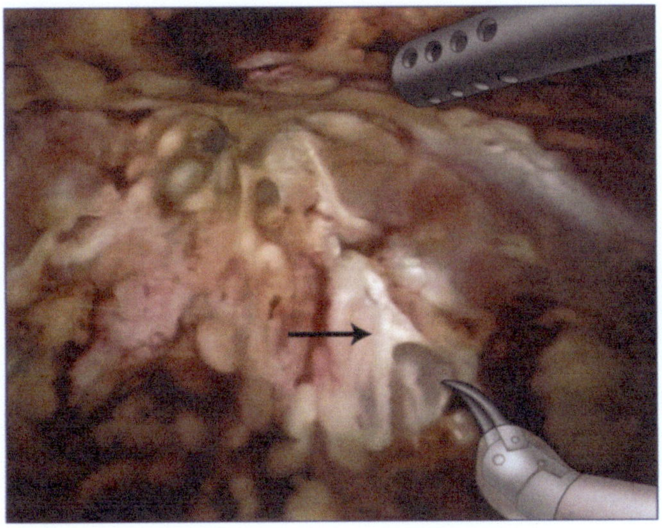

Figure 18-5. At this point, the anterior surface of the prostate along with the puboprostatic ligaments can be optimally visualized. The prostate is defatted in order to clearly identify the endopelvic fascia. This is then sparingly incised medially via the Gap of Guy (arrow), displaying the arcus tendineus and the lateral prostatic fascia.

Preservation of the Anterior Fibrotendinous Pelvic Supports

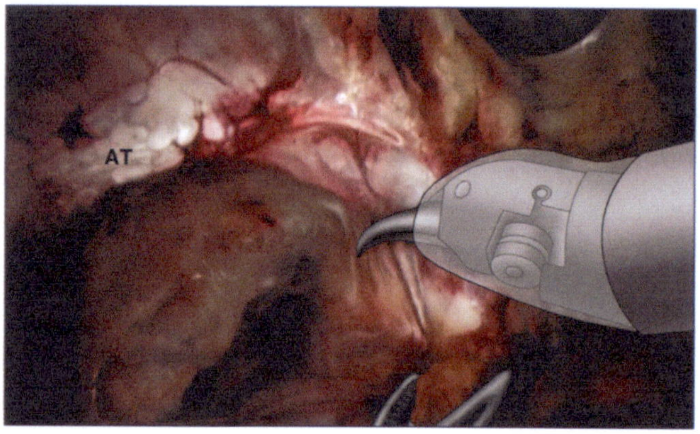

Figure 18-6. As the lateral dissection of the endopelvic fascia proceeds medially to the prostatic apex, the arcus tendineus is preserved along the course of the pelvic rim, as shown.

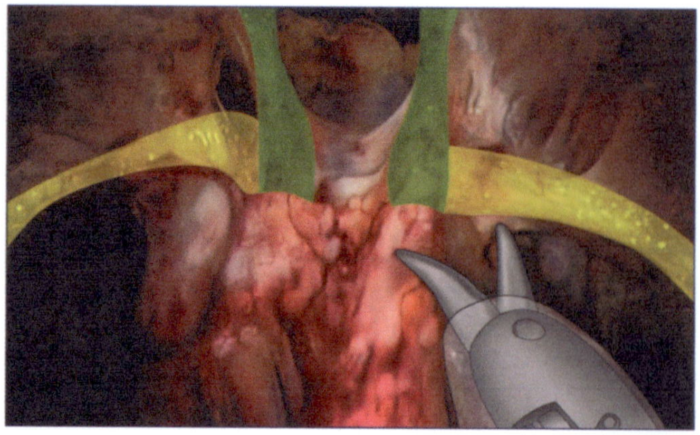

Figure 18-7. After the arcus tendineus (AT) (*yellow*) is completely dissected, the anterior support structures are visualized. The puboprostatic ligaments (*green*) are then clearly identified and dissected out. Together with the AT, the puboprostatic collar consists of the puboprostatic ligaments in continuity with the AT, which looks like a splayed H.

Control of the Dorsal Venous Complex

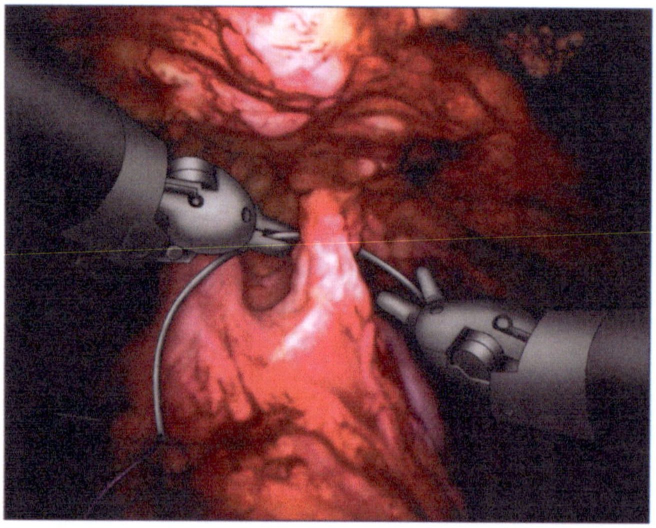

Figure 18-8. It is important to preserve the puboprostatic ligaments during control of the dorsal venous complex (DVC). The DVC is ligated using a 0 Vicryl suture on a CT-1 needle. We pass the needle medially to the right puboprostatic ligament, then behind the venous plexus, to obtain adequate vascular control while avoiding injuring the proximal urethra.

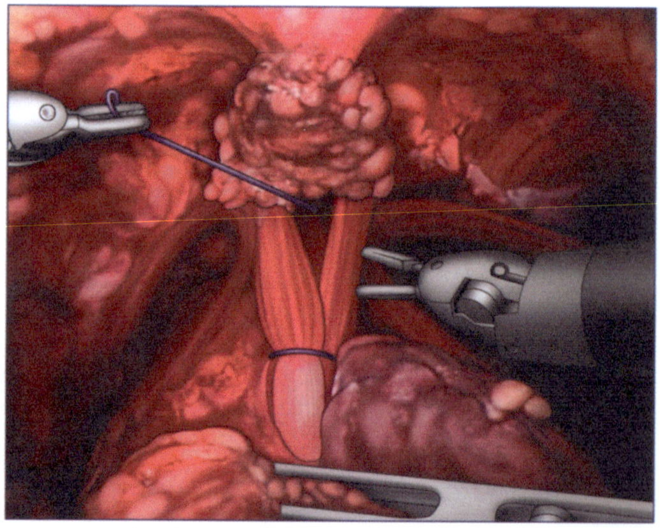

Figure 18-9. The CT-1 needle is then guided inferiorly, encompassing the deep and superficial dorsal veins while sparing the urethra. The suture is then passed medially to the left puboprostatic ligament and the dorsal venous complex is secured with a slipknot.

Bladder Neck Transection

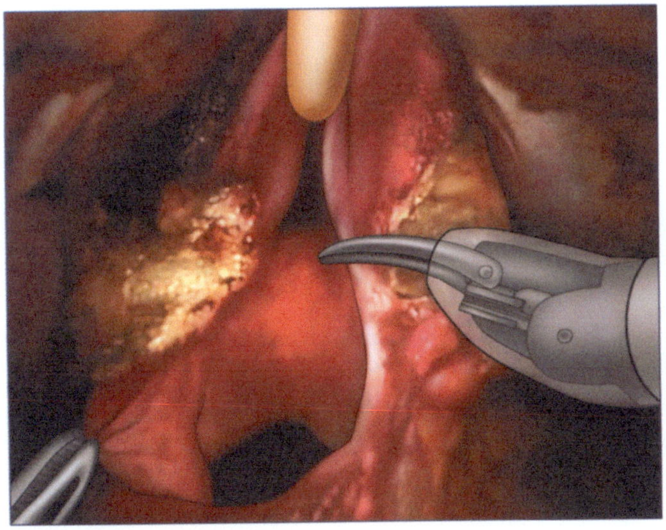

FIGURE 18-10. To better appreciate the prostatovesical junction, we employ the bimanual robotic prostate pinch, wherein both robotic arms are placed at the suspected base of the prostate, with gentle downward pressure applied toward the bladder. At the same time, the indwelling Foley urethral catheter is retracted inferiorly by the assistant, lodging the inflated catheter balloon against the bladder neck. This helps in both distinguishing the prostate/bladder neck junction and in preventing injury to the internal sphincter and the ureteric orifices during bladder neck transection. The bladder neck incision is commenced in the midline using bipolar cautery and is then developed laterally on both sides as the urethra is exposed. The ureteric orifices may be seen as the bladder neck transection is extended laterally, as shown.

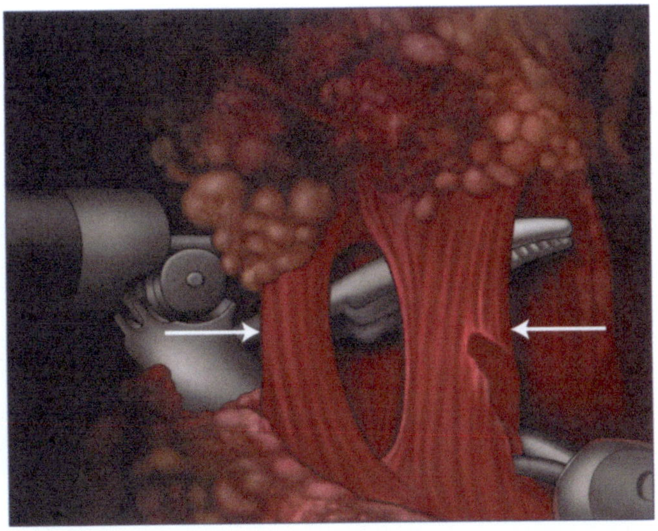

FIGURE 18-11. As the bladder neck transection is completed posteriorly, the retrotrigonal fibromuscular layer (RFL) is visualized (*arrows*). This structure eventually becomes an important tenet for subsequent reconstruction of the posterior musculofascial plate after the completion of prostatectomy. After dividing the RFL, the surgeon arrives at the posterior base of the prostate.

Posterior Dissection of the Prostate

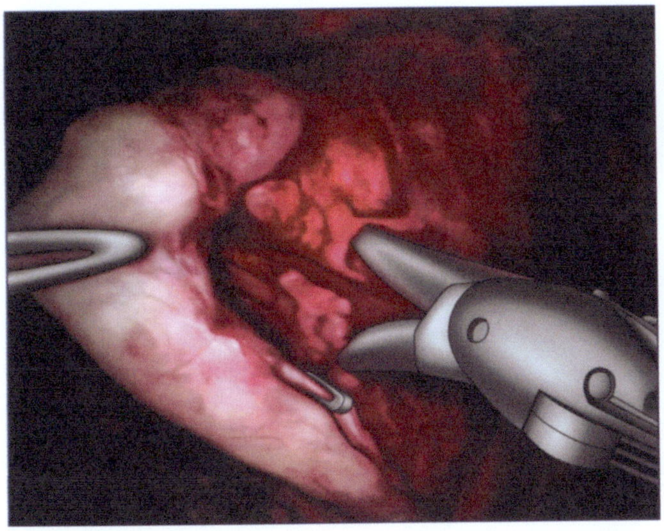

FIGURE 18-12. From this point onward, a strictly athermal approach using robotic scissors is adopted to minimize cautery injury to the erectogenic nerves surrounding the prostate. Dissection commences in the midline to avoid injury to the predominant neurovascular bundles situated at the posterolateral aspects of the prostate. Both vasa deferentia are identified and divided between clips, as shown, followed by delivery of the seminal vesicles.

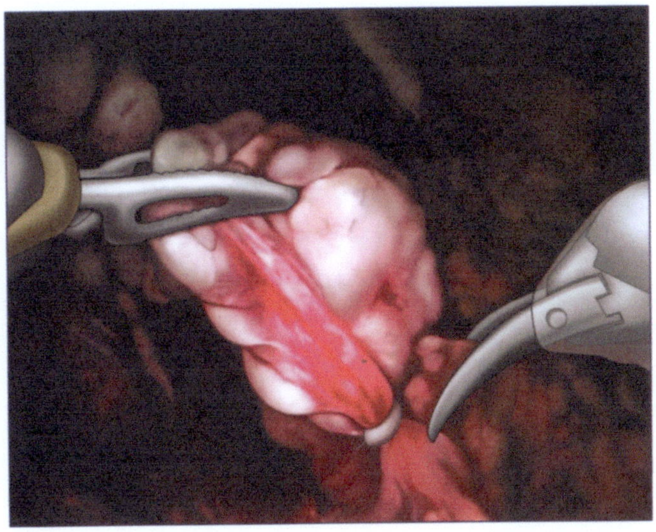

FIGURE 18-13. The seminal vesicles are approached in the midline. As the dissection planes are developed laterally, the seminal vesicle arteries are often encountered and should be controlled athermally with surgical clips, as shown.

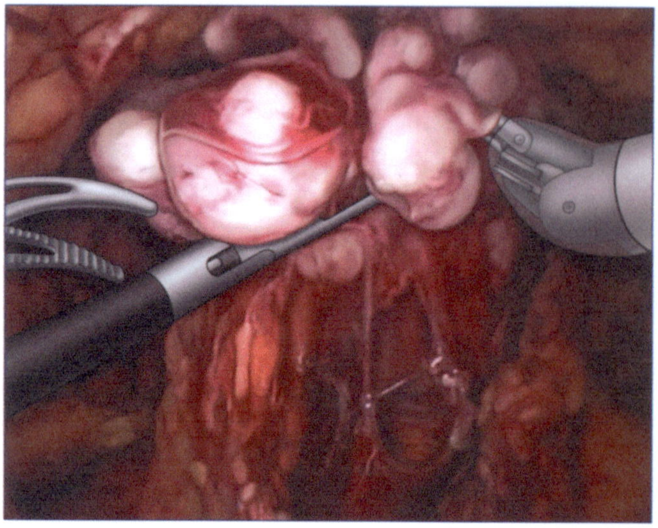

Figure 18-14. Upon division and mobilization of the vas deferentia and seminal vesicles, the dissection is continued posterior–inferiorly down to the apex of the prostate. Care is taken not to breach the posterior musculofascial plate of Denonvilliers fascia. Rectal injury during this portion of the procedure is a rare complication and can often be repaired intraoperatively if it is recognized and promptly addressed.

Risk-stratified Approach to Nerve Preservation

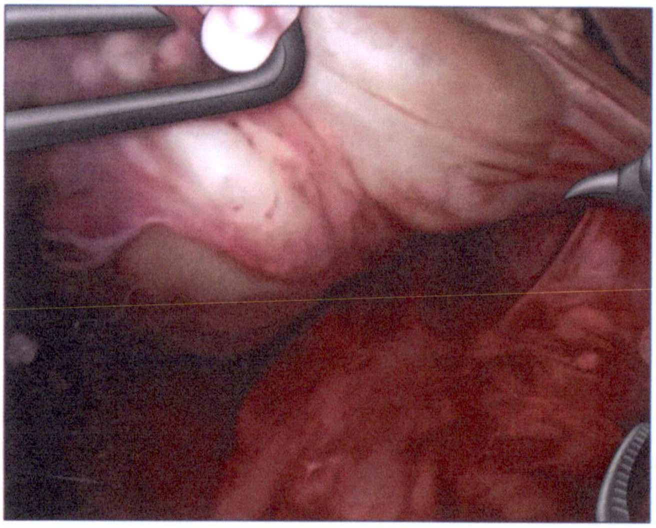

Figure 18-15. Both lateral vascular pedicles are carefully dissected athermally and are ligated with 5-mm Hemolock plastic clips. During posterolateral dissection, the surgeon has to decide on the extent of aggressiveness for nerve preservation. The desire to preserve maximal periprostatic fascial tissue containing the delicate erectogenic nerves must be carefully weighed against the need for complete clearance of cancerous tissue, bearing in mind that a significant proportion of patients have microscopic extracapsular extension (ECE) of prostate cancer. For most surgeons, the extent of nerve sparing is based on the patient's preoperative clinicopathologic characteristics, as well as visual cues of ECE encountered during athermal dissection, *eg*, induration over prostatic capsule and difficulty establishing fascial planes for dissection.

Handling the Prostatic Apex

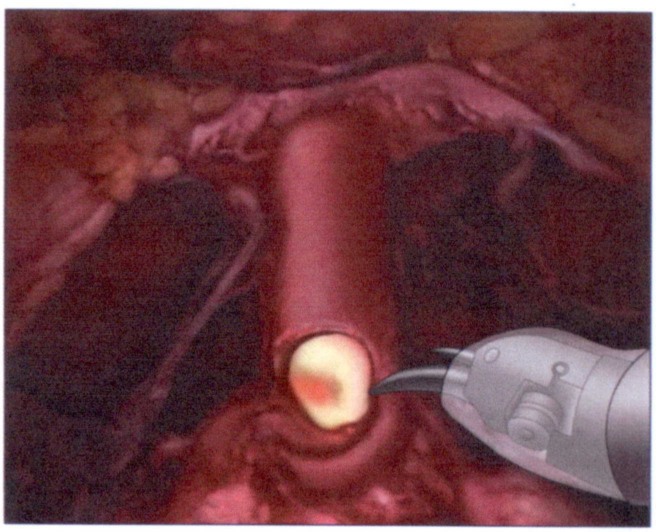

Figure 18-16. Dissection now proceeds toward the prostate apex in the anterior plane. The pubovesical aspect of the puboprostatic ligaments are divided sharply with cold scissors and anterior dissection continues through the puboprostatic components of the anterior fibromuscular stroma. The pubourethral attachments are then identified and divided, bringing the anterior surface of the prostate apex into view.

Once the prostate and the proximal urethra are dissected free, our goal then turns toward preserving maximal functional urethral length. The prostatectomy is completed upon dividing the prostatic apex. A segment of distal prostatic tissue from the apex is sent for frozen section to confirm the absence of residual cancer at the proximal urethral stump.

Approach to Posterior Reconstruction

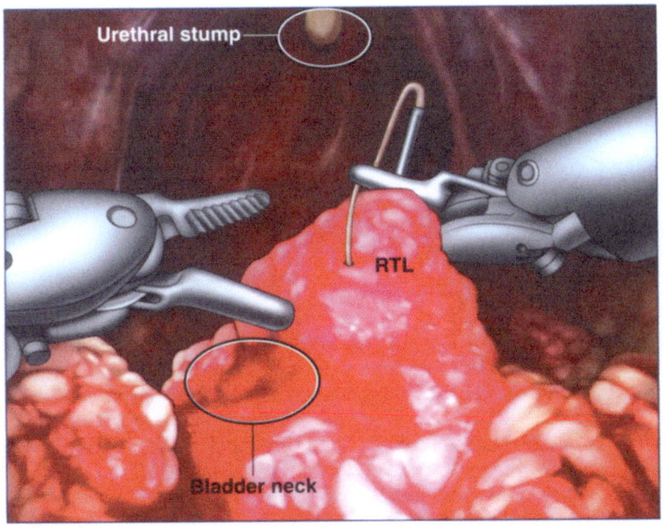

Figure 18-17. Our approach to posterior reconstruction of the bladder neck has evolved in a stepwise approach, to integrate recent advances in our understanding of the anatomy and physiology of the urethral rhabdosphincter. We have identified three areas of posterior structural deficiency resulting from excision of the prostate from its fossa. First, excision of seminal vesicles results in hypermobility and instability of the posterior bladder neck in the unsupported retrotrigonal fossa. Second, the Ω-shaped remnant urethral sphincteric complex is deficient posteriorly, with minimal suspensory support if left on its own. Third, the remnant urethral stump has a natural tendency to retract inferiorly into the pelvic floor, putting a strain on the vesico-urethral anastomosis.

To address these areas of structural deficiency, we begin by posteriorly reinforcing the bladder neck with buttressing sutures using a 0-Vicryl suture on a CT-1 needle, as shown.

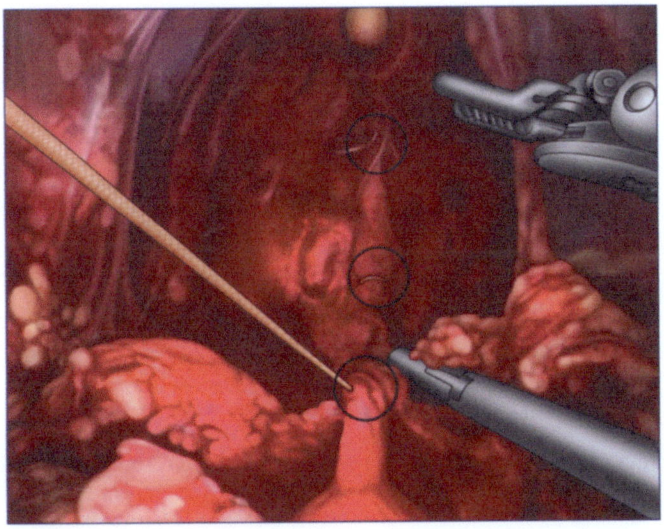

Figure 18-18. To reinforce the posteriorly deficient Ω-shaped urethral rhabdosphincter, we then suture the distal flap of Denonvilliers fascia to the reinforced posterior bladder neck close to the urethral stump to provide maximal suspensory support. The circles demonstrate points where the suture was passed through the Denonvilliers musculofascial plate.

Fashioning the Vesico-urethral Anastomosis

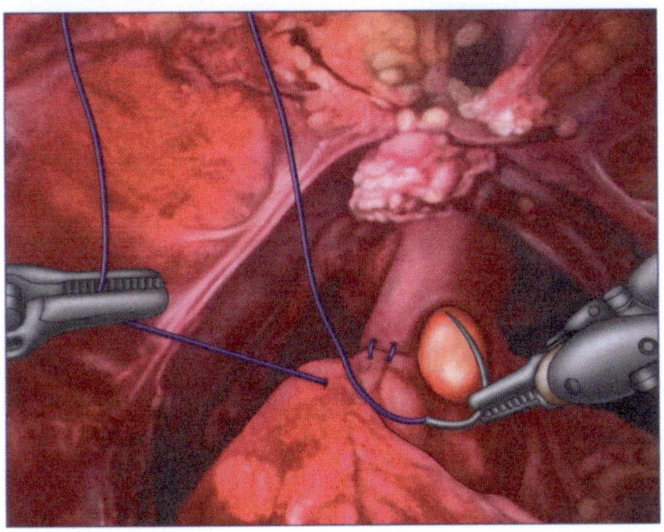

Figure 18-19. Reconstruction of the vesico-urethral anastomosis is performed using a 3-0 Monocryl continuously running suture. The previous steps of reconstructing the posterior bladder neck and Denonvilliers musculofascial plate now serve to offset tension on the anastomosis and to optimize mucosal coaptation during its construction. They also serve to dissipate downward pelvic pressure on the anastomosis during micturition in the postoperative phase. The continuous running suture is passed through the posterior Denonvilliers musculofascial plate to prevent urethral stump recession.

Approach to Anterior Reconstruction

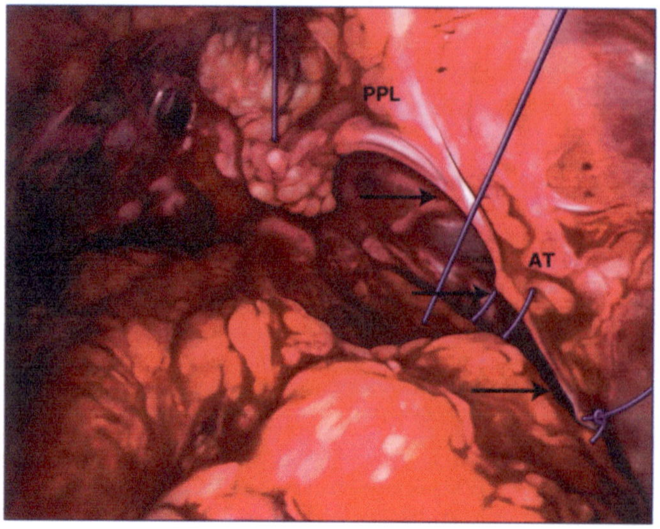

FIGURE 18-20. To provide full circumferential suspensory support to the newly fashioned anastomosis, we now suture the anterior fibrotendinous pelvic supports (chiefly, the arcus tendineus and puboprostatic ligaments) that were previously preserved to the anterior bladder neck using partial-thickness sutures. This segment of anterior reconstruction serves to both prevent pelvic descent of the bladder neck and to dissipate the downward pressure of the bladder on the vesico-urethral anastomosis during micturition.

Conclusion

Comparing our experience of the total anatomic restoration technique in 530 patients versus a cohort of 215 patients receiving conventional vesico-urethral anastomosis, the continence rate following robotic-assisted prostatectomy at 1, 6, 12, and 24 weeks following robotic-assisted radical prostatectomy was 38.6% versus 13.0%, 82.6% versus 35.0%, 90.5% versus 50.0%, and 97.5% versus 62.0%, respectively. We postulate that the overall biomechanical effects of our composite approach are threefold. First, it provides circumferential dynamic suspensory support for the urethral sphincter complex. Second, it avoids pelvic prolapse and downward pressure of the bladder on the healing anastomosis during micturition. Third, tension at the anastomosis is relieved with improved mucosal apposition [16].

References

1. Jemal A, Siegel R, Ward E, *et al.*: Cancer statistics, 2009. *CA Cancer J Clin* 2009, 59:225–249.
2. Grönberg H: Prostate cancer epidemiology. *Lancet* 2003, 361:859–864.
3. Quinn M, Babb P: Patterns and trends in prostate cancer incidence, survival, prevalence and mortality. Part 1: International comparisons. *BJU Int* 2002, 90:162–173.
4. Han M, Partin AW, Chan DY, Walsh PC: An evaluation of the decreasing incidence of positive surgical margins in a large retropubic prostatectomy series. *J Urol* 2004, 171:23–26.
5. Berryhill R Jr, Jhaveri JK, Yadav RA, *et al.*: Robotic prostatectomy: a review of outcomes compared with laparoscopic and open approaches. *Urology* 2008, 72:15–23.
6. Parsons JK, Bennett JL: Outcomes of retropubic, laparoscopic and robotic-assisted prostatectomy. *Urology* 2008, 72:412–416.
7. Coakley FV, Eberhardt S, Kattan MW, *et al.*: Urinary continence after radical retropubic prostatectomy: relationship with membranous urethral length on preoperative endorectal magnetic resonance imaging. *J Urol* 2002, 168:1032–35.
8. Burnett AL, Mostwin JL: In situ anatomical study of the male urethral sphincteric complex: relevance to continence preservation following major pelvic surgery. *J Urol* 1998, 160:1301–1306.
9. Stolzenburg JU, Schwalenberg T, Horn L-C, *et al.*: Anatomical landmarks of radical prostatectomy. *Eur Urol* 2007, 51:629–639.
10. Tewari A, El-Hakim A, Rao S, Raman JD: Identification of the retrotrigonal layer as a key anatomical landmark during robotically assisted radical prostatectomy. *BJU Int* 2006, 98:829–832.
11. Tewari AK, Bigelow K, Rao S, *et al.*: Anatomic restoration technique of continence mechanism and preservation of puboprostatic collar: a novel modification to achieve early urinary continence in men undergoing robotic prostatectomy. *Urology* 2007, 69:726–731.
12. Takenaka A, Tewari AK, Leung RA, *et al.*: Preservation of the puboprostatic collar and puboperineoplasty for early recovery of urinary continence after robotic prostatectomy: anatomic basis and preliminary outcomes. *Eur Urol* 2007, 51:433–440.
13. Tewari A, Jhaveri J, Rao S, *et al.*: Total reconstruction of the vesico-urethral junction. *BJU Int* 2008, 101:871–877.
14. Nguyen L, Jhaveri J, Tewari A: Surgical technique to overcome anatomical shortcoming: balancing post-prostatectomy continence outcomes of urethral sphincter lengths on preoperative magnetic resonance imaging. *J Urol* 2008, 179:1907–1911.
15. Tewari A, Peabody J, Sarle R, *et al.*: Technique of da Vinci robot-assisted anatomic radical prostatectomy. *Urology* 2002, 60:569–572.
16. Tan GY, Jhaveri JK, Tewari AK: Anatomic restoration technique (ART): a biomechanics based approach for early continence recovery following minimally invasive radical prostatectomy. *Urology* 2009, Epub July 7. DOI: 10.1016/j.urology.2009.02.005.
17. Pagano F, Prayer-Galetti T, d'Arrigo L, *et al.*: Radical surgery for clinically confined prostate cancer. *Ann N Y Acad Sci* 1996, 784:85–92.
18. Rocco F, Carmignani L, Acquati P, *et al.*: Restoration of posterior aspect of rhabdosphincter shortens continence time after radical retropubic prostatectomy. *J Urol* 2006, 175:2201–2206.
19. Rocco B, Gregori A, Stener S, *et al.*: Posterior reconstruction of the rhabdosphincter allows a rapid recovery of continence after transperitoneal videolaparoscopic radical prostatectomy. *Eur Urol* 2007, 51:996–1003.
20. Nguyen MM, Kamoi K, Stein RJ, *et al.*: Early continence outcomes of posterior musculofascial plate reconstruction during robotic and laparoscopic prostatectomy. *BJU Int* 2008, 101:1135–1139.

19 Sacral Neuromodulation for Voiding Dysfunction

Travis L. Bullock and Steven W. Siegel

Urinary urgency, frequency, nocturia, urge urinary incontinence, and voiding dysfunction are common disorders affecting the quality of life of millions of men and women. Treatment with behavioral interventions and pelvic floor muscle rehabilitation are appropriate initial treatments, but may be limited by patient compliance and an inability to control symptoms sufficiently. Pharmacotherapy focuses mainly on anticholinergic medications that reduce acetylcholine-mediated detrusor contractions, but in many cases a lack of efficacy or intolerable side effects limit their therapeutic usefulness. When a patient is refractory to the therapies listed previously, other options must be considered. Sacral neuromodulation (SNM) has gained increased acceptance as the standard of care for these individuals [1,2].

SNM for the treatment of refractory voiding dysfunction was first described by Tanagho and Schmidt [3] in 1988. A commercially available device for SNM, InterStim (Medtronic; Minneapolis, MN), was approved by the Food and Drug Administration (FDA) for the treatment of urge urinary incontinence in 1997, and for urgency–frequency syndrome and idiopathic nonobstructive urinary retention in 1999. Later, the labeling was changed to include "overactive bladder" as an appropriate diagnostic category. Patients from these groups are appropriate for SNM when they have chronic symptoms that significantly affect quality of life and conservative treatments have proven unsuccessful. Currently, over 50,000 individuals worldwide have been implanted with the device.

The observation that sacral nerve stimulation may reduce or eliminate symptoms of voiding dysfunction implies an alteration of the pelvic neuromuscular environment and derangement in organ function, as opposed to an anatomic disorder. This pathologic state represents an imbalance of the reflexes between the bladder, sphincter, and pelvic floor, and SNM improves or restores this balance. The fact that the same treatment may be effective for symptoms of overactive bladder and retention implies that the therapy is modulating the central nervous system at the level where switching between bladder emptying and storage occurs.

SNM has proven to be effective and enduring. Initial investigations reported 6-month clinical success (> 50% improvement in baseline voiding symptoms) in 56%, 76%, and 83% of patients with urgency–frequency syndrome, urge urinary incontinence, and nonobstruction urinary retention, respectively. Siegel *et al.* [4] demonstrated that after 3 years of therapy, 59% of urge-incontinent patients showed a greater than 50% reduction in leaking episodes per day, with 46% completely dry. After 2 years, 56% of urgency–frequency syndrome patients showed a greater than 50% reduction in voids per day. At 1.5 years followup, 70% of nonobstructive retention patients showed a greater than 50% reduction in catheterized volumes or eliminated the need for catheterization all together [5]. Furthermore, results from a 5-year prospective, multicenter trial have recently been published, showing that at 5 years postimplantation, 68% of patients with urge incontinence, 56% with urgency–frequency syndrome, and 71% with retention have successful outcomes [6].

The procedure is performed in two phases; the first is a screening test. If this test is successful, it will be followed by conversion to the permanent form of therapy with implantation of the programmable pulse generator. At the time of inception, the screening test was performed via a percutaneous nerve evaluation followed by a sacral laminectomy to access the appropriate nerve roots with implantation of the chronic lead and implantable pulse generator. With the advent of the tined lead, approved by the FDA in 2002, the procedure has evolved to become significantly less invasive, making it possible to complete the procedure under intravenous sedation with local anesthesia. The patient may be alert in order to provide sensory feedback, which may facilitate more accurate placement and comfortable positioning of the lead. In addition, the advent of the tined lead staged trial, first described by Spinelli *et al.* [7], has in many ways improved the screening process and increased therapeutic successes.

In many cases we perform a two-staged procedure with a tined lead implant as the initial therapeutic trial. One benefit of this approach is the ability to place a potentially permanent lead under minimal anesthesia. Additionally, it is our impression that this technique results in a lower rate of false positives and the more accurate placement of the potentially permanent lead, which may also result in a higher rate of appropriate patient selection and decrease the need for future revision surgery. We typically conduct the staged lead implant over a 3- to 4-week time period and if there is at least a 50% improvement of the target symptoms implantation of the neurostimulator is justified. Detailed explanations of the steps involved in the two-stage implantation of a sacral nerve stimulator (InterStim; Medtronic; Minneapolis, MN) are descried in this chapter.

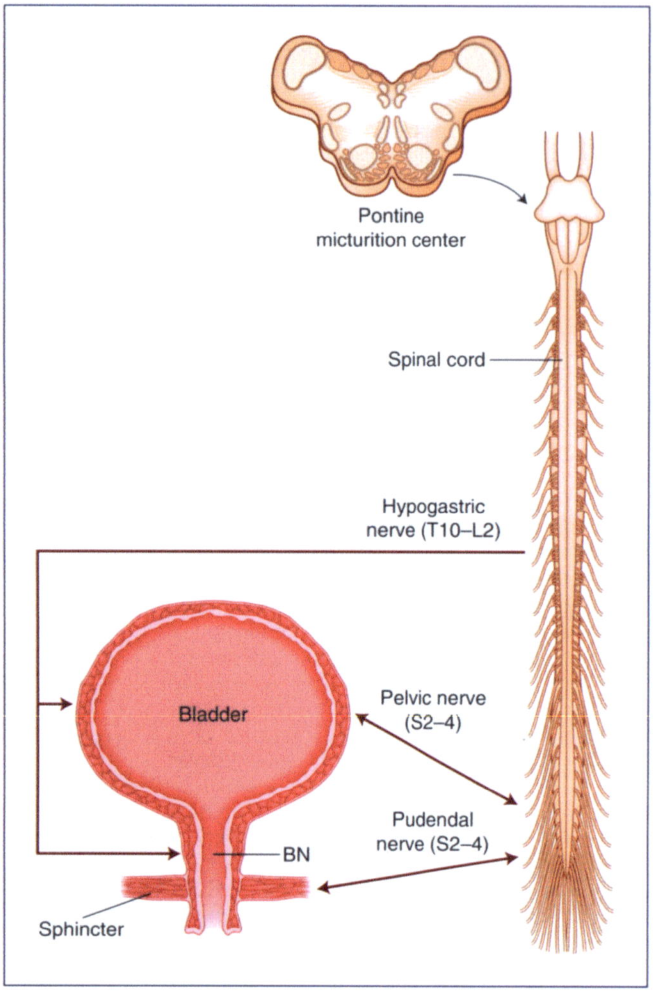

FIGURE 19-1. Neurologic control over voiding. Under nonpathologic conditions, the bladder stores urine under low pressure. The pontine micturition center coordinates elimination though a complex interplay of the sympathetic, parasympathetic, and somatic nervous system. During storage afferent, sympathetic activity is transmitted via the hypogastric nerve (T10–L2), resulting in detrusor relaxation and bladder neck (BN) contraction. Stimulation of the somatic nervous system via the pudendal nerve results in external sphincter contraction, further facilitating storage. During voiding, increased parasympathetic activity via the pelvic nerve results in acetylcholine-mediated detrusor contraction, while the somatic pudendal nerve affects sphincter relaxation and results in a coordinated voiding reflex [8,9].

Possible Mechanisms of Action of Sacral Nerve Stimulation

Direct inhibition of afferent detrusor stimulation through spinal pathways

Stimulation of sensory afferents from the pelvic floor leading to the inhibition of motor neurons

Inhibition of afferent pudendal nerve signaling

Inhibition of the micturition reflex via complex interactions in the central nervous system

Suppression of the guarding reflex by turning off the bladder afferent input to the internal or external urethral sphincter

Activation of bladder efferents to stimulation voiding while simultaneously inhibiting excitatory pathways to the urethra

FIGURE 19-2. Possible mechanisms of sacral nerve stimulation. The true mechanism of action of sacral neuromodulation (SNM) has yet to be fully elucidated, although various hypotheses have been suggested. In patients with urgency–frequency syndrome and urge urinary incontinence, it is likely that the modulatory effects take place via afferent nerve stimulation at the level of the sacral nerve root or the pudendal nerve. In patients with idiopathic retention, SNM is thought to work through inhibition of the guarding reflex, thereby allowing for coordinated voiding [9,10].

Stage 1: Placement of the Sacral Lead

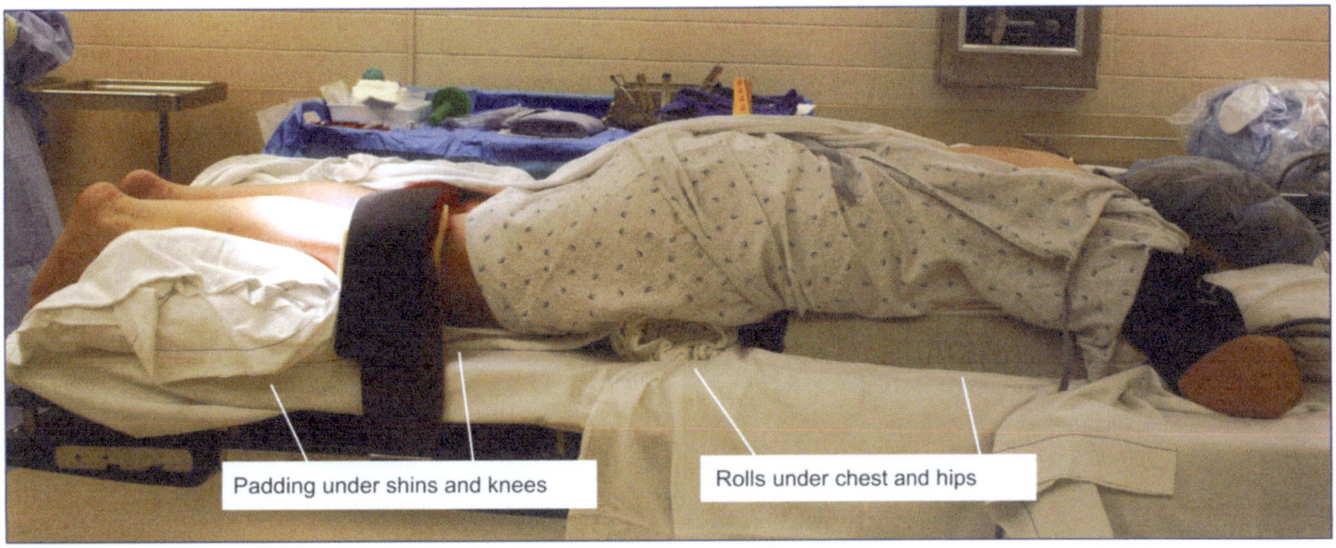

Figure 19-3. Patient positioning. We commonly perform the sacral neuromodulation procedure under monitored anesthesia care with local anesthesia, which allows the patient to give sensory feedback while the lead is being positioned, if desired. In addition, the quick patient recovery allows for immediate programming of the device postoperatively. A cocktail of propofol (Diprivan; AstraZeneca, Wilmington, DE), fentanyl (Sublimaze; Akorn, Somerset, NJ; Janssen, Titusville, NJ), and midazolam (Versed; Hoffmann-La Roche, Nutley, NJ) are often used with bupivacaine (Marcaine; AstraZeneca, Wilmington, DE) at the skin level. In rare cases in which general anesthesia is preferred, it is imperative that only short-acting paralytics are used in order to not obscure motor responses during intra-operative stimulation. The patient is positioned on the operative table in the prone position so that fluoroscopy can be utilized to obtain anterior–posterior and lateral views of the sacrum. Rolls are placed under the chest and pelvis, and pillows are used beneath the knees and shins to pad pressure points. The feet must remain uncovered to allow for direct observation during the procedure. The lower back and buttocks are prepped with an antiseptic solution and draped into the operative field. Before the start of the procedure, a prophylactic dose of an antibiotic that is effective against skin flora, such as cephazolin (Ancef; GlaxoSmith-Kline, Philadelphia, PA), is administered.

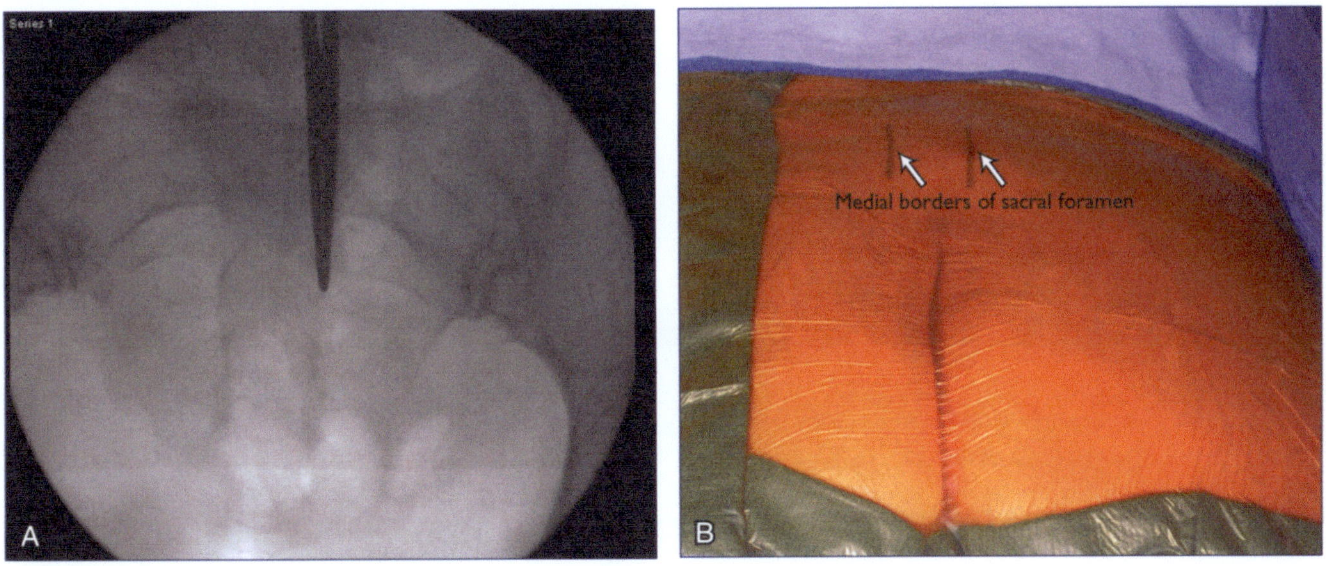

Figure 19-4. Selecting the appropriate spinal foramen. In general, the target spinal foramen is the one that corresponds to the third sacral nerve root (S3). In rare circumstances, the fourth sacral nerve (S4) is preferable. The second sacral nerve (S2) generally is not appropriate for chronic stimulation. If the patient has a lateralizing pain component, the S3 nerve root on that side is usually chosen for lead placement. Initially, an anterior–posterior fluoroscopic view is obtained to determine the medial edge of the sacral foramina and a mark is made on the skin (**A**). An imaginary line parallel to the spine at the level of either mark is where the foramina "line up." The distance between the foramen is usually two finger breadths across the midline. Skin marks corresponding to the medial border of the foramen are made to use as a guide for needle placement (**B**).

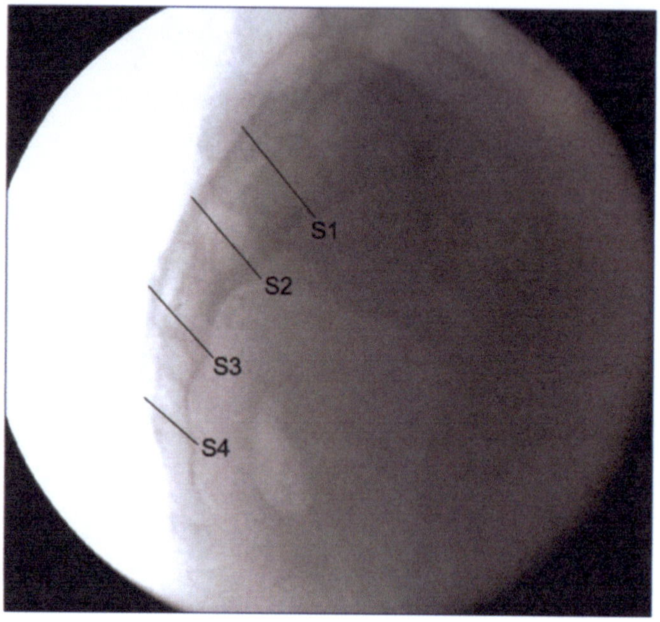

FIGURE 19-5. A lateral fluoroscopic view is obtained to locate the target foramen (S3). On the lateral view, the S2 level is readily identified as where the sacro-iliac joint fuses, forming a characteristic shadow. The first anterior protrusion or "hillock" from the surface of the sacrum below this shadow is typically S3.

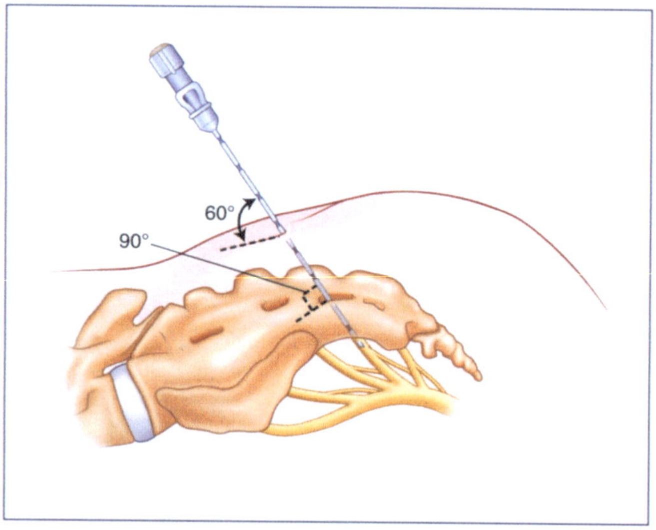

FIGURE 19-6. Once the starting point has been estimated with the aid of fluoroscopy, the skin is anesthetized with 0.25% bupivacaine (Marcaine; AstraZeneca, Wilmington, DE) in order to create a dime-sized wheel. It may also be necessary to numb the sacral periosteum if the patient exhibits discomfort. It is not usually necessary to numb the intervening subcutaneous fat and tissues, as they are devoid of nerve fibers. At a 60-degree angle to the skin, a specialized foramen needle is then "walked" up or down along the line of the foramina, which was determined on the anterior–posterior view, until it drops into the S3 foramen. The course of the needle's passage can be monitored with fluoroscopy to aid in rapid placement. As the aim of the needle is adjusted up or down, it is important to pull it out and reinsert it, rather than torquing or bending it. Once it enters the foramen, fluoroscopy is used to gauge the depth so that the needle tip is just beyond the posterior surface of the bone table. The foramen needle is then stimulated with the screening device to check sacral root responses.

Sacral Root Motor and Sensory Responses

Level	Motor
S2	Bellows (inward rolling of intergluteal fold), clamp (A-P pinching of perineum/coccyx), dorsiflexion of foot, heel rotation, calf cramping
S3	Bellows, dorsiflexion of great toe
S4	Bellows

FIGURE 19-7. Sacral root motor responses. A bellows response (rolling inward and deepening of the intergluteal fold due to levator contraction) and dorsiflexion of the ipsilateral great toes confirms that the S3 nerve is being stimulated. If responses are not appropriate at this level (*ie*, consistent with S2 or S4), the point of introduction at the skin level is reestimated in order to aim for the next foramen either above or below to correctly enter the S3 spinal foramen. In general, S2 is not suitable for chronic stimulation due to significant lower extremity motor responses [9].

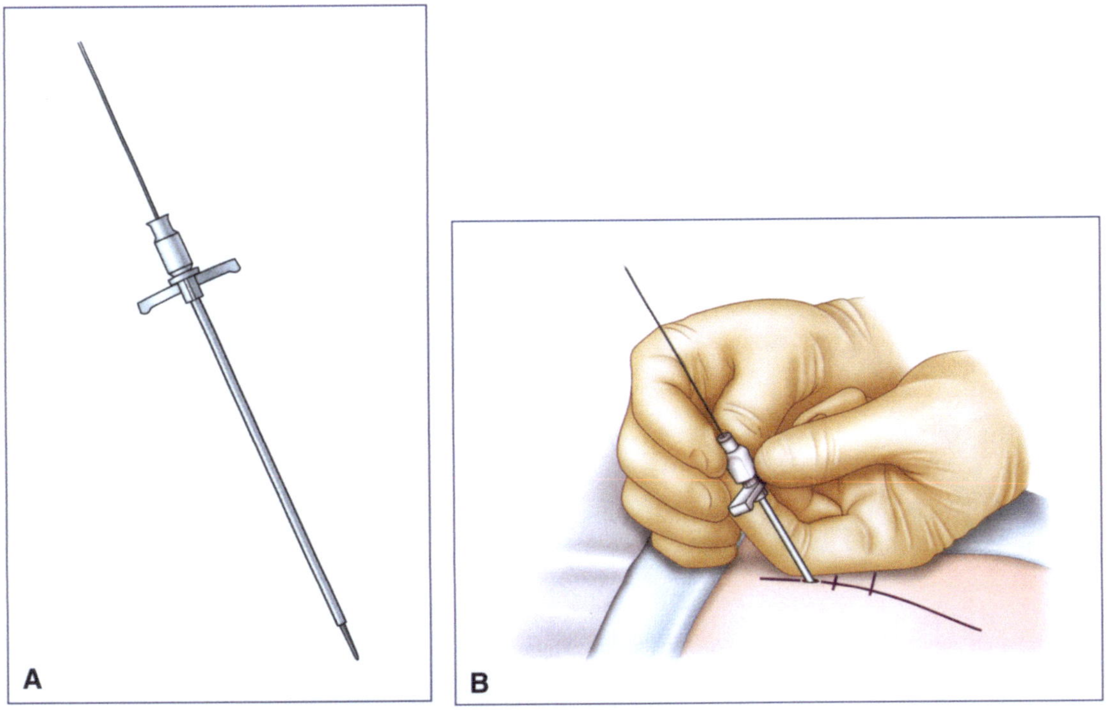

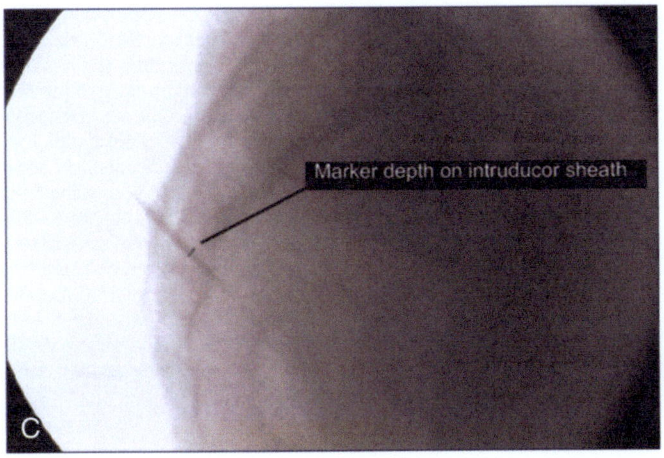

FIGURE 19-8. Placement of the lead introducer sheath. Once the course of the nerve has been fathomed by using the foramen needle, a skin nick is made at this insertion point, the metal stylet is placed through the foramen needle, and the needle is exchanged for the lead introducer sheath (**A** and **B**). The tip of the introducer sheath has a radio opaque marker and its depth should be about one-half to two-thirds through the bone table (**C**). Deployment of the lead at this level allows it to be released in a fatty plane surrounding the neurovascular bundle. It is also very helpful to use the curved stylet, which is included in an accessory kit (Medtronic Dual Lead-Extension Accessory Kit; Medtronic, Minneapolis, MN), as it is softer than the one currently packaged with the lead and is less likely to force the electrode out of the proper plane.

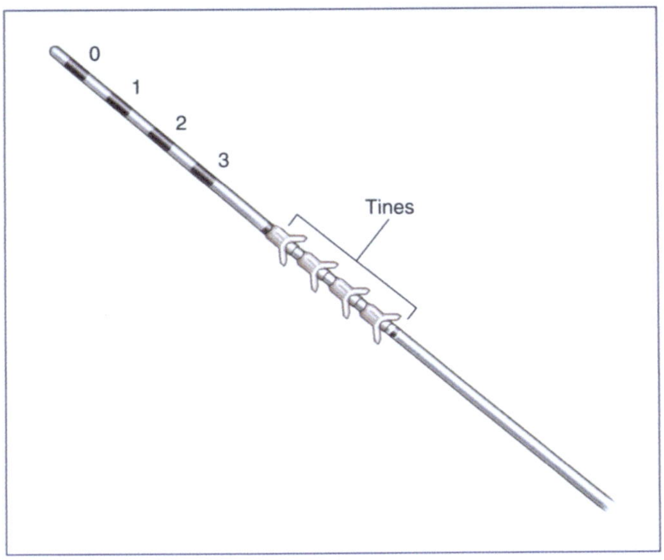

FIGURE 19-9. Tined lead. Approved by the Food and Drug Administration in 2002, the tined lead has allowed lead implantation to evolve from a sacral laminectomy to a minimally invasive procedure performed percutaneously under minimal anesthesia. Instead of direct anchoring of the permanent lead to the periosteum of the sacrum, lead dislodgement is now avoided by utilizing a series of four tines that, after appropriate healing, secure themselves in the subcutaneous tissues. The lead contains four electrodes that ideally parallel and interface with the sacral nerve. These contact points are numbered 0 to 3 and allow for a variation in the site of stimulation.

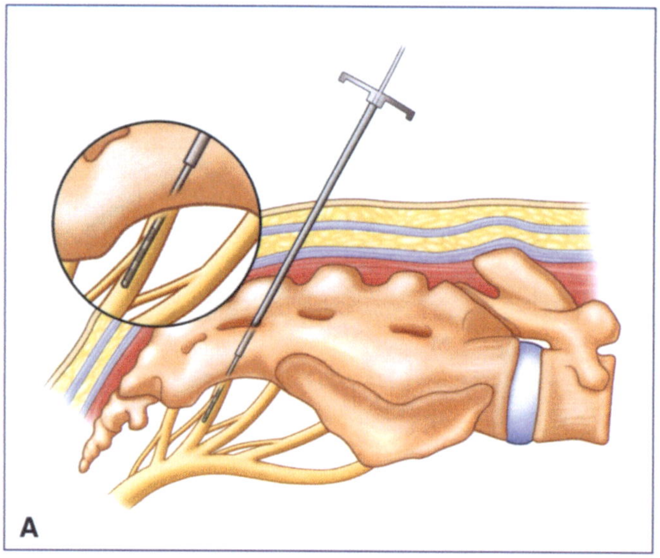

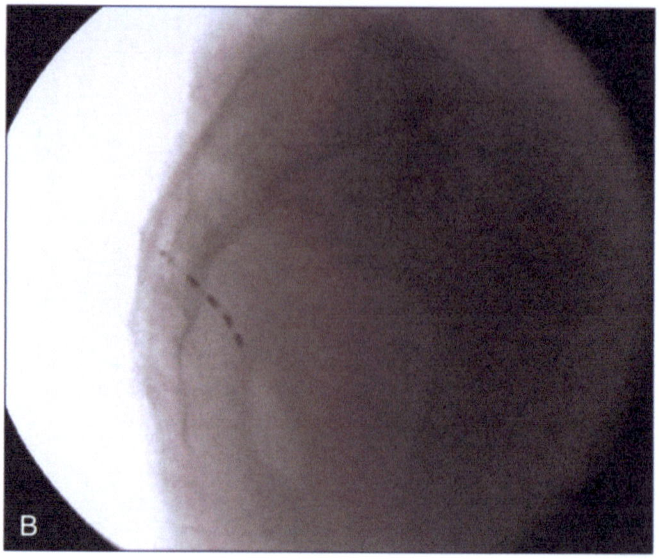

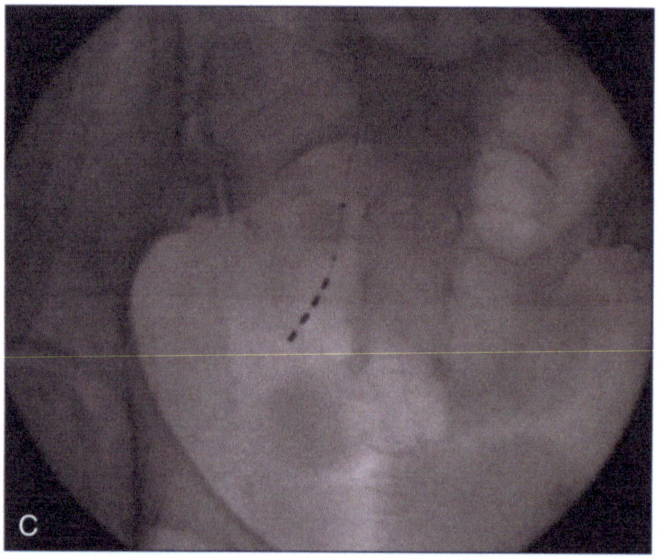

FIGURE 19-10. Deployment of the tined lead. After proper placement of the introducer sheath has been confirmed by fluoroscopy, the tined lead can be placed through its lumen (**A**). When deployed properly, the lead should always point caudally and laterally. We always straddle the bone table with lead sites 2 and 3 (**B**) because this allows for a consistent lead depth, prevents premature deployment of the tines, and provides a point of reference in the future. Once a satisfactory trajectory of the lead has been obtained, each lead site is stimulated and the threshold of response is measured. If each site elicits an appropriate response at a relatively low threshold, the position of the nerve has been appropriately paralleled by the lead. If not, the lead should be pulled back, repositioned under fluoroscopic control, and retested at each contact point. The goal is to get all four contact points yielding an appropriate response at a relatively low threshold. Once the ideal position has been determined, the tines are deployed by pulling the introducer sheath back under fluoroscopic guidance. When viewed in the anterior–posterior orientation, the lead should be seen to sweep laterally, paralleling the course of the nerve (**C**).

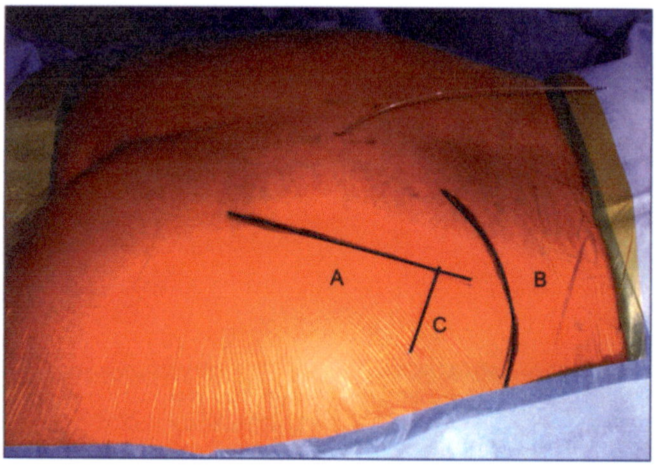

FIGURE 19-11. Once the lead is deployed, the right lateral edge of the sacrum (*A*) and the posterior–superior iliac crest (*B*) are marked. The future site of the implantable pulse generator (IPG) incision is marked (*C*) so that it may be placed in a plane of fat away from boney prominences should the trial be successful and the patient proceed to the permanent implant. After infiltration with a local anesthetic, a 1–2-cm incision at the lateral aspect of the future IPG incision is made and will be the placement site of the connection hub. Care must be taken to deepen the incision completely through the skin into fat, preventing the lead from getting caught too superficially.

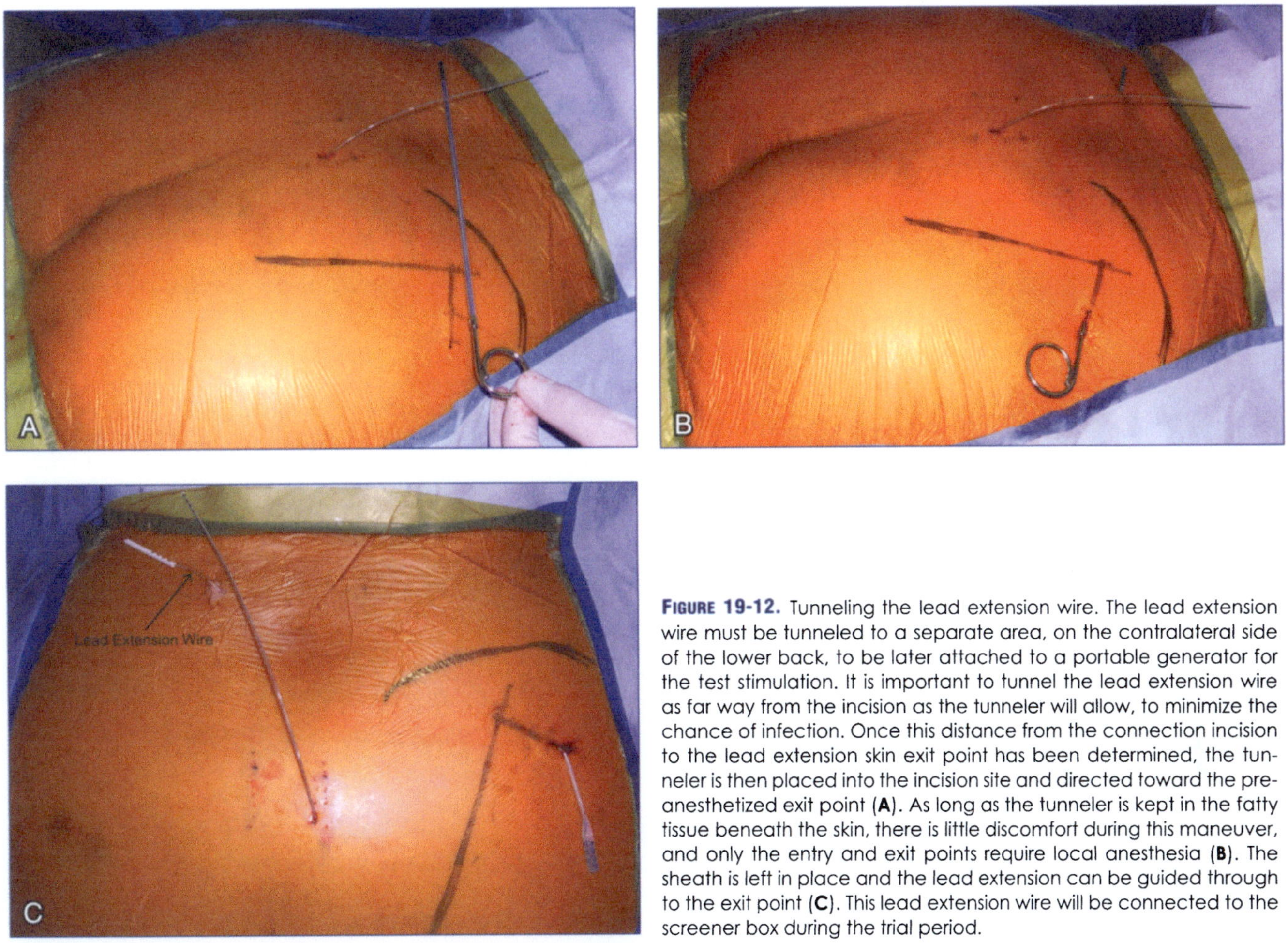

Figure 19-12. Tunneling the lead extension wire. The lead extension wire must be tunneled to a separate area, on the contralateral side of the lower back, to be later attached to a portable generator for the test stimulation. It is important to tunnel the lead extension wire as far way from the incision as the tunneler will allow, to minimize the chance of infection. Once this distance from the connection incision to the lead extension skin exit point has been determined, the tunneler is then placed into the incision site and directed toward the preanesthetized exit point (**A**). As long as the tunneler is kept in the fatty tissue beneath the skin, there is little discomfort during this maneuver, and only the entry and exit points require local anesthesia (**B**). The sheath is left in place and the lead extension can be guided through to the exit point (**C**). This lead extension wire will be connected to the screener box during the trial period.

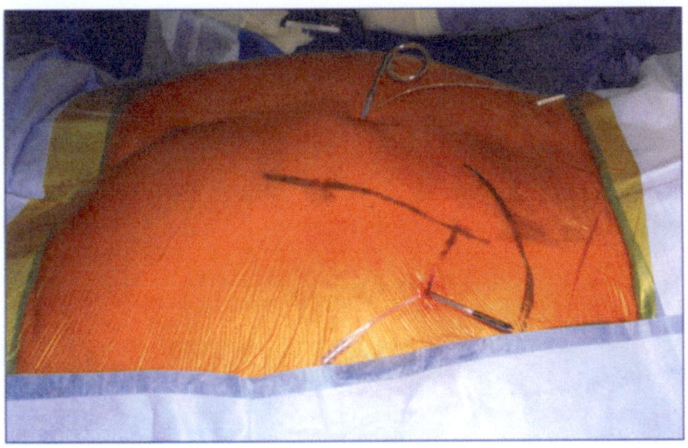

Figure 19-13. Tunneling the tined lead to the connection site. The tined lead is tunneled to the connection incision again, using the tunneling device. We typically curve the tunneling device to cause the lead to sweep down and back up toward the incision, to take up some of the redundant lead length and also to allow for the lead to be placed in a predictable position. The connection hub between the tined lead and lead extension wire is formed and placed in the subcutaneous fat underneath the future implantable pulse generator (IPG) incision site. This allows for the connecting hub to be immediately located during the second phase of the procedure, in which the lead extension wire can be removed or the incision extended medially to allow for IPG placement.

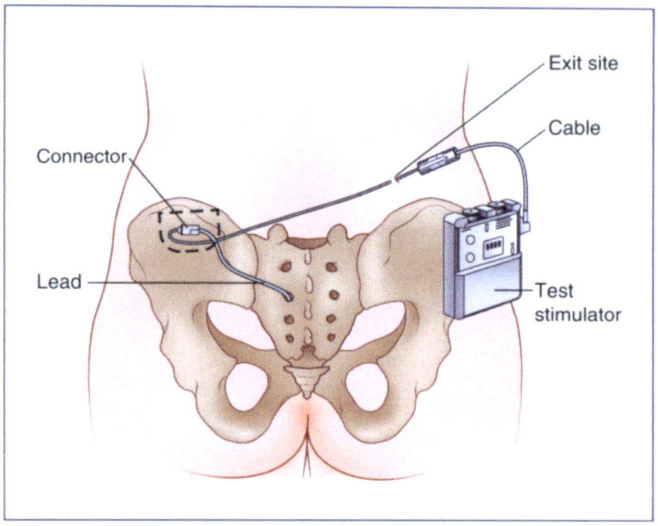

FIGURE 19-14. Completion of stage 1. The procedure is completed by irrigating the wound with an antibiotic solution, achieving final hemostasis, and closing the incisions. It is important that water, rather than saline, is used as an irrigating solution because charged ions may interfere with the electrical connections. Patients are discharged after programming and return in 1 week for reprogramming, as needed. A 3- to 4-week trial period is used routinely, as this is helpful in making sure programming is optimized and for evaluating the response in terms of the target symptoms. At the end of the trial period, the second stage of the procedure is performed, in which the implantable pulse generator can be inserted if appropriate efficacy is achieved or the tined lead and lead extension wire can be explanted if urinary symptoms are not improved to a point that justifies permanent implantation.

Voiding Diary

Date	AM	AM	AM	AM	AM	AM	AM
Fluid intake (oz)	PM	PM	PM	PM	PM	PM	PM
Volume voided into measuring cup (oz or cc)							
Voiding measured by catheter (oz or cc; if applicable)							
Please rate any leaking you experienced (slight = a few drops; moderate = 1–2 tablespoons; heavy = soaks pad/diaper or outer clothing)	None	None	None	None	None	None	None
	Slight	Slight	Slight	Slight	Slight	Slight	Slight
	Moderate	Moderate	Moderate	Moderate	Moderate	Moderate	Moderate
	Heavy	Heavy	Heavy	Heavy	Heavy	Heavy	Heavy
What were you doing at the time of the leaking?							
If leaking caused you to change your pad/diaper/clothing, put an **X** in the box							
Did you feel empty after voiding? **Yes** or **No**							
Rate the force of the stream. For example, **strong, fair, poor, intermittent, etc.**							
Degree of urgency prior to voiding	Normal	Normal	Normal	Normal	Normal	Normal	Normal
	Moderate	Moderate	Moderate	Moderate	Moderate	Moderate	Moderate
	Severe	Severe	Severe	Severe	Severe	Severe	Severe
Pelvic/bladder pain. For example, **mild, moderate, severe, etc.**							

Pre-operatively, the patient should have completed baseline diaries documenting their specific voiding dysfunction or incontinence. These include quantification of urinary frequency, voided volumes, degree of urgency, number and severity of incontinence episodes, and the number and type of pads used daily.

FIGURE 19-15. Voiding diary. During the trial period, the patient should again complete several days of voiding diaries. If an improvement greater than 50% is noted in urinary symptoms, conversion to the permanent therapy and placement of the implantable pulse generator is justified. If improvement is not obtained, the lead is removed at the second-stage procedure.

Stage 2: Explantation of the Sacral Lead

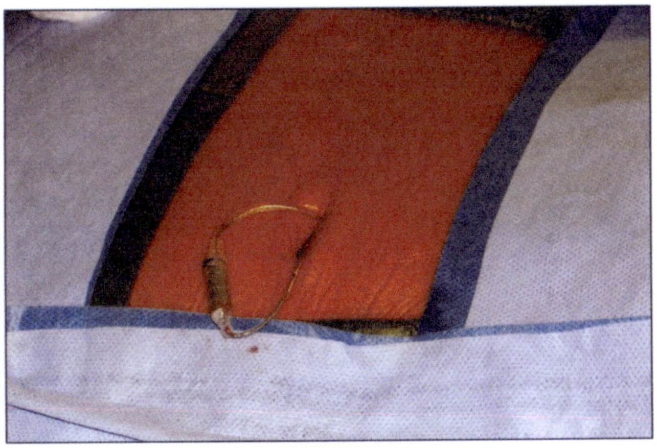

Figure 19-16. If symptoms have not been sufficiently improved, the tined lead and lead extension wire are removed under monitored anesthesia care and local anesthesia by infiltrating the connection site incision with 0.25% bupivacaine (Marcaine; AstraZeneca, Wilmington, DE), opening the incision, and discovering the connection hub. It is pulled into the incision and the lead extension wire is cut and removed at the end of the procedure. The tined lead is then pulled sharply from the connection incision; it will usually move without resistance. If it is pulled slowly, it tends to elongate and thin out, potentially increasing the risk of lead fracture. There is no risk of nerve injury if the lead is deployed as discussed, since the tines are all outside of the foramen.

Stage 2: Placement of an Implantable Pulse Generator

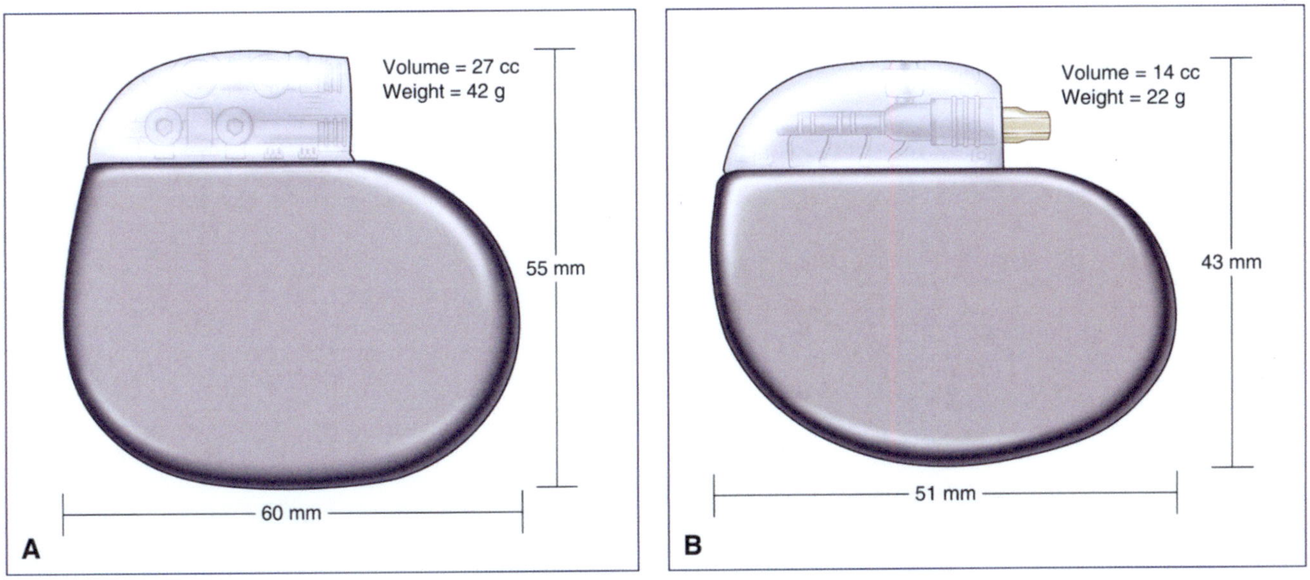

Figure 19-17. The implantable pulse generator (IPG). If the trial proves to be successful and there is sufficient symptom improvement, the therapy can be converted to its permanent form with the implantation of the IPG. The selection of IPG is dependent on the patient's body habitus, pelvic pain component, and stimulation parameters. Patients with settings requiring a high voltage will likely benefit from the larger IPG with its superior battery life (**A**). In thin patients or those with a significant pelvic pain component to their symptoms, we prefer the InterStim II device (Medtronic; Minneapolis, MN) with its smaller profile (**B**). In general, the original InterStim IPG has a battery life of 6 to 10 years, with the InterStim II device lasting 3 to 5 years.

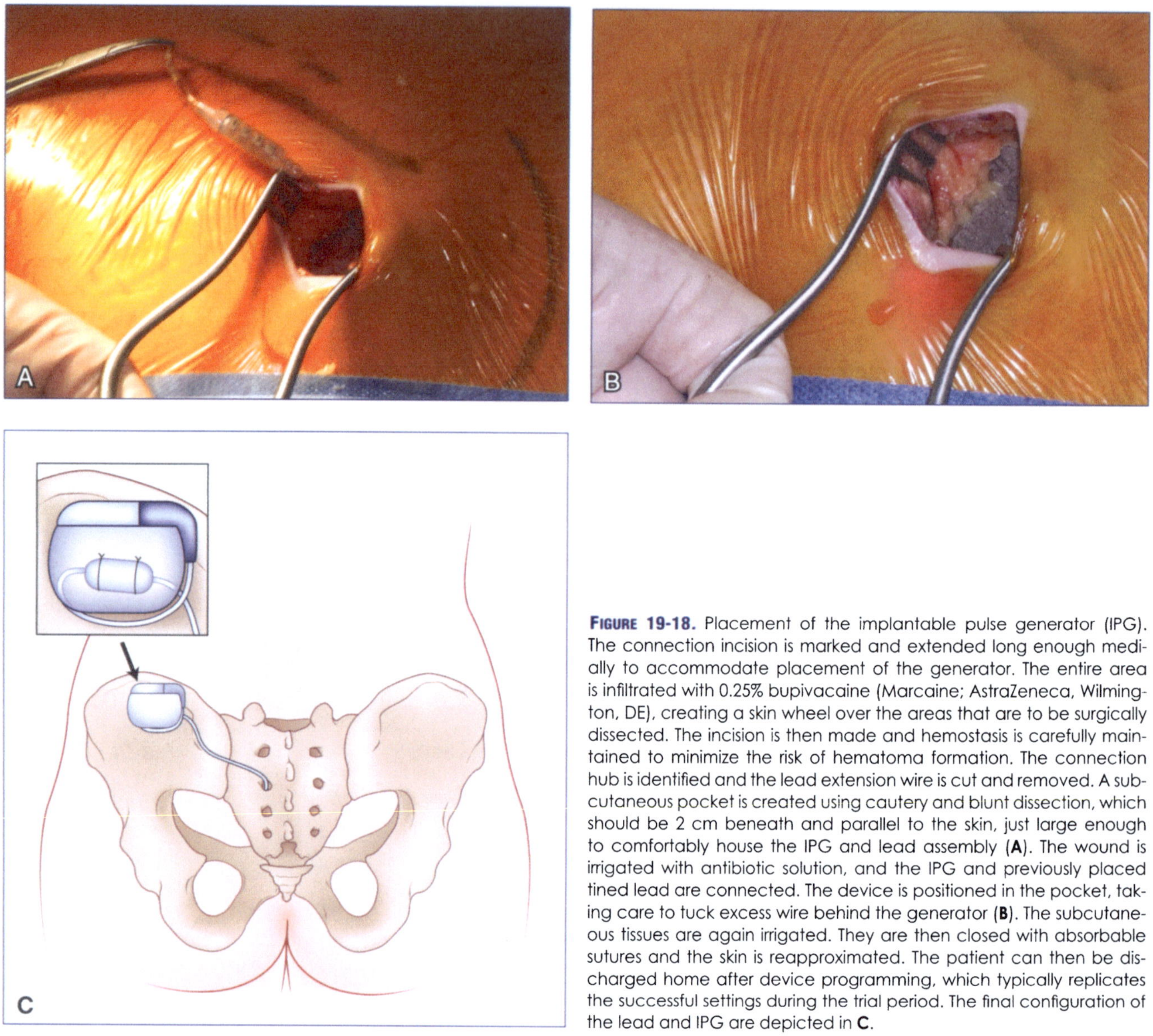

FIGURE 19-18. Placement of the implantable pulse generator (IPG). The connection incision is marked and extended long enough medially to accommodate placement of the generator. The entire area is infiltrated with 0.25% bupivacaine (Marcaine; AstraZeneca, Wilmington, DE), creating a skin wheel over the areas that are to be surgically dissected. The incision is then made and hemostasis is carefully maintained to minimize the risk of hematoma formation. The connection hub is identified and the lead extension wire is cut and removed. A subcutaneous pocket is created using cautery and blunt dissection, which should be 2 cm beneath and parallel to the skin, just large enough to comfortably house the IPG and lead assembly (**A**). The wound is irrigated with antibiotic solution, and the IPG and previously placed tined lead are connected. The device is positioned in the pocket, taking care to tuck excess wire behind the generator (**B**). The subcutaneous tissues are again irrigated. They are then closed with absorbable sutures and the skin is reapproximated. The patient can then be discharged home after device programming, which typically replicates the successful settings during the trial period. The final configuration of the lead and IPG are depicted in **C**.

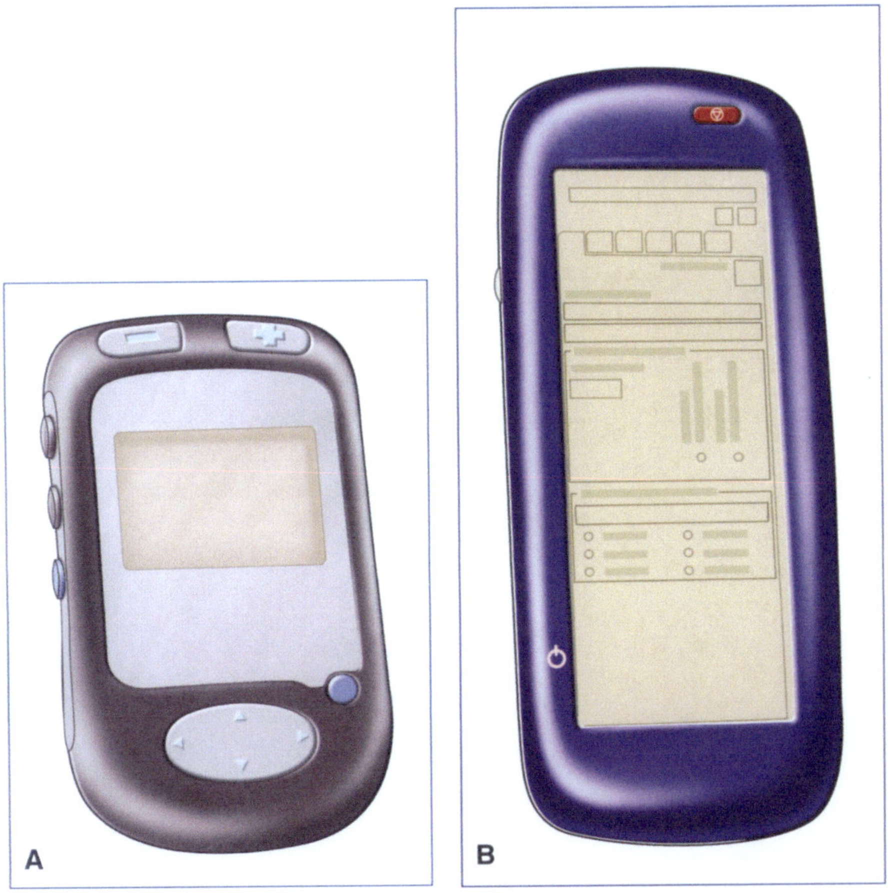

Figure 19-19. The patient has control of their stimulation parameters via telemetry with the usage of the InterStim iCon Patient Programmer (Medtronic; Minneapolis, MN) (**A**). The patient can cycle through up to four separate programs and increase or decrease the intensity of stimulation. If the patient experiences a change in efficacy or abnormal stimulation, the physician can perform dialogistic assessment and reprogramming via telemetry with the N'Vision Clinician Programmer (Medtronic; Minneapolis, MN) (**B**). Typical programming parameters include a rate between 10 and 20 Hz and a pulse width between 180 and 240 μsec. Patients should note sensation (usually a thump, flutter, or pulling) in the perineum, vagina, base of the penis, rectum, or buttock. The sensation should be comfortable and prominent without being distracting.

Clinical Results

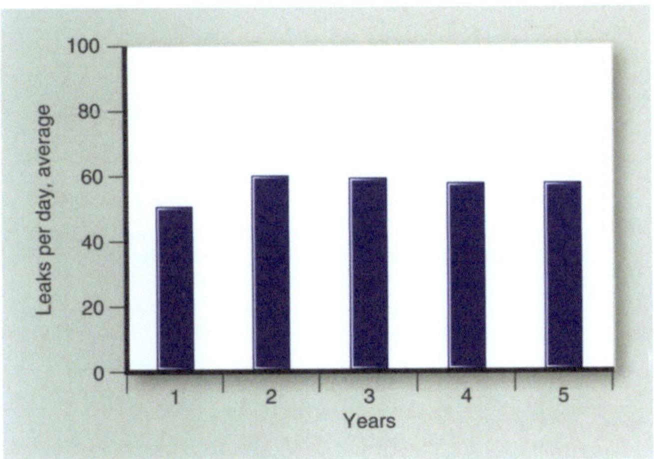

Figure 19-20. The maintained clinical success (> 50% improvement in symptoms) in urge-incontinent patients for the average number of leaks per day is shown in annual intervals. An overall clinical success of 58% has been observed in the number or leaks per day [9].

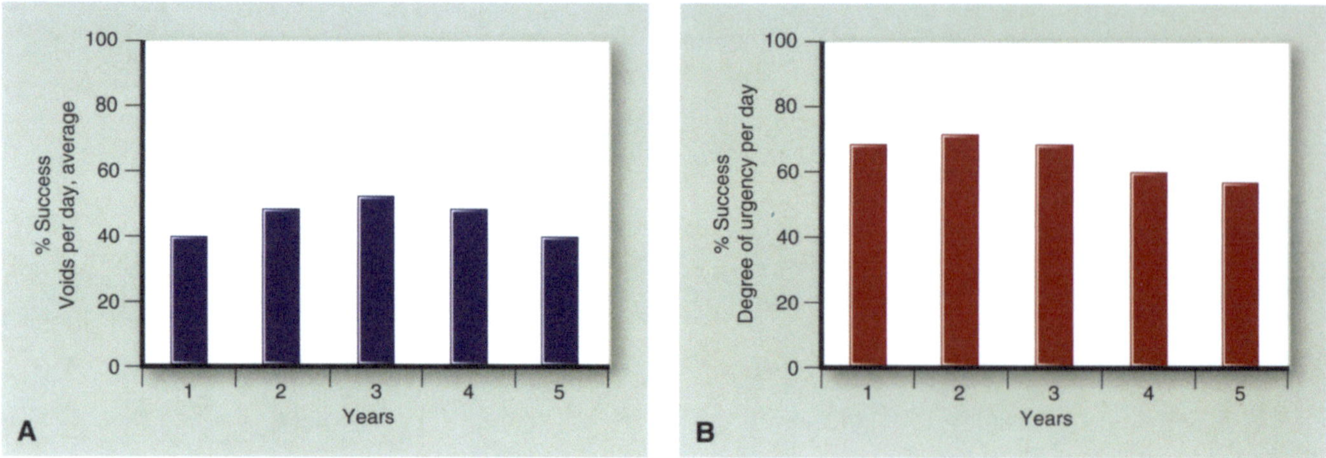

FIGURE 19-21. Percentage of patients with sustained clinical success in the average number of voids per day (**A**) and degree of urgency per day (**B**) for urgency–frequency syndrome patients. Of patients with a successful clinical outcome at 1 year postimplantation, 71% remained successful at 5 years followup [9].

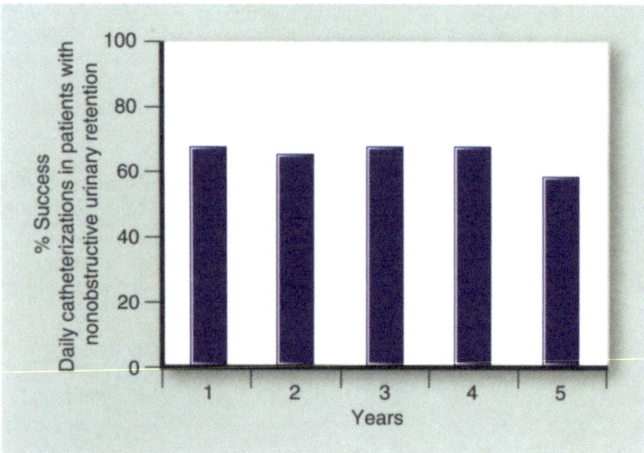

FIGURE 19-22. Sustained efficacy in terms of daily catheterizations (> 50% reduction in the need for catheterization) in patients with nonobstructive urinary retention is shown. A clinical success rate of 71% was observed at 5 years postimplantation [9].

References

1. Abrams P, Blavais JG, Fowler CJ, *et al.*: The role of neuromodulation in the management of urinary urge incontinence. *BJU* 2002, 91:355–359.
2. Siegel SW: Pelvic neuromodulation: s electing patients for sacral nerve stimulation. *Urol Clin N Amer* 2005, 32:19–26.
3. Tanagho EA, Schmidt RA: Electrical stimulation in the clinical management of the neurogenic bladder. *J Urol* 1988, 140:1331–1339.
4. Siegel SW, Catanzaro F, Dijkema HE, *et al.*: Long-term results of a multi-center study on sacral nerve stimulation for treatment of urinary urge incontinence, urgency-frequency, and retention. *Urology* 2000, 56(Suppl 1):87–91.
5. Jonus U, Fowler CJ, Chancellor MB, *et al.*: Efficacy of sacral nerve stimulation for urinary retention: results 18 months after implantation. *J Urol* 2001, 165:15–19.
6. Van Kerrebroeck PE, van Voskulen AC, Heesakkers, JP, *et al.*: Results of sacral neuromodulation therapy for urinary voiding dysfunction: outcomes of a prospective, worldwide clinical study. *J Urol* 2007, 178:2029–2034.
7. Spinelli M, Giardiello G, Gerber M, *et al.*: New sacral neuromodulation lead for percutaneous implantation using local anesthesia: description and first experience. *J Urol* 2003, 170:1905–1907.
8. de Groat WC: Neuroanatomy and neurophysiology: innervation of the lower urinary tract. In *Female Urology*, edn 2. Philadelphia: WB Saunders; 1996:28–42.
9. Siegel SW, Moeller SE: Sacral neuromodulation for the treatment of overactive bladder. In *Female Urology*, edn 3. Edited by Rodriguez L, Raz S. Philadelphia: Saunders-Elsevier; 2008:266–276.
10. Leng WW, Chancellor MB: How sacral nerve stimulation neuromodulation works. *Urol Clin N Amer* 2005, 32:11–18.

20 Percutaneous Tibial Nerve Stimulation and Overactive Bladder

Scott A. MacDiarmid and David R. Staskin

Overactive bladder (OAB) is a chronic syndrome characterized by urinary urgency with or without urge incontinence, usually associated with frequency and nocturia [1]. Approximately 34 million US adults have this condition, representing 16% of the adult population. Prevalence increases with age, with men and women affected almost equally [2]. Patients with OAB may experience a number of adverse effects, including reduced quality of life, impaired mobility, social isolation, sexual function deterioration, and sleep deprivation [3].

The algorithm of care for OAB begins with conservative therapies such as fluid and diet restrictions, pelvic floor muscle strengthening exercises, and scheduled toileting [4]. Pharmacotherapy using anticholinergic drugs has been the backbone of OAB therapy. The effectiveness of pharmacotherapy has been well studied, as have declining patient adherence rates over the course of therapy [5,6,7]. Drug discontinuance is likely due to a number of reasons, including poor or limited efficacy, intolerable side effects, or costs associated with treatment [3].

Neuromodulation therapy uses electrical stimulation to target specific nerves in the sacral plexus that control bladder function [8,9]. Sacral nerve stimulation (SNS) clearly demonstrates the effectiveness of neuromodulation in the management of voiding dysfunction [10,11,12]. Unfortunately the therapeutic impact of SNS is diminished by its invasiveness and associated costs, especially in elderly, frail patients with multiple medical comorbidities [13]. The Urgent® PC system (Uroplasty, Inc.; Minnetonka, MN) uses percutaneous tibial nerve stimulation (PTNS) to target the sacral plexus from an accessible, minimally invasive entry point into the nervous system—the posterior tibial nerve. This chapter will review the clinical effectiveness of PTNS and its incorporation into clinical practice.

Clinical Evidence

The specific mechanism of action of PTNS neuromodulation remains undefined. The posterior tibial nerve contains mixed sensory–motor fibers that originate from L4 through S3 and modulate the innervation to the bladder, urinary sphincter, and pelvic floor. The area superior to the medial malleolus and slightly posterior overlies the posterior tibial nerve. Research since the early 1980s has shown that stimulation of this area results in an improvement in urinary symptoms [14].

A number of studies have demonstrated the efficacy and safety of PTNS in the management of OAB. A prospective multicenter US trial reported a 71% treatment success (25% reduction in mean daytime voids, 21% reduction in mean nighttime voids, 35% improvement in the mean number of urge incontinence episodes, and 20% improvement in quality of life) without significant adverse events [15]. Several studies have demonstrated the beneficial effects of PTNS on bladder function, as measured by urodynamics. Klingler *et al.* [16] reported the elimination of bladder instability in 76.9% of subjects. Mean total bladder capacity increased significantly, from 197 to 252 mL, and the mean volume at first unstable bladder contraction increased from 95 to 133 mL. In responders, the mean increase in total bladder capacity increased from 175 to 266 mL. A urodynamic study of 46 patients by Vandoninck *et al.* [17] demonstrated a 60-mL increase in voiding volume after 12 weeks of PTNS therapy. van der Pal *et al.* demonstrated a 51.8-mL increase in the mean volume voided as an objective measure of PTNS effectiveness [9].

The Overactive Bladder Innovative Therapy (OrBIT) Trial, a multicenter randomized clinical trial, demonstrated comparable effectiveness between PTNS and extended-release tolterodine in reducing OAB symptoms and improving quality of life [18]. To provide a global measurement of treatment response, subjects and investigators were asked to assess OAB symptom improvement after 12 weeks of therapy compared to the baseline. The subject assessments were dramatically improved in the PTNS arm when compared with tolterodine, with 79.5% of PTNS subjects improved or cured versus only 54.8% of those treated with tolterodine ($P = 0.001$). The investigator assessments were similar but did not reach statistical significance ($P = 0.05$) [18].

Thirty-five subjects in the PTNS arm of the OrBIT study who showed symptom improvement were offered ongoing PTNS therapy with longer time intervals between treatments. Thirty and twenty-five subjects completed voiding diaries at 6 and 12 months, respectively, that showed a sustained therapeutic effect similar to results achieved after the initial 12 weeks of therapy. Changes from baseline were statistically significant for frequency ($P < 0.001$), urge incontinence episodes ($P < 0.001$), voids at night ($P = 0.01$), voided volume ($P = 0.04$), and quality of life indices ($P < 0.04$) [19].

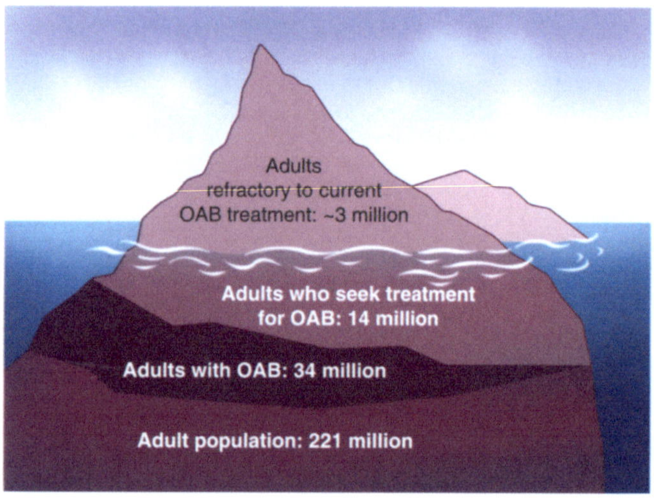

FIGURE 20-1. Prevalence of overactive bladder (OAB). It is estimated that 16% of adults in the United States suffer from OAB, affecting almost 34 million people [2]. The frequency increases with age, with men and women affected almost equally. Women have a higher incidence of urge incontinence and seek treatment at a higher rate than men [3].

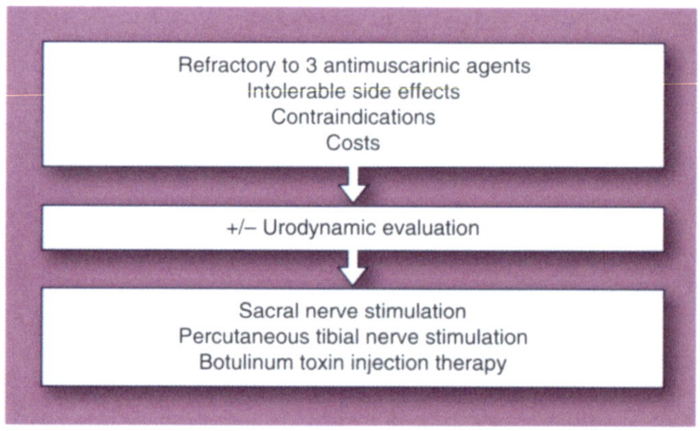

FIGURE 20-2. Overactive bladder (OAB) treatment algorithm. OAB treatment usually begins with conservative therapies such as diet and fluid restrictions, pelvic floor muscle rehabilitation, biofeedback, and bladder training. Pharmacotherapy with antimuscarinics is the mainstay of OAB treatment. Patients who fail three (and sometimes four) antimuscarinic agents are usually considered to be refractory to therapy. Other refractory patients include partial responders, those with intolerable side effects, those in whom antimuscarinics are contraindicated, and those who cannot afford medication. Treatment options for refractory patients include posterior nerve stimulation, sacral nerve stimulation, and the off-label use of botulinum toxin injection therapy. It is the authors' opinion that urodynamics play an important role in the assessment of patients with refractory OAB.

Of the 16% of the US adult population affected by OAB, only 40% actively seek treatment [20]. Reasons given for not seeking therapy include: a belief that incontinence is considered a normal consequence of aging, embarrassment, a health care provider who does not ask about OAB, and a lack of knowledge regarding effective therapies. Of those who do seek treatment, greater than 20% are refractory to conservative therapies such as dietary and fluid restrictions, pelvic floor rehabilitation, bladder retraining, and pharmacotherapy [20].

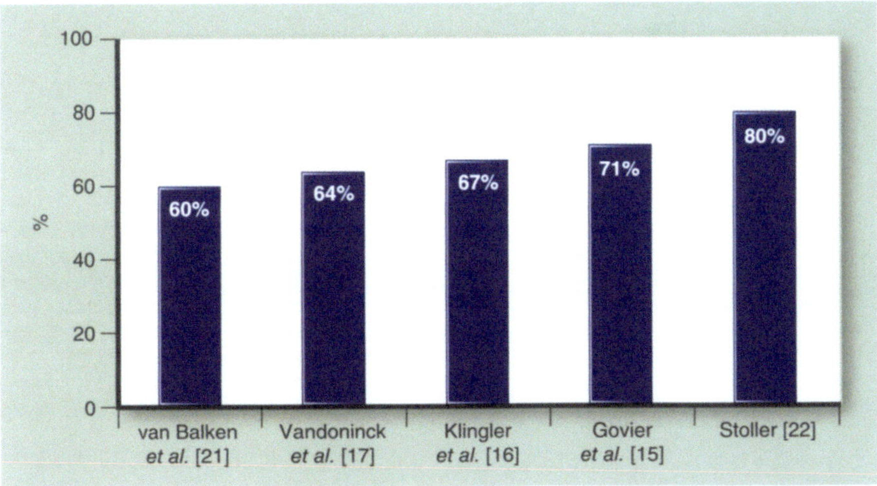

FIGURE 20-3.

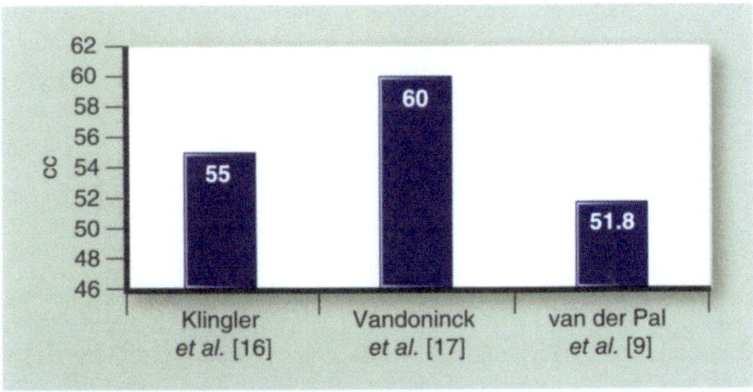

FIGURE 20-4.

Overactive Bladder Innovative Therapy Trial

OrBIT Trial: GRAs				
Subjects' assessment of improvement				
Cured or improved*	PTNS		Extended-release tolterodine	
	Number	%	Number	%
	35	79.5	23	54.8
Investigator assessment of improvement				
Cured or improved**	PTNS		Extended-release tolterodine	
	Number	%	Number	%
	35	79.5	26	60.5

*P = 0.01; **P = 0.05

FIGURE 20-5.

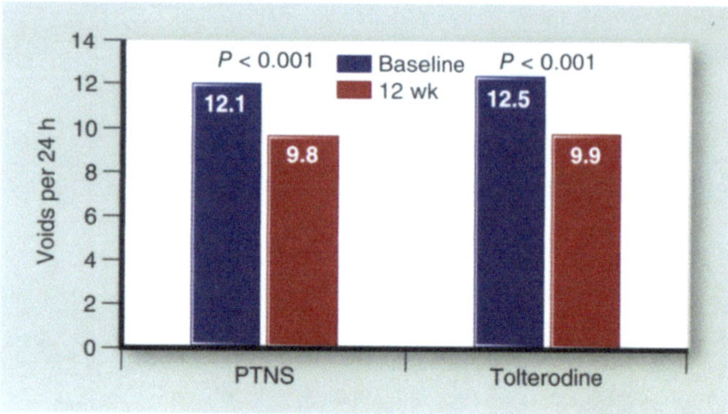

FIGURE 20-6. Overactive Bladder Innovative Therapy (OrBIT) Trial: voids per 24 hours. Using data from a voiding diary, the 24-hour voiding frequency was compared after 12 weeks of therapy with the baseline. Results for 24-hour voiding frequency reductions were statistically significant for both percutaneous tibial nerve stimulation (PTNS) and tolterodine groups, and were comparable between groups.

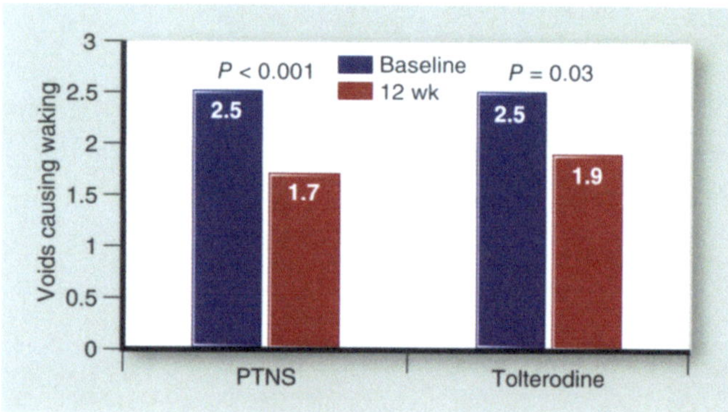

FIGURE 20-7. Overactive Bladder Innovative Therapy (OrBIT) Trial: voids causing waking. Nocturia is often one of the most bothersome symptoms of overactive bladder and increases in frequency with age [23,24]. Subjects in the OrBIT Trial show statistically significant decreases in voids that cause waking ($P < 0.001$). Differences between the groups were not statistically significant. PTNS—percutaneous tibial nerve stimulation.

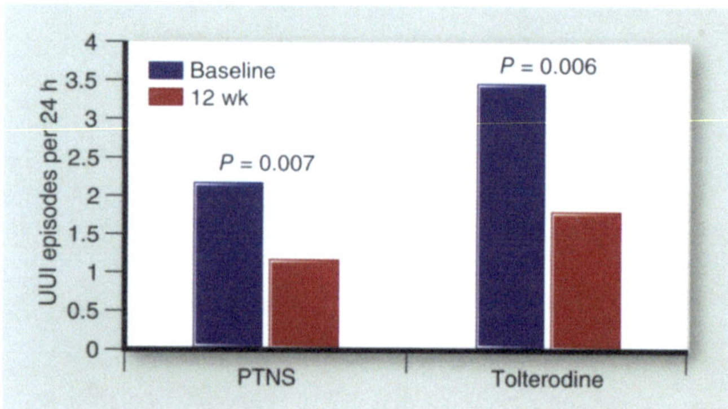

FIGURE 20-8. Overactive Bladder Innovative Therapy (OrBIT) Trial: urge urinary incontinence (UUI) episodes per 24 hours. UUI is the involuntary leakage of urine associated with urgency. Women are more likely to have UUI than men. Both the percutaneous tibial nerve stimulation (PTNS) and tolterodine arms of the OrBIT Trial demonstrated similar statistically significant reductions in UUI episodes in 24 hours ($P = 0.007$ and $P = 0.006$, respectively).

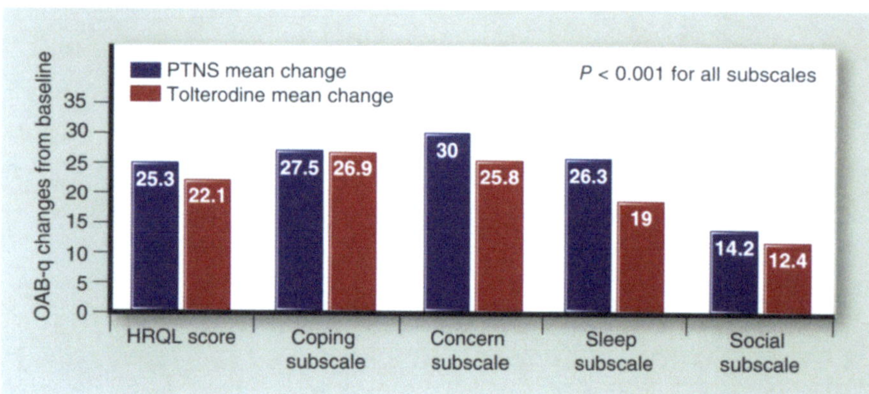

Overactive Bladder Innovative Therapy (OrBIT) Trial: Overactive Bladder Questionnaire (OAB-q) subscale changes. The OAB-q is used extensively in overactive bladder (OAB) drug studies to chart patient improvement and has been shown to be highly responsive to reductions in urinary urgency, frequency, and incontinence and to be a useful outcome measure documenting changes during OAB treatment [6].

OAB-q subscale changes showed a statistically significant improvement from the baseline to 12 weeks for both the percutaneous tibial nerve stimulation (PTNS) and tolterodine group on all subscales ($P < 0.001$). Differences in OAB-q scores were not statistically significant between the two groups. There was a nonsignificant trend of improvement of PTNS over the tolterodine group, primarily in the sleep subscale. HRQL—health-related quality of life.

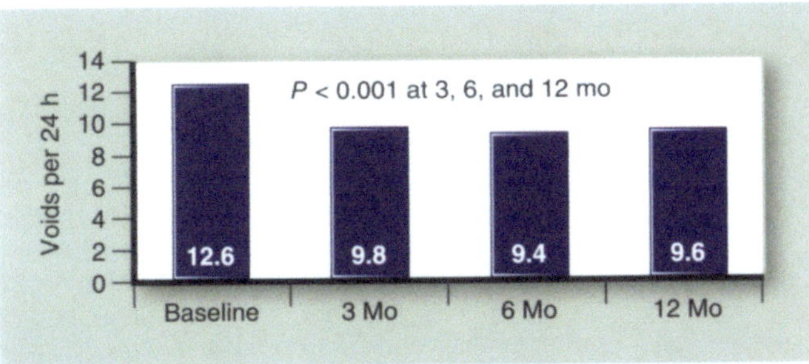

FIGURE 20-10. Overactive Bladder Innovative Therapy (OrBIT) Trial 12-month data: voids per 24 hours. Subjects in the percutaneous tibial nerve stimulation (PTNS) arm of the OrBIT Trial with urinary symptom improvement at 12 weeks were offered ongoing PTNS therapy for up to 12 months. Voiding diary data were collected for 24-hour voiding frequency, urinary urge incontinence episodes, voids causing waking, volume voided, urgency episodes, and quality of life indices [19].

PTNS patients with improved voiding frequency at 12 weeks demonstrated sustained improvement at 6 and 12 months ($P < 0.001$ for each interval). The mean reduction in the number of voids per 24 hours was three, an overall improvement of approximately 20% ($P < 0.001$).

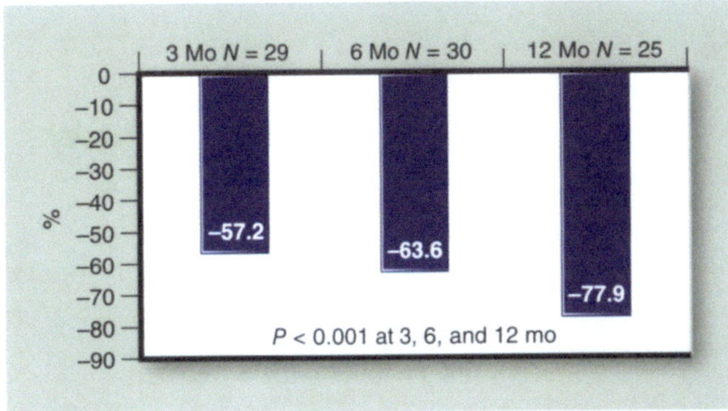

FIGURE 20-11. Overactive Bladder Innovative Therapy (OrBIT) Trial 12-month data: urge urinary incontinence (UUI) episodes per 24 hours. An improvement in mean UUI episodes per 24 hours continued to show statistically significant improvement throughout the 12 months of followup ($P < 0.001$ at 3, 6, and 12 months). As one of the most inconvenient symptoms of overactive bladder, a positive change in UUI episodes is an important parameter of treatment.

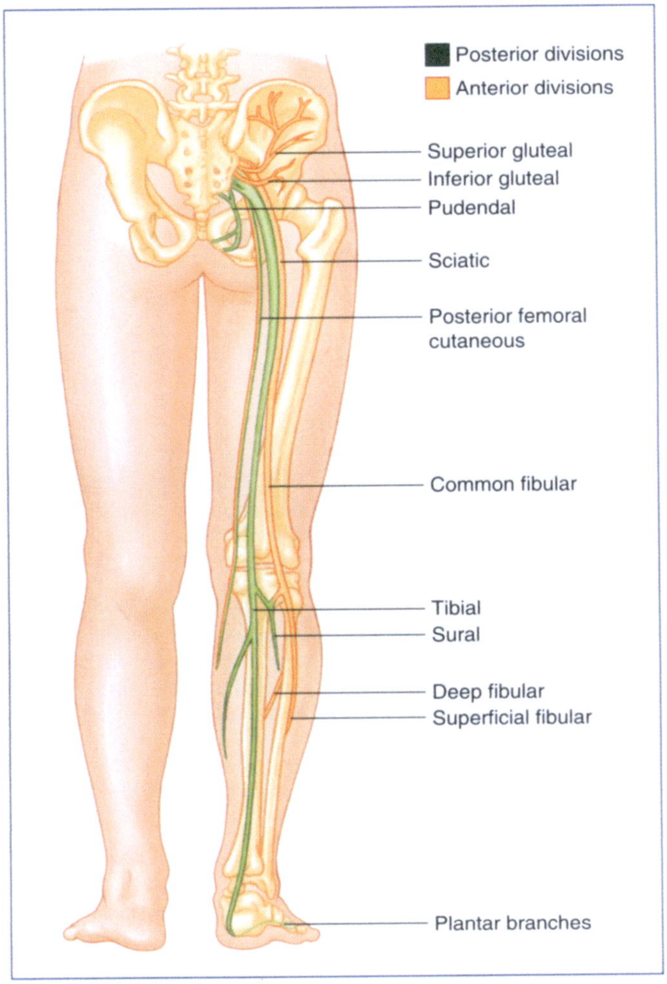

FIGURE 20-12. Tibial nerve route to the sacral plexus. The tibial nerve is a mixed sensory motor nerve that arises from L4 to S3. The posterior tibial nerve can be easily accessed percutaneously at a point slightly superior to the medial malleolus. This minimally invasive access to neural pathways is one advantage of percutaneous tibial nerve stimulation and makes it an ideal procedure to offer within an office practice. (*Courtesy of* Uroplasty, Inc.; Minnetonka, MN.)

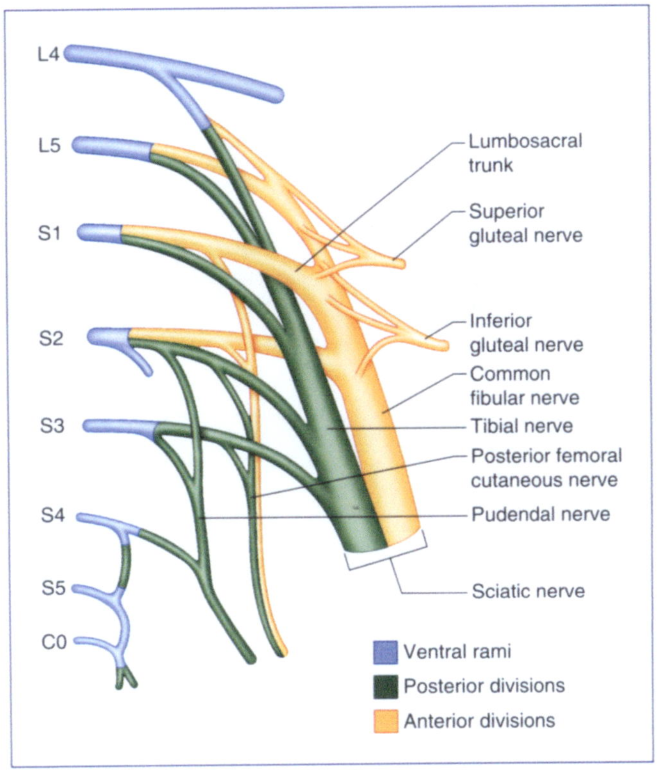

FIGURE 20-13. Tibial nerve and sacral plexus junction. Afferent nerve stimulation uses normal sensory pathways to deliver stimulation to the sacral region. The tibial nerve originates from the same spinal segments that innervate the bladder and pelvic floor, connecting directly to the S2–S3 region of the spine. Stimulating the tibial nerve has been shown to inhibit bladder instability and urge incontinence [22]. (*Courtesy of* Uroplasty, Inc.; Minnetonka, MN.)

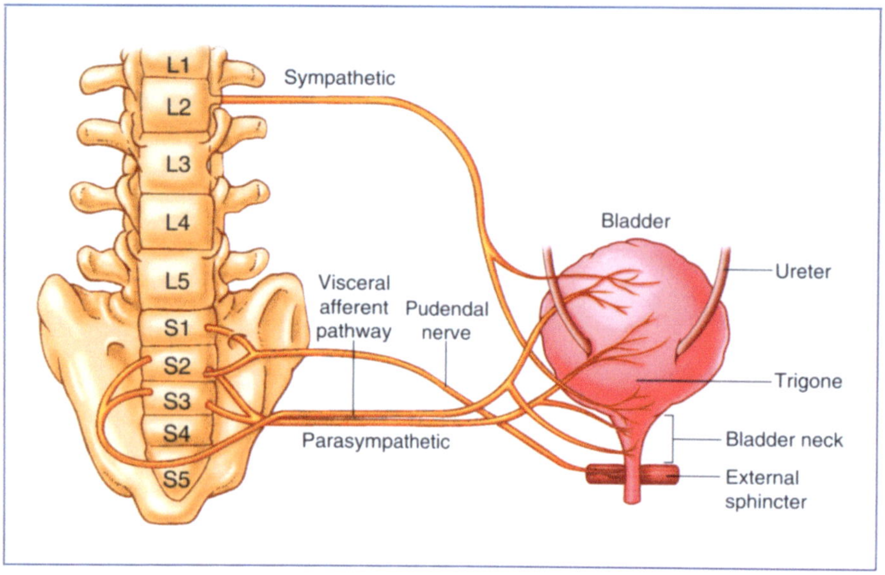

FIGURE 20-14. Sacral plexus and bladder innervation. The physiology and neuroanatomy of the pelvic floor, detrusor mechanism, and micturition reflex are complex and not totally understood. Unlike other viscera, the lower urinary tract is dependent upon neural control storage and elimination, as well as responding to learned behaviors. Neuromodulation targets the nerves that control pelvic floor and bladder function arising from S2–S4, resulting in perineal and pelvic floor muscle reflex responses, inhibition of the detrusor, and interference with visceral afferents. The exact physiological mechanism of electrical stimulation is not fully understood [25]. (*Courtesy of* Uroplasty, Inc.; Minnetonka, MN.)

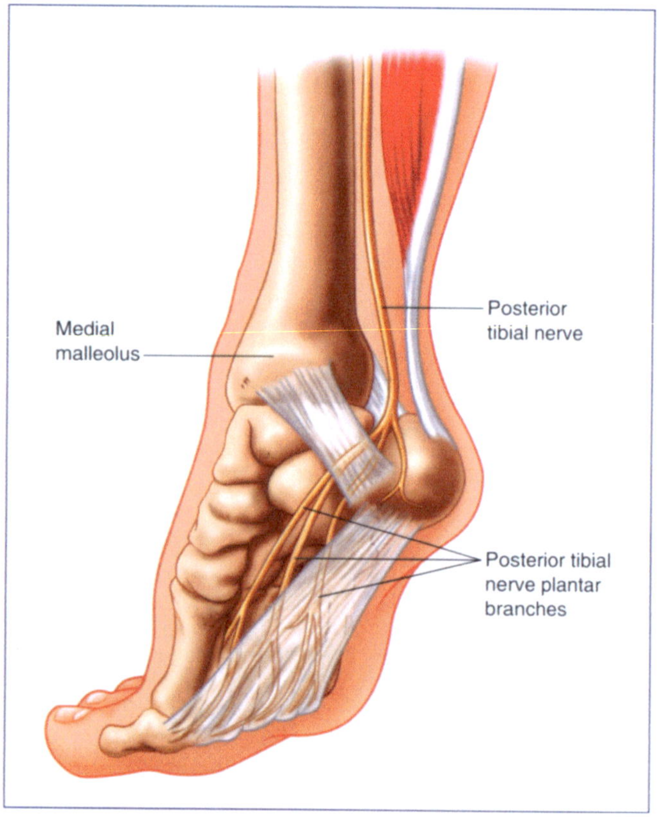

FIGURE 20-15. Posterior tibial nerve access. The posterior tibial nerve provides a minimally invasive access point into the neural pathway, leading to the sacral plexus. A 34-gauge needle electrode inserted approximately 5 cm cephalad to the medial malleolus and slightly posterior to the tibia provides an electrical pathway to the tibial nerve. The patient is typically treated once per week for 30 minutes, for a period of 12 weeks. For patients who are responding to treatment by the end of 12 weeks, the interval between treatment sessions may be slowly increased, with the patient closely monitored for the return of symptoms. If symptoms reappear or increase in severity, the patient's treatment interval should revert to the last previously effective treatment schedule. (*Courtesy of* Uroplasty, Inc.; Minnetonka, MN.)

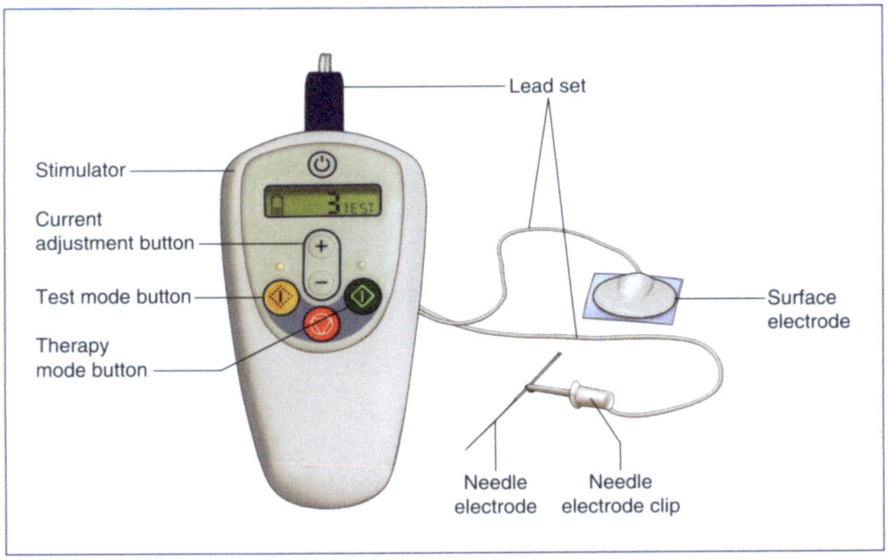

FIGURE 20-16. Urgent PC® system. The Urgent PC system (Uroplasty, Inc.; Minnetonka, MN) consists of a stimulator, a lead set with a surface electrode, and a needle electrode. The stimulator produces an adjustable electrical pulse that travels to the sacral nerve plexus via the tibial nerve. Among other functions, the sacral nerve plexus regulates bladder and pelvic floor function.

Percutaneous Tibial Nerve Stimulation Treatment Protocol

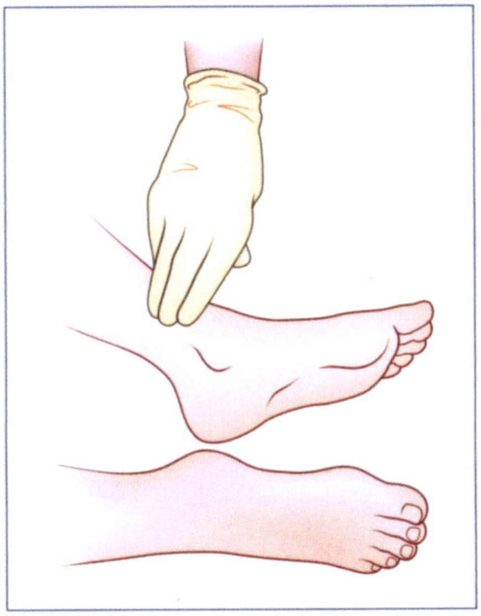

FIGURE 20-17. Percutaneous tibial nerve stimulation: identifying the insertion site. Identifying the insertion site involves two steps. First, place the patient in a comfortable position, either supine or sitting. For example, the patient may sit with the soles of their feet together and their knees abducted and flexed. Then, locate the needle electrode insertion site on the inner aspect of either leg approximately three finger widths (5 cm or 2 in) cephalad to the medial malleolus and approximately one finger width (2 cm or .75 in) posterior to the tibia.

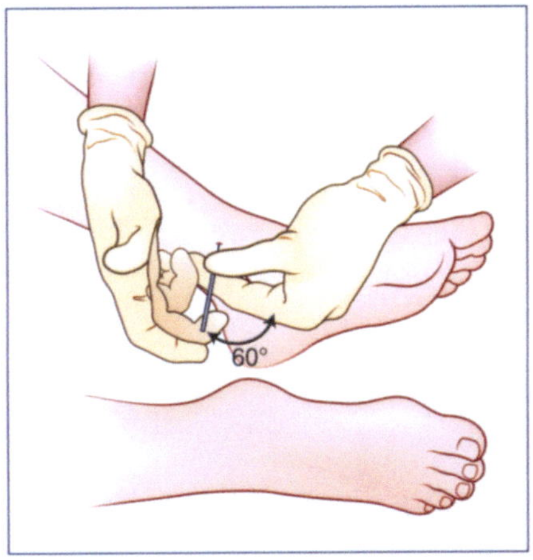

FIGURE 20-18. Percutaneous tibial nerve stimulation: inserting the needle electrode at a 60° angle. First, place the sterile needle electrode/guide tube assembly over the cleaned insertion site at a 60° angle. Then, gently tap the needle electrode head to pierce the skin, maintaining a 60° angle, and insert it to a depth of approximately 2 cm.

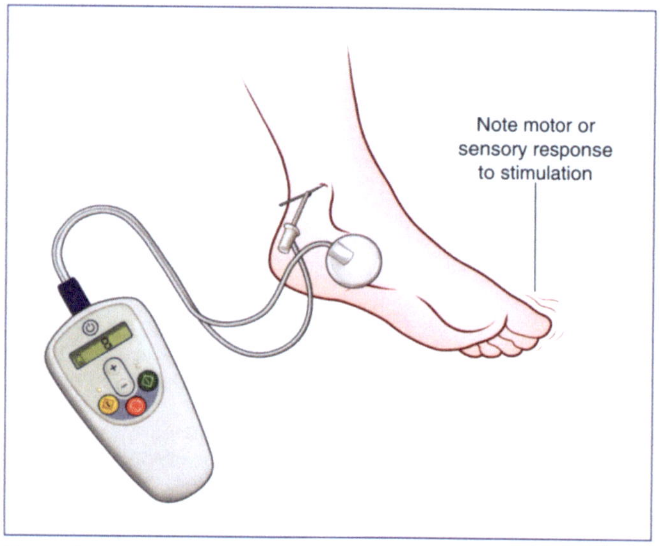

FIGURE 20-19. Percutaneous tibial nerve stimulation: connect the device components and observe the patient response. Adhere the surface electrode near the medial aspect of the calcaneus on the same leg as the needle electrode insertion. The next steps are as follows: 1) plug the lead wire connector into the stimulator; 2) loop the connection hook around the needle electrode and release; 3) turn on the stimulator; 4) press the yellow "test mode" button; and 5) slowly increase the current and observe the patient's foot for a response. The patient's response is generally a toe flex or fan, an extension of the entire foot, or a tingling sensation across the heel or sole. The current setting will be determined based on the patient's sensory and motor responses. Once a patient response is observed, reduce the current setting by one level.

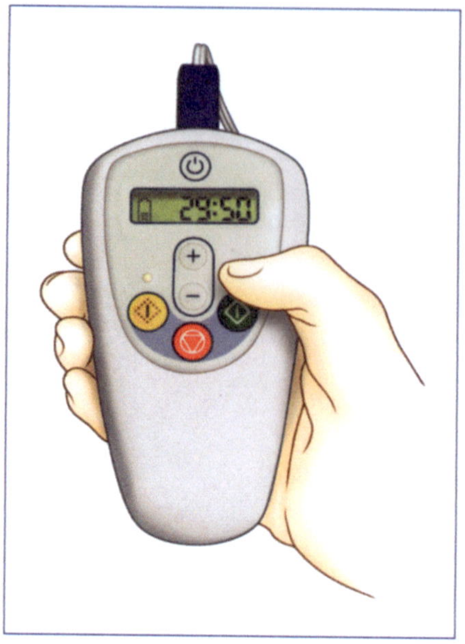

FIGURE 20-20. Percutaneous tibial nerve stimulation: set the current level and conduct therapy. First, press the green "therapy mode" button. The stimulator will automatically deliver the selected current for 30 minutes, then automatically shut off. Next, remove the needle electrode and disconnect all components.

Conduct 12 treatments, typically one per week, documenting voiding parameter changes. After the initial 12 treatments, slowly increase the interval between treatments. Continue to monitor the patient's voiding symptoms. If symptoms reappear or increase in severity, the patient's treatment schedule should revert to the last previously effective treatment interval.

References

1. International Continence Society (ICS): Factsheet 02: overactive bladder. 2005. Available at http://www.icsoffice.org/ASONET_Membership/Membership/Documents?Documents.aspx?FolderID=30. Accessed March 2009.
2. Stewart WF, Van Rooyen JB, Cundiff GW, *et al.*: Prevalence and burden of overactive bladder in the United States. *World J Urol* 2001, 20:327–336.
3. Dmochowski R, Newman D: Impact of overactive bladder on women in the United States: results of a national survey. *Curr Med Res Opin* 2007, 23:65–76.
4. Kohli N, Rosenblatt PL: Neuromodulation techniques for the treatment of overactive bladder. *Clin Obstet Gyn* 2002, 45:218–232.
5. Perfetto EM, Prasan S, Jumadilova Z: Treatment of overactive bladder: a model comparing extended-release formulations of tolterodine and oxybutynin. *Am J Manag Care* 2005, 11:S150–S157.
6. Coyne KS, Elinoff V, Gordon DA, *et al.*: Relationships between improvements in symptoms and patient assessments of bladder condition, symptom bother and health-related quality of life in patients with overactive bladder treated with tolterodine. *Int J Clin Pract* 2008, 62:925–931.
7. Bulmer P, Abrams P: The unstable detrusor. *Urol Int* 2004, 72:1–12.
8. Leng WW, Chancellor MB: How sacral nerve stimulation neuromodulation works. *Urol Clin N Am* 2005, 32:11–18.
9. van der Pal F, van Balken MR, Heesakkers JP, *et al.*: Percutaneous tibial nerve stimulation in the treatment of refractory overactive bladder syndrome: is maintenance treatment necessary. *BJU Int* 2006, 97:113–116.
10. Starkmarn JS, Wolter CE, Scarpero HM, *et al.*: Management of refractory urinary urge incontinence following urogynecological surgery with sacral neuromodulation. *Neurourol Urodyn* 2007, 26:29–35.
11. Schmidt RA, Jonas U, Oleson KA, *et al.*: Sacral nerve stimulation for treatment of refractory urinary urge incontinence. Sacral Nerve Stimulation Study Group. *J Urol* 1999, 162:352–357.
12. Amundsen CL, Romero AA, Jamison MG, Webster GD: Sacral neuromodulation for intractable urge incontinence: are there factors associated with cure? *Urology* 2005, 66:746–750.
13. Zinkgraf K, Quinn AO, Ketterhagen D, *et al.*: Percutaneous tibial nerve stimulation for treatment of overactive bladder and urinary retention in an elderly population. *Urol Nurs* 2009, 29:30–34.
14. McGuire EJ, Zhang SC, Howinski ER, Lytton B: Treatment of motor and sensory detrusor instability by electrical stimulation. *J Urol* 1983, 129:78–79.
15. Govier FE, Litwiller, S, Nitti V, *et al.*: Percutaneous afferent neuromodulation for the refractory overactive bladder: results of a multicenter study. *J Urol* 2001, 165:1193–1198.
16. Klingler HC, Pycha A, Schmidbauer J, Marberger M: Use of peripheral neuromodulation of the S3 region for treatment of detrusor overactivity: a urodynamic-based study. *Urology* 2000, 56:766–771.
17. Vandoninck V, van Balken MR, Finazzi Agro E, *et al.*: Percutaneous tibial nerve stimulation in the treatment of overactive bladder: urodynamic data. *Neururol Urodyn* 2003, 22:227–232.
18. Peters KM, Leong FC, Shobeiri SA, *et al.*: A randomized multicenter study comparing percutaneous tibial nerve stimulation with pharmaceutical therapy for the treatment of overactive bladder. *J Urol* 2009, 182:1055–1061.
19. MacDiarmid SA, Peters KM, Leong FC, *et al.*: Long term durability of percutaneous tibial nerve stimulation for the treatment of overactive blader (OrBIT Trial). *J Urol* 2010; In press.
20. Kinchen KS, Burgio K, Diokno A, *et al.*: Factors associated with women's decisions to seek treatment for urinary incontinence. *J Womens Health* 2003, 12:687–698.
21. van Balken MR, Vandoninck V, Gisolf KWH, *et al.*: Posterior tibial nerve stimulation as neuromodulative treatment of lower urinary tract dysfunction. *J Urol* 2001, 166:914–918
22. Stoller ML: Afferent nerve stimulation for pelvic floor dysfunction. *Eur Urol* 1999, 35(Suppl 2):16.
23. Fitzgerald MP, Letman JH, Link CL, McKinlay JB: BACH Survey Investigators. The association of nocturia with cardiac disease, diabetes, body mass index, age and diuretic use: results from the BACH survey. *J Urol* 2007, 177:1385–1389.
24. Burtsztyn M, Jacob J, Stessman J: Usefulness of nocturia as a mortality risk factor for coronary heart disease among persons born in 1920 or 1921. *Am J Cardiol* 2006, 98:1311–1315.
25. Vodusek DB: Micturition and the sacral reflex arc: lessons from electrophysiological techniques. *Scand J Urol Nephrol* 2002, 6(Suppl):51–54.

21 Lumbar to Sacral Ventral Nerve Rerouting

Benjamin J. Girdler, Juan J. de Benito, and Kenneth M. Peters

There are an estimated 250,000 patients who currently have a spinal cord injury and 70,000 patients who have spina bifida in the United States [1]. The resulting neurogenic bladder and bowel remain a significant source of morbidity. Historically, treatment advances have been mainly aimed at low pressure storage and continence, with the ultimate goal of preserving upper tract function and improving quality of life.

Approximately 12,000 new cases of spinal cord injury occur annually in the United States [2]. Nearly 80% of the cases involve men with an average age of 31.5 years [3]. Improvement in urologic care over the past 40 years has removed renal failure from the major cause of death in this population [4–6]. The characteristic lower urinary tract findings in a complete suprasacral spinal cord injury involve a triad of detrusor overactivity, smooth muscle synergia (for lesions below the sympathetic outflow), and striated sphincter dyssynergia often resulting in incomplete emptying and high intravesical pressures [7–9]. Management focuses on maintaining safe urodynamic pressures, grounded in clean intermittent catheterization and anticholinergic therapy [10–12]. Augmentation cystoplasty or an outlet procedure may be necessary to maintain safe detrusor leak point pressures. Neurostimulation of the anterior roots, most commonly using the Brindley device in combination with sacral posterior rhizotomy, has been used for a select group of spinal cord injury patients, but has not experienced widespread implementation [13,14].

Spina bifida is a congenital defect estimated to impact approximately one in 1000 live births in the United States [15]. Due to the widespread implementation of folic acid supplementation and the early termination of affected pregnancies, this number has been declining over the past 20 years [16–18]. The vast majority of spinal dysraphisms are myelomeningoceles, a herniation of both the meninges as well as neural tissue proper [19]. Sixty-seven percent of myelomeningoceles occur at the lumbosacral or sacral levels [20]. All open defects are traditionally closed neurosurgically shortly after birth. Unfortunately, the impact on lower urinary tract function cannot be reliably predicted based on either the vertebral level of involvement or the extent of lower extremity dysfunction [21]. The lower urinary tract of a myelomeningocele patient can be divided into three characteristic patterns including synnergia, dyssynergia, and complete denervation, each involving approximately a third of the cases [22]. Traditional urologic management has also been based on clean intermittent catheterization and anticholinergics to maintain low pressure storage and continence [11,12]. When these conservative measures fail, surgical intervention is often required to increase bladder capacity and improve outlet resistance. While these advances have dramatically improved the quality of life of spina bifida patients, they have also presented the pediatric and adult urologist with an entirely new realm of challenges.

With the exception of sacral neuroprosthesis implantation, little progress has been made clinically with either disease in the restoration of both lower tract urinary storage and emptying function [13,14]. Xiao and Godoc [23] introduced the concept of the surgical creation of an artificial "skin–central nervous system–bladder" reflex to establish voluntary coordinated bladder emptying, while maintaining low pressure storage and continence. The nerve-rerouting procedure developed has become the standard of care for voiding dysfunction in both patient populations in China [24]. Outside China, the procedure remains largely unproven and continues under experimental protocol at several international centers. Despite widespread interest, adult and pediatric urologists have little experience or understanding of the approach and the relevant anatomy required to perform the procedure. In this chapter, we introduce the concept of nerve rerouting and review our current understanding of the skin–central nervous system–bladder reflex pathway at the basic science level. We then outline the steps required to plan and execute the procedure with an emphasis on the relevant surgical anatomy. Because of the complicated neuroanatomy in spina bifida, we focus the initial discussion on the basic technique in spinal cord injury. Finally, we spend the remainder of the chapter focusing on the fundamental differences of the procedure in spina bifida. Clinical outcomes data are reviewed at the end of each section.

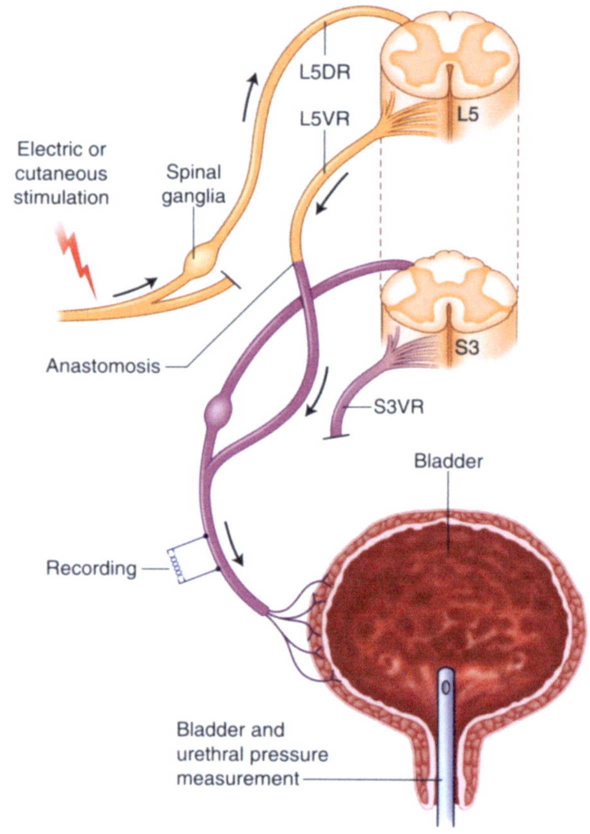

FIGURE 21-1. Nerve-rerouting fundamentals. At its most basic level, nerve rerouting involves exploiting (rewiring) a basic lower extremity knee jerk reflex arc to voluntarily stimulate the bladder to contract [25]. In this example, the ventral motor nerve root to the leg (L5VR) and the ventral motor nerve root to the bladder (S3VR) are isolated and transected. The motor nerve root to the leg is then anastomosed to the nerve root to the bladder. After allowing regenerative time of approximately 1 mm/d, stimulation of the dorsal sensory root of the leg (L5DR) by either scratching the dermatome or electrical depolarization with a transcutaneous electrical nerve stimulation unit sends information to the spinal cord [26]. Instead of that information traveling back down to the leg in the typical reflex arc fashion, it now sends that information to the bladder, causing the bladder to contract. This new reflex arc can subsequently be conceptualized as a bladder jerk instead of a knee jerk. While this oversimplifies both the process of voiding as well as reflex arcs, it illustrates the basic concept. (*Adapted from* Xiao [24].)

Basic Science

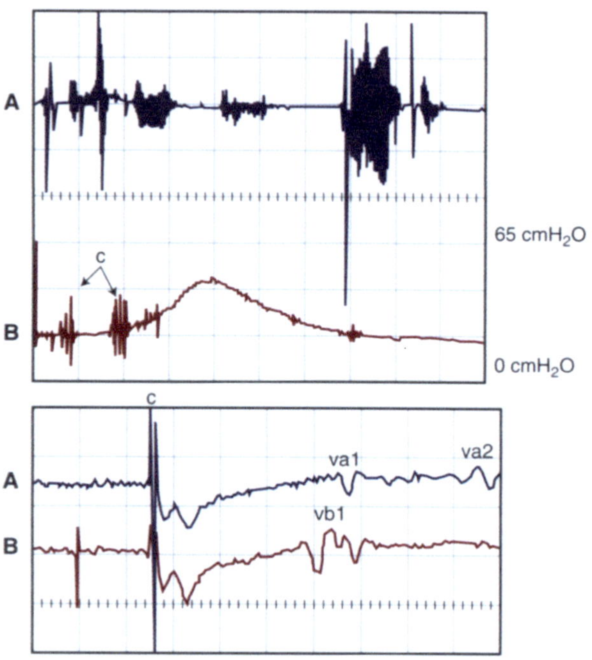

FIGURE 21-2. Electrophysiology. Our fundamental understanding of the ability of the somatic nervous system to assume autonomic control of the lower urinary tract via the skin–central nervous sytem–bladder reflex pathway was established by a series of electrophysiologic, histologic, and pharmacologic animal experiments by Xiao and colleagues beginning in the late 1980s [23–25].

Initial studies in rats established an initial electrophysiologic proof of concept of the procedure [23]. All experimental animals underwent limited laminectomy and intradural microanastomosis of the motor root of L4 to the motor root of L6, which innervates the lower urinary tract in rats. After allowing for regenerative time, stimulation of the L4 sensory root resulted in an evoked potential recorded at the L6 recipient motor root and a coordinated voiding pattern. The contralateral side served as a control in all animals. Similar results were later confirmed in a feline experimental model [25].

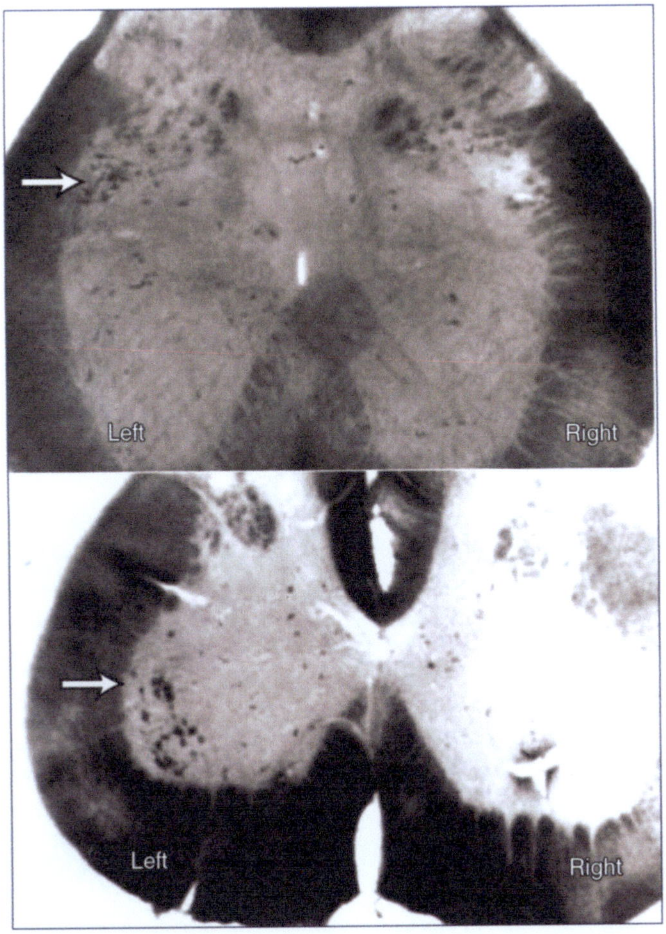

FIGURE 21-3. Histology. Additional rat studies provided histologic evidence of the regeneration of somatic motor axons into a functional autonomic efferent root [23]. When horseradish peroxidase (HRP) was applied to the ipsilateral pelvic ganglia or the nerve distal to the anastamosis, retrograde labeling of the somatic motor neurons from the donor root level was found. The *top* image demonstrates normal bladder innervation by preganglionic neurons in the lateral band of L6/S1 in rat controls. The *bottom* image represents the HRP-labeled somatic neurons in the L4 donor ventral horn of rats after nerve rerouting of L4 to L6.

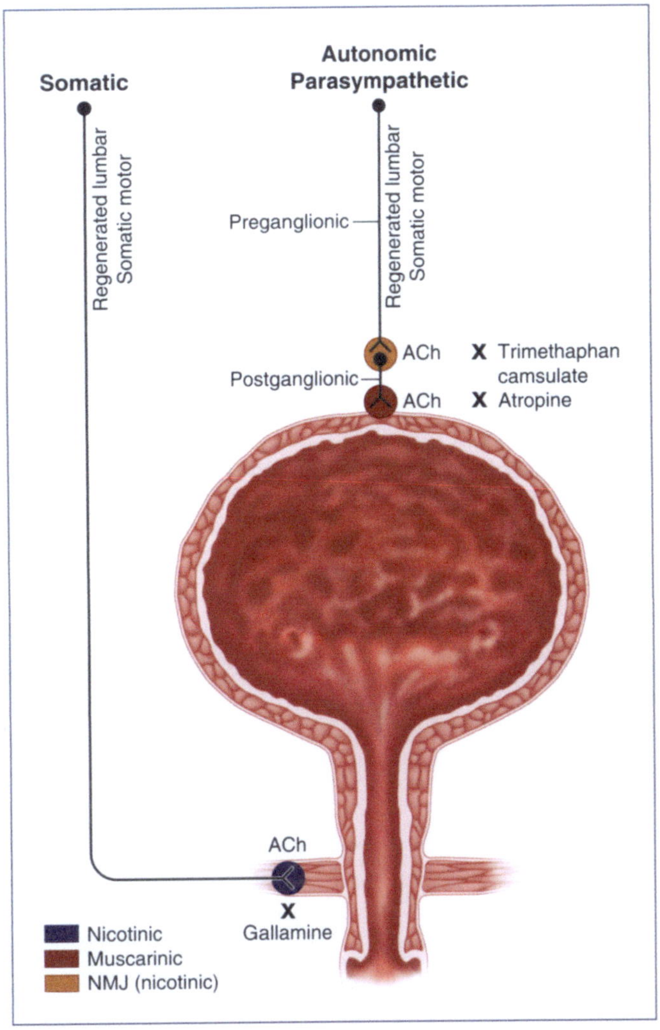

FIGURE 21-4. Pharmacology. Pharmacologic studies were performed in the feline model by Xiao *et al.* [25]. Acetylcholine (Ach) is a common neurotransmitter released at the somatic neuromuscular junction (NMJ), and from both the parasympathetic and sympathetic preganglionic and the parasympathetic postganglionic nerve terminals. Because a regenerated somatic nerve releases the same neurotransmitter as a normal autonomic preganglionic parasympathetic nerve, the somatic nervous system could theoretically assume control over the autonomic nervous system.

Large amplitude bladder contractions were demonstrated in cats during stimulation of the donor dermatome after allowing for regenerative time after nerve rerouting [25]. Indeed, the nicotinic ganglionic inhibitor trimethaphan (5 mg/kg) and antimuscarinic atropine (0.05 mg/kg) both suppressed these large amplitude bladder contractions. On the other hand, the neuromuscular blocking agent gallamine (1 mg/kg) suppressed striated urethral sphincter electromyelogram activity but had no effect on bladder contraction. This pharmacologic data argues for the ability of a somatic nerve to regenerate into the efferent branch of an autonomic parasympathetic nerve and attain control at the ganglionic level.

FIGURE 21-5. **A** and **B**, Coordinated voiding pattern. Controversy remains regarding the mechanism underlying the coordinated voiding patterns that result from dermatomal stimulation. Again, the recipient root contains both preganglionic parasympathetic fibers to the bladder and somatic fibers traveling via the pudendal nerve to the external sphincter. Somatic donor reinnervation should allow stimulation of both systems. In theory, sphincter contraction along with bladder contraction or dyssynergia would be predicted. How could simultaneous stimulation result in coordinated voiding?

First, timing of the reflex activation of the bladder and sphincter are not the same [23]. The smooth muscle of the bladder has slower, more prolonged contractions compared with the striated sphincter. Second, delayed contraction of the bladder compared with the sphincter is theoretically likely because of delayed transmission across the ganglion that is not present in the somatic system [23]. Donor root dermatomal stimulation would likely result in immediate stimulation of the external sphincter followed by gradual contraction of the detrusor. As detrusor pressure rises and dermatomal stimulation ceases, the external sphincter relaxes, resulting in coordinated bladder emptying. Further investigation will be necessary to clarify and confirm synergy between bladder and external sphincter with voiding.

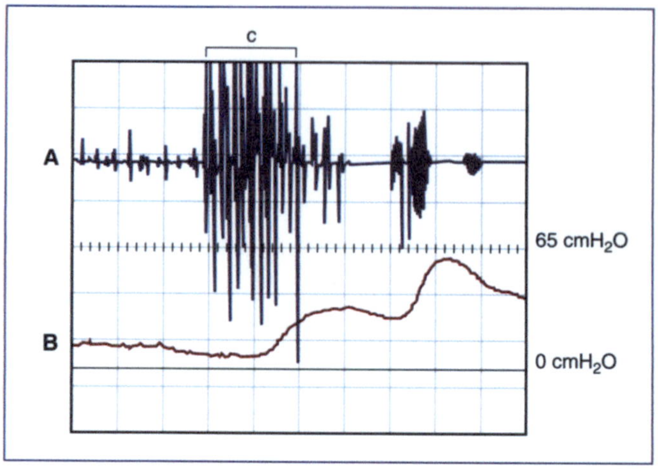

Spinal Cord Injury: The Basic Nerve-Rerouting Procedure and Initial Outcomes

Preoperative Evaluation

Patient selection

Inclusion	**Exclusion**	**Urinary tract**	**Neurological evaluation**
Suprasacral SCI	Bladder capacity < 100 cc	Urodynamics	Neurological examination with reflex testing
At least 1 y postinjury	End-stage storage dysfunction	Flexible cystoscopy	Lower extremity EMG
Stable nerological lesion	Malignant disease	Renal/bladder ultrasound	Nerve conduction studies
Intact donor reflex arc	Bladder neck obstruction	Serum BUN/creatine	Spine MRI
	Urethral stricture		

FIGURE 21-6. Preoperative evaluation. The operative indications for the nerve-rerouting procedure remain in evolution. Published outcomes are limited to suprasacral spinal cord injury (SCI) patients at least 1 year postinjury with a stable neurologic lesion about L2 [24,26]. Exclusion criteria are defined in the figure. They are not yet clear for patients with, for example, previous iliovesicostomy, indwelling spinal hardware, or scoliosis. As the literature matures, the indications and contraindications will become more clear. In theory, the only absolute requirement for the surgery is an undamaged somatic reflex arc in relative proximity to the sacral roots [26,27].

All patients should undergo a comprehensive preoperative evaluation. The status of the patient's urinary tract is evaluated with urodynamics, flexible cystoscopy, renal ultrasound, and serum creatinine. Extensive neurologic evaluation should be performed in conjunction with a neurologist, with the goal of determining the integrity of the lumbar and sacral nerve roots. This evaluation is especially important in patients who have suffered an L1 or T12 bony level injury. At this bony level, injury to the conus medullaris can destroy all roots below the level of the patient's injury. Finally, anatomic information should be obtained from plain films or MRI, depending on the complexity of the case. BUN—blood urea nitrogen; EMG—electromyelogram.

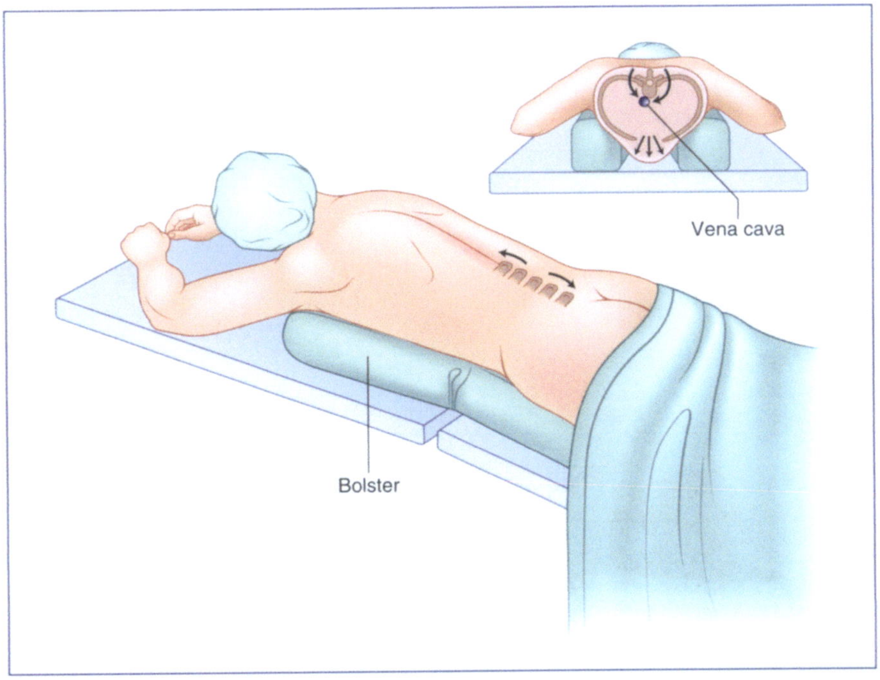

Figure 21-7. Patient positioning. Broad-spectrum parenteral antibiotics (ampicillin and gentamicin) are infused 1 hour prior to incision. While still on the gurney, a general anesthetic is administered and a Foley catheter is placed. The patient is rolled to the prone position on the operating table. Pressure points are padded and extremities are positioned anatomically, as in other prone position surgeries. Foam bolsters are oriented vertically along the patient's sides to elevate the central abdomen and chest off of the table, allowing optimal venous plexus drainage into the vena cava and full chest expansion [28]. This maneuver is critical to minimize intraoperative bleeding and pulmonary complications. By placing the table in the slight jackknife position, the patient's lower back is opened up. Finally, the head of the bed is lowered to position the operative skin surface parallel to the floor.

Next, 13-mm Rhythmlink subdermal electrodes (Rhythmlink International; Columbia, SC) are placed bilaterally to allow for detection of compound muscle action potential activity in, at a minimum, the tibialis anterior (L5), medial gastrocnemius (S1), abductor hallicus (S2), and external anal sphincter muscles (S3) [29]. Additional electrodes can be placed at this time to monitor higher lumbar levels if necessary. (*Adapted from* Hoppenfield and deBoer [28].)

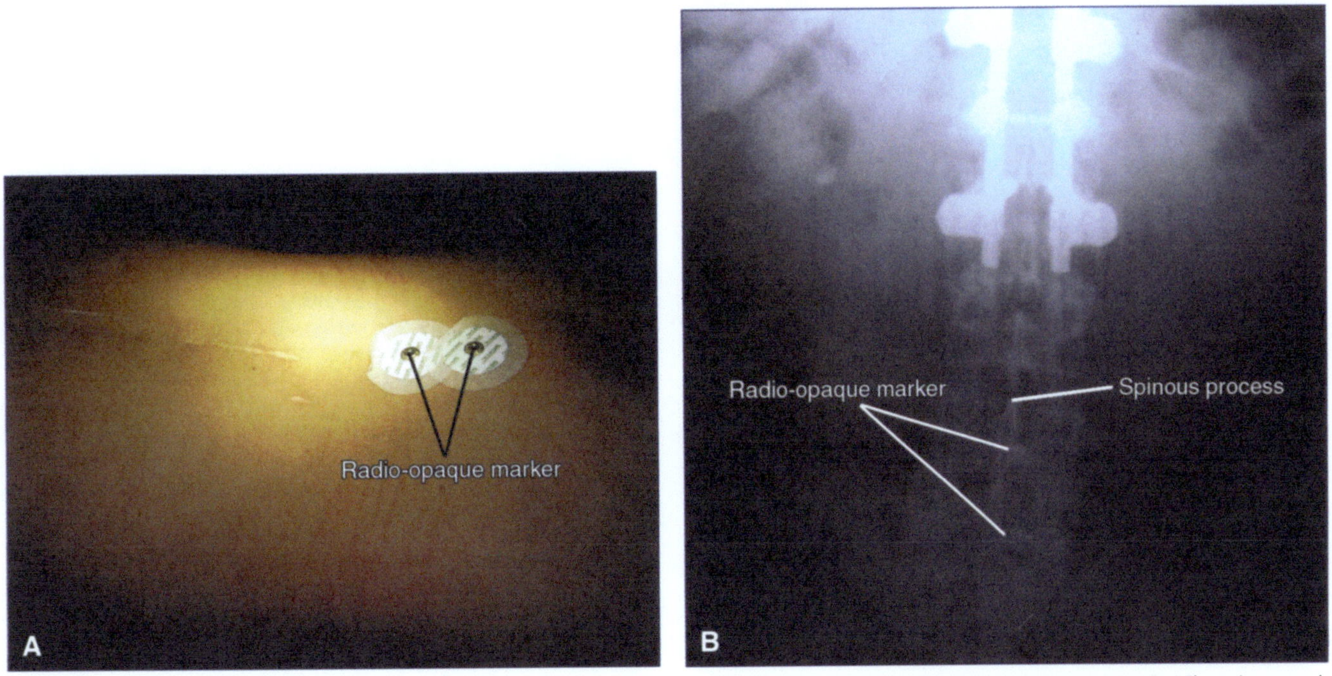

Figure 21-8. Marking the incision. The conus medullaris marks the termination of the spinal cord and is located somewhere between what normally is the T12 and L2 bony levels in humans [29]. The dorsal (sensory) and ventral (motor) nerve roots stretch down from the conus and exit together as a spinal nerve at their respective foramen. Unlike higher levels, where the nerve roots exit the dura almost immediately after leaving the spinal cord, the roots of the cauda equine travel caudally for several bony levels together within the dura before exiting. This relationship leaves more than enough nerve length for the tension-free anastomosis between a lower lumbar ventral root (usually L5) and a sacral ventral root (usually S2 or S3) several levels below. Subsequently, the entire operation can be performed well away from the spinal cord.

With the knowledge of this anatomy, the L5/S1 bony level provides ideal access to expose the relevant roots. A line drawn between the most superior portion of the iliac crests can approximate the L4/L5 interspace [28]. The palpable spinous process below this line is marked as the L5 process. Alternatively, the L5 spinous process can be confirmed preoperatively with a radiography and radio-opaque marker (**A** and **B**).

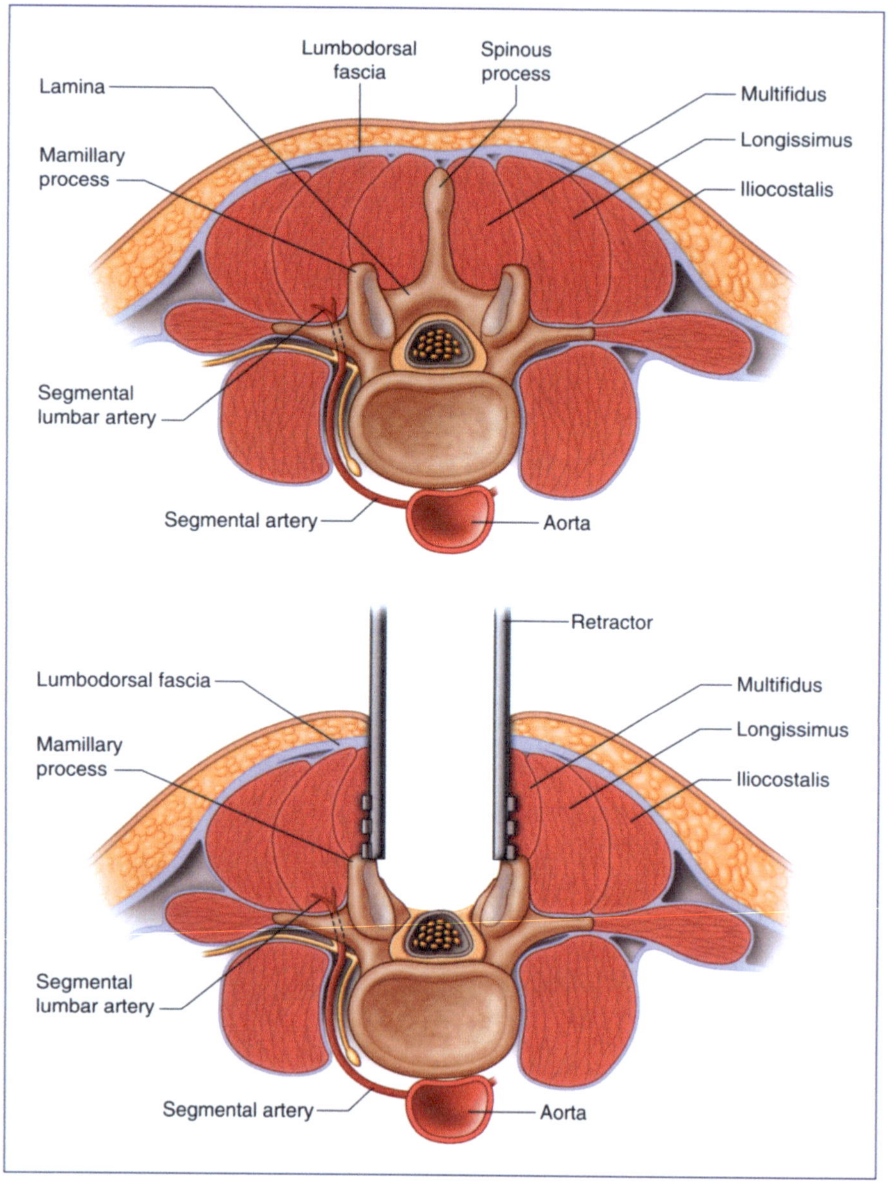

FIGURE 21-9. Incision and initial exposure. A midline vertical incision is extended from the L4/L5 to the S1/S2 interspace. The skin and subcutaneous tissue are dissected using the Bovie unit until the lumbodorsal fascia is encountered. Later, the fascial closure can be facilitated at this point by clearing the fascia from the overlying tissue using Metzenbaum scissors. The fascia is incised sharply in the midline over the spinous processes. To completely free the fascia, it must be incised on both sides of each spinous process.

An avascular, internervous plane lies between the left and right paraspinous muscles [28]. Bilaterally, these muscles are separated below the periosteum as a unit from the spinous process and laminae with very little bleeding using a Cobb elevator and the Bovie unit. However, clearing of the laminae laterally should be limited to be close to the facet joints, where the lumbar segmental paraspinous muscle branch vessels can be encountered. The bony structures protect the underlying dura and cord structures in the midline. At this point, a self-retaining (Taylor or Beckman-Adson) retractor is placed to separate the paraspinous muscles. The spinous processes and laminae are then cleared with a sponge in preparation for laminectomy. (*Adapted from* Hoppenfield and deBoer [28].)

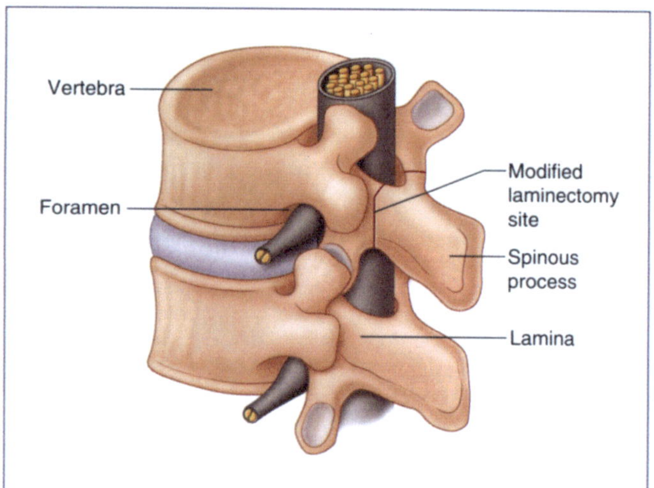

FIGURE 21-10. Multiple laminectomy techniques. Multiple techniques exist for safely removing the laminae and exposing the dura. For good exposure and access to the nerve roots and foramen for the purposes of this procedure, our preference is to use rongeurs to perform a modified laminectomy that removes the spinous process and the medial two-thirds of the bilateral laminae, avoiding bleeding at the facet joints.

The three-column system (anterior, middle, and posterior) proposed by Denis [30] for traumatic injuries is the most popular system to classify spinal integrity. The viability of each of the columns is based on the combined strengths of the bony structures and their corresponding ligamentous attachments. According to Denis's system, the spine is considered unstable when any two of the three columns are disrupted. The bony structures of the posterior column of support consist of paired pedicles and lamina and a single central spinous process that house the dural sac and central nervous system elements. In addition, the supraspinous and interspinous ligaments bind the spinous process of different vertebral levels, while the robust ligamentum flavum bridges the lamina. Assuming viability of the anterior and middle columns, the modified laminectomy should not destabilize the spine because it violates only the posterior column.

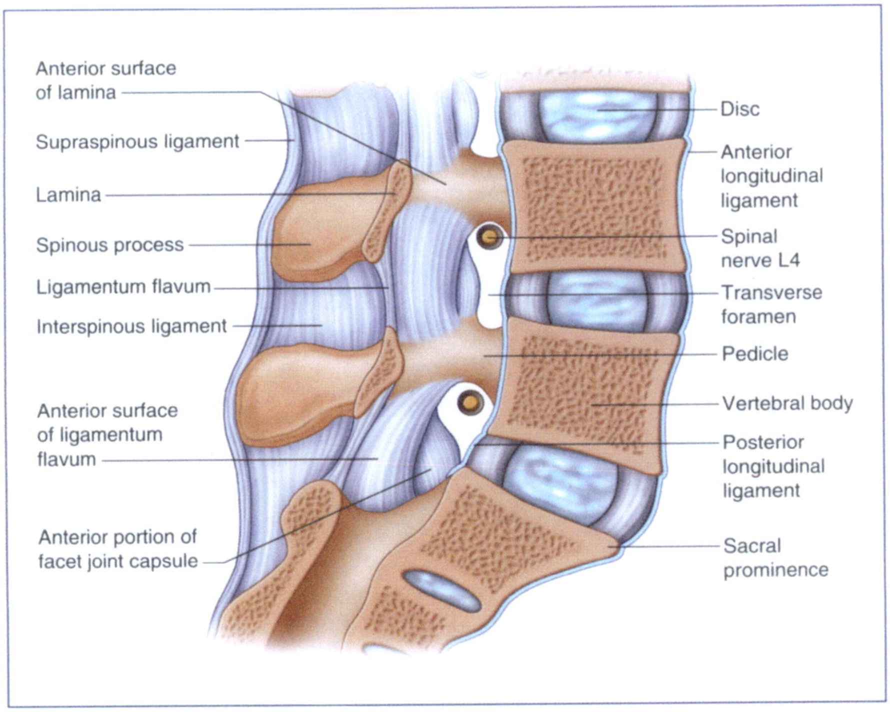

FIGURE 21-11. Laminectomy procedure. To begin the laminectomy, the Luer-Stille or Ruskin rongeurs are used to remove the caudal half of the L5 and the entire S1 spinous process. The ligamentum flavum is incised sharply, providing a window into the epidural space. Throughout this portion of the procedure, great care must be taken to avoid trauma to the underlying dura and root structures. As this window develops, the footplate of a Kerrison rongeur can be slipped under the cranial lamina. Small bites of the lamina are taken initially, until the underlying dural sac is clearly identified. A Freer elevator can be used to gently separate the dura from the overlying lamina. This maneuver provides a space for the safe insertion of the rongeur's footplate without pinching the underlying structures. The blue dural sac and gray-yellow fat of the epidural space become apparent as the laminectomy proceeds. (*Adapted from* Hoppenfield and deBoer [28].)

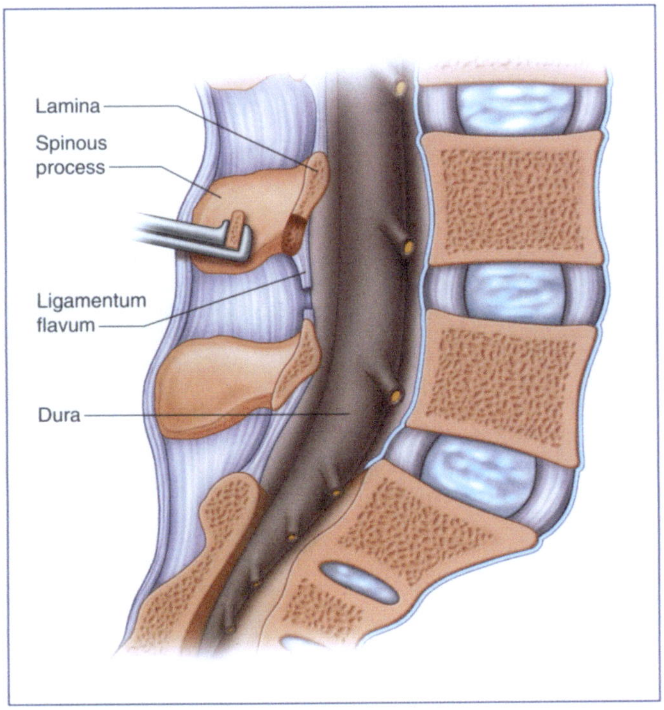

FIGURE 21-12. Rongeur for laminectomy. A rongeur with a larger footplate can be used to complete the removal of the remainder of the medial two-thirds of each lamina. The S1 laminae are removed in a similar fashion, except they are approached from above through the already developed space. At the completion of the modified laminectomy, the cut ends of the lamina should be even with the lateral border of the dural sac.

Occasionally, bleeding can be encountered during this portion of the procedure. The Bovie unit should not be used near the nervous structures. Bleeding from bone that does not respond to pressure usually abates after the application of bone wax. Gel foam and cottonoids can be helpful additions to the troubleshooting algorithm. (*Adapted from* Hoppenfield and deBoer [28].)

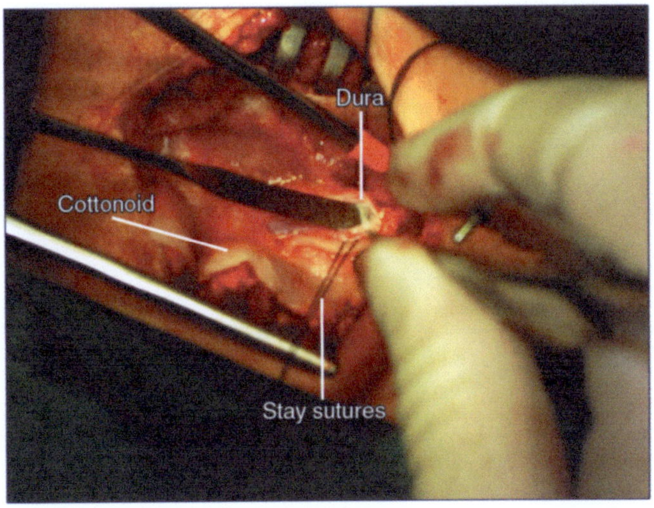

FIGURE 21-13. Dura. Two 3-0 silk stay sutures on a taper needle are passed into the dura just off of the midline, avoiding the inclusion of any underlying nerve fibers. Along the length of the exposure, cottonoids are placed between the dura and cut edge of the lamina, lateral to the stay sutures. An 11 blade is then used to make a small opening between the stay sutures. The immediate return of clear cerebrospinal fluid (CSF) should be noted. The suction tip is changed to a neurosucker with soft tip and the patient is placed in the Trendelenburg position to minimize CSF in the surgical field. The Freer elevator is placed under the dura to protect the nerve roots below and the dura is incised on it cranially and caudally. Alternatively, the dura can be gently split open in the midline proximally and distally by pulling it in opposite directions with nerve hooks. At this point, the numerous roots of the cauda equina become apparent. Additional sutures can be passed through the dura and loosely tied to the adjacent fascia to aid with exposure.

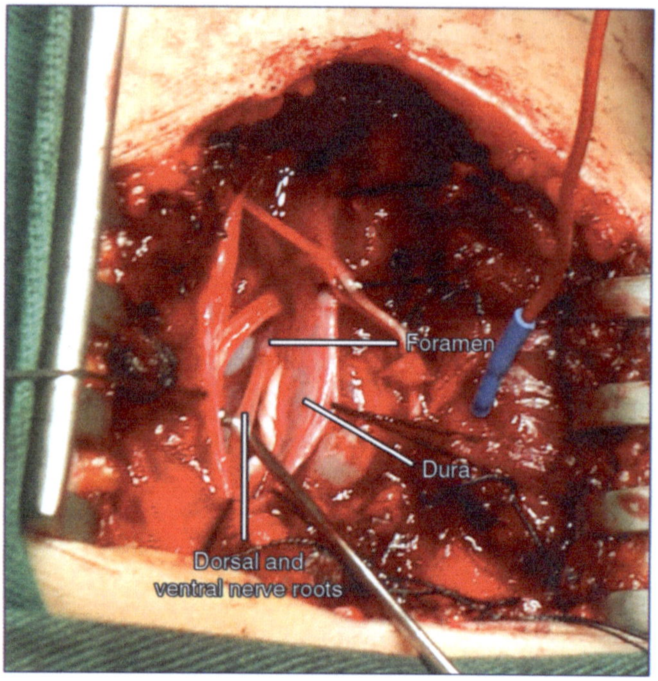

FIGURE 21-14. Nerve root identification. The goal of this portion of the operation is to identify the ventral roots of L5 and S2/S3 on the left. As mentioned above, the dorsal (sensory) and ventral (motor) roots for each level travel together and exit through their respective foramen. At this point, the roots of each segment are not clear because all of the lower lumbar and sacral roots travel in one cluster. By taking advantage of the fact that each segment is relatively fixed at its respective foramen, retraction of the entire bundle to the right with the Freer elevator begins to reveal the individual roots at their exit point. Nerve hooks are then used to complete the separation of the individual root segments on the left.

With the individual roots separated, anatomic relationships can be used to begin to identify the root segments. There is a size discrepancy between the lumbar and sacral roots. Furthermore, the distance between foramen decreases dramatically at the sacral level. Therefore, the L5 donor root can often be identified based on its large size compared with the caudal sacral roots and the decreasing space between the roots below.

Muscle	L3	L4	L5	S1	S2	S3
Vastus medialis	Major	Major				
Tibialis anterior*		Major	Major			
Medial gastrocnemius*				Major	Medium	
Abductor hallicus*				Major	Major	
External anal sphincter*					Major	Major

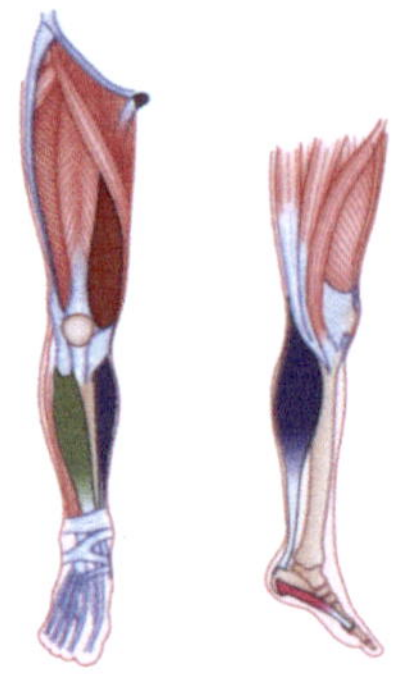

Major contribution
Medium contribution
No contribution

FIGURE 21-15. Nerve root identification. Next, the donor L5 ventral root is separated from its corresponding dorsal root by passing nerve hooks into the visibly identifiable plane that exists between them. The hooks are then pulled in opposite directions, parallel to the nerve fibers, to complete their separation down to the foramen. From this posterior orientation, the smaller ventral root runs beneath the dorsal root. It is essential to keep the dorsal root intact, as it serves as the initiator of the new micturition reflex [24].

Intraoperative monitoring is then used to confirm that the presumed donor L5 ventral root has been isolated. A bipolar stimulator (Cadwell Laboratories, Inc.; Kennewick, WA) is used to elicit compound muscle action potentials (CMAPs), which are acquired from 13-mm subdermal needle electrodes (Rhythmlink International; Columbia, SC) placed in the associated lower extremity muscle groups. Recording CMAPs and altering stimulation output parameters is done using a multimodality Cadwell Cascade. Guidelines for stimulator settings are as follows: current output (0.3–3 mA), duration (0.02–0.2 msec), and frequency (0.5–1 Hz). The stimulation should be accurate and atraumatic, and starting with minimum strength not exceed the upper limit of the given range to prevent neural damage.

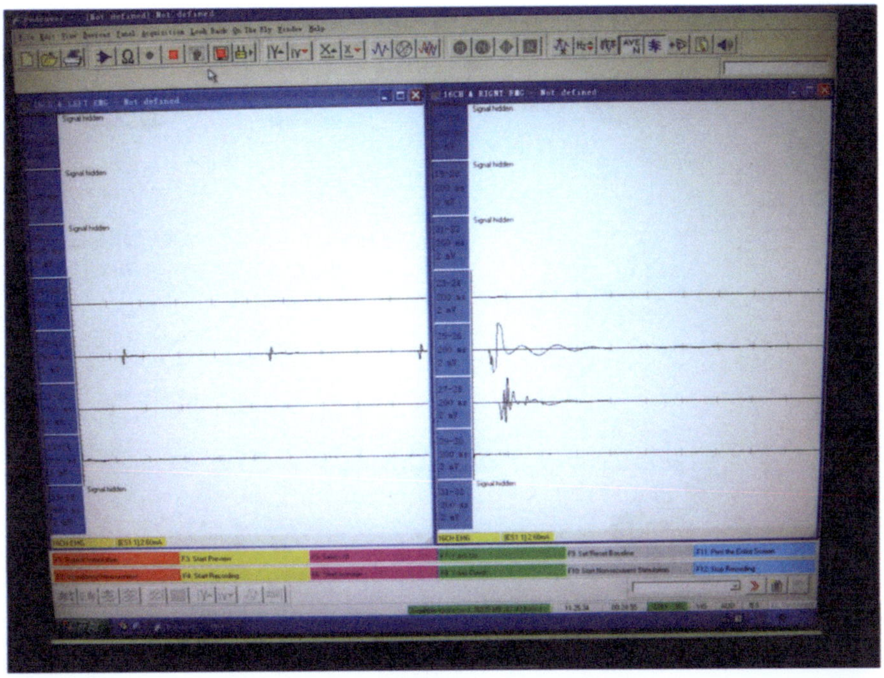

FIGURE 21-16. Nerve root identification. The pattern of muscle group firing is used to confirm the root segment, not the specific activity of a single muscle. For example, the pattern of muscle firing confirming L5 would include compound muscle action potentials (CMAPs) in tibialis anterior and silence in the vastus medialis, medial gastrocnemius, abductor hallices, and external anal sphincter. These characteristic patterns can be used to identify any of the root segments. Furthermore, it is critical to differentiate with certainty the ventral from the dorsal root. CMAP activity will be present with ventral stimulation, but is silent with dorsal stimulation. However, stimulation of what is believed to be the isolated dorsal root will sometimes produce CMAPs. In this situation, the stimulation settings should be minimized to make sure this is not an artifact. As the ventral and dorsal roots are actually comprised of a number of rootlets, it is also possible that a ventral rootlet is included with both packets. In this case, further dissection of the roots will be helpful. If neither root produces CMAP activity, the settings should be increased and the impedances of the recording electrodes should be evaluated or the root may not be functional. EMG—electromyelogram.

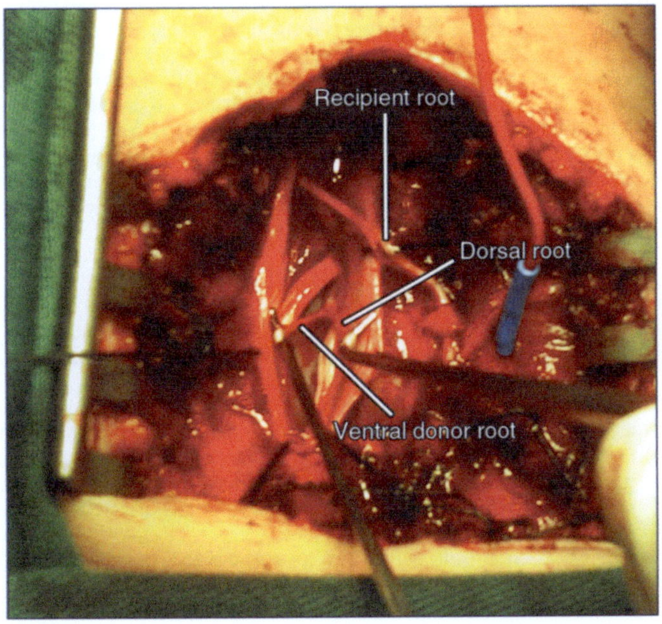

FIGURE 21-17. Nerve root identification. If a functional L5 ventral root cannot be isolated using the standard nerve root identification technique, then an alternative donor root must be localized. Possibilities include the ipsilateral S1, L4, L3, and further ascending lumbar segments. For a tension-free, nongrafted anastomosis, the limiting factor for using higher segments is the distance to the cut end of the recipient root. Alternatively, the corresponding roots on the right side can also be evaluated to serve as the donor root. Preoperative neurophysiological testing can usually define the integrity of the roots reliably and determine the operative plan prior to beginning the case.

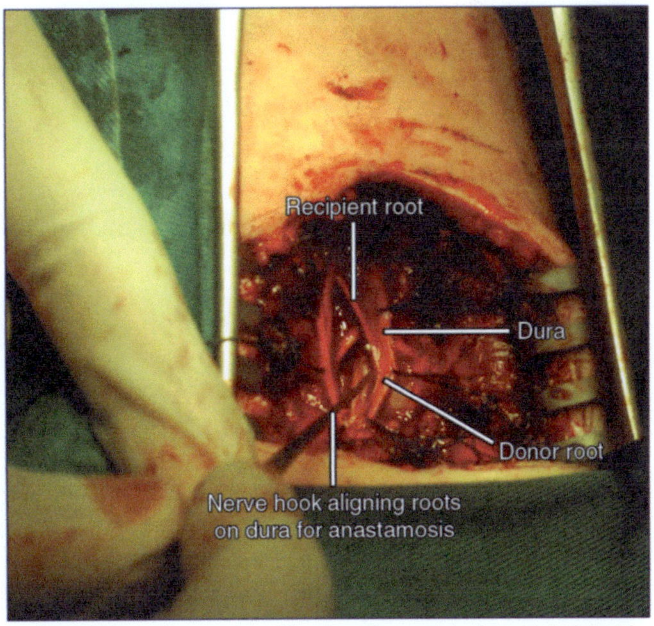

FIGURE 21-18. Nerve root identification. The recipient root is isolated in a similar manner to the donor root. More than one sacral root level can be used because of the size discrepancy with the lumbar donor. The left S2 and S3 ventral roots are preferred when available. The left side is preferred over the right to maximize the reinnervation of both the bladder and bowel [27]. If the ventral root cannot be separated from the dorsal root, then both roots can be included as the recipient. Given the fact that the donor axons only require an intact nerve sheath to serve as a conduit for reinnervation, the recipient root does not need to be functional.

Once the donor and recipient roots have been chosen, they must be transected in preparation for anastomosis. The donor root should be carefully cut using microscissors as distally as possible, near its foramen. On the other hand, the recipient root should be transected as proximally as necessary to assure a tension-free anastomosis. The nerve ends are then aligned along a cleared area of dura.

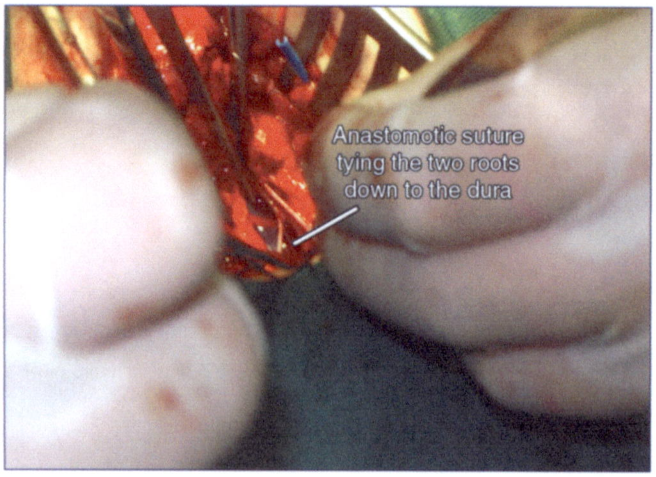

FIGURE 21-19. Anastomosis. The intradural roots are covered only by a thin layer of pia mater [29]. They do not contain the more substantial layer of epineurium, a condensation of the dura surrounding the spinal nerve as it exits its respective foramen. Therefore, the typical epineurial-to-epineurial anastomosis with multiple sutures performed in peripheral nerve surgery is not possible intradurally. Consequently, the delicate anastomosis is performed under loupe magnification using a single 8-0 polyglactin or polyglycolic acid suture on a taper needle. The suture is passed through the donor nerve and 3 to 4 mm of dura in a single motion. Subsequently, the suture is passed through the recipient nerve root and tied down. Tying the knot down to the dura transfers the tension away from the thin pia and provides a fixation point for the anastomosis. Once a secure anastomosis has been performed, suctioning inside the dura should be minimized or avoided completely to prevent its accidental disruption. In preparation for closure, the field is copiously irrigated with saline to aid with visualization of structures and to clear the meninges of irrigative blood.

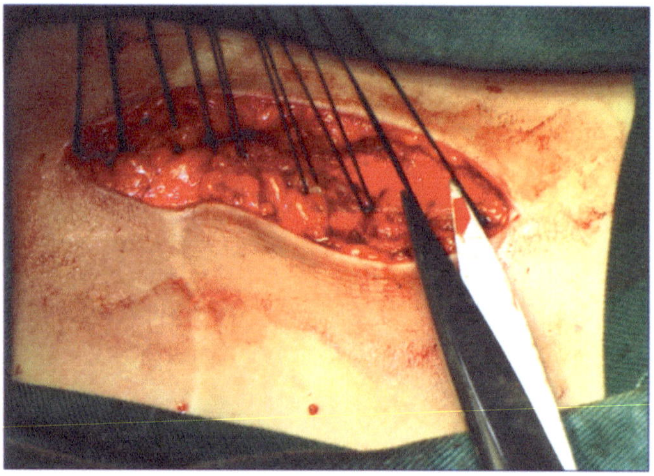

FIGURE 21-20. Closure. The dura is closed with a running 5-0 polyglactin suture on a taper needle. The Freer elevator can be used to protect the anastomosis and nerve roots. The integrity of the closure can be evaluated by taking the patient out of the Trendelenburg position or by performing Valsalva maneuvers. Any significant dural defects that are found can be carefully closed with additional 5-0 polyglactin sutures. DuraSeal (Confluent Surgical; Waltham, MA) can be applied for additional security. The fascia is closed with interrupted 0 polyglactin sutures on a cutting needle. The wound is irrigated and adequate hemostasis is attained. The subcutaneous tissue can be loosely reapproximated with interrupted 3-0 polyglactin sutures. Finally, the skin is closed with simple interrupted 0 silk sutures on a cutting needle and a dressing is applied.

Postoperative Management
Immediately postoperative
Bedrest for 48 h
Clear liquids; advance as tolerated
Foley catheter until off bedrest, then resume the preoperative routine
Parenteral antibiotics until tolerating PO
Narcotics PRN
Discharge
Limited activity for 4–6 wk
Oral antibiotics for 1 wk
PRN pain medication
Suture removal in 7–10 d
Wean anticholinergics 3–6 mo postoperative, as tolerated

FIGURE 21-21. Postoperative management. The patient is admitted postoperatively and maintained on strict bedrest for at least 48 hours. Clear liquids can be started immediately postoperatively and the diet is advanced as tolerated. Parenteral antibiotics are continued until the patient is able to tolerate a regular diet and can be converted to orals. Narcotics are administered as needed. The patient's preoperative bladder-management regimen is resumed once they are no longer on bedrest.

At discharge, activity is limited for 4 to 6 weeks and the patient is sent home on a 1-week course of oral antibiotics (fluoroquinolone or cephalosporin) and pain medications as needed (PRN). Sutures are removed in 7 to 10 days.

Based on a growth rate of approximately 1 mm/d, a nerve-regeneration time of 6 months to 2 years can be expected [26,27]. Once the new reflex arc can be elicited with scratch or stimulation using a transcutaneous electrical nerve stimulation unit of the appropriate dermatome, catheter management and anticholinergics should be gradually discontinued as bladder function recovers. PO—by mouth.

Preoperative and 18-Month Postoperative Urodynamics Data

Variable	Mean preoperative	Mean postoperative	P value (Wilcoxon signed rank test)
Residual urine, *mL*	358.67	60.00	0.0005
Bladder capacity, *mL*	364.17	387.50	0.9374
Maximum detrusor pressure, cmH_2O	82.33	62.83	0.0025
Maximum flow, *mL/s*	2.41	1.33	0.0024

Of the 15 patients, three were not included due to failure in two and loss to followup in one.

Figure 21-22. Xiao spinal cord injury data. Xiao's first human clinic trial involved 15 males with complete suprasacral spinal cord injury who were followed a mean of 3 years postoperatively [26]. All patients had hyperreflexic neurogenic bladders with detrusor external sphincter dyssynergia. At 12 to 18 months after nerve rerouting, 67% of patients gained near-normal storage and synergistic voiding with dermatomal stimulation. Postvoid residual volumes in successful cases decreased from a mean of 332 mL to 31 mL. Partial responses were noted in two additional patients who required a TENS unit to initiate micturition and had postvoid residuals greater than 100 mL. Remarkably, four of the 10 successful patients had nearly normal urodynamic storage and voiding patterns postoperatively, and could empty by either large-volume involuntary reflex voiding or by stimulation of the new micturition pathway. The remaining six successes had improved detrusor pressures, compliance, and capacity, but retained similar urodynamic patterns. Involuntary reflex voiding did not occur, but dermatomal stimulation triggered bladder emptying. Xiao [24] updated his experience in 2005, reporting an 88% success rate in 92 patients with hyperreflexic or acontractile neurogenic bladders secondary to spinal cord injury. Currently, we are enrolling spinal cord injury patients at our institution and have performed the procedure in three patients.

Spina Bifida Operative Considerations and Clinical Outcomes

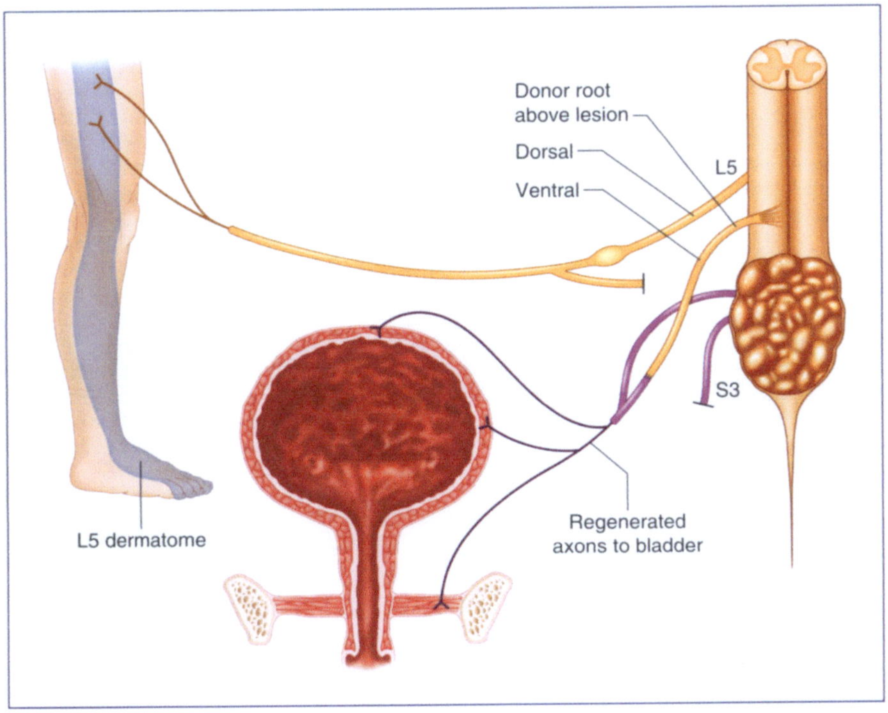

Figure 21-23. Spina bifida general considerations. The concepts behind nerve rerouting that were learned in spinal cord injury were applied to patients with spina bifida by Xiao *et al.* [26]. While the ultimate goal of restoring functional voiding is the same, a few fundamental differences must be considered.

In spina bifida, the donor nerve root is taken from *above* the level of the defect compared to spinal cord injury, where the donor root is taken from below the level of the injury [27]. In spina bifida, there are usually no healthy nerve roots below the level of the defect. Because of this unique anatomy, it may be possible for the new reflex arc to be integrated upstream and processed in the brain [27]. Theoretically, a novel micturition center could develop in the brain after successful spina bifida nerve rerouting [27].

Furthermore, the best candidates for the nerve-rerouting procedure are patients who are ambulatory with or without assistive devices. In spinal cord injury, the transected donor nerve root provided little contribution to a paralyzed lower extremity. However, in spina bifida, the transected donor root contributes functional axons to the lower extremity. Postoperative lower extremity weakness is subsequently of major concern. In fact, initial footdrop rates were reported at 25% [27].

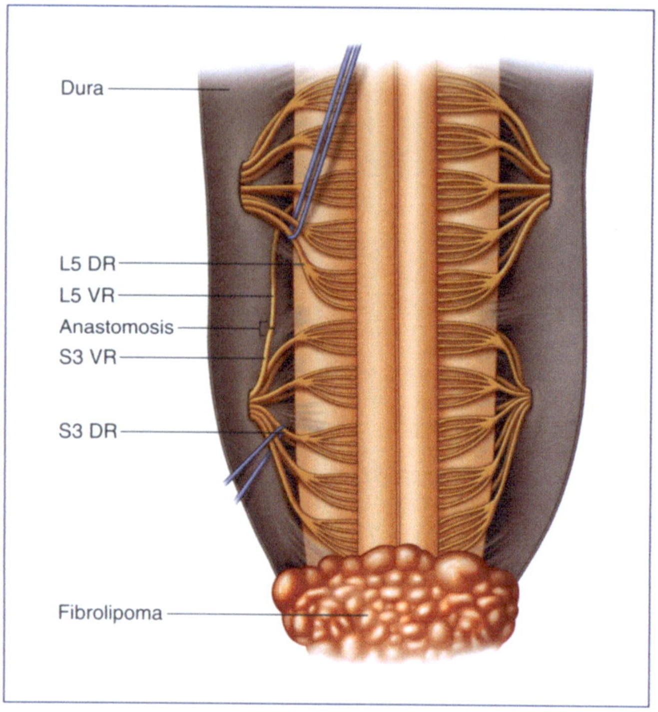

FIGURE 21-24. Spina bifida general considerations. By using only half of the donor root, Xiao reduced the footdrop rate to 5% [24]. Nevertheless, new postoperative deficits in gait can have a devastating impact on quality of life. In addition, the spinal cord in myelomeningocele patients terminates well below the expected upper lumbar vertebral level, often tethered to a thickened filum terminale or to scar tissue. While in a spinal cord injury the spinal cord is well away from the operative site, the cord in spina bifida is often part of the surgical field. Again, this increases the risk of injury to other functional lower extremity motor and sensory fibers.

The expected orderly exit of the roots of a given level through its appropriate foramen is often absent in involved myelomeningocele roots. In fact, some or all of the sacral roots can exit through a single foramen in spina bifida [27]. Furthermore, the recipient sacral root may lack functional axons, which are composed of connective tissue sheaths only [27]. Fortunately, the empty nerve sheaths are sufficient to allow orderly axonal reinnervation, assuming that there is no downstream disruption in scar tissue from a previous surgery. Again, these findings underscore the additional complexity involved in expanding the procedure to this patient population.

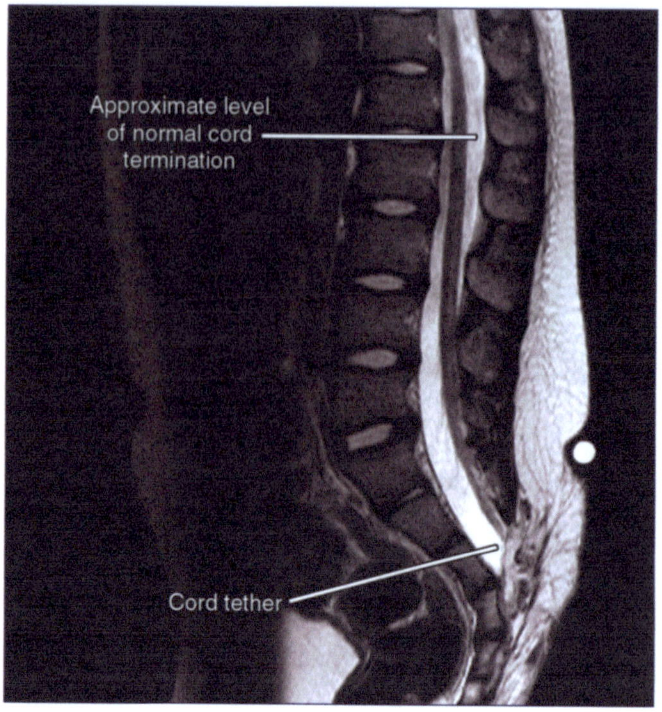

FIGURE 21-25. Spina bifida operative considerations. While the operative procedure involves the same basic steps as for a spinal cord injury, a few important points should be considered in spina bifida. First, the anatomy of each myelomeningocele patient is unique. Preoperative MRI information is critical in planning an uncomplicated procedure. Determining the lowest intact spinous process identifies an area below which normal tissue can be expected. The level of the conus medullaris where the spinal cord is tethered should be studied. Additionally, missing spinous processes and laminae from a prior laminectomy (*ie*, from a prior tethered cord release) should be noted. Finally, the relationship of the dura and the conus medullaris with the surface anatomy and other anomalies, including the extent of any associated lipoma, should be defined.

Having reviewed the MRI in detail, the operative approach should proceed from known to unknown. Usually, scar tissue is present at skin level secondary to the neonatal myelomeningocele closure and other prior spine operations. The initial dissection should be limited through the scar tissue to avoid entering the dura prematurely and injuring underlying nervous tissue.

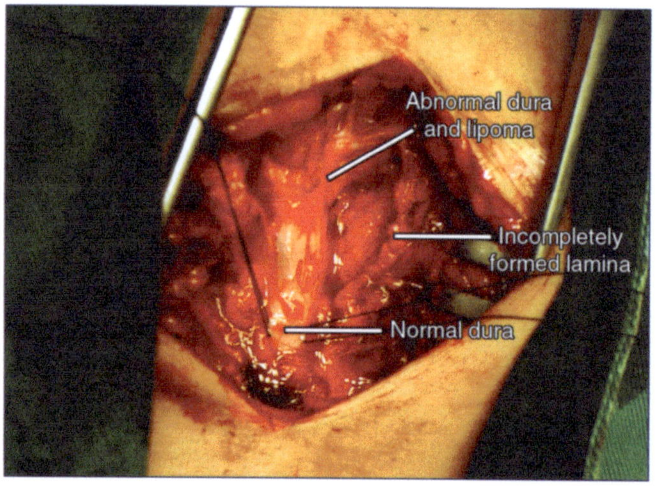

FIGURE 21-26. Spina bifida operative considerations. The initial safe depth of dissection though scar tissue at the skin and subcutaneous tissue level can be estimated on the MRI. However, the focus of the initial dissection should be on the lowest normal spinous process and lamina to safely expose normal dura. In order to maximize exposure prior to performing the laminectomy, the caudal dissection can continue laterally, cauterizing down to the palpable ends of incompletely formed laminae. Any dissection medially to the tips of the laminae at this point risks injury to the nervous tissue. Again, correlation with the MRI findings is important here to allow safe dissection.

The laminectomy is then performed and the normal area of underlying dura is identified. The diseased caudal dura is then carefully exposed along its superolateral surface, dissecting just medially and then inferiorly to the tips of the incompletely formed lamina. Posterolateral dissection should be avoided at this point to prevent injury to the spinal nerves outside the dura. Often, the dura needs to be opened to allow safe confirmation and dissection of the roots both intra- and extradurally.

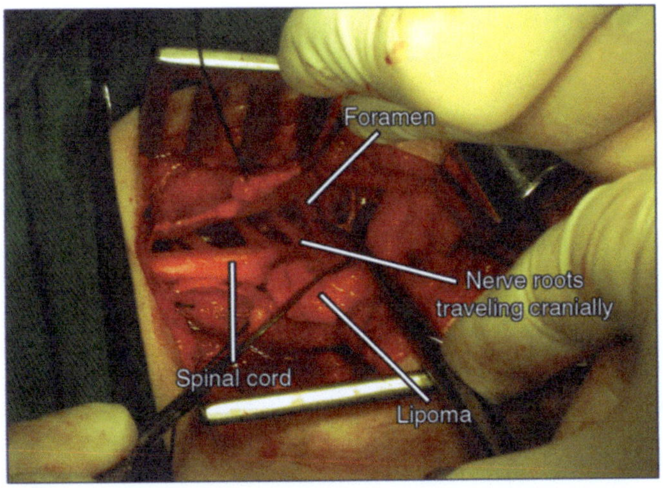

FIGURE 21-27. Spina bifida operative considerations. The dura should be opened cranially at the site of the laminectomy where the anatomy is normal. The nerve roots can then be visualized and separated from the diseased dura caudally before the dura is opened; the dura should be opened as carefully as possible to facilitate later closure and prevent the leakage of cerebrospinal fluid.

Nerve root identification is always more complicated in spina bifida. Depending on the level of the cord tether, the course of the nerve roots can be highly variable with some roots even frequently traveling cranially to exit the dura. Again, many of the sacral nerve roots are really just empty connective tissue sheaths. They are generally more delicate than the corresponding roots in an adult cord patient and are easily avulsed from the adjacent spinal cord. Often, the appropriate sacral recipient root must be determined based on anatomic relationships only because of the frequent lack of compound muscle action potential activity. Nevertheless, it is imperative to identify and confirm a viable donor root with neurophysiological testing. Finally, a DuraSeal (Confluent Surgical; Waltham, MA) application at the time of dural closure is much more critical in these patients to prevent a later cerebrospinal fluid leak.

Urodynamic Data Comparison

		Preoperative/18 mo postoperative		
Patient age/sex	**Bladder capacity, *mL***	**Residual urine, *mL***	**Maximum Pdet, cmH_2O**	**Result**
		Areflexia		Partial recovery
14/F	110/303	70/36	15/25	
12/M	110/180	90/0	16/31	
5/M	106/125	80/60	28/51	
12/M	90/162	80/0	13/39	Partial recovery
13/F	70/317	70/60	13/55	
11/M	75/280	70/25	10/32	No improvement
8/F	80/88	69/27	20/28	
9/F	148/184	80/40	33/41	
7/M	70/70	39/0	28/43	
12/F	85/187	83/0	18/28	
11/M	96/166	85/30	16/31	
13/M	90/210	80/20	14/30	
14/F	355/400	355/350	7/10	
13/F	147/250	140/150	12/12	No improvement
Mean	117.28/208.71	99.36/57	17.35/32.57	No improvement
P value	0.001	0.002	0.0012	
		Hyperreflexia/DESD		
12/M	80/176	72/0	66/60	
13/M	70/160	70/50	89/47	
12/M	134/173	110/12	54/46	
7/F	120/228	50/20	45/43	
10/M	79/250	69/10	67/49	
9/M	83/80	50/50	48/37	
Mean	94.33/177.83	70.17/23.67	61.50/47.00	
P value	0.063	0.045	0.0312	

Due to a small sample size, a nonparametric test (Wilcoxon signed rank) was used to compare preoperative and postoperative residual urine, bladder capacity, and maximum Pdet.

FIGURE 21-28. Spina bifida data. In 2005, Xiao *et al.* published an article about their experience with the nerve-rerouting principle for 20 children with spina bifida and incontinence [27]. Fourteen of the children had areflexic and six had hyperreflexic neurogenic bladder with detrusor–external urethral sphincter dyssynergia (DESD). Overall, 17 of the 20 children gained satisfactory bladder control and continence between 8 and 12 months after the nerve-rerouting procedure. Two additional patients were considered to be partial recoveries because postvoid residuals remained above 50 mL. Remarkably, most children could initiate voiding spontaneously, without the need to scratch the ipsilateral dermatome. Continence was achieved as early as 6 months postoperatively and several children, unexpectedly, appeared to gain bladder sensory function. Unfortunately, five children suffered from variable weakness of muscles of the ipsilateral L4 or L5 lower extremity distribution, two of which had a visible footdrop.

Updated data in 2005 maintained a similar 87% success rate in 110 children with spina bifida [24]. Refinement of the technique, using only half of the donor nerve root, decreased the lower extremity complication rate to 5% [24].

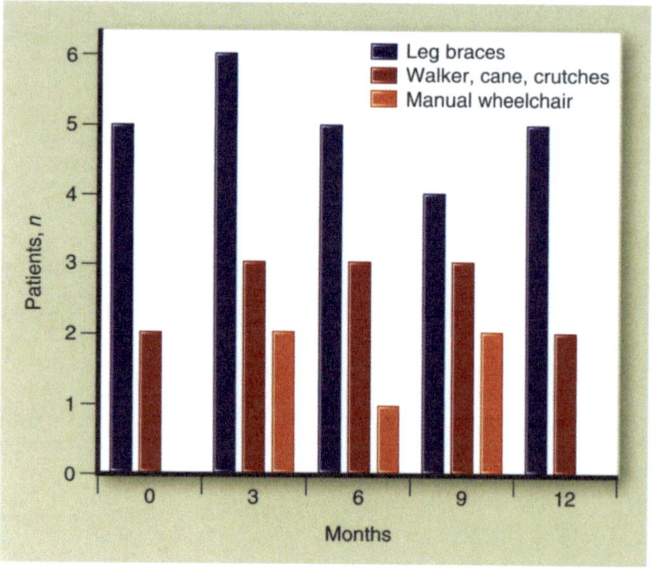

Figure 21-29. Assistive devices for ambulation. In 2006, we obtained institutional review board approval to enroll 20 patients with spina bifida into a pilot study at our institution, William Beaumont Hospital in Royal Oak, Michigan [31]. To date, we have performed the nerve-rerouting procedure in nine patients. One-year outcomes are in press at the time of this publication.

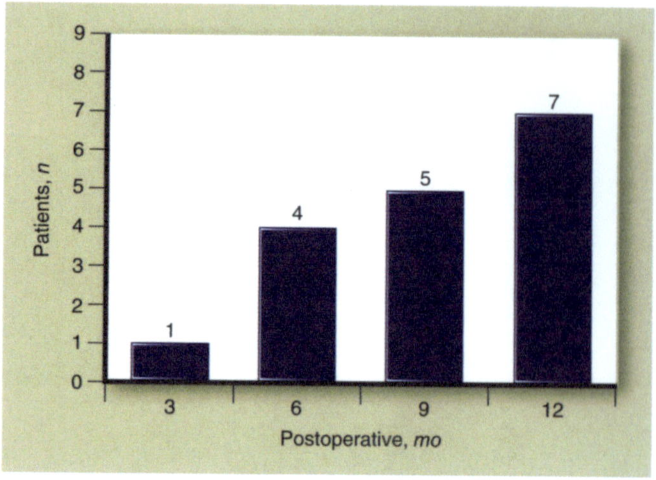

Figure 21-30. Presence of novel reflex arc with stimulation. Postoperatively, there was increased need for use of ankle–foot orthoses; walkers; and, in two cases, wheelchairs, especially for long distances. Fortunately, with physical therapy and time, by 1 year eight of nine patients had returned to or near baseline. However, one patient has a residual footdrop.

Nine patients (three men, six women) with a median age of 8 (range 6–37) years qualified for the procedure following extensive preoperative evaluation. Of the nine patients, five had a prior defect closure within 24 hours of birth, three underwent intrauterine closure, and one had no prior surgery. Mean operative time was 183 (range 127–278) minutes. Mean estimated blood loss was 57 (range 10–100) mL. No intraoperative complications occurred and the length of stay averaged 3.4 (range 2–7) days. Perioperative complications included footdrop in one patient, wound drainage in three patients, and a prolonged inability to bear weight in one patient.

Early in the postoperative course, the lower extremity weakness in some patients was profound. Based on the 1-month neurological examination, eight of nine patients displayed a new variable weakness of one or more lower extremity muscle groups.

There was a gradual increase over time in the number of patients who demonstrated a bladder contraction with dermatomal stimulation until, at 1 year, seven of nine patients had a definitive and reproducible bladder contraction. Preoperatively, two patients were able to void a small amount. By 1-year urodynamic testing, seven children were able to voluntarily void a mean of 133 + 75 cc with an intermittent flow pattern, mean Qmax = 10 + 8 cc/s, and mean postvoid residual = 119 + 125 cc. Overall, all nine of the patients demonstrated a reflex bladder contraction or the ability to initiate voiding by 1 year. However, seven of the nine patients still needed to use their catheter at least once a day to empty their bladder at 1 year. An improvement in bowel function was reported on 1-year global assessment scores in six of the nine patients and 78% reported that they would undergo the procedure again.

Conclusion

Based on the innovative bench-to-bedside pioneering work of CG Xiao and colleagues, nerve rerouting may revolutionize the care of patients with spinal cord injury and spina bifida. While the initial data appear promising, we believe the procedure should remain under strict experimental protocol until confirmatory multi-institutional trials are completed.

Acknowledgements: We would like to thank CG Xiao for his guidance in developing the lumbar-to-sacral nerve-rerouting clinical trial at our institution and for his expertise and willingness to train the surgeons involved.We would like to thank William Nantau from our Department of Clinical Neurophysiology for his expertise, insight, and guidance in intraoperative monitoring.

References

1. Jackson A, Dijkers M, Devivo M, Poczatek R: A demographic profile of new traumatic spinal cord injuries: change and stability over 30 years. *Arch Phys Med Rehabil* 2004; 85:1740–1748.
2. Rabchevsky AG, Smith GM: Therapeutic interventions following mammalian spinal cord injury. *Arch Neurol* 2001, 58:721–726.
3. DeVivo MJ: Causes and costs of spinal cord injury in the United States. *Spinal Cord* 1997, 35:809–813.
4. Hackler R: A 25-year prospective mortality in the spinal cord injured patient: comparison with the long-term living paraplegic. *J Urol* 1977, 117:486–492.
5. Samson G, Cardenas DD: Neurogenic bladder in spinal cord injury. *Phys Med Rehabil Clin N Am* 2007, 18:255–274.
6. Soden RJ, Walsh J, Middleton JW, *et al.*: Causes of death after spinal cord injury. *Spinal Cord* 2000, 38:604–610.
7. Sullivan M, Yalla SV: Spinal cord injury and other forms of myeloneuropathies. *Probl Urol* 1992, 6:643–658.
8. Consortium for Spinal Cord Medicine: *Bladder Management for Adults With Spinal Cord Injury: A Clinical Practice Guideline for Health-Care Providers*. Washington, DC: Paralyzed Veterans of America; 2006.
9. Chancellor MB, Blaivas JG: Spinal cord injury. In *Practical Neurourology*. Boston: Butterworth-Heinemann, 1995:99–118.
10. Lapides J, Diokno AC, Silber SJ, Lowe BS: Clean, intermittent self-catheterization in the treatment of urinary tract disease. *J Urol* 1972, 107:458–461.
11. McGuire EJ, Woodside JR, Borden TA: Upper urinary tract deterioration in patients with myelodysplasia and detrusor hypertonia: a follow-up study. *J Urol* 1983, 129:823–826.
12. McGuire EJ, Woodside JR, Borden TA, Weiss RM: Prognostic value of urodynamic testing in myelodysplastic patients. *J Urol* 1981, 126:205–209.
13. Brinley GS: The first 500 patients with sacral anterior root stimulator implants: general description. *Paraplegia* 1994, 32:795–805.
14. Jezernik S, Craggs M, Grill WM, *et al.*: Electrical stimulation for the treatment of bladder dysfunction: current status and future possibilities. *Neurol Res* 2002, 24:413–430.
15. Sarwark JF: Spina bifida. *Pediatr Clin N Am* 1996, 43:1151–1158.
16. Centers for Disease Control and Prevention: Folic acid and prevention of spina bifida and anencephaly. *MMWR* 2002, 51:9–11.
17. Tulipan N: Intrauterine myelomeningocele repair. *Clin Perinatol* 2003, 30:521–530.
18. MRC Vitamin Study Research Group: Prevention of neural tube defects: results of the Medical Research Council Vitamin study. *Lancet* 1991, 338:131–137.
19. Bowman RM, McLone DG, Grant JA, *et al.*: Spina bifida outcome: a 25-year prospective. *Pediatr Neurosurg* 2001, 34:114–120.
20. Bauer SB, Labib KB, Dieppa RA, Retik AB: Urodynamic evaluation of boys with myelodysplasia and incontinence. *Urology* 1977, 4:354–362.
21. Dator DP, Hatchett L, Dyro EM, *et al.*: Urodynamic dysfunction in walking myelodysplastic children. *J Urol* 1992, 148:362–365.
22. Bauer SB: Early evaluation and management of children with spina bifida. In *Urologic Surgery in Neonates and Young Infants*. Philadelphia: WB Saunders; 1988: 252–264.
23. Xiao CG, Godoc CJ: A possible new reflex pathway for micturition after spinal cord injury. *Paraplegia* 1995, 32:300–307.
24. Xiao CG: Reinnervation for neurogenic bladder: historic review and introduction of a somatic-autonomic reflex pathway procedure for patients with spinal cord injury or spina bifida. *Eur Urol* 2006, 49:22–29.
25. Xiao CG, De Groat WC, Godec CJ, *et al.*: "Skin-CNS-bladder" reflex pathway for micturition after spinal cord injury and its underlying mechanisms. *J Urol* 1999, 162:936–942.
26. Xiao CG, Mao-Xin D, Chengpu D, *et al.*: An artificial somatic-central nervous system-autonomic reflex pathway for controllable micturition after spinal cord injury: preliminary results in 15 patients. *J Urol* 2003, 170:1237–1241.
27. Xiao CG, Mai-Xin D, Li B, *et al.*: An artificial somatic-autonomic reflex pathway procedure for bladder control in children with spina bifida. *J Urol* 2005, 172:2112–2116.
28. Hoppenfield S, deBoer P: The spine. In *Surgical Exposures in Orthopaedics: The Anatomic Approach*, edn 3. Philadelphia: Lippincott Williams & Wilkins; 2003:249–340.
29. Standring S, ed: *Gray's Anatomy*, edn 39. New York: Elsevier Churchill Livingstone; 2005.
30. Denis F: The three column spine and its significance in the classification of acute thoracolumbar spinal injuries. *Spine* 1983, 8:817–831.
31. Girdler B, Turzewski C, Feber K, *et al.*: Six month evaluation of the Beaumont experience with the Xiao "skin-CNS-bladder" reflex in spina bifida [abstract]. *J Urol* 2008:295.

22 Overactive Bladder: Physiology of Normal and Abnormal Urinary Storage and Basis for Pharmacological Therapy

Roger R. Dmochowski and David R. Staskin

Normal voiding is the product of an intricate interaction between the lower urinary tract and the central nervous system. This interface is regulated and potentiated by central nervous system mechanisms and local effects, which result in volitional control of an otherwise primitive reflex arc, the sacral afferent and efferent neuronal circuitry governed by the complex nuclei that reside in Onuf's nucleus. In addition to major input from the sympathetic, parasympathetic, and somatic systems, additional neurotransmitters participate in the normal regulation process [1,2].

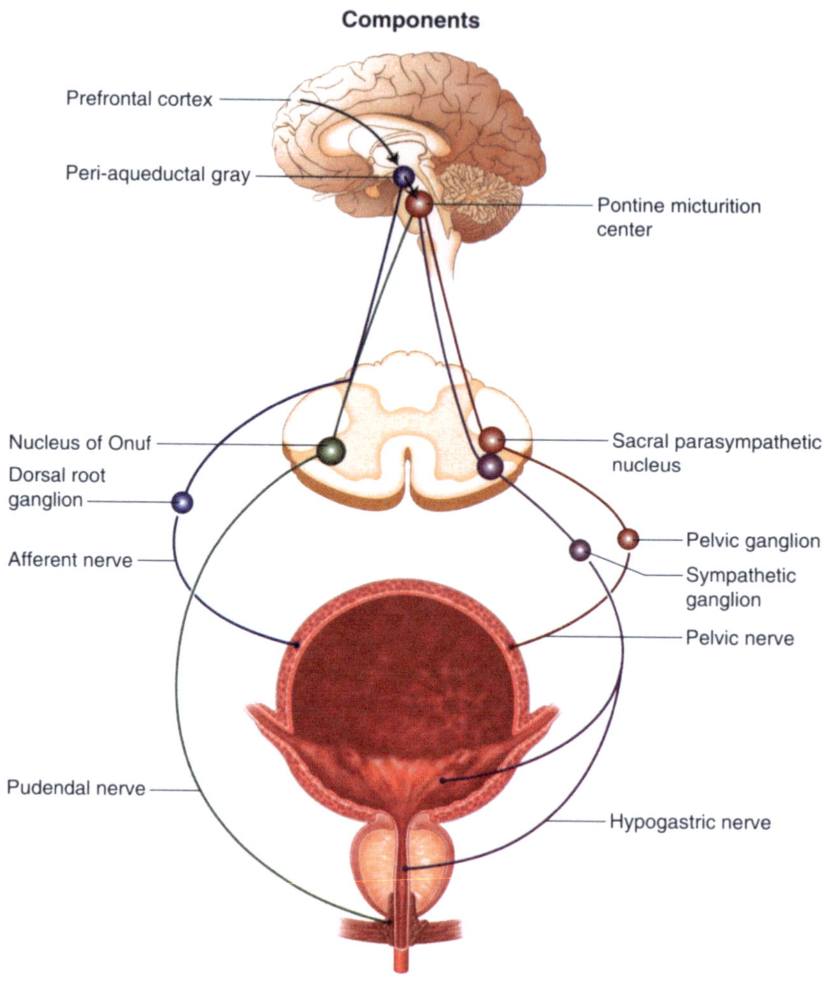

FIGURE 22-1. Control of micturition: the micturition reflexes. Central control of detrusor function is contributed by several areas within the central nervous system (CNS). These include the periaqueductal gray, pons, cingulate, and frontal lobes. The frontal cortex is also actively involved in the perception of urinary events, such as urinary urgency. Neurologic diseases may alter the perception, or lack thereof, of urinary events. Other areas of the CNS involved in micturition include the diencephalon, midbrain, and medulla, and spinal structures [3–5]. Functional MRI has demonstrated the complexity of brain activity during bladder filling. In subjects with detrusor dysfunction, incomplete activation of orbitofrontal cortex has been noted. This also corresponds to the voiding dysfunction associated with frontal cortex pathologies. (*Adapted from* Andersson KE *et al.* [6].)

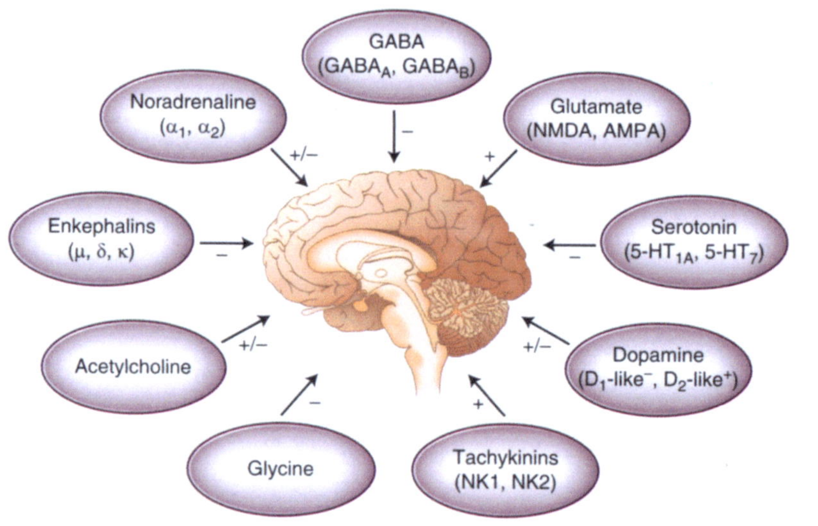

FIGURE 22-2. Control of micturition: central nervous system (CNS) neuro-uropharmacology. The CNS contains a variety of neurotransmitters. These include both inhibitory and excitatory neurotransmitters [7–10]. Glutamic acid provides the excitatory environment in the midbrain and bulbospinal tracts for neural transmission. Other transmitters include glutamic acid, substance P, gamma-aminobutyric acid, and enkephalins. Serotonergic activity is prominent in the sacral cord (Onuf's nuclei) and in the lumbosacral cord. This activity is largely inhibitory to bladder contraction. The 5-HT1A, 5-HT2, and 5-HT7 receptor subtypes appear to be the most prominent for lower urinary tract function [11,12]. The predominant receptor appears to be the 5-HT1A subtype. Several types of opioid peptides and receptors are found in the CNS, especially in the pons and the periaqueductal gray, and these may be important in modulating detrusor activity as well.

Gamma amino butyric receptors (GABA$_A$ and GABA$_B$) are found in the brain and spinal cord, and function in an inhibitory role [13–15]. These receptors appear to inhibit the voiding reflex on a chronic basis.

Dopamine receptors (D$_1^-$ and D$_2$) may also suppress detrusor contraction, as do substance P, and the tachykinins neurokinin A (NKA) and neurokinin B (NKB). Three receptors subtypes (NK1, NK2, and NK3) have been described in the CNS area where micturition is controlled [16,17].

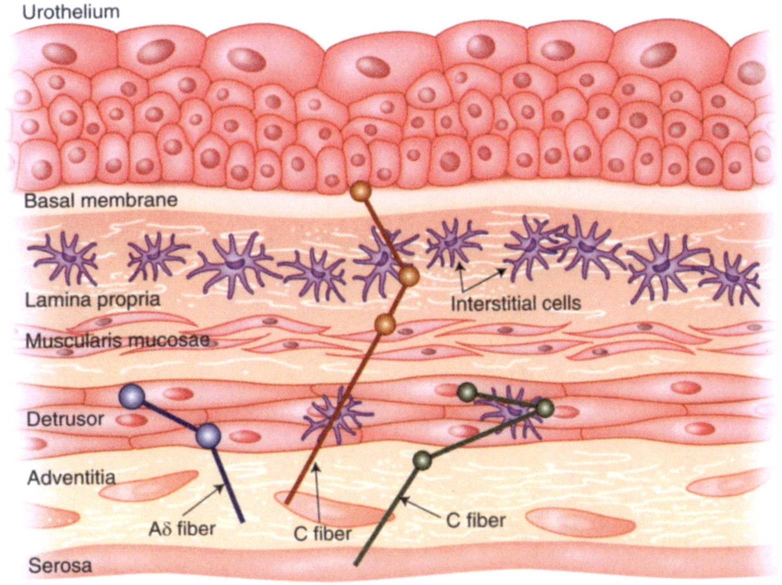

FIGURE 22-3. Control of micturition: role of the urothelium. Recently, increased attention has been focused on the role of the urothelium as an effector organ in the local control of normal regulation of voiding, as well as being a contributor to some aspect of detrusor overactivity manifested in the overactive bladder (OAB) syndrome. Muscarinic receptors have been identified in the urothelium as well as in the lamina propria and muscularis of the detrusor. The muscarinic receptors in the urothelium are thought to modulate the afferent function of the bladder, possibly responding as a result of the stretch of the basal layer of the urothelium associated with bladder filling. Normal bladder activity is perceived by myelinated large axons known A-type fibers that communicate with the pelvic ganglia and the sacral spinal cord.

Bladder storage is associated with quiescence of parasympathetic activity emanating from the sacral spinal cord [18,19]. Apparently, small amounts of acetylcholine are released from the detrusor during this phase of detrusor storage and the likely source is postulated to be the urothelium. As the bladder fills and the detrusor wall stretches, acetylcholine release increases. This increased release of a neurotransmitter has been implicated in part to be a causation of OAB. The interaction between the urothelium and detrusor musculature may be permissive, resulting in diseased bladders in a permissive environment for detrusor overactivity. Increased detrusor activity has been postulated to contribute to subjective urgency and to stimulation of reflex voiding. (*Adapted from* Andersson KE *et al.* [6].)

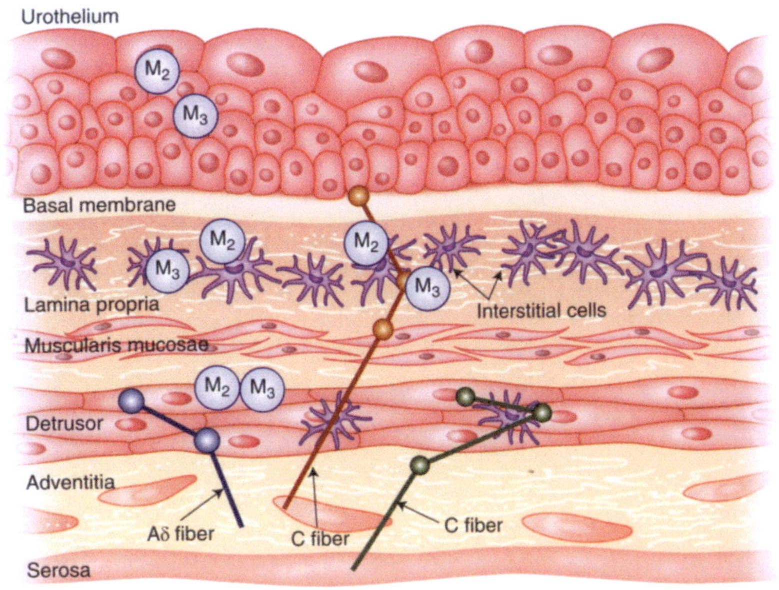

FIGURE 22-4. Control of micturition: role of the urothelium II. The function of another recently appreciated component of the bladder well appears to also be crucial. The interstitial cells of Cajal are interspersed in the lamina propria of the detrusor wall. These cells are complex neural cells that appear to be under the influence of numerous neurotransmitters including ATP, substance P, calcitonin gene related peptide, and possibly acetylcholine. These neurotransmitters may function as the intramural signaling center of the bladder linking local function to the sacral cord and other centers in the central nervous system. In pathologic states, neural transmission appears to occur through smaller unmyelinated neurons known as C fibers. The mechanism by which this transmission conversion occurs is unknown. IC—interstitial cells. (*Adapted from* Andersson KE *et al.* [6].)

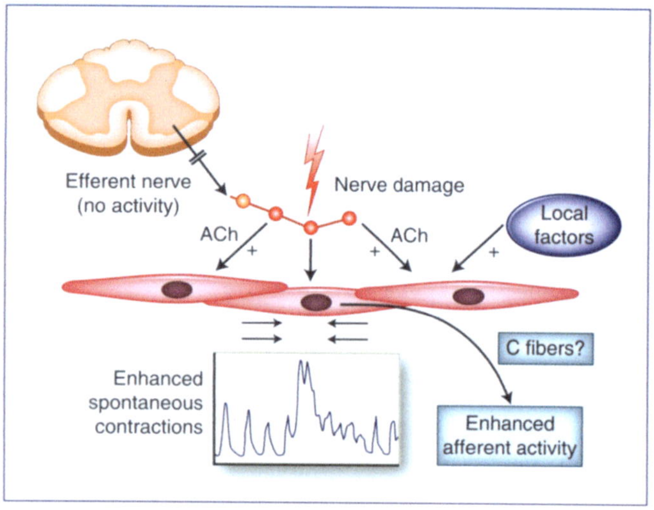

Figure 22-5. Multiple factors may lead to detrusor dysfunction, resulting in overactive bladder syndrome. A leak of acetylcholine has been postulated as one of these factors and provides another possible explanation for the effects of antimuscarinic class of compounds in this syndrome. Other neurotransmitters likely play more or less significant roles in the neural cascade, leading to lower urinary tract symptoms. (*Adapted from* Andersson KE *et al.* [6].)

OAB: Clinical Syndrome
Hallmark symptoms
Urinary urgency
Urinary frequency
Urgency urinary incontinence

Figure 22-6. Overactive bladder (OAB): the clinical syndrome. OAB is a urologic syndrome defined as urinary urgency with or without urge incontinence, usually associated with frequency and nocturia, in the absence of definable pathologic or metabolic factors that could produce these symptoms. The hallmark symptom of this syndrome is urinary urgency, which is defined as a sudden, compelling desire to pass urine that is difficult to defer. As with all symptom syndromes, not all component symptoms may be present for the unique patients. OAB syndrome may consist of only urinary urgency and frequency (OAB dry) or with urgency, frequency, and urge urinary incontinence (OAB wet).

The effect of (anticholinergic) pharmacological therapy purely on the "efferent" system may be referred to as the "old science" with the appreciate of the effects on the "afferent " system. Urinary "urgency" is defined as a pathologic sensation as opposed to the normal increasing "desire" to void, which is (confusingly) referred to as the "urge" to urinate. Normal bladder sensation incrementally increases with bladder filling until the sensation of bladder "fullness" is achieved, representing functional bladder capacity. Normal micturition then is initiated under volitional control until bladder emptying is accomplished.

Pathological "urgency" describes the situation when the afferent reflex arc has increased sensitivity to bladder filling. In effect, the normal bladder afferent reflex arc is "short-circuited" and bladder sensation increases out of proportion to actual bladder volume. Controversy exists as to whether urgency should be described as a rapid "crescendo" (similar to a dimmer switch) or as a precipitant "bolt" (similar to an on–off switch) in contradistinction to the normal sensations associated with increased filling during urinary storage.

The symptoms of OAB often overlap with other lower urinary tract conditions, such as stress incontinence, forming a mixed urinary condition. A key aspect of appreciating the OAB syndrome is that the component symptoms often occur in conjunction with other storage, emptying, and postvoiding complaints. This overlap often confounds the clinical presentation and can significantly impact patient expectations and results of therapy.

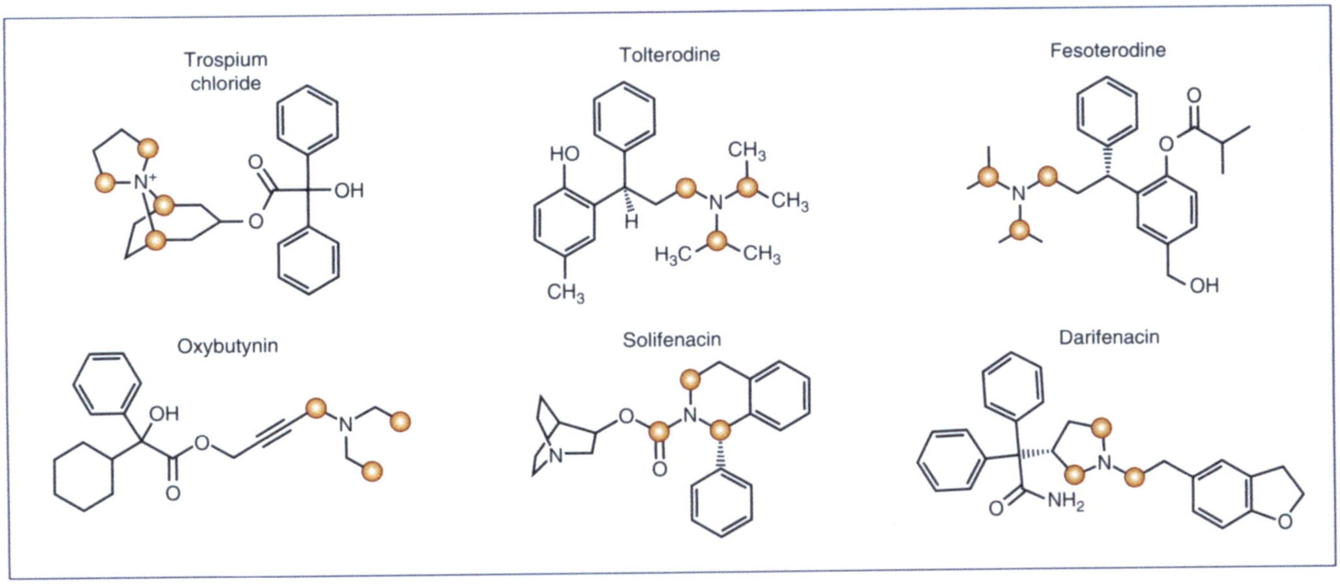

FIGURE 22-7. Antimuscarinic drugs for overactive bladder (OAB). Antimuscarinic drugs for OAB include the following: Gelnique (Watson; Morristown, NJ, 2009); Sanctura XR (Indevus; Lexington, MA, July 2007); Vesicare (GlaxoSmithKline; Research Triangle Park, NC, November 2004); Enablex (Novartis; East Hanover, NJ, February 2006); Detrol LA (Pfizer; New York, NY, December 2006); Toviaz (Pfizer; New York, NY, October 2008).

Muscarinic receptor subtypes have been shown to exist in the urinary bladder with the M_2 and M_3 receptors being predominant on the basis of mRNA analysis. Detrusor contraction is felt to be mediated by the M_3 receptors [20,21]. The rationale for treatment for the OAB syndrome is that detrusor overactivity is driven by muscarinic activity and that by producing a pharmacologic blockade of the muscarinic receptors, a decrease in detrusor activity will occur. Other factors may be involved in detrusor contraction, such as cation channel activation. Also, the activation of Rho-kinase has been postulated to potentiate detrusor contraction. Calcium ion influx appears to be the primary activation stimulant for the M_3 receptors' activity. M_2 receptors may further potentiate this process, providing a counterpoise to sympathetic nervous detrusor relaxation. M_2 receptor stimulation may also activate nonspecific cation channels [22,23]. Signalling pathways such as KATP channels activating protein kinase C may also be involved.

In certain neurogenic disease states, M_2 receptors may contribute to bladder muscle contraction, with less activity of the M_3 subtype. In both rodents and humans, detrusor contractions have been shown to be predominantly mediated by M_2 receptors. Prejunctional muscarinic receptors are known to be involved in the regulation of normal detrusor contraction and the activity of these receptors by increase in spinal cord injury [24,25]. Antimuscarinic drugs may affect C-fiber afferent nerves. Studies have shown that antimuscarinic drugs, when given to animals with central nervous system injury, will decrease detrusor overactivity in animals with intact C-fiber activity but not in those with induced C-fiber blockade. The mediation of detrusor function, previously thought to be just an efferent or motor effect, is now believed to be also an afferent or sensory phenomenon as well. Therefore, the use of drugs with antimuscarinic effects should logically benefit individuals with OAB syndrome.

The major agents are illustrated in Figure 22-5. The presence of an additional carbon molecule around the nitrogen differentiates trospium as a quaternary amine, which has a distinctly lower ability to permeate lipid membranes. Fesoterodine and tolterodine share a common active metabolite (5-HMT), but utilize different metabolic pathways. Oxybutynin, due to the lipophilic nature of the compound at physiologic pH, is available in a transdermal form. All of the agents have shown efficacy for the symptoms of OAB, yet the individual clinical response and the absence of head-to-head trials makes comparison unreliable.

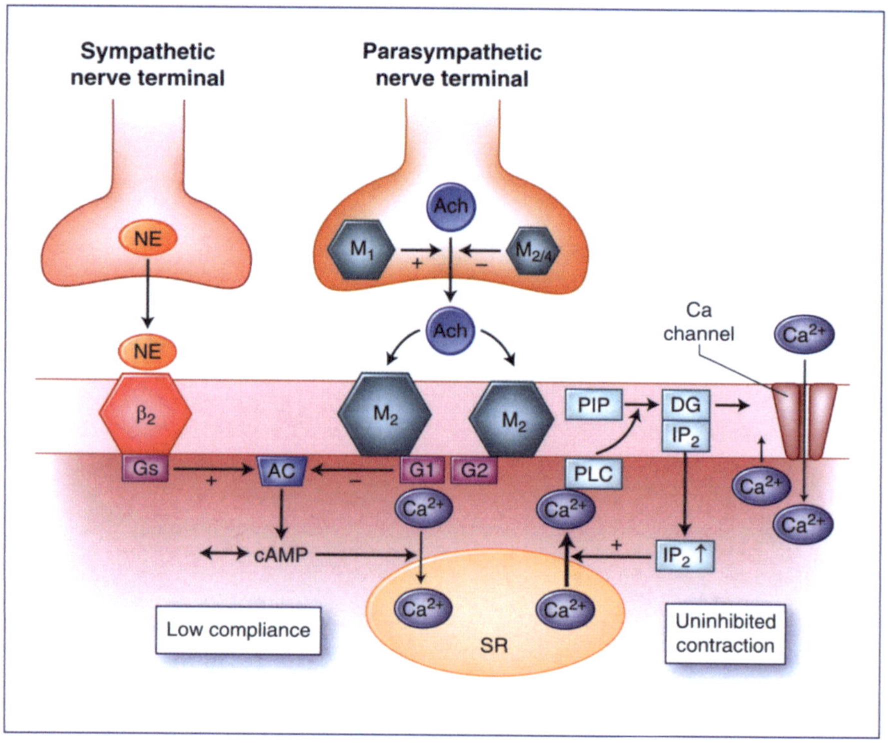

FIGURE 22-8. Future targets for therapy. Many types of receptors participate in normal bladder storage and contraction. The interaction of these receptors is not fully understood, nor is the role of any particular receptor in isolation. In addition to the muscarinic family, sympathetic receptors of the beta class appear to have a role in facilitating storage and may provide a target for pharmacotherapeutic modulation. Potential pharmacologic targets include the detrusor smooth muscle and the neural components involved with afferent and efferent signal transmission. Also, specific ion channels and intracellular signalling cascades may provide putative targets for pharmacologic intervention.

Sympathetically mediated smooth muscle relaxation has been shown to be modulated by β_3-adrenoceptors (ARs) [26]. The most important β_3-AR for bladder relaxation is the β_3-AR [27]. β-AR agonists would stimulate the elaboration of adenylyl cyclase, which in turn increases cAMP. cAMP then activates protein kinase, which results in smooth muscle relaxation. This mechanism has been shown to be effective for detrusor relaxation in animal studies [28]. β_3-ARs also may affect bladder function and are present in the detrusor musculature and the vascular supply of the bladder [29].

Calcium channels are active in generating detrusor contraction; therefore, it would seem logical that calcium channel antagonists would decrease detrusor overactivity. However, clinical trials to date have not shown this effect [30]. Similarly, potassium channels antagonism has been proposed as a possibly therapeutic route. Two types of potassium channels are known to exist in the human detrusor, ATP-sensitive K^+ channels and large conductance calcium-activated K^+ channels. However, modification of these channels has also not produced therapeutic success [31,32].

Afferent signalling from the bladder to the central nervous system is a critical component of normal and abnormal detrusor function. This signalling is accomplished by myelinated Aδ fibers (mechanoreceptor, with stretch sensitivity) and slowly conducting, unmyelinated C fibers (chemoreceptors, with pain sensitivity) [33]. Vanilloid receptors appear to be sensitive to capsaicin. Resiniferatoxin is a much more potent analogue of capsaicin, which also has affects on the C fibers (which are only expressed in detrusor pathologic states). Both agents appear to affect the vanilloid receptors. Therapeutic benefits have been noted with both agents [34,35]. In addition to these agents, botulinum toxin may be utilized to decrease the release of acetylcholine from cholinergic terminals (*see* Chapter 9 on botulinum toxin). DG—diacylglycerol; NE—norepinephrine; PIP—phosphatidylinositol 4,5 biphosphate; PLC—phospholipase C; SR—sarcoplasmic reticulum.

References

1. De Groat WC, Booth AM, Yoshimura N: Neurophysiology of micturition and its modification in animal models of human disease. In *Nervous Control of the Urogenital System*. Edited by Maggi CA. London: Harwood Academic; 1993:227–290.
2. de Groat WC, Yoshimura N: Mechanisms underlying the recovery of lower urinary tract function following spinal cord injury. *Prog Brain Res* 2006, 152:59–84.
3. Griffiths DJ: Cerebral control of bladder function. *Curr Urol Rep* 2004, 5:348–352.
4. Derbyshire S, Stenger A, Resnick N: Brain control of normal and overactive bladder. *J Urol* 2005, 174:1862–1867.
5. Sugaya K, Nishijima S, Miyazato M, Ogawa Y: Central nervous control of micturition and urine storage. *J Smooth Muscle Res* 2005, 41:117–132.
6. Andersson KE, Appell R, Cardozo L, *et al.*: Pharmacological treatment of urinary incontinence. *Incontinence*, edn 4. Edited by Abrams P, Cardozo L, Khoury S, Wein A. Plymouth, UK: Health Publication; 2009:631–700.
7. Andersson KE, Wein AJ. Pharmacology of the lower urinary tract: basis for current and future treatments of urinary incontinence. *Pharmacol Rev* 2004, 56:581–631.
8. Morrison J, Birder L, Craggs M, *et al.* (eds): In *Incontinence*. Edited by Abrams, P, Cardozo, L, Khoury, S, Wein, A. 3rd International Consultation on Incontinence. Plymouth, UK: Health Publication; 2005:811–854.
9. de Groat WC, Yoshimura N: Pharmacology of the lower urinary tract. *Annu Rev Pharmacol Toxicol* 2001, 41:691–721.
10. Andersson KE: Mechanisms of disease: central nervous system involvement in overactive bladder syndrome. *Nat Clin Pract Urol* 2004, 1:103–108.
11. Thor KB, Nickolaus S, Helke CJ: Autoradiographic localization of 5-hydroxytryptamine1A, 5-hydroxytryptamine1B and 5-hydroxytryptamine1C/2 binding sites in the rat spinal cord. *Neuroscience* 1993, 55:235–252.
12. Ramage AG: The role of central 5-hydroxytryptamine (5-HT, serotonin) receptors in the control of micturition. *Br J Pharmacol* 2006, 147(Suppl 2): S120–131.
13. Groat WC: Influence of central serotonergic mechanisms on lower urinary tract function. *Urology* 2002, 59(Suppl 1):30–36.
14. Bowery NG: $GABA_B$ receptor pharmacology. *Annu Rev Pharmacol Toxicol* 1993, 33:109–147.
15. Rudolph U, Crestani F, Möhler H: $GABA_A$ receptor subtypes: dissecting their pharmacological functions. *Trends Pharm Sci* 2001, 22:188–194.
16. Lecci A, Maggi CA: Tachykinins as modulators of the micturition reflex in the central and peripheral nervous system. *Regul Pept* 2001, 101:1–18.
17. Seki S, Erickson KA, Seki M, *et al.*: Elimination of rat spinal neurons expressing neurokinin 1 receptors reduces bladder overactivity and spinal c-fos expression induced by bladder irritation. *Am J Physiol Renal Physiol* 2005, 288:F466–F473.
18. De Groat WC, Booth AM, Yoshimura N: Neurophysiology of micturition and its modification in animal models of human disease. In *Nervous Control of the Urogenital System*. Edited by Maggi CA. London: Harwood Academic; 1993:227–290.
19. Yoshida M, Miyamae K, Iwashita H, *et al.*: Management of detrusor dysfunction in the elderly: changes in acetylcholine and adenosine triphosphate release during aging. *Urology* 2004, 63(Suppl 1):17–23.
20. Hegde SS, Choppin A, Bonhaus D, *et al.*: Functional role of M-2 and M-3 muscarinic receptors in the urinary bladder of rats in vitro and in vivo. *Br J Pharmacol* 1997, 120:1409–1418.
21. Kotlikoff MI, Dhulipala P, Wang YX: M_2 signaling in smooth muscle cells. *Life Sci* 1999, 64:437–442.
22. Bonev AD, Nelson MT: Muscarinic inhibition of ATP-sensitive K^+ channels by protein kinase C in urinary bladder smooth muscle. *Am J Physiol* 1993, 265: C1723–1728.
23. Nakamura T, Kimura J, Yamaguchi O: Muscarinic M_2 receptors inhibit Ca^{2+}-activated K^+ channels in rat bladder smooth muscle. *Int J Urol* 2002, 9:689–996.
24. GT, de Groat WC. Function, signal transduction mechanisms and plasticity of presynaptic muscarinic receptors in the urinary bladder. *Life Sci* 1999, 64:411–418.
25. Yokoyama O, Yusup A, Miwa Y, *et al.*: Effects of tolterodine on an overactive bladder depend on suppression of C-fiber bladder afferent activity in rats. *J Urol* 2005, 174:2032–2036.
26. Hegde SS, Choppin A, Bonhaus D, *et al.*: Functional role of M-2 and M-3 muscarinic receptors in the urinary bladder of rats in vitro and in vivo. *Br J Pharmacol* 1997, 120:1409–1418.
27. Yamaguchi O: $Beta_3$-adrenoceptors in human detrusor muscle. *Urology* 2002, 59(Suppl 1):25–29.
28. Takeda H, Yamazaki Y, Igawa Y, *et al.*: Effects of beta(3)-adrenoceptor stimulation on prostaglandin E(2)-induced bladder hyperactivity and on the cardiovascular system in conscious rats. *Neurourol Urodyn* 2002, 21:558–565.
29. Nomiya M, Yamaguchi O: A quantitative analysis of mRNA expression of alpha 1 and beta-adrenoceptor subtypes and their functional roles in human normal and obstructed bladders. *J Urol* 2003, 170:649–653.
30. Shapiro E, Tang R, Rosenthal E, Lepor H: The binding and functional properties of voltage dependent calcium channel receptors in pediatric normal and myelodysplastic bladders. *J Urol* 1991,146:520–523.
31. Herrera GM, Pozo MJ, Zvara P, *et al.*: Urinary bladder instability induced by selective suppression of the murine small conductance calcium-activated potassium (SK3) channel. *J Physiol* 2003, 551:893–903.
32. Meredith AL, Thorneloe KS, Werner ME, *et al.*: Overactive bladder and incontinence in the absence of the BK large conductance Ca^{2+}-activated K^+ channel. *J Biol Chem* 2004, 279:36746–36752.
33. Szallazi A, Blumberg PM: Vanilloid receptors: new insights enhance potential as a therapeutic target. *Pain* 1996, 68:195–208.
34. Kuo H-C: Inhibitory effect of capsaicin on detrusor contractility: further study in the presence of ganglionic blocker and neurokinin receptor antagonist in the rat urinary bladder. *Urol Int* 1997, 59:95–101.
35. Dasgupta P, Chandiramani V, Parkinson MC, *et al.*: Treating the human bladder with capsaicin: is it safe? *Eur Urol* 1998, 33:28–31.

Index

A

Abdominal hypopressive gymnastics, 114–115
Acellular tissue matrix, 214, 217
α-Adrenergic blockers, 138-139, 143
Adrenergic receptors, 134, 137
Alginate, 214
Altered bladder sensation, 5
Amniotic fluid stem cells, 213
Anatomic restoration radical prostatectomy, 259–266
Androgen suppression therapy, 140–141
Androgens
  in benign prostatic hyperplasia, 139
Anterior colporrhaphy, 161
Anticholinergic agents, 143
Antimuscarinic agents, 309
Appendicovesicostomy, 20–21
Areflexia, 6
Artificial urinary sphincter, 189–194, 201–206
  overview of, 189, 201
  results and complications of, 192
  surgical placement of, 190–194, 202–206
Augmentation ileocystoplasty, 19
Autologous cell sources, 210–212

B

Bacillus Calmette-Guérin immunotherapy
  for bladder cancer, 233–234
Behavior modification
  in nocturia, 30
Benign prostatic hyperplasia
  disease progression in, 141–142
  pathophysiology of, 131–136
  pharmacotherapy of, 138–145
Biofeedback
  in pelvic floor rehabilitation, 107, 109–112, 119, 124
Biomaterials in tissue engineering, 214
Bladder
  botulinum toxin injection in, 152–154, 156–157
  innervation of, 284
  neurogenic, 11–21. *See also* Neurogenic bladder
  overactive. *See* Overactive bladder
  classification of, 1–9
Bladder augmentation
  tissue engineering in, 209–218
Bladder cancer, 221–237, 239–249
  chemoradiation for, 233
  chemotherapy in, 237
  classification and staging of, 221
  diagnosis of, 224–227
  incidence and mortality of, 221, 223
  management by grade/stage of, 230–231
  nodal metastases in, 236
  overview of, 221, 239
  pathologic grading of, 229
  radical cystectomy in, 228, 235, 239–249
  risk factors for, 223
  transurethral resection in, 227
  urinary diversion in, 236–237
  urinary markers for, 235
Bladder capacity
  diminished nocturnal, 25, 27
Bladder diverticula, 68
Bladder hernia, 88
Bladder neck reconstruction
  prostatectomy and, 259–266
Bladder neck suspension, 161–164
Bladder outlet
  anatomy of male, 128–131
Bladder outlet dysfunction
  classification of female, 2, 8
  iatrogenic, 2
  male, 127–145
  neurogenic, 2, 16
  urodynamic studies in, 62–63, 65, 70
Bladder pain syndrome, 35–50
  classification of, 37
  cystoscopy in, 44–45
  detrusor overactivity and, 42
  diseases confused with, 36
  history and physical examination in, 37
  interstitial cystitis and, 35, 40–41
  laboratory tests in, 38
  in male patients, 43
  overactive bladder and, 40
  overview of, 5, 35–36
  potassium-sensitivity testing in, 43–44
  treatment of, 46–50
  voiding diary in, 38–39
Bladder reconstruction
  gastrointestinal segments in, 210, 216
  tissue engineering in, 209–218
Bladder stones, 88
Bladder suspension
  robotic-assisted laparoscopic, 251–257
Bladder tissue engineering, 209–218
  biomaterials in, 214–215
  cell-based therapies in, 211–213
  investigational technologies in, 216–218
  overview of, 209–210
Bladder training, 121
Bladder ultrasound, 81–95
  in bladder hernia, 88
  in bladder neoplasm, 89
  in bladder stones, 88
  fetal, 93
  normal, 82–83, 90–92
  in orthotopic neobladder, 89
  pediatric, 90, 93–94
  in pediatric detrusor hypertrophy, 90
  in prostatic hyperplasia, 84–87
  in stress incontinence, 93
  in urinary retention, 83
  in vesicoureteral reflux, 93
  in voiding dysfunction, 81, 84–95
  of wall thickness, 90–92
Bladder volume assessment, 82–83, 92
Bladder wall thickness assessment, 90-92
Bone-anchored male sling surgery, 189, 195–198
Botulinum toxin, 147–157
  in benign prostatic hyperplasia, 145
  bladder injection of, 152–154, 156–157
  mechanism of action of, 144–145, 152–154
  pathogenic, 148
  structure and subtypes of, 148–151
  tetanus toxin *versus*, 155
Bulbar urethral massage, 119

C

Chemoradiation for bladder cancer, 233
Chemotherapy in bladder cancer, 237
Children
  bladder ultrasound in, 90, 93–94
  detrusor hypertrophy in, 90
  posterior urethral valves in, 94
  vesicoureteral reflux in, 93
Cloning, 212
Clostridium species, 148, 155
Collagen in tissue engineering, 214
Colporrhaphy, 161
Colposuspension, 161–164
Computed tomography urography, 226
Cystectomy, 228, 235, 239–249
Cystometrography, 12, 14, 16, 18
Cystometry
  bladder parameters measured during, 54
  in incontinence, 55–56, 58–59
  in urethral function assessment, 57
Cystoscopy
  in bladder cancer, 225, 227
  in bladder pain syndrome, 44–45
Cytology
  in bladder cancer, 227

D

Detrusor hypertrophy
  from prostatic hyperplasia, 87
  ultrasound in, 90–91
Detrusor overactivity. *See also* Overactive bladder
  in neurogenic bladder, 12, 14, 16–18
  urodynamic assessment of, 56, 64, 123
Dyssynergia, 2, 18

E

Electrical stimulation
  pelvic floor, 112–113, 119, 122–123
Electromyography
  in pelvic floor rehabilitation, 107, 109–110
Embryonic stem cells, 211, 213
Emptying/voiding dysfunction classification, 1–9
EndoWrist instruments, 241
Exercises
  pelvic floor, 108–111

F

Female lower urinary tract dysfunction classification, 1–9
Female stress incontinence surgery, 161–175
Fetal bladder ultrasound, 93
Flowmetry
  in bladder pain syndrome, 42–43
  equipment for, 53
Frequency
  in overactive bladder, 1, 3
  without incontinence, 5
Functional incontinence, 5

G

Gastrointestinal tissue
  in bladder reconstruction, 210, 216
Global polyuria
  in nocturia, 25, 28
Glomerulations, 45

H

Hasson laparoscopic technique, 242
Hematuria, 222, 226
Hinman syndrome, 94
Human embryonic stem cells, 211, 213
Hunner's lesion, 44–45
Hydrodistension, 45, 49
Hyperreflexia, 6
Hyposensitive bladder, 20
Hypropressive gymnastics, 114–115
Hysterectomy sequela, 252

I

Iatrogenic bladder outlet obstruction, 2
Immunotherapy for bladder cancer, 233–234
Implantable pulse generator, 275–277
Incomplete bladder emptying, 14, 16
Incontinence. *See* specific types; Urinary incontinence
Indiana pouch urinary diversion, 79
Interstitial cystitis
  bladder pain syndrome and, 35, 40–41
  treatment of, 50
Intraprostatic protrusion, 85
Intravaginal massage, 105
Intravenous urography, 226
Intravesical therapy
  in bladder cancer, 233–234
  in bladder pain syndrome, 47
Intrinsic male urinary sphincter deficiency, 189–198, 201–206

L

Laminectomy, 294–295
Laparoscopic colposuspension, 164
Laparoscopic radical cystectomy
  robotic-assisted, 239–249
Laparoscopic sacrocolpopexy
  robotic-assisted, 251–257
Low bladder compliance
  urodynamic studies in, 57, 78
Lower urinary tract dysfunction classification
  female, 1–9
Lower urinary tract symptoms
  male bladder outlet, 127–145
  overview of, 52
  urodynamic studies in, 51–79
Lumbar to sacral ventral nerve rerouting therapy, 289–302

M

Magnetic resonance imaging
  of urethral diverticula, 180–184
Male bladder outlet dysfunction
  anatomy in, 128–131
  pathophysiology in, 131–136
  pharmacology of, 127, 132, 136–145
Male incontinence surgery, 189–198, 201–206
Marshall-Marchetti-Krantz procedure, 161
Micturition
  control of, 268, 306–307
  dysfunctional. *See* Voiding dysfunction
Micturition disorders. *See* Voiding disorders
Midurethral sling suspension system, 168–169
Midurethral tape procedures, 165–169
Mixed incontinence
  bladder training in, 121

overview of, 5
pelvic floor rehabilitation in, 121–124
urodynamic study of, 73
Mixed nocturia, 27, 31
Mood disorders
nocturia and, 23
Mucinous bladder adenocarcinoma, 228
Multichannel urodynamic recorder, 52
Multiple sclerosis, 20–21
Multiple systems atrophy, 12
Muscarinic receptors, 132–133

N

Nerve rerouting therapy
overview of, 289
postoperative management in, 298, 302
postoperative urodynamics in, 299, 301
preoperative evaluation in, 292, 299
procedures in, 293–298, 299–301
scientific principles of, 290–292
in spina bifida, 299–302
in spinal cord injury, 292–299
Nerve-preserving radical prostatectomy, 264–266
Neurogenic bladder
classification of, 6
cystometrography in, 12, 14, 16, 18
nerve rerouting therapy in, 289–302
overview of, 11, 289
pelvic floor rehabilitation in, 124–125
posttraumatic, 289
surgical procedures in, 19–21
voiding cystourethrography in, 13–15, 17–18, 20
Neuromodulation therapy
lumbar to sacral ventral nerve rerouting in, 289–302
sacral stimulation in, 269–277
tibial stimulation in, 279–286
Neurotoxin
botulinum, 147–157
Neurotransmitter release, 144
Newborn urethral valves, 94
Nitric oxide, 135
Nocturia, 23–32
case studies of, 29–32
diminished nocturnal bladder capacity in, 25, 27
evaluation of, 24–26
global polyuria in, 25, 28
mixed, 27
nocturnal polyuria in, 25–26
novel treatments for, 31
in overactive bladder, 1, 3
overview of, 23
Nocturnal polyuria, 25–26, 31–32
Nonneurogenic-neurogenic bladder, 94

O

Occult stress incontinence, 59
O'Leary-Sant questionnaire, 41
Orthotopic neobladder, 89
Overactive bladder
bladder pain syndrome and, 40
causes of, 308
classification of, 1–9
effects of, 1, 3–4
future therapy targets in, 310
overview and epidemiology of, 279–280
pelvic floor rehabilitation in, 97, 121–124
percutaneous tibial nerve stimulation for, 279–286
pharmacotherapy of, 309
symptoms of, 308
treatment algorithm for, 280
urodynamic studies in, 66
Overactive Bladder Innovative Therapy Trial, 281–283
Overactive bladder outlet
classification of, 1–9
Overflow incontinence, 5, 20

P

Pad incontinence test, 103
Paraplegia, 18–19
Parkinson's disease, 14
Patient education
in pelvic floor rehabilitation, 104
Pelvic floor dysfunction
classification of, 2, 8–9
in underactive bladder, 1
Pelvic floor rehabilitation, 97–125
biofeedback in, 107, 109–112, 119, 124
electrical stimulation in, 112–113, 119, 122–123
hypopressive techniques in, 114–115
indications for, 97–99
for mixed urinary incontinence, 121–124
muscle training in, 106–115, 119
for neurogenic bladder, 124–125
for overactive bladder, 97, 121–124
overview of, 97–98
pelvic floor assessment in, 100–103
perineal/intravaginal massage in, 105
peripartum/postpartum, 108
for postprostatectomy incontinence, 97, 116–119
referral data for, 100
for stress incontinence, 105–115
treatment planning in, 100, 104–106
for urge incontinence, 106, 120–121
for vaginal prolapse, 125
Pelvic organ prolapse
grading of, 252
overview of, 251–252
pelvic floor rehabilitation in, 125
posthysterectomy, 252
robotic sacrocolpopexy for, 251, 253–257
Percutaneous tibial nerve stimulation
anatomic features of, 283–284
clinical trials of, 280–283
for overactive bladder, 279–286
procedure for, 285–286
Urgent PC system in, 285
Perineal massage, 105
Peripartum pelvic floor exercises, 108
Pharmacotherapy
in bladder cancer, 237
in bladder pain syndrome, 46–47, 50
botulinum toxin in, 145, 147–157
in male bladder outlet dysfunction, 138–145
in overactive bladder, 309
Phosphodiesterase inhibitors
in male bladder outlet dysfunction, 143
Physical therapy
pelvic floor, 97–125. *See also* Pelvic floor rehabilitation
Physical treatments
in bladder pain syndrome, 49

Phytotherapy, 144
Placental stem cells, 213
Polydipsia
nocturia and, 30
Polymer
in tissue engineering, 215
Posterior urethral valves, 94
Postpartum pelvic floor exercises, 108
Postprostatectomy incontinence, 67, 71
artificial urinary sphincter for, 198–194, 201–206
bladder neck reconstruction to prevent, 259–266
pelvic floor rehabilitation in, 97, 116–119
Postvoid male dribbling, 117–119
Potassium-sensitivity testing, 43–44
PRAFAB-Q questionnaire, 103
Pressure-flow nomograms, 69
Pressure-flow studies, 62–64
Prostate anatomy, 128–131
Prostate resection. *See also* Radical prostatectomy
incontinence after, 67, 71, 201, 259.
See also Postprostatectomy incontinence
lower urinary tract symptoms after, 66, 201
Prostatic hyperplasia. *See also* Benign prostatic hyperplasia
bladder ultrasound in, 84–87
nocturia and, 31–32
urodynamic studies in, 62, 65
ProUrge system, 123
Pseudodyssynergia, 2
Pubovaginal sling, 164–165
Pulse generator
implantable, 275–276

Q

Questionnaires
in bladder pain syndrome, 40–41
in interstitial cystitis, 40–41
in nocturia, 23, 26
in urinary incontinence, 103

R

Radical cystectomy, 228
overview of, 239
robotic-assisted laparoscopic, 239–249
survival after, 235
Radical prostatectomy
artificial urinary sphincter after, 201–206
bladder neck reconstruction and, 259–266
minimally invasive, 260–264
5α-Reductase inhibitors, 140–141
Renal failure
from prostatic hyperplasia, 86–87
Retrograde pyelography, 226
Retropubic midurethral tape procedures, 165–169
Robotic-assisted laparoscopic prostatectomy
bladder neck reconstruction and, 259–266
Robotic-assisted laparoscopic radical cystectomy, 239–249
operating room setup for, 241
overview of, 239
patient positioning for, 240
port placement in, 242, 248
procedure for, 242–249
Robotic-assisted laparoscopic sacrocolpopexy, 251–257
equipment for, 254
procedure for, 253–257
results of, 257

S

Sacral dysgenesis, 77
Sacral neuromodulation
implantable pulse generator and, 275–277
instruments for, 271
motor and sensory responses in, 270
in neurogenic bladder, 14
possible mechanisms of, 268
procedure for, 269–275
results of, 277–278
voiding diary during, 274
in voiding dysfunction, 267–278
Sacral plexus anatomy, 283–284
Sacrocolpopexy
robotic-assisted laparoscopic, 251–257
Seeded scaffolding, 215, 218
Sensory disorder classification, 2, 9
Shy-Drager syndrome, 12
Sleep disturbance
from nocturia, 23
Sling surgery
in male patients, 189, 195–198
Somatic cell nuclear transfer, 212
Somatic cell reprogramming, 213
SPARK sling system, 168
Sphincteric dysfunction
intrinsic male, 189–198, 201–206
in stress incontinence, 2
in underactive bladder, 1
Spina bifida
nerve rerouting therapy in, 289, 299–302
neurogenic bladder in, 77, 289
Spinal cord injury
nerve rerouting therapy in, 289, 292–299
neurogenic bladder in, 18–19, 57, 75–76, 289
Squamous cell bladder cancer, 221, 228. *See also* Bladder cancer
Stem cells, 211–213
Storage/filling dysfunction
classification of, 1–9
symptoms of, 52
Stress incontinence
bladder ultrasound in, 93
causes of, 160
overview of, 5, 159–160, 175
pelvic floor rehabilitation in, 105–115
recurrent, 74, 192
surgery for female, 161–175
surgery for male, 189–197, 201–206
in underactive bladder outlet, 1–3
urodynamic assessment of, 55–56, 58–59, 67, 71–74
Stretch reflex
vaginal cones and, 113
Stroke history, 16
Surgical procedures. *See also* specific procedures and conditions
for bladder cancer, 221, 227–232, 235–237, 239–249
in bladder pain syndrome, 48
for female incontinence, 161–175
of lower urinary tract dysfunction, 1, 7
for male incontinence, 189–198, 201–206
prostate, 201–206, 259–266
Synthetic polymer, 215

T

Tension-free vaginal tape procedures, 165–168, 173–175
Tetanus toxin, 155

Tibial nerve
anatomy of, 283–284
percutaneous stimulation of, 279–283, 285–286
Tissue engineering
bladder, 209–218
Tissue expansion techniques, 216
Transitional cell carcinoma, 221. *See also* Bladder cancer
Transobturator sling procedures, 170–173
Transurethral bladder cancer resection, 227
TVT Secur vaginal tape procedures, 173–175

U

Ultrasound
bladder, 81–95. *See also* Bladder ultrasound
Underactive bladder classification, 1–9
Underactive bladder outlet classification, 1–9
Urethral diverticula, 179–188
diverticulectomy technique in, 184–187
imaging of, 180–185, 187
overview of, 179
pathophysiology of, 182
signs and symptoms of, 180
surgical complications in, 187–188
Urethral function assessment, 57
Urge incontinence
in neurogenic bladder, 12, 14, 16
in overactive bladder, 1
overview of, 5
pelvic floor rehabilitation in, 106, 120–121
Urgency
in overactive bladder, 1, 3
without incontinence, 5
Urgent PC system, 285
Urinary diversion procedures, 236–237
Urinary incontinence. *See also* specific types
classification of, 5
pelvic floor assessment in, 100–103
surgery for female, 161–175
surgery for male, 189–197, 201–206
treatment overview of, 98–99
Urinary retention
in benign prostatic hyperplasia, 141–142
bladder ultrasound in, 83
in neurogenic bladder, 14
Urinary sphincter
male artificial, 189–194, 201–206
Urodynamic studies, 51–79. *See also* Videourodynamic studies
in bladder pain syndrome, 42–43
in detrusor activity assessment, 32, 56, 64, 115
equipment and setup for, 52–53
filling cystometry as, 54–59
of lower urinary tract function, 1, 7
overview of, 51
pressure flow, 62–64
pressure-flow nomograms in, 69
uroflow, 60–61
Uroflow studies, 60–61
Urothelial carcinoma, 221, 228–229. *See also* Bladder cancer

V

Vaginal cones, 113
Vaginal prolapse
pelvic floor rehabilitation for, 125
robotic sacrocolpopexy in, 251–252
Vesicovaginal fistula, 1, 7
Videourodynamic studies
in bladder diverticulum, 68
in bladder outlet obstruction, 70
in dyssynergia, 75–76
in incontinence, 71–74, 77
in low bladder compliance, 78
in nocturia and polyuria, 30
with pouch urinary diversion, 79
for prostate-related symptoms, 65–67, 71
setup for, 53
Voiding
control of, 268, 306–307
urodynamic studies of, 60–64
Voiding cystourethrography
in neurogenic bladder, 13–15, 17–18, 20
in urethral diverticulum, 182
Voiding diary
in bladder pain syndrome, 38–39
in nocturia, 23–24, 26–28, 30–32
in pelvic floor assessment, 101
in sacral neuromodulation therapy, 274
Voiding dysfunction
bladder ultrasound in, 81–95
classification of, 1–9
male postvoid dribbling as, 117–119
in neurogenic bladder, 11–20
overview of, 267–268
pathophysiology of, 81
sacral neuromodulation for, 267–278
symptoms of, 52

W

Water deprivation test
in nocturia, 30

MIX
Papier aus verantwortungsvollen Quellen
Paper from responsible sources
FSC® C105338

If you have any concerns about our products,
you can contact us on
ProductSafety@springernature.com

In case Publisher is established outside the EU,
the EU authorized representative is:
Springer Nature Customer Service Center GmbH
Europaplatz 3, 69115 Heidelberg, Germany

Printed by Libri Plureos GmbH
in Hamburg, Germany